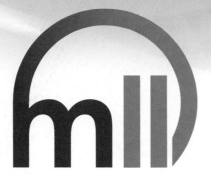

Access the Medical Language Lab

Redeem your ACCESS CODE today.

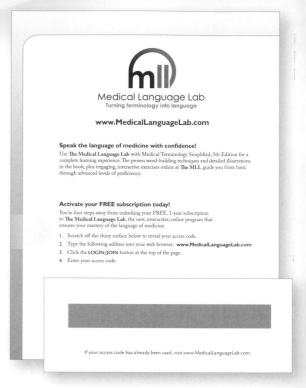

STEP 1

Find the access code on the inside front cover of your new book.

STEP 2

Go to **www.MedicalLanguageLab.com** and click the **Login/Join** button.

STEP 3

Select the "**New Student**" option.
Enter your access code exactly as it appears in your textbook.
Fill in your personal information and create a password.
Then, click "**Submit.**"

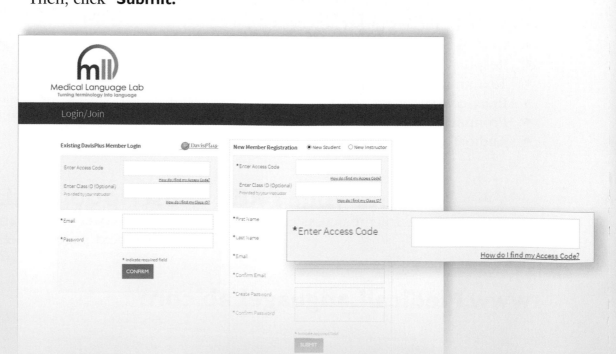

FREE, for one full year!

STEP 4

If you are studying on your own, you are logged in and ready to experience **The MLL**.

If you are studying in class, see your Instructor for your Class ID to enroll in your Instructor's MLL class.

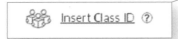

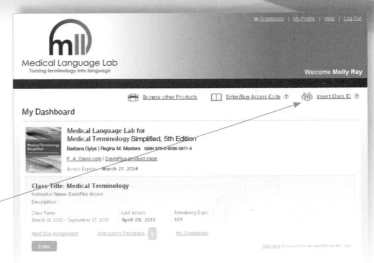

Stay on track

The **Dashboard** is a convenient, central access point. Quickly find your next assignment, receive feedback, and track your progress.

Advance Step by Step

Each **Lesson** organizes concepts from simple to complex to help you build your medical language skills.

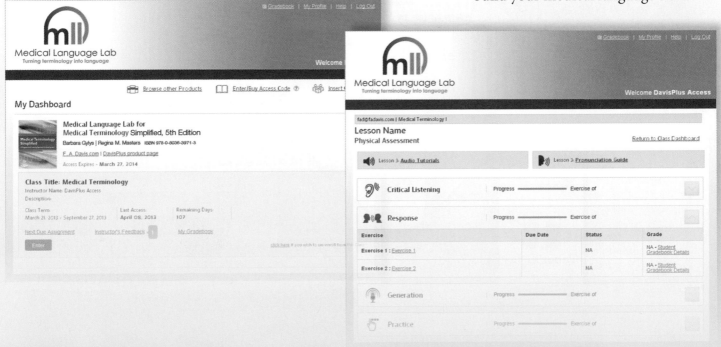

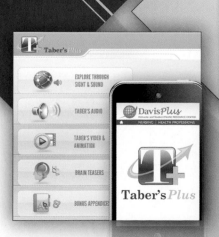
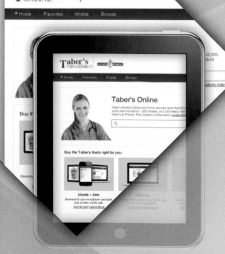
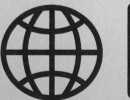
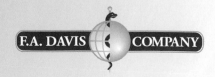

Medical Terminology Simplified

A Programmed Learning Approach by Body System

FIFTH EDITION

Barbara A. Gylys (GĬL-ĭs), BS, MEd, CMA-A (AAMA)
Professor Emerita
College of Health and Human Services
University of Toledo
Toledo, OH

Regina M. Masters, BSN, MEd, RN, CMA (AAMA)
Adjunct Nursing Faculty
Lourdes University
Sylvania, OH

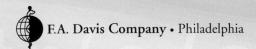
F.A. Davis Company • Philadelphia

F. A. Davis Company
1915 Arch Street
Philadelphia, PA 19103
www.fadavis.com

Copyright © 2014 by F. A. Davis Company

Printed in the United States of America

Last digit indicates print number: 10 9 8 7 6 5 4

Publisher: Quincy McDonald
Manager of Content Development: George W. Lang
Developmental Editor: Brenna H. Mayer
Art and Design Manager: Carolyn O'Brien

As new scientific information becomes available through basic and clinical research, recommended treatments and drug therapies undergo changes. The author(s) and publisher have done everything possible to make this book accurate, up to date, and in accord with accepted standards at the time of publication. The author(s), editors, and publisher are not responsible for errors or omissions or for consequences from application of the book, and make no warranty, expressed or implied, in regard to the contents of the book. Any practice described in this book should be applied by the reader in accordance with professional standards of care used in regard to the unique circumstances that may apply in each situation. The reader is advised always to check product information (package inserts) for changes and new information regarding dose and contraindications before administering any drug. Caution is especially urged when using new or infrequently ordered drugs.

Library of Congress Cataloging-in-Publication Data

Gylys, Barbara A., author.
  Medical terminology simplified: a programmed learning approach by body system/Barbara A. Gylys, Regina M. Masters. — Fifth edition.
    p.; cm.
  Includes index.
  ISBN 978-0-8036-3971-3
  I. Masters, Regina M., 1959- author. II. Title.
  [DNLM: 1. Terminology as Topic—Programmed Instruction. W 15]
  R123
  610.1'4—dc23

                                                                    2014000092

This Book is Dedicated with Love

to my best friend, colleague, and husband, Julius A. Gylys

and

to my children, Regina Maria and Julius A., II

and

to Andrew Masters, Dr. Julia Halm, Caitlin Masters, Anthony Bishop-Gylys, Matthew Bishop-Gylys, Liam Halm, and the little one, Harrison Robert.

    —BARBARA GYLYS

to my mother, best friend, mentor, and co-author, Barbara A. Gylys

and

to my father, Dr. Julius A. Gylys

and

to my husband, Bruce Masters, and my children Andrew, Dr. Julia, and Caitlin, all of whom have given me continuous encouragement and support, and to my grandsons Liam and Harrison who bring me endless joy.

    —REGINA MASTERS

Preface

Building on the success of the past edition, *Medical Terminology Simplified: A Programmed Learning Approach by Body System,* 5th edition, continues to live up to its established track record of reflecting current trends and new approaches to teaching medical terminology. This edition includes a variety of special features to make studying medical terminology a more encompassing and rewarding experience. We have continued to develop new features, based on feedback from instructors and students. A review of the "What's Inside" section provides explanations and illustrations about all of the text's distinctive features, as well as a short introduction to the many resources available to support the text. The design and flexibility of *Simplified,* 5th edition, enables its use as a self-instructional book, as an eBook, or as a text in traditional lecture and classroom environments. The organization and pedagogical devices are designed to help instructors teach and students learn medical terminology easily and quickly. When students use the available learning tool, they will find that the language of medicine stays with them and they can quickly apply the terminology in the clinical field.

This edition also continues to present eponyms without showing the possessive form, such as Alzheimer disease, Down syndrome, and Parkinson disease. Medical dictionaries, as well as the American Association for Medical Transcription and the American Medical Association, support these changes. A summary of common symbols and an updated list of "do-not-use" abbreviations are provided in Appendix E: Abbreviations and Symbols. In addition, all outdated medical terms in the textbook have been replaced with the most recent, state-of-the-art terms.

CHAPTERS

We have enhanced the popular, effective features found in the previous edition, so the learner can easily apply and process the language of medicine correctly in the workplace. The main focus of this edition is to improve retention of medical terms and relate their applications in the clinical setting. The following is a brief summary of chapter content.

- Chapter 1 introduces the programmed learning, medical word-building approach. It also includes summaries and activities to reinforce retention of common suffixes and prefixes used in medical word building.
- Chapter 2 discusses the structural organization of the human body.
- Chapters 3 through 11 are organized according to specific body systems and may be taught in any sequence. These chapters include key anatomical and physiological terms; anatomy and physiology; combining forms, suffixes, and prefixes; terms related to diseases and conditions, as well as diagnostic, surgical, and medical procedures; and abbreviations. Included are section reviews and medical record activities. All activities allow self-assessment and evaluation of competency.

APPENDICES

The appendices offer learning tools to reinforce the information presented in the chapters. Your students will also find the appendices useful for study, review, and reference as they begin their careers in the allied health field.

- *Appendix A: Glossary of Medical Word Elements* contains alphabetical lists of medical word elements with corresponding meanings.
- *Appendix B: Answer Key* provides answers to anatomical labeling and chapter reviews, as well as the medical record activities.
- *Appendix C: Index of Diagnostic, Medical, and Surgical Procedures* summarizes procedures covered in the textbook that establish a diagnosis, as well as various methods of treatment.
- *Appendix D: Drug Classifications* provides information on prescription and nonprescription drugs used for the treatment of various medical conditions.

- *Appendix E: Abbreviations and Symbols* summarizes commonly used medical abbreviations and symbols, including their meanings.
- *Appendix F: Medical Specialties* provides a summary and description of medical specialties.
- *Appendix G: Glossary of English-to-Spanish Translations* is an enhanced appendix of English-to-Spanish vocabulary and phrases relevant to various medical specialties. It is intended to help health-care workers who do not speak Spanish but who encounter Spanish-speaking patients in the medical environment.

LEARNING STYLES

All enhancements in the fifth edition are constructed to improve retention and make the study of medical terminology more enjoyable and engaging. As more and more students identify themselves as visual learners, the authors met this challenge by ensuring that the illustrations in the text and ancillary products are as helpful to students as possible. Many of the figures depicting the toughest topics for students to grasp have been newly developed; others from the previous edition have been enhanced for clarity and ease of understanding. Thus, one of the most extraordinary features of this edition is the collection of visually outstanding full-color illustrations. These illustrations are extremely useful as students learn the association of medical terms to anatomy, physiology, pathology, and medical treatments of the human body. All of the artwork presents precise depictions of medical terms in action. Full-color figures enable students to see a true representation of the body system, pathological condition, or operative procedure.

Programmed Learning Approach

The programmed learning approach presents a word-building method for developing a medical vocabulary in an effective, interesting manner. The book is designed to help students learn skills that will enable them to analyze medical terms by breaking them down into their basic components. By learning and reinforcing this technique, students will master the terms in this book and learn to decipher new medical terms that they encounter in the workplace. It is not a book in which the student simply memorizes a list of vocabulary terms. In addition, the text can be used in a traditional classroom setting or with guidance from an instructor for independent study. The workbook text format is designed to guide the student through exercises that teach and reinforce medical terminology.

The programmed learning technique makes use of frames, or isolated pieces of information that, together, provide the building blocks of learning medical terminology. The frames, each numbered with the chapter number and then the frame number within that chapter, allow students to learn at their own pace and in their own way. Each frame contains not only information about terminology, but also fill-in lines to reinforce understanding of the information. The student can find the answer to each fill-in line in the frame's answer box, located at the left of the page.

The key to using frames wisely is the bookmark included with every book. Students should use it to cover the answer column to verify their understanding of the content provided in the frame. Pronunciation keys for all medical words are also included in the frame answer boxes. Newly designed pronunciation guides in each chapter help students pronounce medical terms correctly.

TEACHING AND LEARNING PACKAGE

Numerous teaching aids are available free of charge to instructors who adopt *Medical Terminology Simplified: A Programmed Learning Approach by Body System,* 5th edition. These teaching aids contain an abundance of information and activities to help students retain what they have learned in a given chapter. Various types of electronic resources are designed to enhance course content and ensure a program of excellence in a medical terminology curriculum. These resources will also help you plan course work and provide you with various types of presentations to reinforce the learning process. These teaching aids include the Web-based *Medical Language Lab* and the Davis*Plus Online Resource Center* for students and instructors.

Medical Language Lab

Included in every new copy of *Medical Terminology Simplified: A Programmed Learning Approach by Body System,* 5th edition, is access to the ultimate online medical terminology resource for students. The *Medical Language Lab* is a rich learning environment using proven language development methods to help students become effective users of medical language. To access the *Medical Language Lab,* students simply go to *http://www.medicallanguagelab.com*

IMAGE RESOURCE

We have enhanced and expanded the *Image Resource,* a popular feature of the past edition, to meet the current demands of numerous instructors. The *Image Resource* is an electronic image bank that contains all illustrations from the textbook. It is fully searchable and allows users to zoom in and out and display a JPG image of an illustration that can be copied into a Microsoft Word document or PowerPoint presentation.

ELECTRONIC TEST BANK

The electronic test bank uses *ExamView Pro,* a powerful, user-friendly test-generation program. It enables instructors to create custom-made or randomly generated tests in a printable format from a test bank of more than 1,230 test items, with 370 new test items for this edition. The test bank includes multiple-choice, matching, true-false, and medical word–building questions. Because of the flexibility of the *ExamView Pro* test-generating program, instructors can edit questions in the test bank to meet their specific educational needs. Therefore, if instructors wish to restate, embellish, or streamline questions or change distractors, they can do so with little effort. They can also add questions to the test bank. The *ExamView Pro* program is available for PC and Macintosh users.

RESOURCE KIT

Learning Management Systems Resource Kit is available for Blackboard, Angel, Moodle, Canvass, and SCORM-compliant systems.

TEACHING AND STUDENT GUIDES

The Teaching and Student Guides are extensive instructional aids matched to every lecture in a common single-term Medical Terminology course. The Teaching Guide is filled with sample homework assignments, in-class activities, and extensive lecture notes with suggested topic durations. When viewed electronically, the Teaching Guide also provides live hyperlinks to the instructor resources on Davis*Plus*. The accompanying Student Guide may be distributed to students at the instructor's discretion. The Student Guide contains study tips, lists of accompanying resources, and a list of the homework assignments from the Teaching Guide.

DAVIS DIGITAL VERSION

Adopters have access to the complete content of the text online in a searchable format that can be bookmarked and accessed wherever you have a browser with a live Internet connection.

Term*Plus*

Term*Plus* 3.0 is a powerful, interactive CD-ROM program that is available for this edition as a separate product. Term*Plus* is a popular competency-based, self-paced, multimedia program that includes graphics, audio, and a dictionary culled from *Taber's Cyclopedic Medical Dictionary,* 22nd edition. Help menus provide navigational support. The software comes with numerous interactive learning activities, including the following:

- Anatomy Focus
- Tag the Elements
- Spotlight the Elements
- Concentration
- Build Medical Words
- Programmed Learning
- Medical Vocabulary
- Chart Notes
- Spelling
- Crossword Puzzles
- Word Scramble
- Terminology Teaser

All activities can be graded and the results printed or e-mailed to an instructor. This feature makes Term*Plus* especially valuable as a distance-learning tool because it provides evidence of student drill and practice in various learning activities.

HOW TO USE THIS BOOK

This self-instructional book is designed to provide the student with skills to learn medical terminology easily and quickly. The book's design and flexibility enable its use as a self-instructional book or one that can be used in traditional lecture and classroom environments. The following distinctive features are included in this learning package:

- The programmed learning approach presents a word-building method for developing a medical vocabulary in an effective, interesting manner. It is designed for use in a traditional classroom setting or for independent study with an instructor.
- The workbook-text format is designed to guide you through exercises that teach and reinforce medical terminology.
- Numerous activities in each unit are designed to enable the student to be interactively involved in the learning process. Writing, reading, listening, visualizing, and keyboarding encompass the various learning styles employed in the book to help the student master medical terminology. With this method, the student will not only understand but also remember the significant concepts of medical word building.
- Students learn by active participation. In this book, students write answers in response to blocks of information, complete section review exercises, and analyze medical reports. If a student is not satisfied with his or her level of comprehension after the review exercises, reinforcement frames direct the student to go back and rework the corresponding informational frames.

- New to this edition is a designated icon in each chapter that directs the student to visit the *Medical Language Lab* for a flash-card review of word elements covered in the chapter.
- The audio exercises provide reinforcement of pronunciation, definitions, and spelling practice of medical terms. The terms and pronunciations are now available by visiting the Davis*Plus* website.
- Pronunciation keys for all medical words are included in the frame answer boxes and help the student pronounce each term correctly. Newly designed pronunciation guides in each chapter give the student a more accurate understanding of the proper pronunciation of medical words.
- The appendices include many tools students can use as references when they begin working in the clinical field.

We hope the pedagogical and visual features of *Medical Terminology Simplified: A Programmed Learning Approach by Body System,* 5th edition, make learning the language of medicine an exciting, rewarding process. We invite instructors and students to continue the tradition of sending their suggestions to the F. A. Davis Company so that we can consider them for the next edition.

—BARBARA A. GYLYS
—REGINA M. MASTERS

Reviewers

JANNA F. EDRINGTON, MSN, RNC, ARNP
Assistant Professor
Nursing
Luther College
Decorah, IA

DAWN HAMMERSCHMIDT, PhD, ATC
Assistant Professor
Health and Physical Education
Minnesota State University
Moorhead, MN

PATRICIA HODSON, PT, DPT
*Clinical Professor and Director of Clinical
    Education*
Health Sciences
East Carolina University
Greenville, NC

MARIE L. KOTTER, PhD
Department Chair
Physical Therapy
Weber State University
Ogden, UT

CATHERINE NOWAK, MS, PA-C
Associate Program Director
Physician Assistant Program
Mercy College
Bronx, NY

CHRISTINE M. PETRAGLIA, RPh, MSEd
Adjunct Faculty
Health and Natural Sciences
Holyoke Community College
Holyoke, MA

CAROLYN SCHEESE, RN, MS
*Director, Simulation Learning Center—Faculty
    Instructor—Clinical*
College of Nursing
University of Utah
Salt Lake City, UT

GLYNDA R. SHERRILL, RN, MS
*Practical Nursing Instructor, Might Medical
    Terminology Instructor*
Practical Nursing
Indian Capital Technology Center
Tahlequah, OK

GINA TICE, MSRS, RT(R)
Clinical Coordinator
Radiologic Technology Program
Gadsden State Community College
Gadsden, AL

Acknowledgments

The fifth edition of *Medical Terminology Simplified: A Programmed Learning Approach by Body System* was greatly improved by comments that the authors received from the many users of previous editions—both educators and students. Although there are too many people to acknowledge individually, we are deeply grateful to each one. As in the past, the editorial and production staffs at F. A. Davis have inspired, guided, and shaped this project. The authors would like to acknowledge the valuable contributions of F. A. Davis's editorial and production team who were responsible for this project:

- Quincy McDonald, Publisher, provided the overall design and layout for the fifth edition. He was instrumental in assisting the authors in designing a wide variety of state-of-the-art pedagogical products within the text to aid students in their learning activities and to help instructors plan course work and presentations. These teaching aids are described in the Teaching and Learning Package section of the Preface.
- Elizabeth Schaeffer, Developmental Editor of Electronics, patiently and enthusiastically addressed our numerous questions and background queries to ensure the textbook was appropriately updated and accurately revised.
- George W. Lang, Manager of Content Development, expertly guided the manuscript through the developmental and production phases of the process.
- Brenna H. Mayer, Developmental Editor, systematically and meticulously read the manuscript, helping it along at every stage of production.
- Margaret Biblis, Publisher, once again provided her support and efforts for the quality of the finished product.

We also acknowledge and thank our exceptionally dedicated publishing partners who helped guide and shape this large project:

- **Alisa Hathaway,** *Editorial Assistant*
- **Robert Butler,** *Production Manager*
- **Kate Margeson,** *Illustrations Coordinator*
- **Carolyn O'Brien,** *Art and Design Manager*
- **Linda Van Pelt,** *Managing Editor*
- **Kirk Pedrick,** *Electronic Product Development Manager, Electronic Publishing*
- **Elizabeth Y. Stepchin,** *Developmental Associate*

We also we extend our sincerest gratitude to Neil Kelly, Director of Sales, and his staff of sales representatives, whose continued efforts have undoubtedly contributed to the success of this textbook.

Contents at a Glance

CHAPTER 1   Introduction to Programmed Learning and Medical Word Building   *1*

CHAPTER 2   Body Structure   *27*

CHAPTER 3   Integumentary System   *63*

CHAPTER 4   Respiratory System   *107*

CHAPTER 5   Cardiovascular and Lymphatic Systems   *155*

CHAPTER 6   Digestive System   *217*

CHAPTER 7   Urinary System   *277*

CHAPTER 8   Reproductive Systems   *329*

CHAPTER 9   Endocrine and Nervous Systems   *393*

CHAPTER 10   Musculoskeletal System   *453*

CHAPTER 11   Special Senses: Eyes and Ears   *507*

APPENDICES

APPENDIX A   Glossary of Medical Word Elements   *548*

APPENDIX B   Answer Key   *558*

APPENDIX C   Index of Diagnostic, Medical, and Surgical Procedures   *604*

APPENDIX D   Drug Classifications   *607*

APPENDIX E   Abbreviations and Symbols   *613*

APPENDIX F   Medical Specialties   *622*

APPENDIX G   Glossary of English-to-Spanish Translations   *624*

     Index   *633*

     Rules for Singular and Plural Suffixes   *Facing the inside back cover*

     Pronunciation Guidelines   *Inside back cover*

Contents

CHAPTER 1 Introduction to Programmed Learning and Medical Word Building   *1*

Objectives   *1*

Instructions   *2*

Word Elements   *3*

   Word Root   4

   Combining Forms   5

   Suffixes   8

   Prefixes   13

Pronunciation Guidelines   *15*

   Pronunciation Tools   15

   Section Review 1–1   16

Common Suffixes   *16*

   Surgical Suffixes   16

   Diagnostic Suffixes   18

   Pathological Suffixes   19

   Plural Suffixes   21

   Section Review 1–2   22

Common Prefixes   *23*

CHAPTER 2 Body Structure   *27*

Objectives   *27*

Word Elements   *29*

   Section Review 2–1   31

Basic Units of Structure   *31*

Directional Terms   *32*

   Section Review 2–2   39

Word Elements   *40*

   Section Review 2–3   41

Body Planes and Cavities   *41*

   Body Planes   41

   Body Cavities   44

Abdominopelvic Quadrants and Regions   45
   Abdominopelvic Quadrants   46
   Abdominopelvic Regions   46
   Section Review 2–4   49
Abbreviations   50
Additional Medical Terms   50
   Diseases and Conditions   50
   Diagnostic Procedures   51
   Medical and Surgical Procedures   54
   Additional Medical Terms Review   55
Body Structure Chapter Review   56
   Word Elements Summary   56
   Word Elements Chapter Review   57
   Quadrants and Regions Review   61

CHAPTER   3   Integumentary System   63
Objectives   63
Medical Specialty   63
   Dermatology   63
Anatomy and Physiology Overview   63
Word Elements   64
   Section Review 3–1   67
Skin and Accessory Organs   67
   Skin   67
   Accessory Organs of the Skin   73
   Section Review 3–2   77
   Combining Forms Denoting Color   78
   Section Review 3–3   83
Abbreviations   84
Additional Medical Terms   84
   Diseases and Conditions   84
   Diagnostic Procedures   90
   Medical and Surgical Procedures   91
Pharmacology   92
   Additional Medical Terms Review   93
   Primary and Secondary Lesions Review   94
Medical Record Activities   95
   Medical Record Activity 3–1: Compound Nevus   95
   Medical Record Activity 3–2: Psoriasis   97
Integumentary System Chapter Review   100
   Word Elements Summary   100
   Word Elements Chapter Review   101
   Vocabulary Review   105

CHAPTER 4   Respiratory System   *107*

Objectives   *107*
Medical Specialty   *107*
    Pulmonology   107
Anatomy and Physiology Overview   *107*
Word Elements   *109*
    Section Review 4–1   111
Respiratory System   *111*
    Upper Respiratory Tract   111
    Section Review 4–2   117
    Lower Respiratory Tract   118
    Section Review 4–3   131
Abbreviations   *132*
Additional Medical Terms   *133*
    Diseases and Conditions   133
    Diagnostic Procedures   136
    Medical and Surgical Procedures   138
Pharmacology   *139*
    Additional Medical Terms Review   141
Medical Record Activities   *142*
    Medical Record Activity 4–1: Upper Airway Obstruction   142
    Medical Record Activity 4–2: Bronchoscopy   144
Respiratory System Chapter Review   *147*
    Word Elements Summary   147
    Word Elements Chapter Review   149
    Vocabulary Review   153

CHAPTER 5   Cardiovascular and Lymphatic Systems   *155*

Objectives   *155*
Medical Specialties   *155*
    Cardiology   155
    Immunology   155
Anatomy and Physiology Overview   *156*
Word Elements   *157*
    Section Review 5–1   159
Cardiovascular System   *159*
    Layers of the Heart Wall   159
    Circulation and Heart Structures   161
    Blood Flow Through the Heart   166
    Heart Valves   171
    Section Review 5–2   173

Conduction Pathway of the Heart 174
Cardiac Cycle and Heart Sounds 176
Lymphatic System *181*
Word Elements *182*
Section Review 5–3 183
Lymphatic Structures *183*
Tonsil, Spleen, and Thymus 186
Section Review 5–4 188
Abbreviations *189*
Additional Medical Terms *190*
Diseases and Conditions 190
Diagnostic Procedures 194
Medical and Surgical Procedures 198
Pharmacology *202*
Additional Medical Terms Review 203
Medical Record Activities *204*
Medical Record Activity 5–1: Myocardial Infarction 204
Medical Record Activity 5–2: Cardiac Catheterization 206
Cardiovascular and Lymphatic Systems Chapter Review *208*
Word Elements Summary 208
Word Elements Chapter Review 210
Vocabulary Review 216

CHAPTER 6   **Digestive System** *217*
Objectives *217*
Medical Specialty *217*
Gastroenterology 217
Anatomy and Physiology Overview *217*
Word Elements *219*
Section Review 6–1 221
Upper GI Tract *221*
Oral Cavity 221
Esophagus, Pharynx, and Stomach 226
Section Review 6–2 232
Word Elements *233*
Section Review 6–3 234
Lower GI Tract *234*
Small and Large Intestine 234
Rectum and Anus 240
Section Review 6–4 243
Word Elements *244*
Section Review 6–5 245
Accessory Organs of Digestion 245
Liver 246

Gallbladder *247*

Pancreas *251*

Section Review 6–6 *254*

Abbreviations 255

Additional Medical Terms 255

Diseases and Conditions *255*

Diagnostic Procedures *260*

Medical and Surgical Procedures *262*

Pharmacology 263

Additional Medical Terms Review *264*

Medical Record Activities 265

Medical Record Activity 6–1: Rectal Bleeding *265*

Medical Record Activity 6–2: Carcinosarcoma of the Esophagus *267*

Digestive System Chapter Review 269

Word Elements Summary *269*

Word Elements Chapter Review *271*

Vocabulary Review *276*

CHAPTER 7   **Urinary System**   277

Objectives 277

Medical Specialties 277

Urology *277*

Nephrology *277*

Anatomy and Physiology Overview 278

Word Elements 280

Section Review 7–1 *282*

Macroscopic Structures 282

Kidneys *282*

Section Review 7–2 *289*

Ureters, Bladder, and Urethra *289*

Section Review 7–3 *296*

Microscopic Structures 296

Section Review 7–4 *304*

Abbreviations 305

Additional Medical Terms 305

Diseases and Conditions *305*

Diagnostic Procedures *307*

Medical and Surgical Procedures *309*

Pharmacology 313

Additional Medical Terms Review *314*

Medical Record Activities 315

Medical Record Activity 7–1: Cystitis *315*

Medical Record Activity 7–2: Dysuria with Benign Prostatic Hypertrophy *317*

Urinary System Chapter Review   *320*

   Word Elements Summary   320

   Word Elements Chapter Review   322

   Vocabulary Review   327

CHAPTER 8   Reproductive Systems   *329*

Objectives   *329*

Medical Specialties   *329*

   Gynecology   329

   Obstetrics   329

   Obstetrics and Gynecology   329

   Urology   330

Anatomy and Physiology Overview   *330*

Female Reproductive System   *330*

Word Elements   *332*

   Section Review 8–1   334

   Section Review 8–2   344

   Section Review 8–3   353

Male Reproductive System   *354*

Word Elements   *354*

   Section Review 8–4   356

   Section Review 8–5   365

Abbreviations   *366*

Additional Medical Terms   *366*

   Diseases and Conditions   366

   Diagnostic Procedures   372

   Medical and Surgical Procedures   375

Pharmacology   *379*

   Additional Medical Terms Review   380

Medical Record Activities   *381*

   Medical Record Activity 8–1: Postmenopausal Bleeding   381

   Medical Record Activity 8–2: Bilateral Vasectomy   383

Reproductive Systems Chapter Review   *385*

   Word Elements Summary   385

   Word Elements Chapter Review   387

   Vocabulary Review   391

CHAPTER 9   Endocrine and Nervous Systems   *393*

Objectives   *393*

Medical Specialties   *393*

   Endocrinology   393

   Neurology   393

Anatomy and Physiology Overview   *394*

Endocrine System   *394*

Word Elements   *396*

   Section Review 9–1   398

   Hormones   398

   Pituitary Gland   400

   Table 9–1: Pituitary Hormones   404

   Thyroid Gland   405

   Table 9–2: Thyroid Hormones   407

   Section Review 9–2   408

   Parathyroid Glands   408

   Table 9–3: Parathyroid Hormone   409

   Adrenal Glands   410

   Table 9–4: Adrenal Hormones   411

   Pancreas (Islets of Langerhans)   411

   Table 9–5: Pancreatic Hormones   413

   Pineal and Thymus Glands   415

   Ovaries and Testes   415

   Section Review 9–3   417

Nervous System   *417*

Word Elements   *419*

   Section Review 9–4   420

   Brain   420

   Spinal Cord   422

   Mental Disorders   426

   Section Review 9–5   428

Abbreviations   *429*

Additional Medical Terms   *429*

   Diseases and Conditions   429

   Diagnostic Procedures   435

   Medical and Surgical Procedures   437

Pharmacology   *438*

   Additional Medical Terms Review   439

Medical Record Activities   *440*

   Medical Record Activity 9–1: Diabetes Mellitus   440

   Medical Record Activity 9–2: Stroke   443

Endocrine and Nervous Systems Chapter Review   *446*

   Word Elements Summary   446

   Word Elements Chapter Review   448

   Vocabulary Review   452

CHAPTER 10   Musculoskeletal System   *453*

Objectives   *453*
Medical Specialties   *453*
    Orthopedics   *453*
    Osteopathy   *453*
    Chiropractic   *454*
Anatomy and Physiology Overview   *454*
Word Elements   *455*
    Section Review 10–1   *457*
Muscles   *457*
    Types of Muscle Fibers   *457*
    Section Review 10–2   *461*
Skeletal System   *462*
Word Elements   *463*
    Section Review 10–3   *466*
    Structure and Function of Bones   *466*
    Section Review 10–4   *473*
    Joints   *474*
    Combining Forms Related to Specific Bones   *476*
    Fractures and Repairs   *479*
    Vertebral Column   *480*
    Section Review 10–5   *485*
Abbreviations   *486*
Additional Medical Terms   *486*
    Diseases and Conditions   *486*
    Diagnostic Procedures   *492*
    Medical and Surgical Procedures   *492*
Pharmacology   *493*
    Additional Medical Terms Review   *494*
Medical Record Activities   *495*
    Medical Record Activity 10–1: Degenerative, Intervertebral Disk Disease   *495*
    Medical Record Activity 10–2: Rotator Cuff Tear, Right Shoulder   *497*
Musculoskeletal System Chapter Review   *500*
    Word Elements Summary   *500*
    Word Elements Chapter Review   *502*
    Vocabulary Review   *506*

CHAPTER 11   Special Senses: Eyes and Ears   *507*

Objectives   *507*
Medical Specialties   *507*
    Ophthalmology   *507*
    Otolaryngology   *507*
Anatomy and Physiology Overview   *508*

Eyes   *508*

Word Elements   *508*

   Section Review 11–1   510

   Fibrous Tunic   511

   Vascular Tunic   512

   Sensory Tunic   512

Ears   *517*

Word Elements   *518*

   Section Review 11–2   519

   Section Review 11–3   524

Abbreviations   *525*

Additional Medical Terms   *525*

   Diseases and Conditions   525

   Diagnostic Procedures   530

   Medical and Surgical Procedures   533

Pharmacology   *535*

   Additional Medical Terms Review   536

Medical Record Activities   *537*

   Medical Record Activity 11–1: Retinal Detachment   537

   Medical Record Activity 11–2: Otitis Media   539

Special Senses: Eyes and Ears Chapter Review   *541*

   Word Elements Summary   541

   Word Elements Chapter Review   543

   Vocabulary Review   547

APPENDICES

APPENDIX A   Glossary of Medical Word Elements   *548*

APPENDIX B   Answer Key   *558*

APPENDIX C   Index of Diagnostic, Medical, and Surgical Procedures   *604*

APPENDIX D   Drug Classifications   *607*

APPENDIX E   Abbreviations and Symbols   *613*

APPENDIX F   Medical Specialties   *622*

APPENDIX G   Glossary of English-to-Spanish Translations   *624*

Index   *633*

Rules for Singular and Plural Suffixes   *Facing inside back cover*

Pronunciation Guidelines   *Inside back cover*

Introduction to Programmed Learning and Medical Word Building

OBJECTIVES

Upon completion of this chapter, you will be able to:

• Learn medical terminology by using the programmed learning technique.

• Identify and define four elements used to build medical words.

• Analyze and define the various parts of a medical term.

• Apply the rules learned in this chapter to pronounce medical words correctly.

• Define and provide examples of surgical, diagnostic, pathological, and related suffixes.

• Apply the rules learned in this chapter to write singular and plural forms of medical words.

• Locate and apply guidelines for pluralizing terms.

• Practice pronouncing the medical terms presented in this chapter.

• Demonstrate your knowledge of this chapter by successfully completing the frames and learning activities.

INSTRUCTIONS

In the first few pages, you will learn the most efficient use of this self-instructional programmed learning approach. *First remove the sliding card and cover the left-hand answer column with it.*

answer	**1-1** This text is designed to help you learn medical terminology effectively. The principal technique used throughout the book is known as *programmed learning,* which consists of a series of teaching units called *frames.* Each frame presents information and calls for an answer on your part. When you complete a sentence by writing an answer on the blank line, you are learning information by using the programmed learning technique. A frame consists of a block of information and a blank line. The purpose of the blank line is to write an _____.
	1-2 Slide the card down in the left column to see the correct answer. After you correct the answer, read the next frame.
answer	**1-3** It is important to keep the left-hand answer column covered until you write your _____.
learning	**1-4** This book employs several methods to help you master medical terminology, but the main technique used is called *programmed* _____.
answer(s)	**1-5** After you write your answer, it is important to verify that it is correct. To do so, compare your answer with the one listed in the left-hand answer column. To obtain immediate feedback on your responses, you must verify your _____.

Study frames in sequence because each frame builds on the previous one. Words are reviewed and repeated throughout the book to reinforce your learning. Consequently, you do not need to memorize every word that is presented.

one	**1-6** The number of blank lines in a frame determines the number of words you write for your answer. Review the number of blank lines in Frame 1-5. It has _____ blank line(s). Therefore, the answer requires one word.
two, lines	**1-7** A frame that requires two answers will have _____ blank _____.
	1-8 In some frames, you will be asked to write the answer in your own words. In these instances, there will be one or more blank lines across the entire frame. List at least two reasons why you want to learn medical terminology. Keep these objectives in mind as you work through the book. _____ _____

Do not look at the answer column before you write your response and do not move ahead in a chapter. Progress in developing a medical vocabulary depends on your ability to learn the material presented in each frame.

frame	**1–9** Completing one frame at a time is the most effective method of learning. To achieve your goal of learning medical terminology, complete one _____ at a time.
back	**1–10** Whenever you make an error, it is important to go back and review the previous frame(s). You need to determine why you wrote the wrong answer before proceeding to the next frame. You may always go _____ and review information you have forgotten. Just remember, do not look ahead.
correct, check, or verify	**1–11** Do not be afraid to make a mistake. In programmed learning, you will learn and profit by your mistakes if you correct them immediately. Always _____ your answer immediately after you write it.
answer	**1–12** Because accurate spelling is essential in medicine, correct all misspelled words immediately. Do so by comparing your answer with the one in the left-hand _____ column.
correctly, or accurately	**1–13** In medicine, it is important to spell correctly. Correct spelling can be a crucial component in determining the validity of evidence presented in a malpractice lawsuit. A physician can lose a lawsuit because of misspelled words that result in a misinterpreted medical record. To provide correct information, medical words must be spelled _____ in a medical record.

WORD ELEMENTS

A medical word consists of some or all of the following elements:

- Word root
- Combining form
- Suffix
- Prefix

How you combine these elements and whether all or some of them are present in a medical word determine the meaning of a word. The purpose of this chapter is to help you learn to identify these elements and use them to form medical terms.

suffix, prefix	**1–14** The four elements that are used to build a medical word are the word root, combining form, _____, and _____.
elements, or parts	**1–15** Medical terminology is not difficult to learn when you understand how the elements are combined to form a word. To develop a medical vocabulary, you must understand the _____ that form medical words.

Word Root

A word root (WR) is the main part, or foundation, of a word. All medical words have at least one word root.

teach	**1-16** In the words *teach*er, *teach*es, *teach*ing, the word root is _____.

speak	**1-17** In the words *speak*er, *speak*s, *speak*ing, the word root is _____.

1-18 Identify the roots in the following words:

read
spend
play

Word	Root
reader	_____
spending	_____
playful	_____

 A word root, also called a *root*, may be used alone or combined with other elements to form another word with a different meaning.

1-19 Review the following examples to see how roots are used alone or with other elements to form words. The meaning of each term in the right-hand column is also provided.

Root as a Complete Word	Root as Part of a Word
alcohol	**alcohol**ism (condition marked by impaired control over alcohol use)
sperm	**sperm**icide (agent that kills sperm)
thyroid	**thyroid**ectomy (excision of the thyroid gland)

1-20 Throughout the book, a slash is used to separate word elements, as shown in the following examples.

alcohol
dent
lump
insulin
gastr

Write the roots in the right-hand column for each of these terms:

alcohol/ic	_____
dent/ist	_____
lump/ectomy	_____
insulin/ism	_____
gastr/itis	_____

cardi	**1–21** In medical words, the root usually indicates a body part (anatomical structure). For example, the root in cardi/al, cardi/ac, and cardi/o/gram is _____ and it means heart.

dent/al DĚN-tăl **pancreat/itis** păn-krē-ă-TĪ-tĭs **dermat/o/logist** děr-mă-TŎL-ō-jĭst	**1–22** You will find that the roots in medical words are usually derived from Greek or Latin words. Some examples include *dent* in the word dent/ist, *pancreat* in the word pancreat/itis, and *dermat* in the word dermat/o/logist. Underline the roots in the following words: dent/al pancreat/itis dermat/o/logist

part	**1–23** In Frame 1–22, the root *dent* means *tooth,* *pancreat* means *pancreas,* and *dermat* means *skin.* All three roots indicate a body _____.

Combining Forms

A combining form (CF) is created when a word root is combined with a vowel. This vowel is usually an *o*. The vowel has no meaning of its own, but enables two word elements to be linked.

combining form	**1–24** Like the word root, the CF is the basic foundation on which other elements are added to build a complete word. In this text, a combining form will be listed as *word root/vowel,* such as *dent/o* and *gastr/o.* A word root + a vowel (usually an *o*) forms a new element known as a _____ _____.

therm/o **gastr/o**	**1–25** The CF in therm/o/meter is _____ / _____. The CF in gastr/o/scope is _____ / _____.

combining form **gastr, o**	**1–26** *Gastr/o* is an example of the word element called a _____ _____. The root in *gastr/o* is _____; the combining vowel is _____.

o **o** **o**	**1–27** List the combining vowel in each of the following elements: arthr/o: _____ phleb/o: _____ lith/o: _____

therm/o **abdomin**/o **nephr**/o	**1–28** Underline the word root in the following combining forms: therm/o abdomin/o nephr/o

---

1–29 Use the combining vowel *o* to change the following roots to combining forms, and separate the elements with a slash.

cyst/o **arthr**/o **leuk**/o **gastr**/o	**Root** **Combining Form (Root + Vowel)** cyst _____ arthr _____ leuk _____ gastr _____

---

o	**1–30** Usually, the combining vowel is an *o*, although other vowels may be encountered occasionally. The combining vowel is usually an _____.

1–31 Instead of joining the two elements *chem* and *-therapy* directly, the combining vowel *o* is attached to the root to form the word chem/o/therapy. The vowel has no meaning of its own, but enables two elements to be connected to each other. Use the combining vowel to build medical terms below. Chem/o/therapy is given as an example.

chem/o/therapy kē-mō-THĔR-ă-pē **dermat/o/logy** dĕr-mă-TŎL-ō-jē **encephal/o/graphy** ĕn-sĕf-ă-LŎG-ră-fē **neur/o/logy** nū-RŎL-ō-jē **therm/o/meter** thĕr-MŎM-ĕ-tĕr	**Word Root** **Suffix** **Medical Term** chem therapy *becomes* *chem/o/therapy* dermat -logy *becomes* _____ / ____ / _____ encephal -graphy *becomes* _____ / ____ / _____ neur -logy *becomes* _____ / ____ / _____ therm -meter *becomes* _____ / ____ / _____

---

vowel	**1–32** The words in Frame 1–31 are easier to pronounce because the word roots are linked with the combining vowel *o*. To make a word easier to pronounce, attach a combining _____ to the word root.

---

elements, or parts	**1–33** Although you may not know the meaning of all the words in this unit, you have already started to learn the word-building system by identifying the basic _____ of a medical word.

medical	**I–34** Understanding the word-building system will help you decipher the meanings of medical terms. Using the word-building system to identify basic elements of a medical word will help you learn _____ terminology.
dermat, dermat/o	**I–35** In the word dermat/o/logy, the root is _____; the combining form is _____ / _____.

A combining vowel is used to link a root to another root to form a compound word. This rule holds true even if the next root begins with a vowel, as in gastr/o/enter/itis.

o	**I–36** In the word gastr/o/enter/itis, the roots *gastr* (stomach) and *enter* (intestine) are linked together with the combining vowel _____.
leuk, cyt **-penia**	**I–37** The roots in leuk/o/cyt/o/penia are _____ and _____. The suffix is _____.
leuk/o, cyt/o	**I–38** Identify the CFs in leuk/o/cyt/o/penia: _____ / _____ and _____ / _____.
electr/o, cardi/o	**I–39** List the CFs in electr/o/cardi/o/gram: _____ / _____ and _____ / _____.
back	**I–40** You are now using the programmed learning method. If you are experiencing difficulty writing the correct answers, go back to Frame 1–1 and rework the frames. To master material that has been covered, you can always go _____ to review the frames.

Throughout the textbook, all word roots and combining forms that stand alone are set in **boldface**.

Suffixes

A suffix is a word element located at the end of a word. Substituting one suffix for another suffix changes the meaning of the word. In medical terminology, a suffix usually indicates a procedure, condition, disease, or part of speech. In this text, a suffix that stands alone is preceded by a hyphen.

suffix	**1–41** The element at the end of a word is called the _____.

play/er **read/er** **speak/er**	**1–42** **Play, read,** and **speak** are complete words and also roots. Add the suffix *-er* (meaning *one who*) to each root to modify its meaning. **Play** *becomes* _____ / _____. **Read** *becomes* _____ / _____. **Speak** *becomes* _____ / _____.

one who **one who** **one who**	**1–43** By attaching the suffix *-er (one who)* to **play, read,** and **speak,** we create nouns that mean the following: **Play**/*er* means _____ _____ *plays.* **Read**/*er* means _____ _____ *reads.* **Speak**/*er* means _____ _____ *speaks.*

A word root links a suffix that begins with a vowel.

1–44   Link the following roots with suffixes, each of which begins with a vowel. Then practice pronouncing the terms aloud by referring to the pronunciations in the left-hand answer column.

tonsill/itis
tŏn-sĭl-Ī-tĭs

gastr/ectomy
găs-TRĔK-tō-mē

arthr/itis
ăr-THRĪ-tĭs

Word Root	Suffix		Medical Term
tonsill	-itis	*becomes*	_____ / _____
gastr	-ectomy	*becomes*	_____ / _____
arthr	-itis	*becomes*	_____ / _____

root, suffix	**1–45** Changing the suffix modifies the meaning of the word. In the word dent/al, *dent* is the word _____ and *-al* is the _____.

-ist **-al**	**1-46** A dent/ist is a specialist in teeth. *Dent/al* means *pertaining to teeth*. Simply changing the suffix gives the word a new meaning. The suffix in *dent/ist* is _____. It means *specialist*. The suffix in *dent/al* is _____. It means *pertaining to*.

A combining form (root + **o**) links a suffix that begins with a consonant.

scler/o/derma sklĕr- ō-DĔR-mă **mast/o/dynia** măst-ō-DĬN-ē-ă **arthr/o/plasty** ĂR-thrō-plăs-tē	**1-47** Change the following roots to combining forms and link them with suffixes that begin with a consonant. Then practice pronouncing the terms aloud by referring to the pronunciations in the left-hand answer column.

Word Root	Suffix		Medical Term
scler	-derma	*becomes*	_____ / ____ / _____
mast	-dynia	*becomes*	_____ / ____ / _____
arthr	-plasty	*becomes*	_____ / ____ / _____

hyphen	**1-48** Throughout the book, whenever a suffix stands alone, it will be preceded by a hyphen, as in *-oma (tumor)*. The hyphen indicates that another element is needed to transform the suffix into a complete word. A suffix that stands alone will be preceded by a _____.

Pronouncing medical words correctly is crucial, because mispronunciations can result in incorrect medical interpretations and treatments. In addition, misspelled terms in a medical report may become a legal issue. Learning how to pronounce and spell medical terms is a matter of practice. To familiarize yourself with medical words, make it a habit to pronounce a word aloud each time you see the pronunciation listed in the answer column.

dent/ist DĔN-tĭst **arthr/o/centesis** ăr-thrō-sĕn-TĒ-sĭs **neur/algia** nū-RĂL-jē-ă **angi/oma** ăn-jē-Ō-mă **gastr/ic** GĂS-trĭk **nephr/itis** nĕf-RĪ-tĭs **scler/o/derma** sklĕr-ō-DĔR-mă	**1-49** Underline the suffixes in the following words: dent/ist arthr/o/centesis neur/algia angi/oma gastr/ic nephr/itis scler/o/derma

arthr/o, scler/o **dent, neur, angi,** **gastr, nephr**	**1–50** Elements preceding a suffix can be a root or a combining form. Review Frame 1–49 and list the combining forms preceding suffixes: _____ / _____ and _____ / _____ roots preceding suffixes: _____, _____, _____, _____, and _____.

1–51   Analyze the following medical terms by identifying their elements. The first is completed as an example. The vowel has no meaning of its own, but enables two elements to be connected. Refer to Appendix A: Glossary of Medical Word Elements, if needed.

Medical Term	Combining Form (root + o)	Word Root	Suffix
arthr/o/scop/ic ăr-thrōs-KŌP-ĭk	_arthr_ / _o_	_scop_	_-ic_
erythr/o/cyt/osis ĕ-rĭth-rō-sī-TŌ-sĭs	_____ / _____	_____	_____
append/ix ă-PĔN-dĭks	_____ / _____	_____	_____
dermat/itis dĕr-mă-TĪ-tĭs	_____ / _____	_____	_____
gastr/o/enter/itis găs-trō-ĕn-tĕr-Ī-tĭs	_____ / _____	_____	_____
orth/o/ped/ic or-thō-PĒ-dĭk	_____ / _____	_____	_____
oste/o/arthr/itis ŏs-tē-ō-ăr-THRĪ-tĭs	_____ / _____	_____	_____
vagin/itis văj-ĭn-Ī-tĭs	_____ / _____	_____	_____

Find answers to this frame in Appendix B: Answer Key, page 558.

suffixes	**1–52** The examples in Frame 1–51 show how medical words can be formed by various combinations of combining forms, roots, and _____.

Three Rules of Word Building

There are three important rules of word building:

- **Rule 1:** A root links a suffix that begins with a vowel.
- **Rule 2:** A combining form (root + *o*) links a suffix that begins with a consonant.
- **Rule 3:** A combining form (root + *o*) links a root to another root to form a compound word. (This rule holds true even if the next root begins with a vowel.)

leuk/emia
loo-KĒ-mē-ă

cephal/algia
sĕf-ă-LĂL-jē-ă

gastr/itis
găs-TRĪ-tĭs

append/ectomy
ăp-ĕn-DĔK-tō-mē

1–53 Rule 1: In the following examples, use a word root to link suffixes that begin with a vowel.

Word Root	Suffix		Medical Word
leuk	-emia	*becomes*	_____ / _____ / _____
cephal	-algia	*becomes*	_____ / _____ / _____
gastr	-itis	*becomes*	_____ / _____ / _____
append	-ectomy	*becomes*	_____ / _____ / _____

---

gastr/o/scope
GĂS-trō-skōp

men/o/rrhea
mĕn-ō-RĒ-ă

angi/o/rrhexis
ăn-jē-ō-RĔK-sĭs

ureter/o/lith
ū-RĒ-tĕr-ō-lĭth

1–54 Rule 2: In the following examples, use a combining form (root + *o*) to link the suffixes that begin with a consonant.

Word Root	Suffix		Medical Term
gastr	-scope	*becomes*	_____ / _____ / _____
men	-rrhea	*becomes*	_____ / _____ / _____
angi	-rrhexis	*becomes*	_____ / _____ / _____
ureter	-lith	*becomes*	_____ / _____ / _____

---

oste/o/chondr/itis
ŏs-tē-ō-kŏn-DRĪ-tĭs

oste/o/chondr/oma
ŏs-tē-ō-kŏn-DRŌ-mă

oste/o/arthr/itis
ŏs-tē-ō-ăr-THRĪ-tĭs

gastr/o/enter/itis
găs-trō-ĕn-tĕr-Ī-tĭs

1–55 Rule 3: In the following four examples, apply the rule, "Use a combining form (root + *o*) to link a root to another root to form a compound word." (This rule holds true even if the next root begins with a vowel.)

oste + chondr + *-itis* becomes _____ / _____ / _____ / _____.

oste + chondr + *-oma* becomes _____ / _____ / _____ / _____.

oste + arthr + *-itis* becomes _____ / _____ / _____ / _____.

gastr + enter + *-itis* becomes _____ / _____ / _____ / _____.

---

word root

1–56 Would you use a word root or a combining form as a link to the suffixes

-algia, -edema, and *-uria?* _____ _____

---

cardi/o/gram
KĂR-dē-ō-grăm

Rule 2: A combining form (root + *o*) links a suffix that begins with a consonant.

1–57 Refer to the three rules of word building on page 10 to complete Frames 1–57 to 1–62.

Form a word with **cardi** and *-gram:* _____ / _____ / _____
                                                         (root)   (suffix)

Summarize the rule that applies in this frame.

Rule 2: _____

_____

prefix **root** **suffix**	**1–68** Whenever a prefix stands alone, it is identified with a hyphen after it, as in *hyper-*. When it is part of a word, the prefix is not highlighted, but a slash separates it from the next element, as in *hyper/tension.* Analyze hyper/insulin/ism by identifying the elements. *hyper-* is a _____. *insulin* is a _____. *-ism* is a _____.
prefixes	**1–69** *Hypo-, intra-, super-,* and *homo-* are examples of word elements called _____.
post/operative pōst-ŎP-ĕr-ă-tĭv **after**	**1–70** Pre/operative designates the time before a surgery. By changing the prefix, you alter the meaning of the word. Build a word that designates the time after surgery. _____ / _____. Can you remember what *post-* in *post/operative* means? _____
post-, after **after**	**1–71** You will recognize many prefixes in medical terms because they are the same ones found in the English language. In the term *post/mortem,* the prefix is _____ and means _____. *Post/mortem* means _____ death.
pre-, before **before**	**1–72** In the term pre/mature, the prefix is _____ and means _____. *Pre/mature* means _____ maturity.

Defining Medical Words

When defining a medical word, first define the suffix. Second, define the beginning of the word; finally, define the middle of the word. Here is an example using the term *osteoarthritis.*

oste/o/arthr/itis
(2)   (3)   (1)

1. Define the suffix first: *-itis* means *inflammation.*
2. Define the beginning of the word: *oste/o* means *bone.*
3. Define the middle of the word: *arthr* means *joint.*

Therefore, *oste/o/arthr/itis* is an inflammation of the bone and joint.

suffix **beginning** **last**	**1–73** The element that is defined first is the _____. The element that is defined next is the _____ of the word. The middle or rest of the word is defined _____.

-itis gastr/o enter	**1–74** Use the technique for defining medical words, described on page 14, to break the word gastr/o/enter/itis into its parts in order to define it. Write the element that is defined first: _____. Write the element that is defined next: _____ / _____. Write the element that is defined last: _____.
intestine (usually small)	**1–75** Appendix A: Glossary of Medical Word Elements on page 548 summarizes word elements and their meanings. Use this reference whenever you need to define an element. For example, look up the meaning of the CF *enter/o* and list it here. _____
inflammation of the stomach and intestine (usually small intestine)	**1–76** Define gastr/o/enter/itis using the technique for defining medical words as described above. _____ _____ _____

   In addition to word roots and CFs in **boldface** and suffixes in **boldface blue** in subsequent frames, all prefixes that stand alone will be set in **boldface pink** type.

PRONUNCIATION GUIDELINES

Although pronunciation of medical words usually follows the same rules that govern pronunciation of English words, you may have difficulty pronouncing some medical terms when you first encounter them. Selected terms in this book include phonetic pronunciation. In addition, you can find pronunciation guidelines on the inside back cover of this book. Use them whenever you need help with the pronunciation of medical words. Locate and study the pronunciation guidelines before proceeding with Section Review 1–1.

Pronunciation Tools

At appropriate times in each chapter you will be directed to use the following pronunciation tools:

- Visit the *Medical Terminology Simplified* online resource center at Davis*Plus* for an audio exercise of terms from the Word Elements tables. Other activities are also available to reinforce content.
- Visit the *Medical Terminology Simplified* online resource center at Davis*Plus* to hear pronunciation and meanings of selected terms from the medical reports sections.
- Visit the Medical Language Lab at *medicallanguagelab.com*. Use the "flash-card–word elements" exercises to reinforce your study of word elements. We recommend you complete the flash-card activity before starting the Word Elements Chapter Reviews.

SECTION REVIEW 1–1

Review the pronunciation guidelines (located in the inside back cover of this book). Use them as a reference when needed. Then, in the exercise below, underline one of the items within the parentheses to complete each sentence.

1. The diacritical mark ˘ is called a (breve, macron).

2. The diacritical mark ⁻ is called a (breve, macron).

3. The macron (⁻) above a vowel is used to indicate (short, long) vowel pronunciations.

4. The breve (˘) above a vowel is used to indicate the (short, long) vowel pronunciations.

5. When *pn* is in the middle of a word, pronounce (only *p, n, pn*). Examples are ortho*pn*ea, hyper*pn*ea.

6. The letters *c* and *g* have a (hard, soft) sound before the letters *a* and *o*. Examples are *c*ardiac, *c*ast, *g*astric, *g*onad.

7. When *pn* is at the beginning of a word, pronounce (only *p, n, pn*). Examples are *pn*eumonia, *pn*eumotoxin.

8. When *i* is at the end of a word (to form a plural), it is pronounced like (*eye, ee*). Examples are bronch*i*, fung*i*, nucle*i*.

9. For *ae* and *oe*, only the (first, second) vowel is pronounced. Examples are burs*ae*, pleur*ae*, r*oe*ntgen.

10. When *e* and *es* form the final letter or letters of a word, they are commonly pronounced as (combined, separate) syllables. Examples are syncop*e*, systol*e*, appendic*es*.

Competency Verification: Check your answers in Appendix B: Answer Key, page 558. If you are not satisfied with your level of comprehension, review the pronunciation guidelines (on the inside back cover of this book) and retake the review.

Correct Answers _____ × 10 = _____% Score

COMMON SUFFIXES

In previous frames, you learned that a combining form (CF) is a word root + vowel and that the CF is the main part, or foundation, of a medical term. Examples of CFs are ***gastr/o*** (stomach), ***dermat/o*** (skin), and ***nephr/o*** (kidney). When you see ***gastr/o*** in a medical term, you will know the term refers to the stomach. You also learned that a suffix is an element located at the end of a word. The following sections introduce common surgical, diagnostic, and pathological suffixes as well as plural suffixes. Some of these elements have already been introduced in previous frames, but they are reinforced below.

 Combinations of four elements are used to form medical words. These four elements are the word root, combining form, suffix, and prefix. Some words may also be used as suffixes. Other words may consist of just a prefix and a word root.

Surgical Suffixes

Common suffixes associated with surgical procedures, their meanings, and an example of a related term are presented in the table that follows. First, study the suffix as well as its meaning and practice pronouncing the term aloud. Then use the information to complete the meaning of the term. The first is completed for you. You may also refer to Appendix A: Glossary of Medical Word Elements, page 548. To build a working vocabulary of medical terms and understand how those terms are used in the health-care industry, it is important that you complete these exercises.

Suffix	Term	Meaning
-centesis surgical puncture	arthr/o/**centesis** ăr-thrō-sĕn-TĒ-sĭs *arthr/o:* joint	*surgical puncture of a joint* _____ _____
-desis binding, fixation (of a bone or joint)	arthr/o/**desis** ăr-thrō-DĒ-sĭs *arthr/o:* joint	_____ _____
-ectomy excision, removal	append/**ectomy** ăp-ĕn-DĔK-tō-mē *append:* appendix	_____ _____
-lysis separation; destruction; loosening	thromb/o/**lysis** thrŏm-BŎL-ĭ-sĭs *thromb/o:* blood clot	_____ _____ *Drug therapy is usually used to dissolve a blood clot.*
-pexy fixation (of an organ)	mast/o/**pexy** MĂS-tō-pĕks-ē *mast/o:* breast	_____ *Mastopexy is performed to affix sagging breasts in a more elevated position, commonly improving their shape.*
-plasty surgical repair	rhin/o/**plasty** RĪ-nō-plăs-tē *rhin/o:* nose	_____ _____
-rrhaphy suture	my/o/**rrhaphy** mī-OR-ă-fē *my/o:* muscle	_____ _____
-stomy forming an opening (mouth)	trache/o/**stomy** trā-kē-ŎS-tō-mē *trache/o:* trachea (windpipe)	_____ *Tracheostomy may be performed to bypass an obstructed upper airway.*
-tome instrument to cut	oste/o/**tome** ŎS-tē-ō-tōm *oste/o:* bone	_____ _____
-tomy incision	trache/o/**tomy** trā-kē–ŎT-ō–mē *trache/o:* trachea (windpipe)	_____ *Tracheotomy may be performed to gain access to an airway below a blockage.*
-tripsy crushing	lith/o/**tripsy** LĬTH-ō-trĭp-sē *lith/o:* stone, calculus	_____ _____

Pronunciation Help	Long sound	ā in rāte	ē in rēbirth	ī in īsle	ō in ōver	ū in ūnite
	Short sound	ă in ălone	ĕ in ĕver	ĭ in ĭt	ŏ in nŏt	ŭ in cŭt

Competency Verification: Check your answers in Appendix B: Answer Key, page 559. If you are not satisfied with your level of comprehension, review the surgical suffixes and their meanings.

Diagnostic Suffixes

Common suffixes associated with diagnostic procedures, their meanings, and an example of a related term are presented in the table that follows. First, study the suffix as well as its meaning and practice pronouncing the term aloud. Then use the information to complete the meaning of the term. You may also refer to Appendix A: Glossary of Medical Word Elements, page 548. To build a working vocabulary of medical terms and understand how those terms are used in the health-care industry, it is important that you complete these exercises.

Suffix	Term	Meaning
-gram	electr/o/cardi/o/**gram**	_____
record, writing	ē-lĕk-trō-KĂR-dē-ō-grăm *electr/o:* electricity *cardi/o:* heart	*An electrocardiogram allows diagnosis of specific cardiac abnormalities.*
-graph	cardi/o/**graph**	_____
instrument for recording	KĂR-dē-ō-grăf *cardi/o:* heart	_____
-graphy	angi/o/**graphy**	_____
process of recording	ăn-jē-ŎG-ră-fē *angi/o:* vessel (usually blood or lymph)	_____
-meter	pelv/i/**meter***	_____
instrument for measuring	pĕl-VĬM-ĕ-tĕr *pelv/i:* pelvis	_____
-metry	pelv/i/**metry***	_____
act of measuring	pĕl-VĬM-ĕ-trē *pelv/i:* pelvis	_____
-scope	endo/**scope**	_____
instrument for examining	ĔN-dō-skōp *endo-:* in, within	_____
-scopy	endo/**scopy**	_____
visual examination	ĕn-DŎS-kō-pē *endo-:* in, within	_____

Pronunciation Help	Long sound	ā in rāte	ē in rēbirth	ī in īsle	ō in ōver	ū in ūnite
	Short sound	ă in ălone	ĕ in ĕver	ĭ in ĭt	ŏ in nŏt	ŭ in cŭt

*The *i* in *pelv/i/meter* is an exception to the rule of using the connecting vowel *o.*

Competency Verification: Check your answers in Appendix B: Answer Key, page 560. If you are not satisfied with your level of comprehension, review the diagnostic suffixes and their meanings.

Pathological Suffixes

Common suffixes associated with pathological (disease) conditions, their meanings, and an example of a related term are presented in the table that follows. First, study the suffix as well as its meaning and practice pronouncing the term aloud. Then use the information to complete the meaning of the term. You may also refer to Appendix A: Glossary of Medical Word Elements, page 548. To build a working vocabulary of medical terms and understand how those terms are used in the health-care industry, it is important that you complete these exercises.

Suffix	Term	Meaning
-algia, -dynia	neur/**algia**	_____
pain	nū-RĂL-jē-ă *neur:* nerve	_____
	ot/o/**dynia**	_____
	ō-tō-DĬN-ē-ă *ot/o:* ear	_____
-cele	hepat/o/**cele**	_____
hernia, swelling	hĕ-PĂT-ō-sēl *hepat/o:* liver	_____
-ectasis	bronchi/**ectasis**	_____
dilation, expansion	brŏng-kē-ĔK-tă-sĭs *bronchi:* bronchus (plural, bronchi)	*Bronchiectasis is associated with various lung conditions and is commonly accompanied by chronic infection.*
-edema	lymph/**edema**	_____
swelling	lĭmf-ĕ-DĒ-mă *lymph:* lymph	*Lymphedema may be caused by a blockage of the lymph vessels.*
-emesis	hyper/**emesis**	_____
vomiting	hī-pĕr-ĔM-ĕ-sĭs *hyper-:* excessive, above normal	_____
-emia	an/**emia**	_____
blood condition	ă-NĒ-mē-ă *an-:* without, not	_____
-iasis	chol/e/lith/**iasis***	_____
abnormal condition (produced by something specific)	kō-lē-lĭ-THĪ-ă-sĭs *chol/e:* bile, gall *lith:* stone, calculus	_____
-itis	gastr/**itis**	_____
inflammation	gās-TRĪ-tĭs *gastr:* stomach	_____
-lith	chol/e/**lith***	_____
stone, calculus	KŌ-lē-lĭth *cho/e:* bile, gall	

Continued

Suffix	Term	Meaning
-malacia softening	chondr/o/**malacia** kŏn-drō-mă-LĀ-shē-ă *chondr/o:* cartilage	_____
-megaly enlargement	cardi/o/**megaly** kăr-dē-ō-MĔG-ă–lē *cardi/o:* heart	_____
-oma tumor	neur/**oma** nū-RŌ-mă *neur:* nerve	_____
-osis abnormal condition; increase (used primarily with blood cells)	cyan/**osis** sī-ă-NŌ-sĭs *cyan:* blue	_____
-pathy disease	my/o/**pathy** mī-ŎP-ă-thē *my/o:* muscle	_____
-penia decrease, deficiency	erythr/o/**penia** ĕ-rĭth-rō-PĒ-nē-ă *erythr/o:* red	_____
-phobia fear	hem/o/**phobia** hē-mō-FŌ-bē-ă *hem/o:* blood	_____
-plegia paralysis	hemi/**plegia** hĕm-ē-PLĒ-jē-ă *hemi-:* one half	_____ *Hemiplegia affects the right or left side of the body and is caused by a brain injury or stroke.*
-rrhage, -rrhagia bursting forth (of)	hem/o/**rrhage** HĔM-ĕ-rĭj *hem/o:* blood men/o/**rrhagia** mĕn-ō-RĀ-jē-ă *men/o:* menses, menstruation	_____ _____
-rrhea discharge, flow	dia/**rrhea** dī-ă-RĒ-ă *dia-:* through, across	_____
-rrhexis rupture	arteri/o/**rrhexis** ăr-tē-rē-ō-RĔK-sĭs *arteri/o:* artery	_____
-stenosis narrowing, stricture	arteri/o/**stenosis** ăr-tē-rē-ō-stĕ-NŌ-sĭs *arteri/o:* artery	_____

Suffix	Term	Meaning
-toxic	hepat/o/**toxic**	_____
poison	HĔP-ă-tō-tŏk-sĭk	_____
	hepat/o: liver	
-trophy	dys/**trophy**	_____
nourishment, development	DĬS-trō-fē	_____
	dys-: bad; painful; difficult	

Pronunciation Help	Long sound	ā in rāte	ē in rēbirth	ī in īsle	ō in ōver	ū in ūnite
	Short sound	ă in ălone	ĕ in ĕver	ĭ in ĭt	ŏ in nŏt	ŭ in cŭt

*The e in *chol/e/lithiasis* and *chol/e/lith* is an exception to the rule of using the connecting vowel *o.*

Competency Verification: Check your answers in Appendix B: Answer Key, page 560. If you are not satisfied with your level of comprehension, review the pathological suffixes and their meanings.

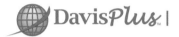 Visit the *Medical Terminology Simplified* online resource center at Davis*Plus* for an audio exercise of the terms in the Word Elements tables. It will help you master pronunciations and meanings of the medical terms.

Plural Suffixes

Because many medical words have Greek or Latin origins, there are a few unusual rules you need to learn to change a singular word into its plural form. When you begin learning these rules, you will find that they are easy to apply. You will also find that some English word endings have been adopted for commonly used medical terms. When a word changes from a singular to a plural form, the suffix of the word is the part that changes. A summary of the rules for changing a singular word into its plural form is located opposite the inside back cover of this book. Use it to complete Section Review 1–2 below and whenever you need help forming plural words.

SECTION REVIEW 1–2

Write the plural form for each of the following words and state the rule that applies. The first word is completed for you.

Singular	Plural	Rule
sarcoma săr-KŌ-mă	*sarcomata*	*Retain the* ma *and add* ta.
thrombus THRŎM-bŭs		
appendix ă-PĔN-dĭks		
diverticulum dī-vĕr-TĬK-ū-lŭm		
ovary Ō-vă-rē		
diagnosis dī-ăg-NŌ-sĭs		
lumen LŪ-mĕn		
vertebra VĔR-tĕ-bră		
thorax THŌ-răks		
spermatozoon pĕr-măt-ō-ZŌ-ŏn		

Competency Verification: Check your answers in Appendix B: Answer Key, page 562. If you are not satisfied with your level of comprehension, review the rules for changing a singular word into its plural form (opposite the inside back cover of this book) and retake the review.

Correct Answers _____ x 10 = _____% Score

COMMON PREFIXES

Common prefixes, their meanings, and an example of a related term are presented in the table that follows. First, study the prefix as well as its meaning and practice pronouncing the term aloud. Then use the information in the following table to complete the meaning of the term. You may also refer to Appendix A: Glossary of Medical Word Elements, page 548. To build a working vocabulary of medical terms and understand how those terms are used in the health-care industry, it is important that you complete these exercises.

Prefix	Term	Meaning

a-*, an-†
 	
without, not
	a/mast/ia
	ă-MĂS-tē-ă
	   mast: breast
	     -ia: condition
	
	an/esthesia
	ăn-ĕs-THĒ-zē-ă
	   -esthesia: feeling
		_____
		
		_____
		Amastia may be the result of a congenital defect, an endocrine disorder, or mastectomy.
		
		_____
		
		_____

circum-, peri-
 	
around
	circum/duction
	sĕr-kŭm-DŬK-shŭn
	   -duction: act of leading,
	           bringing, conducting
	
	peri/odont/al
	pĕr-ē-ō-DŎN-tăl
	   odont: teeth
	     -al: pertaining to
		_____
		
		_____
		
		_____
		
		_____

dia-, trans-
 	
through, across
	dia/rrhea
	dī-ă-RĒ-ă
	-rrhea: discharge, flow
	
	trans/vagin/al
	trăns-VĂJ-ĭn-ăl
	   vagin: vagina
	     -al: pertaining to
		_____
		
		Diarrhea is a condition of abnormally frequent discharge or flow of fluid fecal matter from the bowel.
		
		_____
		
		_____

dipl-, diplo-
 	
double
	dipl/opia
	dĭp-LŌ-pē-ă
	-opia: vision
	
	diplo/bacteri/al
	dĭp-lō-băk-TĒR-ē-ăl
	   bacteri: bacteria
	     -al: pertaining to
		_____
		
		_____
		
		_____
		
		Diplobacteria reproduce in such a manner that they are joined together in pairs.

endo-, intra-
 	
in, within
	endo/crine
	ĔN-dō-krīn
	   -crine: secrete
	
	intra/muscul/ar
	ĭn-tră-MŬS-kū-lăr
	   muscul: muscle
	     -ar: pertaining to
		_____
		
		_____
		Endocrine refers to a gland that secretes directly into the bloodstream.
		
		_____
		
		_____

Continued

Prefix	Term	Meaning
homo-, homeo-	**homo**/graft	_____
same	HŌ-mō-grăft	
	-graft: transplantation	*A homograft is also called an allograft.*
	homeo/plasia	_____
	hō-mē-ō-PLĀ-zē-ă	_____
	-plasia: formation, growth	
hypo-	**hypo**/derm/ic	_____
under, below, deficient	hī-pō-DĔR-mĭk	_____
	derm: skin	
	-ic: pertaining to	
macro-	**macro**/cyte	_____
large	MĂK-rō-sīt	_____
	-cyte: cell	
micro-	**micro**/scope	_____
small	MĪ-krō-skōp	_____
	-scope: instrument for examining	
mono-, uni-	**mono**/cyte	_____
one	MŎN-ō-sīt	_____
	-cyte: cell	
	uni/nucle/ar	_____
	ū-nĭ-NŪ-klē-ăr	_____
	nucle: nucleus	
	-ar: pertaining to	
post-	**post**/nat/al	_____
after, behind	pōst-NĀ-tăl	_____
	nat: birth	
	-al: pertaining to	
pre-, pro-	**pre**/nat/al	_____
before, in front of	prē-NĀ-tăl	_____
	nat: birth	
	-al: pertaining to	
	pro/gnosis	_____
	prŏg-NŌ-sĭs	_____
	-gnosis: knowing	
primi-	**primi**/gravida	_____
first	prī-mĭ-GRĂV-ĭ-dă	_____
	-gravida: pregnant woman	

Prefix	Term	Meaning
retro-	**retro**/version	_____
backward, behind	rĕt-rō-VĚR-shŭn	_____
	-version: turning	
super-	**super**/ior	_____
upper, above	soo-PĒ-rē-or	_____
	-ior: pertaining to	

Pronunciation Help	Long sound	ā in rāte	ē in rēbirth	ī in īsle	ō in ōver	ū in ūnite
	Short sound	ă in ălone	ĕ in ĕver	ĭ in ĭt	ŏ in nŏt	ŭ in cŭt

*The prefix *a-* is usually used before a consonant.

†The prefix *an-* is usually used before a vowel.

Competency Verification: Check your answers in Appendix B: Answer Key, page 562. If you are not satisfied with your level of comprehension, review the common prefixes tables. You may also visit the *medicallanguagelab.com* to review the chapter's flash-card exercises of suffixes and prefixes before proceeding to Chapter 2.

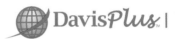 **DavisPlus** | Visit the *Medical Terminology Simplified* online resource center at Davis*Plus* for an audio exercise of the terms in the Word Elements tables. It will help you master pronunciations and meanings of the medical terms.

Body Structure

OBJECTIVES

Upon completion of this chapter, you will be able to:

• List and describe the basic structural units of the body.

• Describe the anatomical position of the body.

• Locate the body cavities and abdominopelvic regions of the body.

• Describe terms related to position, direction, and planes of the body and their applications during radiographic examinations.

• Describe common diseases, conditions, and procedures related to several body systems.

• Recognize, define, pronounce, and spell terms correctly.

• Demonstrate your knowledge of this chapter by successfully completing the frames and reviews.

The human body consists of several structural and functional levels of organization. The complexity of each level increases from one to the next, because the higher level incorporates the structures and functions of the previous level or levels. Eventually, all levels contribute to the structure and function of the entire organism. (See Fig. 2–1.) The levels of organization from the least to the most complex are the

- **cellular level,** the smallest structural and functional unit of the body;
- **tissue level,** groups of cells that perform a specialized function;
- **organ level,** groups of tissues that perform a specific function;
- **system level,** groups of organs that are interconnected or that have similar or interrelated functions; and
- **organism level,** collection of body systems that makes up the most complex level—a living human being.

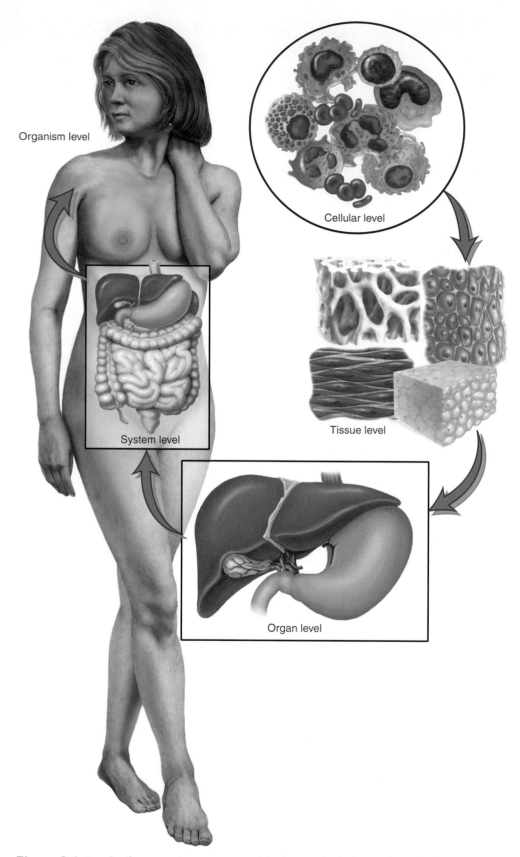

Organism level

Cellular level

Tissue level

Organ level

System level

Figure 2-1 Levels of structural organization of the human body shown from the basic unit of structure, the cellular level, to the most complex, the organism level—a living human being. The body system illustrated is the digestive system.

WORD ELEMENTS

This section introduces combining forms (CFs) related to the basic structural units of the body and those that describe a particular location or direction in the body. Key suffixes are also summarized. Other word elements are defined in the right-hand column as needed. Review the table and pronounce each word in the word analysis column aloud before you begin to work in the frames.

Word Element	Meaning	Word Analysis
Combining Forms Basic Structural Units		
chondr/o	cartilage	**chondr**/oma (kŏn-DRŌ-mă): tumor composed of cartilage *-oma:* tumor
cyt/o	cell	**cyt**/o/meter (sī-TŎM-ĕ-ter): instrument for counting and measuring cells *-meter:* instrument for measuring *A cytometer counts and measures cells within a specified amount of fluid, such as blood, urine, or cerebrospinal fluid.*
hist/o	tissue	**hist**/o/lysis (hĭs-TŎL-ĭ-sĭs): separation, destruction, or loosening of tissue *-lysis:* separation; destruction; loosening
nucle/o	nucleus	**nucle**/ar (NŪ-klē-ăr): pertaining to a nucleus *-ar:* pertaining to
Directional		
anter/o	anterior, front	**anter**/ior (ăn-TĒ-rē-ōr): pertaining to the front (of the body, organ, or structure) *-ior:* pertaining to
caud/o	tail	**caud**/ad (KAW-dăd): toward the tail *-ad:* toward
dist/o	far, farthest	**dist**/al (DĬS-tăl): pertaining to the farthest (point of attachment) *-al:* pertaining to
dors/o	back (of body)	**dors**/al (DŌR-săl): pertaining to the back (of the body) *-al:* pertaining to
infer/o	lower, below	**infer**/ior (ĭn-FĒ-rē-or): pertaining to below or lower (structure or surface) *-ior:* pertaining to
later/o	side, to one side	**later**/al (LĂT-ĕr-ăl): pertaining to the side *-al:* pertaining to
medi/o	middle	**medi**/al (MĒ-dē-ăl): pertaining to the middle *-al:* pertaining to
poster/o	back (of body), behind, posterior	**poster**/ior (pŏs-TĒ-rē-or): pertaining to the back (of the body, organ, or structure) *-ior:* pertaining to
proxim/o	near, nearest	**proxim**/al (PRŎK-sĭm-ăl): pertaining to the nearest (point of attachment) *-al:* pertaining to
super/o	upper, above	**super**/ior (soo-PĒ-rē-or): pertaining to above or upper (part of the body organ or structure) *-ior:* pertaining to
ventr/o	belly, belly side	**ventr**/al (VĔN-trăl): pertaining to the belly side (front of the body) *-al:* pertaining to

Continued

Word Element	Meaning	Word Analysis
Suffixes		
-ad	toward	medi/**ad** (MĒ-dē-ăd): toward the middle or center *medi/o-:* middle
-logist	specialist in the study of	hist/o/**logist** (hĭs-TŎL-ō-jĭst): specialist in the study of tissue *hist/o:* tissue
-logy	study of	cyt/o/**logy** (sī-TŎL-ō-jē): study of cells *cyt/o:* cell
-lysis	separation; destruction; loosening	cyt/o/**lysis** (sī-TŎL-ĭ-sĭs): destruction, dissolution, or separation of a cell *cyt/o:* cell

Pronunciation Help	Long sound	ā in rāte	ē in rēbirth	ī in īsle	ō in ōver	ū in ūnite
	Short sound	ă in ălone	ĕ in ĕver	ĭ in ĭt	ŏ in nŏt	ŭ in cŭt

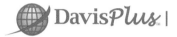 Visit the *Medical Terminology Simplified* online resource center at Davis*Plus* for an audio exercise of the terms in this table. It will help you master pronunciations and meanings of medical terms.

S E C T I O N   R E V I E W   2 - 1

For the following medical terms, first write the suffix and its meaning. Then translate the meaning of the remaining elements starting with the first part of the word. For example, the first word is completed for you.

Term	Meaning
1. dist/al	-al: pertaining to; far, farthest
2. poster/ior	
3. hist/o/logist	
4. dors/al	
5. anter/ior	
6. later/al	
7. medi/ad	
8. chondr/oma	
9. proxim/al	
10. ventr/al	

Competency Verification: Check your answers in Appendix B: Answer Key, page 564. If you are not satisfied with your level of comprehension, review the vocabulary and retake the review.

Correct Answers _____ x 10 = _____% Score

BASIC UNITS OF STRUCTURE

nucle/o

2–1   Cells are the smallest living units of structure and function in the human body. Every tissue and organ in the body is composed of cells. Review the illustration depicting the cellular level in Figure 2–1.

Note the nucleus, the darkened area in the center. The nucleus is the control center of the cell and is responsible for reproduction. This spherical unit contains genetic codes for maintaining life systems of the organism and for issuing commands for growth and reproduction.

The CF for nucleus is _____ / _____.

-toxic

nucle/o

2–2   Any chemical substance, such as a drug, that interferes with or destroys the cellular reproductive process in the nucleus is referred to as a nucle/o/toxic substance. Examples of nucle/o/toxic drugs are those administered to cancer patients during chemotherapy.

Identify the elements in this frame that mean

pertaining to poison: _____

nucleus: _____ / _____

cell	**2-3** Recall that *cyt/o* and *-cyte* are used to form words that refer to a _____.
cyt/o/logy sī-TŎL-ō-jē	**2-4** A cyt/o/logist is usually a biologist who specializes in the study of cells, especially one who uses cyt/o/log/ic techniques to diagnose neoplasms. Using *cyt/o,* build a word that means *study of cells:* _____ / _____ / _____.
cyt/o/logist sī-TŎL-ō-jĭst **cyt/o/lysis** sī-TŎL-ĭ-sĭs	**2-5** Use *cyt/o* to form words that mean *specialist in the study of cells:* _____ / _____ / _____ *dissolution or destruction of a cell:* _____ / _____ / _____
-logist **hist/o**	**2-6** At the tissue level, the structural organization of the human body consists of groups of cells working together to carry out a specialized activity. (See Fig. 2–1.) The medical scientist who specializes in the study of microscopic structures of tissues is called a *hist/o/logist.* Identify word elements in *hist/o/logist* that mean *specialist in the study of:* _____ *tissue:* _____ / _____

 When defining a medical word, first define the suffix. Second, define the beginning of the word; finally, define the middle of the word. Here is an example of the term

super/medi/al
(2) (3) (1)

1. Define the suffix first: *-al* means *pertaining to.*

2. Define the beginning of the word: *super-* means *upper, above.*

3. Define the middle of the word: *medi* means *middle.*

DIRECTIONAL TERMS

The following frames introduce terms that describe regions of the body. Included are directional terms that describe a structure in relation to some defined center or reference point.

dors/al DŌR-săl **later/al** LĂT-ĕr-ăl **ventr/al** VĔN-trăl	**2-7** The suffixes *-ac, -al, -ar, -iac, -ic,* and *-ior* are adjective endings that mean *pertaining to.* You will find them used throughout this book. These suffixes help describe position, direction, body divisions, and body structures. Use the adjective ending *-al* to form words that mean *pertaining to the* *back (of body):* dors / _____ *side, to one side:* later / _____ *belly, belly side:* ventr / _____

Boldface indicates a word root or combining form. Blue indicates a suffix. Pink indicates a prefix.

dors/al DŌR-săl **later/al** LĂT-ĕr-ăl **ventr/al** VĔN-trăl	**2–8** Practice building medical terms with *dors/o, later/o,* and *ventr/o.* Form medical terms that mean *pertaining to the* *back (of body):* _____ / _____ *side, to one side:* _____ / _____ *belly, belly side:* _____ / _____

-ac **-al** **-ar** **-ary** **-eal** **-iac** **-ic** **-ior** **-ous** **-tic**	**2–9** Frame 2–7 reviews six adjective suffixes that mean *pertaining to.* Four additional adjective suffixes meaning *pertaining to* that are common in medical terms are *-ary, -eal, -ous,* and *-tic.* You may want to summarize these suffixes on a 5″ × 3″ index card and keep it in your book as a reference until you commit all of them to memory. However, if you are in doubt about meanings of any word elements, refer to Appendix A: Glossary of Medical Word Elements. List in alphabetical order the 10 adjective suffixes that mean *pertaining to.* _____ _____ _____ _____ _____ _____ _____ _____ _____ _____

cardi/ac KĂR-dē-ăk	**2–10** Underline the suffixes in the following terms that mean *pertaining to:* cardi/ac
umbilic/al ŭm-BĬL-ĭ-kăl	umbilic/al
nucle/ar NŪ-klē-ăr	nucle/ar
pulmon/ary PŬL-mō-nĕ-rē	pulmon/ary
tox/ic TŎKS-ĭk	tox/ic
anter/ior ăn-TĒ-rē-or	anter/ior
cutane/ous kū-TĀ-nē-ŭs	cutane/ous
acous/tic ă-KOOS-tĭk	acous/tic

2–11   The human body is capable of being in many different positions, such as standing, kneeling, and lying down. To guarantee consistency in descriptions of location, the anatomic/al position is used as a reference point to describe the location or direction of a body structure. In anatomic/al position, the body is erect and the eyes are looking forward. The arms hang to the sides, with palms facing forward; the legs are parallel with the toes pointing straight ahead.

Review Figure 2–2 and study the terms to become acquainted with their usage in denoting positions of direction when the body is in the anatomic/al position. Refer to this figure to complete the following frames.

anatomic/al position
ăn-ă-TŎM-ĭk-ăl

2–12   When a person is standing upright, facing forward, arms at his or her sides, palms facing forward, legs parallel, and feet slightly apart with the toes pointing

forward, he or she is in the standard position called the _____ /

_____ _____.

anter/ior, ventr/al
ăn-TĒ-rē-or, VĔN-trăl

poster/ior, dors/al
pŏs-TĒ-rē-or, DŌR-săl

2–13   Health-care professionals use a common language of special terms when referring to body structures and their functions. However, their descriptions of any region or part of the human body assume that it is in anatomic/al position.

In anatomical position, the terms anter/ior and ventr/al refer to the *front of the body* or the *front of any body structure.* The terms poster/ior and dors/al refer to the *back of the body* or the *back of any body structure.*

Identify the elements in this frame that refer to the

front of the body: _____ / _____ and

_____ / _____

back of the body: _____ / _____ and

_____ / _____

Boldface indicates a word root or combining form. Blue indicates a suffix. Pink indicates a prefix.

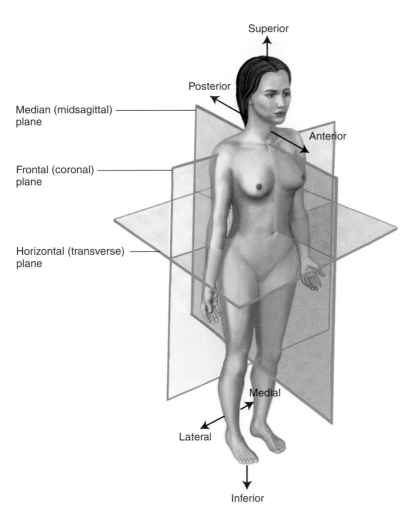

Figure 2-2 Body planes. (Note that the body is in the anatomical position.)

front **back**	**2-14** What position of the body do the terms anter/ior and ventr/al refer to? _____ (of the body) What position of the body do the terms poster/ior and dors/al refer to? _____ (of the body)
-ior **poster/o** **anter**	**2-15** The term poster/o/anter/ior refers to the back and front of the body. Identify the word elements in this frame that mean *pertaining to:* _____ *back:* _____ / _____ *front:* _____

posterior, anterior pŏs-TĒ-rē-or, ăn-TĒ-rē-or **or** **back, front**	**2-16** Directional terms are commonly used in radi/o/logy to describe the direction of the x-ray beam from its source and its point of exit. In an anter/o/poster/ior projection, the beam enters the body anteriorly and exits posteriorly. A poster/o/anter/ior projection indicates that the beam enters the body on the _____ side and exits on the _____ side.
anter/ior ăn-TĒ-rē-or **poster/ior** pŏs-TĒ-rē-or	**2-17** Use anter/ior or poster/ior to complete the following statements, which refer to the position of body structures. The stomach is located on the _____ / _____ side of the body. The shoulder blades are located on the _____ / _____ side of the body.
infer/ior ĭn-FĒ-rē-or	**2-18** The term inferior in the English language refers to something of little or no importance. However, when used in a medical report, it designates a position or direction meaning *lower, below.* Combine ***infer/o*** (lower, below) +-*ior* (pertaining to) to form a directional term that literally means *pertaining to lower or below.* _____ / _____
above	**2-19** In medical terms, the prefix *super-* designates an upper position. When you say "the head is superior to the stomach," you mean it is located above the stomach. When you say "the eyes are superior to the mouth," you mean they are located _____ the mouth.
side	**2-20** The word element **later/o** means *side, to one side.* A radiographic projection that enters through the left or right side of the body is referred to as a *later/al projection.* The term later/al *position* refers to the _____ (of the body).

Review the three basic rules for building medical words.
- **Rule 1:** Word root links a suffix that begins with a vowel.
- **Rule 2:** CF (root + **o**) links a suffix that begins with a consonant.
- **Rule 3:** CF (root + **o**) links a root to another root to form a compound word. (This rule holds true even if the next root begins with a vowel.)

later/al LĂT-ĕr-ăl **anter/o/later/al** ăn-tĕr-ō-LĂT-ĕr-ăl **poster/o/later/al** pŏs-tĕr-ō-LĂT-ĕr-ăl	**2-21** Here is a review of terms in radi/o/logy that specify the direction of the x-ray beam from its source to its exit surface before striking the film. Build directional terms that mean *pertaining to the side or to one side (of the body):* _____ / _____ *pertaining to the anterior, or front, and the side (of the body):* _____ / _____ / _____ / _____ *pertaining to the posterior, or back, and the side (of the body):* _____ / _____ / _____ / _____

Boldface indicates a word root or combining form. Blue indicates a suffix. Pink indicates a prefix.

medi **-al**	**2-22** The term medi/al is used to describe the midline of the body or a structure. The medi/al portion of the face contains the nose. From the term medi/al, determine the root meaning *middle*: _____ suffix meaning *pertaining to*: _____
-ad, medi **medi/ad** MĒ-dē-ăd	**2-23** The suffix for *toward* is _____. The word root for *middle* is _____. Combine *medi* + *-ad* to form a word that means *toward the middle*. _____ / _____
medi/ad MĒ-dē-ăd	**2-24** Use *-ad* to form a directional term that means *toward the middle (or center of the body)*. _____ / _____ .
infer/ior ĭn-FĒ-rē-or **infer/ior** ĭn-FĒ-rē-or	**2-25** Anatomists use the term infer/ior to refer to a body structure located below another body structure or the lower part of a structure. For example, your chin is situated infer/ior to your mouth. The rectum is the infer/ior portion of the colon. To indicate that a structure is below another structure, use the directional term _____ / _____ . To indicate the lower part of a structure, use the directional term _____ / _____ .
infer/ior ĭn-FĒ-rē-or **later/al** LĂT-ĕr-ăl	**2-26** Practice using the directional terms later/al and infer/ior to describe the following positions. The legs are _____ / _____ to the trunk. The eyes are _____ / _____ to the nose.
cephal/ad SĔF-ă-lăd	**2-27** Anatomists and other health-care professionals use the term super/ior to refer to a body structure that is above another body structure or toward the head, because the head is the most superior structure of the body. Cephal/ad is a term that refers to the direction toward the head. When referring to the direction going toward the head, use the term _____ / _____ .
pertaining to **upper, above**	**2-28** Define the word elements in super/ior. *-ior:* _____ *super:* _____

super/ior soo-PĒ-rē-or **infer/ior** ĭn-FĒ-rē-or **super/ior** soo-PĒ-rē-or	**2-29** Use super/ior or infer/ior to complete the following statements that refer to the relative position of one body structure to another body structure. The chest is _____ / _____ to the stomach. The stomach is _____ / _____ to the lungs. The head is _____ / _____ to the neck.
caud/al KAWD-ăl	**2-30** The CF *caud/o* means *tail*. In this sense, *tail* designates a position toward the end of the body, away from the head. In humans, it also refers to an infer/ior position in the body or within a structure. Combine *caud* + *-al* to build a word that means *pertaining to the tail*. _____ / _____
proxim/al PRŎK-sĭm-ăl **dist/al** DĬS-tăl	**2-31** The terms proxim/al and dist/al are used as positional and directional terms. Proxim/al describes a structure as being nearest the point of attachment to the trunk or near the beginning of a structure. Dist/al describes a structure as being far from the point of attachment to the trunk or from the beginning of a structure. Identify the terms in this frame that mean *nearest the point of attachment:* _____ / _____ *farthest from the point of attachment:* _____ / _____
proxim/al PRŎK-sĭm-ăl **dist/al** DĬS-tăl	**2-32** The directional element *proxim/o* means *near or nearest the point of attachment*; *dist/o* means *far or farthest from the point of attachment*. The knee is proxim/al to the foot; the palm is dist/al to the elbow. To describe a structure nearest the point of attachment, use the directional term _____ / _____. To describe a structure as being farthest from the point of attachment, use the directional term _____ / _____.
ad/duction ă-DŬK-shŭn	**2-33** Some directional terms, such as ab/duction and ad/duction, indicate movement away from the body and movement toward the body. The prefix *ab-* means *from, away from*; the suffix *-duction* means *act of leading, bringing, conducting*. Thus, *ab/duction* means *movement away from the body*. Can you determine the directional term in this frame that means movement toward the body? _____ / _____

Boldface indicates a word root or combining form. Blue indicates a suffix. Pink indicates a prefix.

SECTION REVIEW 2-2

Using the word elements in the table that follows, write the CF or suffix that matches its definition in the space provided to the left of the definition. There may be more than one word element that matches a definition.

Combining Form

caud/o	later/o
cyt/o	medi/o
dist/o	proxim/o
hist/o	ventr/o
infer/o	

Suffix

-ad	-lysis
-al	-toxic
-ior	
-logist	
-logy	

1. _____ tissue

2. _____ pertaining to

3. _____ middle

4. _____ near, nearest

5. _____ study of

6. _____ cell

7. _____ belly, belly side

8. _____ poison

9. _____ toward

10. _____ tail

11. _____ specialist in study of

12. _____ far, farthest

13. _____ lower, below

14. _____ separation; destruction; loosening

15. _____ side, to one side

Competency Verification: Check your answers in Appendix B: Answer Key, page 565. If you are not satisfied with your level of comprehension, go back to Frame 2–1 and rework the frames.

Correct Answers _____ × 6.67 = _____ % Score

WORD ELEMENTS

This section introduces word elements that describe a body structure. When these elements are attached to positional prefixes or suffixes, they form words that describe a region or position in the body. Review the following table and pronounce each word in the word analysis column aloud before you begin to work in the frames.

Word Element	Meaning	Word Analysis
Combining Forms		
abdomin/o	abdomen	**abdomin**/al (ăb-DŎM-ĭ-năl): pertaining to the abdomen *-al:* pertaining to
cephal/o	head	**cephal**/ad (SĔF-ă-lăd): toward the head *-ad:* toward
cervic/o	neck; cervix uteri (neck of uterus)	**cervic**/al (SĔR-vĭ-kăl): pertaining to the neck of the body or the neck of the uterus *-al:* pertaining to
crani/o	cranium (skull)	**crani**/al (KRĀ-nē-ăl): pertaining to the cranium or skull *-al:* pertaining to
gastr/o	stomach	**gastr**/ic (GĂS-trĭk): pertaining to the stomach *-ic:* pertaining to
ili/o	ilium (lateral, flaring portion of hip bone)	**ili**/ac (ĬL-ē-ăk): pertaining to the ilium *-ac:* pertaining to
inguin/o	groin	**inguin**/al (ĬNG-gwĭ-năl): pertaining to the groin *-al:* pertaining to
lumb/o	loins (lower back)	**lumb**/ar (LŬM-băr): pertaining to the loin area or lower back *-ar:* pertaining to
pelv/i*	pelvis	**pelv**/i/meter (pĕl-VĬM-ĕ-tĕr): instrument for measuring the pelvis *-meter:* instrument for measuring
spin/o	spine	**spin**/al (SPĪ-năl): pertaining to the spine or spinal column *-al:* pertaining to
thorac/o	chest	**thorac**/ic (thō-RĂS-ĭk): pertaining to the chest *-ic:* pertaining to
umbilic/o	umbilicus, navel	peri/**umbilic**/al (pĕr-ē-ŭm-BĬL-ĭ-kăl): pertaining to the area around the umbilicus *peri-:* around *-al:* pertaining to

*The *i* in *pelv/i/meter* is an exception to the rule of using the connecting vowel *o*.

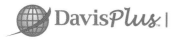

Visit the *Medical Terminology Simplified* online resource center at Davis*Plus* for an audio exercise of the terms in this table. It will help you master pronunciations and meanings of the selected medical terms.

SECTION REVIEW 2-3

For the following medical terms, first write the suffix and its meaning. Then translate the meaning of the remaining elements starting with the first part of the word. The first word is completed for you.

Term	Meaning
1. ili/ac	-ac: pertaining to; ilium: lateral, flaring portion of hip bone
2. abdomin/al	
3. inguin/al	
4. spin/al	
5. peri/umbilic/al	
6. cephal/ad	
7. gastr/ic	
8. thorac/ic	
9. cervic/al	
10. lumb/ar	

Competency Verification: Check your answers in Appendix B: Answer Key, page 565. If you are not satisfied with your level of comprehension, review the vocabulary and retake the review.

Correct Answers _____ × 10 = _____ % Score

BODY PLANES AND CAVITIES

To visualize structural arrangements of various organs, the body may be sectioned (cut) according to planes of reference. The three major planes are the frontal, median, and horizontal planes, as shown in Figure 2–2. In addition, body cavities, as shown in Figure 2–3, contain internal organs and are used as a point of reference to locate structures within body cavities.

Body Planes

2-34 Review Figures 2–2 and 2–3 before proceeding with the next frame. You may refer to the two figures to complete the following frames.

---

body plane

2-35 A body plane is an imaginary flat surface that divides the body into two sections. Different planes divide the body into different sections, such as front and back, left side and right side, and top and bottom. These planes serve as points of reference for describing the direction from which the body is being observed. Planes are particularly useful to describe views in which radiographic images are taken.

An imaginary flat surface that divides the body into two sections is a

_____ _____.

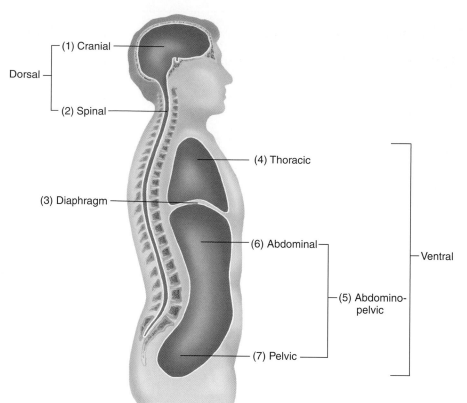

Figure 2-3 Body cavities, with the ventral (anterior) cavities located in the front of the body and the dorsal (posterior) cavities located in the back of the body.

---

median (midsagittal) mĭd-SĂJ-ĭ-tăl	**2–36** Examine Figure 2–2 and list the three major planes of the body. _____ (_____) _____ (_____) _____ (_____)
frontal (coronal) kŏ-rō-năl	
horizontal (transverse) trăns-VĔRS	

 When in doubt about the meaning of a word element, refer to Appendix A, page 548.

---

midsagittal plane mĭd-SĂJ-ĭ-tăl	**2–37** The median (midsagittal) plane lies exactly in the middle of the body and divides the body into two equal halves. (See Fig. 2–2.) When the chest is divided into equal right and left sides, it is divided by the median plane, also known as the _____ _____.

Boldface indicates a word root or combining form. Blue indicates a suffix. Pink indicates a prefix.

median plane	**2–38** When the lungs are divided into equal right and left sides, they are divided by the midsagittal plane, also known as the _____ _____.
infer/ior, super/ior ĭn-FĒ-rē-or, soo-PĒ-rē-or	**2–39** The horizontal (transverse) plane runs across the body from the right side to the left side and divides the body into upper (superior) and lower (inferior) portions. Figure 2–2 shows the division of this plane. Recall the term super/ior. It is a point of reference that refers to a structure above or oriented toward a higher place. For example, the head is superior to the heart. Infer/ior is a point of reference that refers to a structure situated below or oriented toward a lower place. For example, the feet are inferior to the legs. Because the head is located superior to the heart, the heart is located _____ / _____ to the head. Because the feet are located inferior to the legs, the legs are located _____ / _____ to the feet.
transverse plane trăns-VĔRS	**2–40** The plane that divides the body into superior and inferior portions is the horizontal plane. This plane is also called the _____ _____.
cross-sectional	**2–41** Many different trans/verse planes exist at every possible level of the body, from head to foot. A trans/verse section is also called a *cross-sectional plane.* Some radiographic imaging devices produce cross-sectional images. Cross-sectioning of the body or of an organ along different planes results in different views. In radiography, the horizontal, or trans/verse, plane is also known as the _____ plane.
-graph **radi/o** **trans-** **-verse**	**2–42** A radi/o/graph of the liver along a trans/verse plane results in a different view than a radiograph along the frontal plane. That is why a series of x-rays is commonly taken using different planes. Views along different planes result in a complete and comprehensive image of a body structure. Identify the elements in this frame that mean *instrument for recording:* _____ *radiation, x-ray; radius (lower arm bone on thumb side):* _____ / ____ *through, across:* _____ *turning:* _____
coronal plane CŎR-ŏ-năl	**2–43** Locate the frontal plane in Figure 2–2. The frontal plane is also called the _____ _____.

poster/ior pŏs-TĒ-rē-or	**2-44** The frontal (coronal) plane is commonly used to take an anter/o/poster/ior (AP) chest radiograph, indicating that the x-ray beam enters the body on the anterior side and exits the body on the _____ / _____ side. The radiograph produced shows a view from the front of the chest toward the back (of the body).
study of	**2-45** In the previous frame, you learned that anter/o/poster/ior is used in radi/o/logy to describe the direction or path of an x-ray beam. The CF *radi/o* means *radiation; x-ray; radius (lower arm bone on thumb side)*. The suffix *-logy* means _____ _____.
radi/o/logy rā-dē-ŎL-ō-jē	**2-46** Use *radi/o* to form a word that means *study of radiation or x-rays*: _____ / _____ / _____.
AP	**2-47** Identify the abbreviation in Frame 2–44 that designates the path of an x-ray beam from the anterior to the posterior part of the body: _____.

Body Cavities

	2-48 **Body cavities** are hollow spaces within the body that help protect, separate, and support internal organs. There are four body cavities: two dors/al cavities, which are located in the back (posterior) part of the body, and two ventr/al cavities, which are located in the front (anterior) part of the body. The thorac/ic and abdominal cavities are separated by a muscular wall known as the **diaphragm.** Because the abdominal and pelvic cavities are not separated by a wall, they are commonly referred together as the **abdominopelvic cavity.** Review Figure 2–3 to study the location of the dors/al cavities.
crani/al KRĀ-nē-ăl **spin/al** SPĪ-năl	**2-49** The dors/al cavity is subdivided into the (1) **crani/al** and (2) **spin/al** cavities. The crani/al cavity is encased by the skull and contains the brain; the spin/al cavity contains the spinal cord. Practice building words that refer to the body cavities by building a term that means *pertaining to the cranium (skull):* _____ / _____ *pertaining to the spine:* _____ / _____
	2-50 The (3) **diaphragm** is a dome-shaped muscle that plays an important role in breathing. It separates the thorac/ic cavity from the abdomin/o/pelv/ic cavity. Locate the diaphragm in Figure 2–3.
pelv **thorac** **abdomin**	**2-51** Let us review some of the elements in the previous frame. Indicate the root that refers to the *pelvis:* _____ *chest:* _____ *abdomen:* _____

Boldface indicates a word root or combining form. Blue indicates a suffix. Pink indicates a prefix.

2–52 The major body cavities of the trunk are the thorac/ic and abdomin/o/pelv/ic cavities. The (4) **thoracic cavity** contains the heart and lungs, and the (5) **abdominopelvic** cavity contains the digestive and reproductive organs. The abdomin/o/pelv/ic cavity contains by far the greatest number of organs of any of the body cavities and is further subdivided into the (6) **abdominal** and (7) **pelvic** cavities. Locate these cavities in Figure 2–3.

ventr/al cavity VĔN-trăl	**2–53** Review Figure 2–3 to identify the largest cavity in the body that incorporates the abdomin/o/pelv/ic and thorac/ic cavities: _____ / _____ _____
super/ior soo-PĒ-rē-or **infer/ior** ĭn-FĒ-rē-or	**2–54** Medical personnel locate a structure of interest by referring to the body cavity in which it can be found. Use the terms super/ior and infer/ior to describe locations, or positions, of body cavities. The thoracic cavity is located _____ / _____ to the abdominopelvic cavity. The spinal cavity is located _____ / _____ to the cranial cavity.

ABDOMINOPELVIC QUADRANTS AND REGIONS

The abdominopelvic cavity is further divided into quadrants and regions. (See Figs. 2–4A and B.)

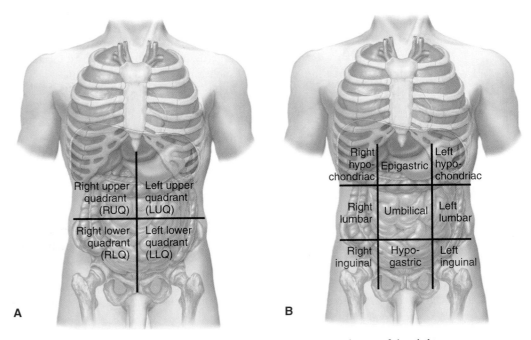

Figure 2-4 Abdominopelvic quadrants and regions. (**A**) Four quadrants of the abdomen. (**B**) Nine regions of the abdomen showing superficial organs.

Abdominopelvic Quadrants

2-55   Because the abdomin/o/pelv/ic cavity is a large area and contains many organs, it is useful to divide it into smaller sections. One method divides the abdomin/o/pelv/ic cavity into quadrants. A second method divides the abdomin/o/pelv/ic cavity into regions. Physicians and other health-care professionals use quadrants or regions as a point of reference.

The larger division of the abdomin/o/pelv/ic cavity consists of four quadrants: right upper quadrant (RUQ), left upper quadrant (LUQ), right lower quadrant (RLQ), and left lower quadrant (LLQ). Locate these quadrants in Figure 2–4A.

right upper quadrant

left upper quadrant

right lower quadrant

left lower quadrant

2-56   After you have located and reviewed the quadrants, determine the meaning of the following abbreviations.

RUQ: _____ _____ _____

LUQ: _____ _____ _____

RLQ: _____ _____ _____

LLQ: _____ _____ _____

RLQ

2-57   Quadrants are useful in describing the location in the body in which a surgical procedure will be performed. They are also useful in denoting incision sites or the location of abnormal masses such as tumors.

A tumor located in the right lower quadrant will most likely be denoted in the medical record with the abbreviation _____.

RLQ
LLQ

2-58   Quadrants may also be used to describe the location of a patient's symptoms. The physician may pinpoint a patient's abdominal pain in the RLQ. Such a finding could indicate a diagnosis of appendicitis, because the appendix is located in that quadrant. Pain in another quadrant, such as the LLQ, would indicate a different diagnosis.

Identify the abbreviation for the

right lower quadrant: _____

left lower quadrant: _____

left upper quadrant,
LUQ

2-59   Locate the quadrant that contains a major part of the stomach.

This quadrant is the _____ _____ _____

and its abbreviation is _____.

Abdominopelvic Regions

2-60   Whereas larger sections of the abdomin/o/pelv/ic cavity are divided into four quadrants, the smaller sections are divided into nine regions, each of which corresponds to a region near a specific point in the body. As with quadrants, body region designation is also used to describe the location of internal organs and the origin of pain. Review Figure 2–4B to see the location of various organs within these regions.

Boldface indicates a word root or combining form. Blue indicates a suffix. Pink indicates a prefix.

hypo/chondr/iac hī-pō-KŎN-drē-ăk **epi/gastr/ic** ĕp-ĭ-GĂS-trĭk **inguin/al** ĬNG-gwĭ-năl **lumb/ar** LŬM-băr **umbilic/al** ŭm-BĬL-ĭ-kăl	**2–61** Now that you have examined the nine regions, let us review some of the terms within each region. These terms are commonly used to describe a location of organs within the abdominal cavity. Although the CFs in the left-hand column below denote a body structure, when attached to directional elements, they form terms denoting specific regions of the abdomen. Study the meaning of each regional term, then divide each one in the right-hand column into its basic elements. The first term is completed for you.

Combining Form	Meaning	Regions of the Abdomen
chondr/o	cartilage	h y p o / c h o n d r / i a c*
gastr/o	stomach	e p i g a s t r i c
inguin/o	groin	i n g u i n a l
lumb/o	loins (lower back)	l u m b a r
umbilic/o	umbilicus, navel	u m b i l i c a l

*Although *chondr/o* means *cartilage*, *hypo/chondr/iac* also refers to the right and left regions below the ribs (see Fig. 2–4B).

adjectives	**2–62** Suffixes *-ac, -ic, -ous* and *-ior* mean *pertaining to*. Can you identify the parts of speech of these suffixes? _____

hypo/gastr/ic hī-pō-GĂS-trĭk **epi/gastr/ic** ĕp-ĭ-GĂS-trĭk	**2–63** Use *gastr/o* to develop medical words that pertain to the area under or below the stomach: _____ / _____ / _____ above or on the stomach: _____ / _____ / _____

epi/gastr/ic ĕp-ĭ-GĂS-trĭk	**2–64** The epi/gastr/ic region may be the location of "heartburn" pain. Pain in this area could be symptomatic of many abnormal conditions, including indigestion or heart attack. The area of heartburn pain may be felt in the _____ / _____ / _____ region.

-iac **hypo-** **chondr**	**2–65** The right and left hypo/chondr/iac* regions are located on each side of the epi/gastr/ic region and directly under the cartilage of the ribs. Identify the elements in *hypo/chondr/iac* that mean *pertaining to:* _____ *under, below, deficient:* _____ *cartilage:* _____

 Refer to Figure 2–4B to answer the following frames. If needed, use Appendix A: Glossary of Medical Word Elements.

loins (lower back)	**2–66** The lumbar regions consist of the middle right and middle left regions, located near the waistline of the body. The term *lumb/ar* means *pertaining to the* _____ (_____ _____)
lumb/o/abdomin/al lŭm-bō-ăb-DŎM-ĭ-năl	**2–67** Combine *lumb/o +abdomin +-al* to form a term that means *pertaining to the loins and abdomen.* _____ / _____ / _____ / _____
umbilic/al region ŭm-BĬL-ĭ-kăl	**2–68** The center of the umbilic/al region marks the point where the umbilic/al cord of the mother enters the fetus. This point is called the *navel* or, in layman's terms, the "belly button." The region that lies between the right and left lumbar regions is designated as the _____ / _____.
umbilic/al ŭm-BĬL-ĭ-kăl	**2–69** CF *umbilic/o* refers to the *umbilicus,* or *navel.* The region that literally means *pertaining to the navel* is the _____ / _____ region.
inguin/al ĬNG-gwĭ-năl	**2–70** A hernia is a protrusion or projection of an organ through the wall of the cavity that normally contains it. A common type of hernia that may occur, particularly in males, is an inguin/al hernia. This hernia would be located in the right or left _____ / _____ region.
right inguin/al hernia ĬNG-gwĭ-năl HĔR-nē-ă	**2–71** Locate the right inguin/al region and the left inguin/al region in Figure 2–4B. A hernia on the right side of the groin is called a _____ _____ / _____ _____.
hypo/gastr/ic hī-pō-GĂS-trĭk	**2–72** The area between the right and left inguin/al regions is called the hypo/gastr/ic region. This region contains the large intestine (colon), which is involved in the removal of solid waste from the body. Identify the name of the region below the stomach that literally means *pertaining to below the stomach.* _____ / _____ / _____

Boldface indicates a word root or combining form. Blue indicates a suffix. Pink indicates a prefix.

SECTION REVIEW 2-4

Using the table below, write the combining form, suffix, or prefix that matches its definition in the space provided to the left of the definition. There may be more than one word element that matches a definition.

Combining Forms		Suffixes	Prefixes
abdomin/o	lumb/o	-ac	epi-
chondr/o	pelv/i, pelv/o	-ad	hypo-
crani/o	poster/o	-al	
gastr/o	spin/o	-ic	
inguin/o	thorac/o	-ior	
	umbilic/o		

1. _____ toward

2. _____ groin

3. _____ stomach

4. _____ pelvis

5. _____ cartilage

6. _____ above, on

7. _____ pertaining to

8. _____ loins, (lower back)

9. _____ chest

10. _____ under, below, deficient

11. _____ cranium (skull)

12. _____ spine

13. _____ umbilicus, navel

14. _____ back (of body), behind, posterior

15. _____ abdomen

Competency Verification: Check your answers in Appendix B: Answer Key, page 565. If you are not satisfied with your level of comprehension, go back to Frame 2–34 and reword the frame.

Correct Answers _____ × 6.67 = _____ % Score

ABBREVIATIONS

This section introduces body structure and abbreviations related to radiology and their meanings.

Abbreviation	Meaning	Abbreviation	Meaning
Body Structure and Related			
AP	anteroposterior	LUQ	left upper quadrant
Bx, bx	biopsy	PA	posteroanterior; pernicious anemia; pulmonary artery; physician assistant
LAT, lat	lateral	RLQ	right lower quadrant
LLQ	left lower quadrant	RUQ	right upper quadrant
Radiology			
CT	computed tomography	PET	positron emission tomography
CXR	chest x-ray, chest radiograph	US	ultrasound; ultrasonography
MRI	magnetic resonance imaging	SPECT	single-photon emission computed tomography

ADDITIONAL MEDICAL TERMS

The following are additional terms related to the structure of the body. Recognizing and learning these terms will help you understand the connection between a pathological condition, its diagnosis, and the rationale behind the method of treatment selected for a particular disorder.

Diseases and Conditions

adhesion
ăd-HĒ-zhŭn

Band of scarlike tissue that forms between two surfaces inside the body and causes them to stick together (See Fig. 2–5.)

Adhesions develop when the body's repair mechanisms respond to any tissue disturbance, such as surgery, infection, trauma, or radiation. Although adhesions can occur anywhere in the body, they form most commonly in the abdomen after abdominal surgery, inflammation, or injury.

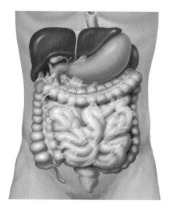

Figure 2-5 Abdominal adhesions.

inflammation ĭn-flă-MĀ-shun	Protective response of body tissues to irritation, infection, or allergy *Signs of inflammation include redness, swelling, heat, and pain, commonly accompanied by loss of function.*

septicemia
sĕp-tĭ-SĒ-mē-ă
  septic: infection
  -emia: blood
	Systemic disease caused by infection with microorganisms and their toxins in circulating blood; also called *sepsis* and *blood poisoning*
	
	If a patient becomes "septic," he or she will likely have low blood pressure leading to poor circulation. This condition can develop as a result of the body's own defense system or from toxic substances made by the infecting agent (such as a bacterium, virus, or fungus).

Diagnostic Procedures

culture & sensitivity **(C&S)**	Laboratory test of a body fluid placed on a culture medium to identify the cause of an infection (usually a bacterium) and a sensitivity test that determines which antibiotic drug will work best to treat the infection *A C&S test may be done on many different body fluids, such as urine, mucus, blood, pus, saliva, spinal fluid, or a discharge from the vagina or penis.*

endoscopy
ĕn-DŎS-kō-pē
  endo-: in, within
  -scopy: visual
         examination
	Visual examination of the interior of organs and cavities with a specialized lighted instrument called an *endoscope*
	
	Endoscopy can also be used to obtain tissue samples for biopsy, perform surgery, and follow the course of a disease, as in the assessment of the healing of gastric ulcers. The cavity or organ examined dictates the name of the endoscopic procedure, such as gastroscopy and bronchoscopy. A camera and video recorder are commonly used during this procedure to provide a permanent record. (See Fig. 2–6.)

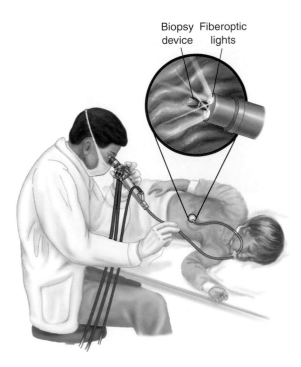

Biopsy   Fiberoptic
device   lights

Figure 2-6 Endoscopy of the stomach.

fluoroscopy
floo-or-ŎS-kō-pē
fluor/o: luminous,
        fluorescence
-scopy: visual
        examination
	Radiographic procedure that uses a fluorescent screen instead of a photographic plate to produce a visual image from x-rays that pass through the patient, resulting in continuous imaging of the motion of internal structures and immediate serial images
	
	Fluoroscopy is invaluable in diagnostic and clinical procedures. It permits the radiographer to observe organs, such as the digestive tract and heart, in motion. It is also used during intrauterine fetal transfusion, biopsy surgery, nasogastric tube placement, and cardiac catheterization.

magnetic resonance imaging (MRI) măg-NĚT-ĭc RĚZ-ĕn-ăns ĬM-ĭj-ĭng	Radiographic procedure that uses electromagnetic energy to produce multiplanar cross-sectional images of the body *MRI does not require a contrast medium; however, one may be used to enhance visualization of internal structures. (See Fig. 2–7E.) MRI is regarded as superior to CT for most abnormalities of the central nervous system (particularly of the brainstem and spinal cord), musculoskeletal system, and pelvic area.*

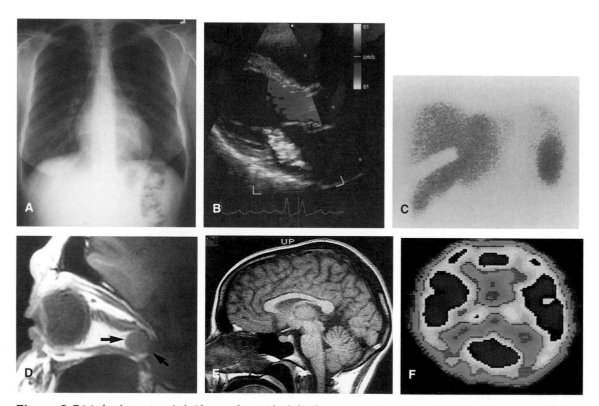

Figure 2-7 Medical imaging. (**A**) Chest radiograph. (**B**) Ultrasonography of blood flow with color indicating direction. (**C**) Nuclear scan of the liver and spleen. (**D**) Computed tomography (CT) scan of the eye showing a tumor below the optic nerve (*arrow*). (**E**) Magnetic resonance imaging (MRI) scan of the head. (**F**) PET scan of the brain. (A) From McKinnis, L. *Fundamentals of Orthopedic Radiology,* page 149. F. A. Davis, 1997, with permission. (B) Courtesy of Suzanne Wambold, PhD, University of Toledo. (C) From Pittiglio, D. H., and Sacher, R. A. *Clinical Hematology and Fundamentals of Hemostasis,* page 302. F. A. Davis, 1987, with permission. (D, E, F) From Mazziotta, J. C., and Gilman, S. *Clinical Brain Imaging: Principles and Applications,* pages 27 and 298. Oxford University Press, 1992, with permission.

nuclear scan NŪ-klē-ăr	Radiographic procedure that produces images of an organ or area of the body by introducing a radionuclide substance (*tracer* or *radiopharmaceutical*) that releases a low level of radiation; also called *nuclear scanning, radionuclide imaging,* and *nuclear medicine scan* (See Fig. 2–7C.) *Nuclear scan uses a very small amount of radioactivity and is not known to cause harm.*

tomography
tō-MŎG-ră-fē
   tom/o: to cut, slice
-graphy: process of
      recording
	Any of several radiographic procedures in which specialized machines produce a film representing a detailed cross section, or *slice* (cut), of an area, tissue, or organ
	
	Tomography is a valuable diagnostic tool for identifying space-occupying lesions, such as those found in the liver, brain, pancreas, and gallbladder. Types of tomography include computed tomography (See Fig. 2–8), positron emission tomography (See Fig. 2–7F), and single-photon emission computed tomography (SPECT).

computed tomography (CT)
   cŏm-PŪ-tĕd
   tō-MŎG-ră-fē
   tom/o: to cut
   -graphy: process of
        recording
	Tomography in which a narrow beam of x-rays rotates in a full arc around the patient to acquire multiple views of the body, which a computer interprets to produce cross-sectional images of an internal organ or tissue; also called *computerized axial tomography (CAT) scanning*
	
	CT scans help detect tumor masses, accumulations of fluid, and bone displacements. CT scans may be performed with or without a contrast medium. (See Figs. 2–7D and 2–8).

ultrasonography (US)
ŭl-tră-sŏn-ŎG-ră-fē
   ultra-: excess, beyond
   son/o: sound
   -graphy: process of
      recording
	Radiographic procedure in which a small transducer passed over the skin transmits high-frequency sound waves (ultrasound) that bounce off body tissues and are then recorded to produce an image of an internal organ or tissue (See Fig. 2–9.)
	
	In contrast to other imaging techniques, US does not use ionizing radiation (x-ray). It is used to evaluate fetal development; examine internal structures of the abdomen, brain, and heart; diagnose musculoskeletal disorders; and evaluate blood flow. (See Fig. 2–7B.) The record produced by US is called a sonogram or echogram.

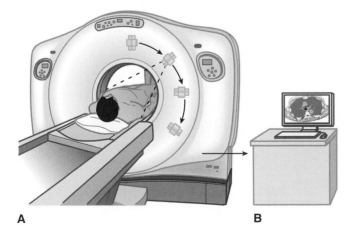

A   B

Figure 2-8 Computed tomography (CT) scan. with motorized table (**A**) and computer (**B**).

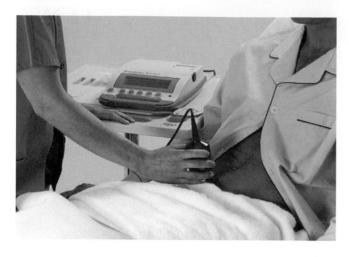

Figure 2-9 Ultrasonography of the bladder. This bladder scan is performed at bedside and may be used instead of catheterization after the patient urinates to determine the amount of urine remaining in the bladder.

x-ray	High-energy electromagnetic waves (x-rays) pass through the body onto a photographic film to produce an image of internal structures of the body for diagnosis and therapeutic purposes; also called *radiograph* *Soft body tissues, such as the stomach or liver, appear black or gray on the x-ray; dense body tissues, such as bone, appear white, making it useful in diagnosing fractures. Figure 2–7A is a chest radiograph showing widening of the mediastinum.*

Medical and Surgical Procedures

anastomosis ă-năs-tō-MŌ-sĭs	Connection between two vessels, such as the surgical joining of two ducts, blood vessels, or bowel segments to allow flow from one to the other (See Fig. 2–10.)
cauterize KAW-tĕr-īz	Process of burning abnormal tissue with electricity, freezing, heat, or chemicals (silver nitrate) *Cauterization is usually performed to destroy damaged or diseased tissues or coagulate blood vessels.*

Pronunciation Help	Long sound Short sound	ā in rāte ă in ălone	ē in rēbirth ĕ in ĕver	ī in īsle ĭ in ĭt	ō in ōver ŏ in nŏt	ū in ūnite ŭ in cŭt

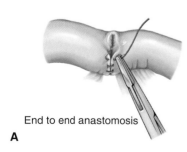

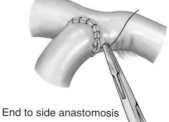

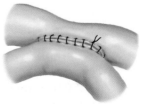

A   End to end anastomosis

B   End to side anastomosis

C   Side to side anastomosis

Figure 2-10 Anastomosis.

ADDITIONAL MEDICAL TERMS REVIEW

Match the medical terms with the definitions in the numbered list.

adhesion   CT   inflammation   radiopharmaceutical
anastomosis   endoscope   MRI   septicemia
C&S   endoscopy   nuclear scan   tomography
cauterize   fluoroscopy   radiography   US

1. _____ uses a narrow beam of x-rays, which rotates in a full arc around the patient to image the body in cross-sectional slices.

2. _____ directs x-rays through the body to a fluorescent screen to view the motion of organs, such as the digestive tract and heart.

3. _____ employs high-frequency sound waves to produce images of internal structures of the body.

4. _____ employs magnetic energy (without ionizing x-rays) to produce cross-sectional images.

5. _____ is a laboratory test performed on a body fluid to identify the causative agent and its antibiotic susceptibility.

6. _____ is a specialized lighted instrument to view the interior of organs and cavities.

7. _____ surgically joins two ducts, blood vessels, or bowel segments to allow flow from one to the other.

8. _____ is a protective response of body tissue that includes symptoms of redness, swelling, heat, and pain.

9. _____ is any of several radiographic techniques, such as CT, PET, or SPECT, that produces a film representing a detailed cross section of tissue structure.

10. _____ is a drug that contains a radioactive substance that travels to an area or a specific organ to be scanned.

11. _____ is a procedure to enable visualization of the interior of organs and cavities with a lighted instrument.

12. _____ is a procedure to burn abnormal tissue with electricity, freezing, heat, or chemicals.

13. _____ is a band of scar tissue that binds anatomical surfaces that normally are separate from each other.

14. _____ is a production of shadow images on photographic film.

15. _____ is a severe bacterial infection in the blood in which toxins circulating in the blood cause severe systemic symptoms.

Competency Verification: Check your answers in Appendix B: Answer Key, page 565. If you are not satisfied with your level of comprehension, review the pathological, diagnostic, and therapeutic terms and retake the review.

Correct Answers _____ x 6.67 = _____ % Score

BODY STRUCTURE CHAPTER REVIEW

WORD ELEMENTS SUMMARY

The following table summarizes CFs, suffixes, and prefixes related to body structure.

Word Element	Meaning	Word Element	Meaning
Combining Forms			
abdomin/o	abdomen	infer/o	lower, below
anter/o	anterior, front	inguin/o	groin
caud/o	tail	later/o	side, to one side
cephal/o	head	lumb/o	loins (lower back)
cervic/o	neck; cervix uteri (neck of uterus)	medi/o	middle
chondr/o	cartilage	nucle/o	nucleus
crani/o	cranium (skull)	pelv/o, pelv/i	pelvis
cutane/o	skin	poster/o	back (of the body), behind, posterior
cyt/o	cell	proxim/o	near, nearest
dist/o	far, farthest	radi/o	radiation, x-ray; radius (lower arm bone on the thumb side)
dors/o	back (of the body)	spin/o	spine
fluor/o	luminous, fluorescence	super/o	upper, above
gastr/o	stomach	thorac/o	chest
hist/o	tissue	umbilic/o	umbilicus, navel
ili/o	ilium (lateral, flaring portion of the hip bone)	ventr/o	belly, belly side
Suffixes			
-ac, -al, -ar, -ary, -ous, -iac, -ic, -ior	pertaining to	-meter	instrument for measuring
-ad	toward	-lysis	separation; destruction; loosening
-graphy	process of recording	-scopy	visual examination
-logist	specialist in the study of	-toxic	poison
-logy	study of	-verse	turning
Prefixes			
endo-	in, within	medi-	middle
epi-	above, upon	super-	upper, above
hypo-	under, below; deficient	trans-	through, across

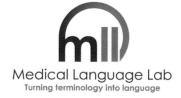

Medical Language Lab
Turning terminology into language

Visit the Medical Language Lab at *medicallanguagelab.com*. Use the flash-card word elements exercise to reinforce your study of word elements. We recommend you complete the flash-card activity before starting the Word Elements Review that follows.

WORD ELEMENTS CHAPTER REVIEW

This review provides a verification of your knowledge of the word elements covered in this chapter. Write the meaning of the word element in the space provided. To reinforce your understanding of the word parts that comprise a medical term, each word element is identified as a prefix (P), word root (WR), combining form (CF), or suffix (S). The first word is completed for you.

Medical Term	Word Element	Meaning
1. anterior	anter (WR)	anterior, front
	-ior (S)	pertaining to
2. cephalad		
3. cervical		
4. chondroma		
5. craniometer		

Continued

Medical Term	Word Element	Meaning
6. cutaneous		
7. cytology		
8. cytolysis		
9. distal		
10. dorsal		
11. endoscopy		

Medical Term	Word Element	Meaning
12. epigastric		
13. histologist		
14. hypochondriac*		
15. inferior		
16. lumbar		
17. periumbilical		

Continued

Medical Term	Word Element	Meaning
18. proximal		
19. radiography		
20. transverse		

*Refers to the right and left regions below the ribs (see Fig. 2–4B).

Competency Verification: Check your answers in Appendix B: Answer Key, page 565. If you are not satisfied with your level of comprehension, review the chapter's flash-card activity at the MLL online resource center and retake the review.

Correct Answers _____ × 5 = _____ % Score

QUADRANTS AND REGIONS REVIEW

In Figure A, label the four abdominopelvic quadrants; in Figure B, label the nine abdominopelvic regions.

Right upper quadrant (RUQ)
Left upper quadrant (LUQ)
Right lower quadrant (RLQ)
Left lower quadrant (LLQ)

A

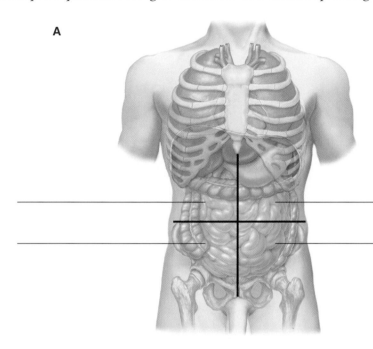

Right hypochondriac
Epigastric
Right lumbar
Right inguinal
Left hypochondriac
Umbilical
Left lumbar
Left inguinal
Hypogastric

B

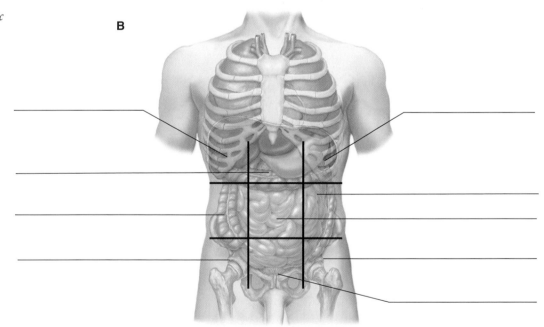

Competency Verification: Compare your answers by referring to Figure 2–4, page 45.

Integumentary System

OBJECTIVES

Upon completion of this chapter, you will be able to:

• Describe the type of medical treatment the dermatologist provides.

• Identify the integumentary system structures by labeling the anatomical illustrations.

• Describe the primary functions of the integumentary system.

• Describe diseases, conditions, and procedures related to the integumentary system.

• Apply your word-building skills by constructing various medical terms related to the integumentary system.

• Describe common abbreviations and symbols related to the integumentary system.

• Recognize, define, pronounce, and spell terms correctly.

• Demonstrate your knowledge of this chapter by successfully completing the frames, reviews, and medical report evaluations.

MEDICAL SPECIALTY

Dermatology

Dermatology is the medical specialty concerned with diagnosis and treatment of diseases involving the skin and the relationship of skin lesions to systemic diseases. The physician who specializes in diagnosis and treatment of skin diseases is called a **dermatologist.** The dermatologist's scope of practice includes management of skin cancers, moles, and other skin tumors. This specialist also uses various techniques for the enhancement and correction of cosmetic skin defects and prescribes measures to maintain the skin in a state of health.

ANATOMY AND PHYSIOLOGY OVERVIEW

The integumentary system consists of the skin and its accessory organs: the hair, nails, sebaceous glands, and sweat glands. The skin is the largest organ in the body and protects the body from the external environment. It shields the body against injuries, infection, dehydration, harmful ultraviolet rays, and toxic compounds. Beneath the skin's surface is an intricate network of sensory receptors that register sensations of temperature, pain, and pressure. The millions of sensory receptors and a vascular network aid the functions of the entire body in maintaining homeostasis, which is the stable internal environment of the body. (See Fig. 3–1.)

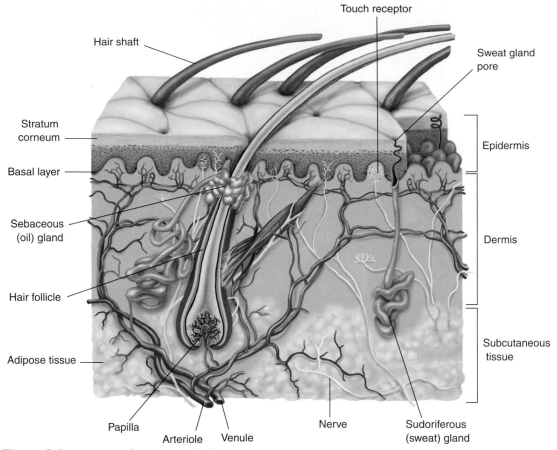

Figure 3-1 Structure of the skin and subcutaneous tissue.

WORD ELEMENTS

This section introduces combining forms (CFs) related to the integumentary system. Included are key suffixes; prefixes are defined in the right-hand column as needed. Review the following table, and pronounce each word in the word analysis column aloud before you begin to work the frames.

Word Element	Meaning	Word Analysis
Combining Forms		
adip/o	fat	**adip/o/cele** (ĂD-ĭ-pō-sēl): hernia containing fat or fatty tissue *-cele:* hernia, swelling
lip/o		**lip/o/cyte** (LĬP-ō-sīt): fat cell *-cyte:* cell
steat/o		**steat/itis** (stē-ă-TĪ-tĭs): inflammation of fatty tissue *-itis:* inflammation
cutane/o	skin	**cutane/ous** (kū-TĀ-nē-ŭs): pertaining to the skin *-ous:* pertaining to
dermat/o		**dermat/o/logist** (dĕr-mă-TŎL-ō-jĭst): physician specializing in treating skin disorders *-logist:* specialist in the study of
derm/o		hypo/**derm**/ic (hī-pō-DĔR-mĭk): under or inserted under the skin, as in a hypodermic injection *hypo-:* under, below, deficient *-ic:* pertaining to

Word Element	Meaning	Word Analysis

hidr/o	sweat	**hidr**/aden/itis (hī-drăd-ĕ-NĪ-tĭs): inflammation of a sweat gland
		  aden: gland
		  -itis: inflammation
		
		Do not confuse hidr/o (sweat) with hydr/o (water).

sudor/o		**sudor**/esis (sū-dō-RĒ-sĭs): condition of profuse sweating; also called *diaphoresis* and *hyperhidrosis* *-esis:* condition
ichthy/o	dry, scaly	**ichthy**/osis (ĭk-thē-Ō-sĭs): any of several dermatologic conditions characterized by noninflammatory dryness and scaling of the skin and commonly associated with other abnormalities of lipid metabolism *-osis:* abnormal condition; increase (used primarily with blood cells) *A mild form of ichthyosis, called winter itch, is commonly seen on the legs of older patients, especially during the dry winter months.*
kerat/o	horny tissue; hard; cornea	**kerat**/osis (kĕr-ă-TŌ-sĭs): any condition of the skin characterized by an overgrowth and thickening of the skin *-osis:* abnormal condition; increase (used primarily with blood cells)
melan/o	black	**melan**/oma (mĕl-ă-NŌ-mă): malignant tumor of melanocytes that commonly begins in a darkly pigmented mole and can metastasize widely *-oma:* tumor *Melanomas are caused by intense exposure to sunlight and commonly metastasize throughout the body.*

myc/o	fungus (plural, *fungi*)	dermat/o/**myc**/osis (dĕr-mă-tō-mī-KŌ-sĭs): fungal infection of the skin
		
		  dermat/o: skin
		  -osis: abnormal condition; increase (used primarily with blood cells)

onych/o	nail	**onych**/o/malacia (ŏn-ĭ-kō-mă-LĀ-shē-ă): abnormal softening of the nails *-malacia:* softening

pil/o	hair	**pil**/o/nid/al (pī-lō-NĪ-dăl): growth of hair in a dermoid cyst or in a sinus opening on the skin
		  nid: nest
		  -al: pertaining to
		
		A pilonidal cyst commonly develops in the sacral region (fourth segment of the lower spinal column) of the skin. The cystic tumor contains elements derived from the ectoderm, such as hair, skin, sebum, or teeth.

trich/o		**trich**/o/pathy (trĭk-ŎP-ă-thē): any disease of the hair *-pathy:* disease
scler/o	hardening; sclera (white of eye)	**scler**/o/derma (sklĕr-ō-DĔR-mă): chronic disease with abnormal hardening of the skin caused by formation of new collagen *-derma:* skin
seb/o	sebum, sebaceous	**seb**/o/rrhea (sĕb-or-Ē-ă): increase in the amount and, commonly, an alteration of the quality of the fats secreted by the sebaceous glands *-rrhea:* discharge, flow
squam/o	scale	**squam**/ous (SKWĀ-mŭs): covered with scales or scalelike *-ous:* pertaining to
xer/o	dry	**xer**/o/derma (zē-rō-DĔR-mă): chronic skin condition characterized by excessive roughness and dryness *-derma:* skin *Xeroderma is a mild form of ichthyosis.*

Continued

Word Element	Meaning	Word Analysis
Suffixes		
-derma	skin	py/o/**derma** (pī-ō-DĔR-mă): any pyogenic infection of the skin *py/o:* pus
-oid	resembling	derm/**oid** (DĔR-moyd): resembling skin *derm:* skin
-phoresis	carrying, transmission	dia/**phoresis** (dī-ă-fō-RĒ-sĭs): condition of profuse sweating, also called *sudoresis* and *hyperhidrosis* *dia-:* through, across
-plasty	surgical repair	dermat/o/**plasty** (DĔR-mă-tō-plăs-tē): surgical repair of the skin *dermat/o:* skin
-therapy	treatment	cry/o/**therapy** (krī-ō-THĔR-ă-pē): treatment using cold as a destructive medium *cry/o:* cold *Warts and actinic keratosis are some of the common skin disorders treated with cryotherapy.*
Pronunciation Help	Long sound	ā in rāte ē in rēbirth ī in īsle ō in ōver ū in ūnite
	Short sound	ă in ălone ĕ in ĕver ĭ in ĭt ŏ in nŏt ŭ in cŭt

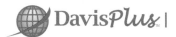

Visit the *Medical Terminology Simplified* online resource center at Davis*Plus* for an audio exercise of the terms in this table. It will help you master pronunciations and meanings of the selected medical terms.

SECTION REVIEW 3-1

For the following medical terms, first write the suffix and its meaning. Then translate the meaning of the remaining elements starting with the first part of the word. The first word is an example that is completed for you.

Term	Meaning
1. hypo/derm/ic	-ic: pertaining to; under, below, deficient; skin
2. melan/oma	
3. kerat/osis	
4. cutane/ous	
5. lip/o/cyte	
6. onych/o/malacia	
7. scler/o/derma	
8. dia/phoresis	
9. dermat/o/myc/osis	
10. cry/o/therapy	

Competency Verification: Check your answers in Appendix B: Answer Key, page 567. If you are not satisfied with your level of comprehension, review the vocabulary and retake the review.

Correct Answers _____ x 10 = _____ % Score

SKIN AND ACCESSORY ORGANS

The skin is a sensory organ that also provides protection for the body. The accessory organs of the skin include the hair, nails, sebaceous glands, and sweat glands.

Skin

3-1   The skin is considered an organ and is composed of two layers of tissue: the outer epidermis, which is visible to the naked eye, and the inner layer, the dermis.

Identify and label the (1) **epidermis** and the (2) **dermis** in Figure 3–2.

epi/derm/is
ĕp-ĭ-DĔR-mĭs

derm/is
DĔR-mĭs

3–2   The epi/derm/is forms the protective covering of the body and does not have a blood or nerve supply. It is dependent on the dermis's network of capillaries for nourishment. As oxygen and nutrients flow out of the capillaries in the dermis, they pass through tissue fluid, supplying nourishment to the deeper layers of the epidermis.

When you talk about the outer layer of skin, you are referring to the

_____ / _____ / _____.

When you talk about the deeper layer of skin, consisting of nerve and blood vessels, you are talking about the _____ / _____.

---

epi-
-is

3–3   The epi/derm/is is thick on the palms of the hands and the soles of the feet, but relatively thin over most other areas.

Identify the element in epi/derm/is that means

above or upon: _____

a part of speech (noun): _____.

---

skin

3–4   The CF *derm/o* refers to the skin. Derm/o/pathy is a disease of the

_____.

3–5   Although the epidermis is composed of several layers, the (3) **stratum corneum** and the (4) **basal layer** are of greatest importance.

The stratum corneum is composed of dead, flat cells. Its thickness is correlated with normal wear of the area it covers. Only the basal layer is composed of living cells. It is where new cells are continuously reproduced. Label these two structures in Figure 3–2.

3–6   As new cells form in the basal layer, they move toward the stratum corneum. Eventually, they die and become filled with a hard protein material called keratin. The relatively waterproof characteristic of keratin prevents body fluids from evaporating and moisture from entering the body. These keratinized cells gradually flake away and are replaced in a continuous cycle. The entire process by which a cell forms in the basal layers, rises to the surface, becomes keratinized, and sloughs off takes about 1 month.

Check the basal layer in Figure 3–1 to see the single row of newly formed cells in the deepest layer of the epi/derm/is.

---

skin

study, skin

3–7   In addition to *derm/o,* two other CFs for skin are *cutane/o* and *dermat/o.*

Cutane/ous means pertaining to the _____.

Dermat/o/logy is the _____ of the _____.

---

dermat/o/logist
dĕr-mă-TŎL-ō-jĭst

3–8   A physician who specializes in treating skin diseases is called a

_____ / _____ / _____.

---

dermat/itis
dĕr-mă-TĪ-tĭs

3–9   Use *dermat* to build a word meaning *inflammation of the skin.*

_____ / _____.

Boldface indicates a word root or combining form. Blue indicates a suffix. Pink indicates a prefix.

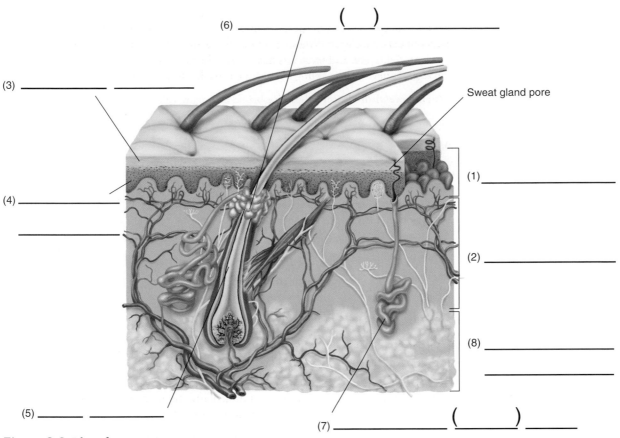

(6) _____ (___) _____

(3) _____ _____

Sweat gland pore

(4) _____

_____

(1) _____

(2) _____

(5) _____ _____

(8) _____

_____

(7) _____ (___) _____

Figure 3-2 Identifying integumentary structures.

skin skin	**3-10** The prefix *sub-* means under or below; the prefix *hypo-* means *under, below, deficient.* A sub/cutane/ous injection occurs beneath the _____. A hypo/derm/ic needle is inserted under the _____.
skin	**3-11** Sub/cutane/ous literally means pertaining to under the _____.
skin	**3-12** When you see the terms derm/a, derm/is, and derm/oid, you will know the roots refer to the _____.
skin	**3-13** As discussed previously, suffixes *-al, -ic, -ior,* and *-ous* are adjective endings that mean *pertaining to.* Terms such as derm/al and derm/ic mean *pertaining to the* _____.

melan/o/cyte MĔL-ăn-ō-sīt **melan/oma** mĕl-ă-NŌ-mă	**3-14** In the basal layer, specialized cells, called melan/o/cytes, produce a black pigment called melanin. Production of melanin increases with exposure to strong ultraviolet light. This exposure creates a suntan that provides a protective barrier from damaging effects of the sun. The CF *melan/o* refers to the color black. Build a word that literally means *black cell:* :_____ / _____ / _____ *black tumor:* :_____ / _____
	3-15 Activity of melan/o/cytes is genetically regulated and inherited. Local accumulations of melanin are seen in pigmented moles and freckles. Environmental and physiological factors also play a role in skin color. Locate the basal layer in Figure 3–1.
albin/ism ĂL-bĭn-ĭzm	**3-16** Absence of pigment in the skin, eyes, and hair is most likely due to an inherited inability to produce melanin. This lack of melanin results in the condition called albin/ism. A person with this condition is called an albino. Deficiency or absence of pigment in the skin, hair, and eyes due to an abnormality in production of melanin is known as _____ / _____.
melanin MĔL-ă-nĭn	**3-17** The number of melan/o/cytes is about the same in all races. Differences in skin color are attributed to production of melanin. In people with dark skin, melan/o/cytes continuously produce large amounts of melanin. In people with light skin, melan/o/cytes produce less _____.

When defining a medical word, first define the suffix. Second, define the beginning of the word; finally, define the middle of the word. Below is an example of a term, which is translated as *abnormal condition of a skin fungus.*

dermat / o / myc / osis
(2)   (3)   (1)

adjective **adjective**	**3-18** The term derm/is is a noun that means *pertaining to the skin.* Identify the part of speech in *derm/ic:* _____ *derm/al:* _____
	3-19 Label Figure 3–2 as you learn about the parts of the dermis. The second layer of skin, the derm/is, contains the (5) **hair follicle**, (6) **sebaceous (oil) gland**, and (7) **sudoriferous (sweat) gland.**
inflammation, skin	**3-20** Dermat/itis is an _____ of the _____.
disease, skin	**3-21** Derm/o/pathy is a disease of the skin; dermat/o/pathy is also a _____ of the _____.

Boldface indicates a word root or combining form. Blue indicates a suffix. Pink indicates a prefix.

aden/oma ăd-ĕ-NŌ-mă	**3–22** An aden/oma is a benign (not malignant) neo/plasm in which the tumor cells form glands or glandlike structures. The tumor is usually well circumscribed, tending to compress rather than infiltrate or invade adjacent tissue. Build a word that means tumor composed of glandular tissue. _____ / _____
adip/ectomy ăd-ĭ-PĔK-tō-mē	**3–23** Lip/o and adip/o are CFs that mean *fat*. A lip/ectomy is *excision of fat or adipose tissue.* Use *adip/o* to form another surgical term that means excision of fat. _____ / _____
adip/o, lip/o **steat/o**	**3–24** Adip/oma and lip/oma are terms that mean *fatty tumor.* Both are benign tumors consisting of fat cells. The CFs in this frame that mean fat are _____ / _____ and _____ / _____. A third CF that refers to fat is _____ / _____.
	3–25 The dermis is attached to underlying structures of the skin by (8) **subcutaneous tissue.** Identify and label the layer of subcutaneous tissue in Figure 3–2.
sub/cutane/ous sŭb-kū-TĀ-nē-ŭs **lip/o/cytes** LĬP-ō-sītz	**3–26** Sub/cutane/ous tissue forms lip/o/cytes, also known as fat cells. Determine words in this frame that mean *pertaining to under or below the skin:* _____ / _____ / _____ *fat cells:* _____ / _____ / _____
cell, tumor	**3–27** Whereas a lip/o/cyte is a fat _____, an adip/oma is a fatty _____.

Competency Verification: Check your labeling of Figure 3–2 in Appendix B: Answer Key, page 567.

	3–28 Suction lip/ectomy, also called lip/o/suction, is removal of sub/cutane/ous fat tissue using a blunt-tipped cannula (tube) introduced into the fatty area through a small incision. Suction is applied and fat tissue is removed. Locate the sub/cutane/ous tissue in Figure 3–1.
sub/cutane/ous sŭb-kū-TĀ-nē-ŭs **lip/ectomy** *or* **lip/o/suction** lĭ-PĔK-tō-mē, LĬP-ō-sŭk-shŭn	**3–29** Identify terms in Frame 3–28 that mean *under the skin:* _____ / _____ / _____ *excision of fat:* _____ / _____ or _____ / _____ / _____.

fat	**3–30** Lip/o/suction is performed for cosmetic reasons and used primarily to remove or reduce localized areas of fat around the abdomen, breasts, legs, face, and upper arms. Lip/o/suction literally means *suction of* _____.
derm/o, dermat/o, cutane/o	**3–31** List three CFs that refer to the skin. _____ / _____, _____ / _____, and _____ / _____
dermat/o/plasty DĔR-mă-tō-plăs-tē **dermat/itis** dĕr-mă-TĪ-tĭs	**3–32** Use *dermat/o* to form a word meaning *surgical repair (of) skin:* _____ / _____ / _____ *inflammation (of the) skin:* _____ / _____
log **-ist** **-y**	**3–33** The noun suffixes *-logy* and *-logist* contain the same root, **log/o,** which means *study of.* The *y* at the end of a term means *condition or process* and denotes a noun ending. The definitions of both suffixes are easier to remember if you analyze their components: *-logy* means *study of; -logist* means *specialist in the study of.* The root in each suffix that means *study of* is _____. The element in the suffix *-logist* that means specialist is _____. The element in the suffix *-logy* that means *condition or process* is _____.
dermat/o/logy dĕr-mă-TŎL-ō-jē **dermat/o/logist** dĕr-mă-TŎL-ō-jĭst	**3–34** Refer to Frame 3–33 and use *dermat/o* to develop words that mean *study of the skin:* _____ / _____ / _____ *specialist who treats skin disorders:* _____ / _____ / _____
dermat/oma dĕr-mă-TŌ-mă **dermat/o/pathy** dĕr-mă-TŎP-ă-thē **dermat/o/logy** dĕr-mă-TŎL-ō-jē	**3–35** Use *dermat/o* to practice forming words that mean *tumor of the skin:* _____ / _____ *disease of the skin:* _____ / _____ / _____ *study of the skin:* _____ / _____ / _____
hardening	**3–36** Scler/osis is an abnormal condition of _____.
skin	**3–37** Scler/o/derma, a chronic hardening and thickening of the skin, is caused by new collagen formation. It is characterized by inflammation that ultimately develops into fibrosis (scarring), then sclerosis (hardening) of tissues. Systemic scler/o/derma can be defined as hardening of the _____.

Boldface indicates a word root or combining form. Blue indicates a suffix. Pink indicates a prefix.

system/ic scler/osis sĭs-TĔM-ĭk sklĕ-RŌ-sĭs **hardening**	**3–38** System/ic scler/osis, a form of scler/o/derma, is characterized by formation of thickened collagenous fibrous tissue, thickening of the skin, and adhesion to underlying tissues. The disease progresses to involve tissues of the heart, lungs, muscles, genit/o/urin/ary tract, and kidneys. A form of scler/o/derma that causes fibr/osis and scler/osis of multiple body systems is known as _____ / _____ _____ / _____. If you check *scler/o* in Appendix A: Glossary of Medical Word Elements, you will see that *scler/o* means *hardening; sclera (white of eye)*. In the integumentary system, however, *scler/o* specifically refers to _____.
horny tissue, hard **cornea**	**3–39** The CF *kerat/o* means *horny tissue; hard; cornea.* (The cornea of the eye is covered in Chapter 11.) When *kerat/o* is used in discussions of the skin, it refers to _____ _____ or _____. When *kerat/o* is used in discussions of the eye, it refers to the _____.
kerat/osis kĕr-ă-TŌ-sĭs	**3–40** Kerat/osis, a skin condition, is characterized by hard, horny tissue. A person with a skin lesion in which there is overgrowth and thickening of the epidermis most likely would be diagnosed with _____ / _____.
tumor	**3–41** A kerat/oma is a horny _____, also called *kerat/osis*.

Accessory Organs of the Skin

sebaceous sē-BĀ-shŭs **sudoriferous** sū-dŏr-ĬF-ĕr-ŭs	**3–42** Accessory organs of the skin include the sebaceous (oil) glands, sudoriferous (sweat) glands, hair, and nails. Refer to Figure 3–1 to complete this frame. Oil-secreting glands of the skin are called _____ glands. Sweat glands are called _____ glands.
comedos KŎM-ē-dōs **pustules** PŬS-tūlz	**3–43** Sebaceous glands are found in all areas of the body that have hair. The oily material, called sebum, is secreted by the sebaceous gland. It keeps hair and skin soft and pliable and inhibits growth of bacteria on the skin. Increased activity of sebaceous glands at puberty may block the hair follicle and form blackheads (comedos). As bacteria feed on the sebum, they release irritating substances that produce inflammation. Large numbers of bacteria produce infection, forming whiteheads (pustules). Identify the medical term for *blackheads:* _____ *whiteheads:* _____
sebaceous sē-BĀ-shŭs	**3–44** Comedos and pustules are the result of hypersecretion of sebum by the _____ (oil) glands.

sudoriferous sū-dŏr-ĬF-ĕr-ŭs	**3–45** Sweat glands that are not associated with hair follicles open to the surface of the skin through pores, as illustrated in Figure 3–1. These glands are stimulated by temperature increases or emotional stress and produce perspiration that evaporates on the surface of the skin and provides a cooling effect. Sweat, or perspiration, is produced by the _____ (sweat) glands.
hidr/osis hī-DRŌ-sĭs	**3–46** The CF for sweat is **hidr/o**. Use *-osis* to form a word that means *abnormal condition of sweat:* _____ / _____
sweat **gland** **inflammation** **excessive, above normal** **sweat** **abnormal condition**	**3–47** The term dia/phoresis denotes a condition of profuse or excessive sweating. The following two terms also refer to sweating. The term hidr/aden/itis means *hidr:* _____ *aden:* _____ *-itis:* _____ The term hyper/hidr/osis means *hyper-:* _____, _____ _____ *hidr:* _____ *-osis:* _____ _____
sweat, water	**3–48** Although **hidr/o** and **hydr/o** sound alike, they have different meanings. *Hidr/o* refers to _____. *Hydr/o* refers to _____.
an/hidr/osis ăn-hī-DRŌ-sĭs	**3–49** An/hidr/osis is an abnormal condition characterized by inadequate perspiration. When a person suffers from an absence of sweating, you would say the person has a condition called _____ / _____ / _____.
myc/osis mī-KŌ-sĭs	**3–50** The CF **myc/o** refers to a fungus (plural, *fungi*). Combine **myc/o** and *-osis* to form a word that means abnormal condition caused by fungi. _____ / _____
skin	**3–51** Dermat/o/myc/osis, a fungal infection of the skin, is caused by dermato-phytes, yeasts, and other fungi. When you see this term in a medical report, you will know it refers to a fungal infection of the _____.
fungus FŬN-gŭs	**3–52** Myc/o/dermat/itis, an inflammation of the skin, is caused by a _____.

Boldface indicates a word root or combining form. Blue indicates a suffix. Pink indicates a prefix.

derm/o/pathy dĕr-MŎP-ă-thē	**3–53** Use *derm/o* to form a medical term that means disease of the skin. _____ / _____ / _____
trich/o/pathy trĭk-ŎP-ă-thē **trich/osis** trĭ-KŌ-sĭs	**3–54** The CF *trich/o* refers to the hair. Construct medical terms that mean *disease of the hair:* _____ / _____ / _____ *abnormal condition of the hair:* _____ / _____
trich/o/myc/osis trĭk-ō-mī-KŌ-sĭs	**3–55** Combine *trich/o* + *myc* + *-osis* to form a medical term that means *abnormal condition of the hair caused by a fungus.* _____ / _____ / _____ / _____
hair	**3–56** Another CF for hair is *pil/o.* Whenever you see *pil/o* or *trich/o* in a word, you will know it refers to the _____.
pil/o, -oid	**3–57** Pil/o/cyst/ic refers to a *derm/oid cyst containing hair.* The element in this frame that means hair is _____ / _____. The element in this frame that means resembling is _____.

3–58 Label the structures of the fingernail in Figure 3–3 as you read the following material. Each nail is formed in the (1) **nail root** and is composed of keratin, a hard fibrous protein, which is also the main component of hair. As the nail grows from a (2) **matrix** of active cells beneath the (3) **cuticle,** it stays attached and slides forward over the epithelial layer called the (4) **nail bed**. Most of the (5) **nail body** appears pink because of the underlying blood vessels. The (6) **lunula** is the crescent-shaped area at the base of the nail. It has a whitish appearance because the vascular tissue underneath does not show through.

Here is a review of the three basic rules of word building:
- **Rule 1:** Word root links a suffix that begins with a vowel.
- **Rule 2:** Combining form (root + *o*) links a suffix that begins with a consonant.
- **Rule 3:** Combining form (root + *o*) links a root to another root to form a compound word. (This rule holds true even if the next root begins with a vowel.)

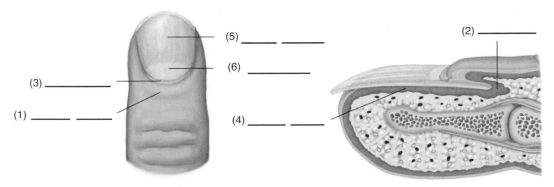

Figure 3-3 Structure of a fingernail.

onych/oma ŏn-ĭ-KŌ-mă **onych/o/pathy** ŏn-ĭ-KŎP-ăth-ē	**3-59** The CF *onych/o* refers to the nail(s). Form medical words that mean *tumor of the nail (or nail bed):* _____ / _____ *disease of the nail:* _____ / ____ / _____
onych/o/malacia ŏn-ĭ-kō-mă-LĀ-shē-ă	**3-60** The term malacia means *abnormal softening of tissue.* This term is also used in words as a suffix. Build a word with *-malacia* that means *softening of the nail(s).* _____ / ____ / _____
onych/o **myc** **-osis**	**3-61** Nails become white, opaque, thickened, and brittle when a person has a disease called onych/o/myc/osis. Identify elements in onych/o/myc/osis that mean *nail:* _____ / ____ *fungus:* _____ *abnormal condition:* _____
nail(s)	**3-62** When you see the term onych/o/myc/osis in a medical chart, you will know it means an infection of the _____ caused by a fungus.
xer/o	**3-63** The noun suffix *-derma* denotes *skin.* A person with excessive dryness of the skin has a condition called xer/o/derma. From xer/o/derma, identify the CF that means dry. _____ / ____
hernia, swelling	**3-64** The suffix *-cele* refers to a _____ or _____.
lip/o/cele LĬP-ō-sēl	**3-65** A hernia containing fat or fatty tissue is called an adip/o/cele or _____ / ____ / _____.

Competency Verification: Check your labeling of Figure 3–3 in Appendix B: Answer Key, page 567.

Boldface indicates a word root or combining form. Blue indicates a suffix. Pink indicates a prefix.

SECTION REVIEW 3-2

Using the following table, write the CF, suffix, or prefix that matches its definition in the space provided to the left of the definition. There may be more than one word element that matches a definition.

Combining Forms		Suffixes	Prefixes
adip/o	pil/o	-cele	epi-
cutane/o	scler/o	-derma	hypo-
derm/o	steat/o	-logist	
dermat/o	trich/o	-malacia	
hidr/o	xer/o	-osis	
lip/o		-pathy	
onych/o		-rrhea	

1. _____ disease

2. _____ dry

3. _____ fat

4. _____ discharge, flow

5. _____ hair

6. _____ hardening; sclera (white of the eye)

7. _____ hernia, swelling

8. _____ nail

9. _____ skin

10. _____ softening

11. _____ specialist in the study of

12. _____ above, upon

13. _____ abnormal condition; increase (used primarily with blood cells)

14. _____ sweat

15. _____ under, below; deficient

Competency Verification: Check your answers in Appendix B: Answer Key, page 567. If you are not satisfied with your level of comprehension, go back to Frame 3–1 and rework the frames.

Correct Answers _____ × 6.67 = _____ % Score

 When defining a medical word, first define the suffix. Second, define the beginning of the word. Finally, define the middle of the word. Here is an example using the term

sub / cutane / ous
(2)   (3)   (1)

Combining Forms Denoting Color

Skin

albin/ism
ĂL-bĭn-ĭzm

cyan/o/derma
sī-ă-nō-DĔR-mă

erythr/o/derma
ĕ-rĭth-rō-DĔR-mă

leuk/o/derma
loo-kō-DĔR-mă

melan/o/derma
mĕl-ăn-ō-DĔR-mă

xanth/oma
zăn-THŌ-mă

3–66 Examine the CFs that denote color and their meanings in the left-hand column of the table below. Examples of medical terms with their definitions are provided in the middle column. In the right-hand column, use a slash to break down each word into its basic elements.

Combining Form	Medical Term	Word Breakdown
albin/o: white	albinism: white condition	a l b i n i s m
cyan/o: blue	cyanoderma: blue skin	c y a n o d e r m a
erythr/o: red	erythroderma: red skin	e r y t h r o d e r m a
leuk/o: white	leukoderma: white skin	l e u k o d e r m a
melan/o: black	melanoderma: black skin	m e l a n o d e r m a
xanth/o: yellow	xanthoma: yellow tumor	x a n t h o m a

nouns

3–67 The -*a* ending in cyan/o/derma, erythr/o/derma, leuk/o/derma, and melan/o/derma designates that these words are (adjectives, nouns)

_____.

erythr/o/derma
ĕ-rĭth-rō-DĔR-mă

melan/o/derma
mĕl-ăn-ō-DĔR-mă

xanth/o/derma
zăn-thō-DĔR-mă

xer/o/derma
zē-rō-DĔR-mă

3–68 Use -*derma* to build medical words that mean

skin that is red: _____ / _____ / _____

skin that is black: _____ / _____ / _____

skin that is yellow: _____ / _____ / _____

skin that is dry: _____ / _____ / _____

Cells

cells

cell

3–69 You already learned that a cell is the smallest basic unit of the human organism and that every tissue and organ in the human body is made up of cells.

Cyt/o/logy is the study of _____.

The word elements **cyt/o** and -*cyte* are used to build words that refer to a

_____.

Boldface indicates a word root or combining form. Blue indicates a suffix. Pink indicates a prefix.

cells	**3-70** Cyt/o/logy is the study of _____.

erythr/o/cyte ĕ-RĬTH-rō-sīt **leuk/o/cyte** LOO-kō-sīt **melan/o/cyte** mĕl-ĂN-ō-sīt **xanth/o/cyte** ZĂN-thō-sīt	**3-71** Use *-cyte* (cell) to form words that mean *cell that is red:* _____ / _____ / _____ *cell that is white:* _____ / _____ / _____ *cell that is black:* _____ / _____ / _____ *cell that is yellow:* _____ / _____ / _____

-penia **leuk/o** **cyt/o**	**3-72** Leuk/o/cyt/o/penia, an abnormal decrease in white blood cells (WBCs), may be caused by an adverse drug reaction, radiation poisoning, or a path/o/logic/al condition. The term leuk/o/cyt/o/penia is formed from the *suffix that means decrease or deficiency:* _____ *CF that means white:* _____ / _____ *CF that means cell:* _____ / _____

leuk/o/cyt/o/penia loo-kō-sī-tō-PĒ-nē-ă	**3-73** A deficiency in white blood cell production may be a sign of a path/o/logic/al condition known as leuk/o/penia or _____ / _____ / _____ / _____ / _____

WBC	**3-74** The abbreviation for white blood cell is _____.

blood	**3-75** The suffix *-emia* is used in words to mean *blood condition.* Xanth/emia, an occurrence of yellow pigment in the blood, literally means *yellow* _____.

xanth/omas zăn-THŌ-măz	**3-76** High cholesterol levels may cause small yellow tumors called _____ / _____.

blood **white**	**3-77** Leuk/emia is a progressive malignant disease of the blood-forming organs. It is characterized by proliferation and development of immature leuk/o/cytes in the blood and bone marrow. Leuk/emia literally means *white* _____. Leuk/o/cytes are _____ blood cells.

leuk/emia loo-KĒ-mē-ă	**3-78** A disease of unrestrained growth of immature white blood cells is called _____ / _____.

melan/o/cyte mĕl-ĂN-ō-sīt **melan/oma** mĕl-ă-NŌ-mă	**3-79** Melan/oma is a malignant neo/plasm (new growth) that originates in the skin and is composed of melan/o/cytes. Form medical words that literally mean *black cell:* _____ / _____ / _____ *black tumor:* _____ / _____
melan/oma mĕl-ă-NŌ-mă	**3-80** The lesion of melan/oma is characterized by its asymmetry, irregular border, and lack of uniform color. Malignant melan/oma is the most dangerous form of skin cancer because of its tendency to metastasize rapidly. The medical term that literally means *black tumor* is _____ / _____.
cyan/o/derma sī-ă-nō-DĔR-mă	**3-81** Cyan/osis, also called *cyan/o/derma,* is caused by a deficiency of oxygen and an excess of carbon dioxide in the blood. A person who is rescued from drowning exhibits a dark bluish or purplish discoloration of the skin. This condition is known as *cyan/osis* or _____ / _____ / _____.
cyan/osis sī-ă-NŌ-sĭs **erythr/osis** ĕr-ĭ-THRŌ-sĭs **melan/osis** mĕl-ăn-Ō-sĭs **xanth/osis** zăn-THŌ-sĭs	**3-82** Use *-osis* to develop medical words that mean *abnormal condition of blue (skin):* _____ / _____ *abnormal condition of red (skin):* _____ / _____ *abnormal condition of black (pigmentation):* _____ / _____ *abnormal condition of yellow (skin):* _____ / _____
increase **leuk/o/cyt/osis** loo-kō-sī-TŌ-sĭs	**3-83** The suffix *-osis* is used in words to mean *abnormal condition.* However, when *-osis* is used in a word related to blood, it means *increase.* The complete meaning of *-osis* is *abnormal condition; increase (used primarily with blood cells).* The term *erythr/o/cyt/osis* is an _____ in red blood cells. Use **leuk/o** (white) to build a term that means *increase in white blood cells:* _____ / _____ / _____ / _____.
melan/oma mĕl-ă-NŌ-mă	**3-84** The most common skin cancers are **basal cell carcinoma** and **squamous cell carcinoma.** According to the American Cancer Society (ACS), the annual rates of all forms of skin cancer are increasing at an alarming rate due to repeated overexposure to the ultraviolet rays of the sun. ACS estimates that nearly half of all Americans who live to age 65 will develop skin cancer at least once. Sun exposure, especially excessive tanning of the skin, can cause the lethal black tumor called _____ / _____.

Boldface indicates a word root or combining form. Blue indicates a suffix. Pink indicates a prefix.

carcin/oma kăr-sĭ-NŌ-mă	**3-85** Basal cell carcin/oma is a skin cancer of the basal cell layer (deepest layer) of the epidermis. Metastasis is rare, but local invasion destroys underlying and adjacent tissue. This condition occurs most commonly on areas of the skin exposed to the sun. (See Fig. 3–4.) A type of skin cancer that affects the deepest layer of the epidermis is called basal cell _____ / _____.
carcin/oma kăr-sĭ-NŌ-mă	**3-86** Squamous cell carcin/oma is a skin cancer of the squamous cells (top layer) of the epidermis. It is an invasive tumor with potential for metastasis and occurs most commonly in fair-skinned white men over age 60. Repeated overexposure to the sun's ultraviolet rays greatly increases the risk of squamous cell carcin/oma. (See Fig. 3–5.) A carcin/oma that affects the top layer of the epidermis is called squamous cell _____ / _____.

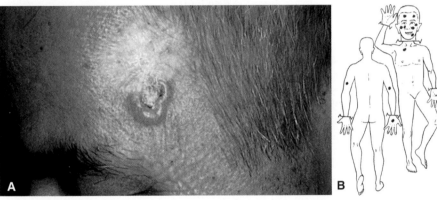

Figure 3-4 Basal cell carcinoma. **(A)** Pearly, flesh-colored papule with depressed center and rolled edge. **(B)** Common sites of basal cell carcinoma. From Goldsmith, Lazarus, and Tharp: *Adult and Pediatric Dermatology: A Color Guide to Diagnosis and Treatment.* F. A. Davis, Philadelphia, 1997, p 157, with permission.

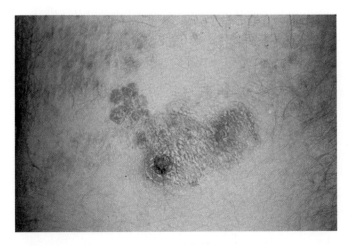

Figure 3-5 Squamous cell carcinoma, in which the surface is fragile and bleeds easily. From Goldsmith, Lazarus, and Tharp: *Adult and Pediatric Dermatology: A Color Guide to Diagnosis and Treatment.* F. A. Davis, Philadelphia, 1997, p 237, with permission.

AIDS **Kaposi sarc/oma** KĂP-ō-sē săr-KŌ-mă	**3–87** The CF **sarc/o** means *flesh (connective tissue)*. Kaposi sarc/oma, a malignant skin tumor commonly associated with patients who are diagnosed with acquired immunodeficiency syndrome (AIDS), is usually fatal. Initially, the tumor appears as a purplish brown lesion. The abbreviation for acquired immunodeficiency syndrome is _____. The type of skin cancer associated with the AIDS virus is _____ _____ / _____.
death	**3–88** The CF **necr/o** is used in words to denote death or necr/osis. Necr/o/tic is a word that means *pertaining to necr/osis or* _____.
dead	**3–89** The term necr/osis is used to denote the death of areas of tissue or bone surrounded by healthy tissue. Cellular necr/osis means that the *cells are* _____.
necr/osis nĕ-KRŌ-sĭs	**3–90** Bony necr/osis occurs when dead bone tissue results from the loss of blood supply (for example, after a fracture). The term that means abnormal condition of death is _____ / _____.
gangrene GĂNG-grēn	**3–91** Gangrene is a form of necr/osis associated with loss of blood supply. Before healing can take place, the dead matter must be removed. When there is an injury to blood flow, a form of necr/osis may develop that is known as _____.
self **self** **self**	**3–92** In the English language, an auto/graph is a signature written by oneself. In medical words, **auto-** is used as a prefix and means *self, own*. Auto/hypnosis is hypnosis of one's _____. Auto/examination is an examination of one's _____. An auto/graft is skin transplanted from one's _____.
auto/grafts AW-tō-grăfts	**3–93** A graft is tissue transplanted or implanted in a part of the body to repair a defect. Grafts done with tissue transplanted from the patient's own skin are called _____ / _____.
derm/a/tome DĔR-mă-tōm	**3–94** A derm/a/tome* is an instrument used to incise or cut. When there is a need to graft a thin slice of skin, the physician asks for an instrument called a _____ / _____ / _____.
auto/graft AW-tō-grăft	**3–95** Skin transplanted from another person does not survive very long. Thus, a graft is typically performed using tissue transplanted from the patient's own skin. This surgical procedure is called an _____ / _____.

*The use of *a* as the connecting vowel is an exception to the rule of using an *o*.

Boldface indicates a word root or combining form. Blue indicates a suffix. Pink indicates a prefix.

SECTION REVIEW 3-3

Using the following table, write the CF, suffix, or prefix that matches its definition in the space provided to the left of the definition. There may be more than one word element that matches a definition.

Combining Forms		**Suffixes**		**Prefixes**
cyan/o	melan/o	-cyte	-osis	auto-
cyt/o	necr/o	-derma	-pathy	
erythr/o	xanth/o	-emia	-penia	
leuk/o		-oma	-rrhea	

1. _____ black

2. _____ blue

3. _____ blood condition

4. _____ cell

5. _____ decrease, deficiency

6. _____ disease

7. _____ discharge, flow

8. _____ red

9. _____ self, own

10. _____ skin

11. _____ tumor

12. _____ white

13. _____ yellow

14. _____ death, necrosis

15. _____ abnormal condition; increase (used primarily with blood cells)

Competency Verification: Check your answers in Appendix B: Answer Key, page 567. If you are not satisfied with your level of comprehension, go back to Frame 3–66 and rework the frames.

Correct Answers _____ x 6.67 = _____ % Score

ABBREVIATIONS

This section introduces abbreviations related to the integumentary system and their meanings.

Abbreviation	Meaning	Abbreviation	Meaning
AIDS	acquired immune deficiency syndrome	Dx	diagnosis
BCC	basal cell carcinoma	FH	family history
Bx, bx	biopsy	I&D	incision and drainage; irrigation and débridement
Derm	dermatology	PE	physical examination; pulmonary embolism; pressure-equilizing tube

ADDITIONAL MEDICAL TERMS

The following terms are additional terms related to the integumentary system. Recognizing and learning these terms will help you understand the connection between common signs, symptoms, and diseases and their diagnoses, as well as the rationale behind methods of treatment selected for a particular disorder.

Diseases and Conditions

abrasion ă-BRĀ-zhŭn	Scraping, or rubbing away of a surface, such as skin, by friction *Abrasion may be the result of trauma, such as a skinned knee; therapy, as in dermabrasion of the skin to remove scar tissue; or normal function, such as wearing down of a tooth by mastication.*
abscess ĂB-sĕs	Localized collection of pus at the site of an infection (characteristically, a staphylococcal infection) *An abscess can occur in any body part. Treatment includes oral antibiotics and I&D to drain the purulent material. (See Fig. 3–6.)*
furuncle FŪ-rŭng-kl	Abscess that originates in a hair follicle; also called boil
carbuncle KĂR-bŭng-kl	Cluster of furuncles in the subcutaneous tissue *Large furuncles with connecting channels to the skin surface form a carbuncle.*
acne ĂK-nē	Inflammatory disease of sebaceous follicles of the skin, marked by comedos (blackheads), papules, and pustules *Acne is especially common in puberty and adolescence. It usually affects the face, chest, back, and shoulders. (See Fig. 3–7.)*

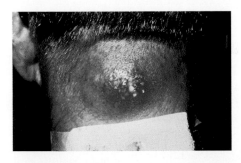

Figure 3-6 Abscess that has formed a furuncle in hair follicles of the neck. From Goldsmith, Lazarus, and Tharp: *Adult and Pediatric Dermatology: A Color Guide to Diagnosis and Treatment.* F. A. Davis, Philadelphia, 1997, p 364, with permission.

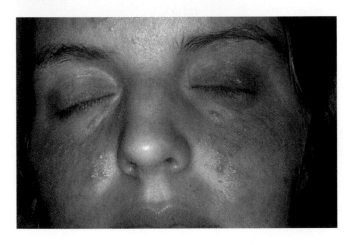

Figure 3-7 Acne. From Goldsmith, Lazarus, and Tharp: *Adult and Pediatric Dermatology: A Color Guide to Diagnosis and Treatment.* F. A. Davis, Philadelphia, 1997, p 227, with permission.

alopecia ăl-ō-PĒ-shē-ă	Absence or loss of hair, especially of the head; also known as *baldness*
comedo KŎM-ē-dō	Discolored, dried sebum plugging an excretory duct of the skin; also called *blackhead*
cyst SĬST	Closed sac or pouch in or under the skin with a definite wall that contains fluid, semifluid, or solid material *The cyst may enlarge as sebum collects and may become infected.*
sebaceous sē-BĀ-shŭs	A cyst filled with sebum (fatty material) from a sebaceous gland
eczema ĔK-zě-mă	Redness of the skin caused by swelling of the capillaries *Eczematous rash may result from various causes, including allergies, irritating chemicals, drugs, scratching or rubbing the skin, or sun exposure. It may be acute or chronic. (See Fig. 3–8.)*

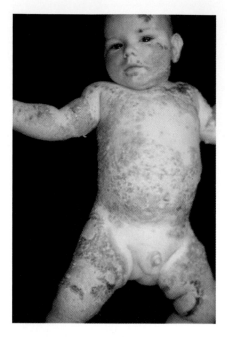

Figure 3-8 Scattered eczema of the trunk of an infant. Goldsmith, Lazarus, and Tharp: *Adult and Pediatric Dermatology: A Color Guide to Diagnosis and Treatment.* F. A. Davis, Philadelphia, 1997, p 243, with permission.

hemorrhage HĔM-ĕ-rĭj	Loss of a large amount of blood in a short period, externally or internally *Hemorrhage may be arterial, venous, or capillary.*
contusion kŏn-TOO-zhŭn	Hemorrhage of any size under the skin in which the skin is not broken; also known as a *bruise*
ecchymosis ĕk-ĭ-MŌ-sĭs	Skin discoloration consisting of a large, irregularly formed hemorrhagic area with colors changing from blue-black to greenish brown or yellow; commonly called a *bruise* (See Fig. 3–9.)
petechia pē-TĒ-kē-ă	Minute, pinpoint hemorrhagic spot on the skin *A petechia is a smaller version of an ecchymosis.*

hematoma hĕm-ă-TŌ-mă	Elevated, localized collection of blood trapped under the skin that usually results from trauma

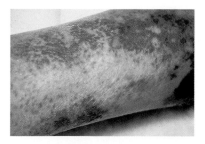

Figure 3-9 Ecchymosis. From Harmening: *Clinical Hematology and Fundamentals of Hemostasis,* 4th ed. F. A. Davis, Philadelphia, 2001, p 489, with permission.

hirsutism HŬR-sūt-ĭzm	Condition characterized by excessive growth of hair or presence of hair in unusual places, especially in women *Hirsutism may be caused by hypersecretion of testosterone, or it may be due to an adrenal neoplasm.*
impetigo ĭm-pĕ-TĪ-gō	Bacterial skin infection characterized by isolated pustules that become crusted and rupture
psoriasis sō-RĪ-ă-sĭs	Autoimmune disease characterized by itchy red patches covered with silvery scales (See Fig. 3–10.) *Psoriasis seems to be genetically determined and is typically a lifelong condition. Various treatments help control symptoms, including topical treatments (lubricants, retinoids, corticosteroids, and saltwater immersions) and systemic treatments (ultraviolet [UV] light therapy and excimer light therapy).*
scabies SKĀ-bēz	Contagious skin disease transmitted by the itch mite
skin lesion LĒ-zhŭn	Area of pathologically altered tissue caused by disease, injury, or a wound due to external factors or internal disease *Evaluation of skin lesions, injuries, or changes to tissue helps establish the diagnosis of skin disorders. Lesions are described as primary or secondary. (See Fig. 3–11.)*
primary lesion	Skin lesion caused directly by a disease process *A primary lesion is the initial reaction to pathologically altered tissue and may be flat or elevated.*
secondary lesion	Skin lesion that evolves from a primary lesion or that is caused by external forces, such as infection, scratching, trauma, or the healing process

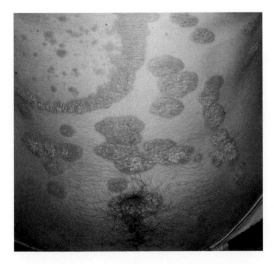

Figure 3-10 Psoriasis. From Goldsmith, Lazarus, and Tharp: *Adult and Pediatric Dermatology: A Color Guide to Diagnosis and Treatment.* F. A. Davis, Philadelphia, 1997, p 258, with permission.

PRIMARY LESIONS

FLAT LESIONS
Flat, discolored, circumscribed lesions of any size

Macule
Flat, pigmented, circumscribed area less than 1 cm in diameter.
Examples: freckle, flat mole, or rash that occurs in rubella.

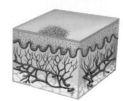

- -

ELEVATED LESIONS

Solid   *Fluid-filled*

Papule
Solid, elevated lesion less than 1 cm in diameter that may be the same color as the skin or pigmented.
Examples: nevus, wart, pimple, ringworm, psoriasis, eczema.

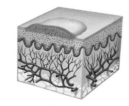

Vesicle
Elevated, circumscribed, fluid-filled lesion less than 0.5 cm in diameter.
Examples: poison ivy, shingles, chickenpox.

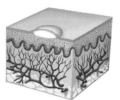

Nodule
Palpable, circumscribed lesion; larger and deeper than a papule (0.6 to 2 cm in diameter); extends into the dermal area.
Examples: intradermal nevus, benign or malignant tumor.

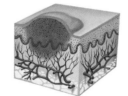

Pustule
Small, raised, circumscribed lesion that contains pus; usually less than 1 cm in diameter.
Examples: acne, furuncle, pustular psoriasis, scabies.

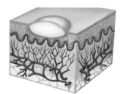

Tumor
Solid, elevated lesion larger than 2 cm in diameter that extends into the dermal and subcutaneous layers.
Examples: lipoma, steatoma, dermatofibroma, hemangioma.

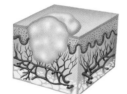

Bulla
A vesicle or blister larger than 1 cm in diameter.
Examples: second degree burns, severe poison oak, poison ivy.

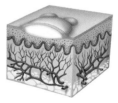

Wheal
Elevated, firm, rounded lesion with localized skin edema (swelling) that varies in size, shape, and color; paler in the center than its surrounding edges; accompanied by itching.
Examples: hives, insect bites, urticaria.

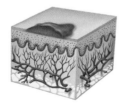

- -

SECONDARY LESIONS

DEPRESSED LESIONS
Depressed lesions caused by loss of skin surface

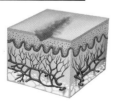

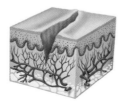

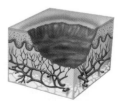

Excoriations
Linear scratch marks or traumatized abrasions of the epidermis.
Examples: scratches, abrasions, chemical or thermal burns.

Fissure
Small slit or cracklike sore that extends into the dermal layer; could be caused by continuous inflammation and drying.

Ulcer
An open sore or lesion that extends to the dermis and usually heals with scarring.
Examples: pressure sore, basal cell carcinoma.

Figure 3-11 Primary and secondary skin lesions.

tinea TĬN-ē-ă	Fungal infection whose name commonly indicates the body part affected; also called *ringworm* *Examples of tinea include tinea barbae (beard), tinea corporis (body), tinea pedis (athlete's foot), tinea versicolor (skin), and tinea cruris (jock itch).*
ulcer ŬL-sĕr	Lesion of the skin or mucous membranes marked by inflammation, necrosis, and sloughing of damaged tissues *Ulcers may be the result of trauma, caustic chemicals, intense heat or cold, arterial or venous stasis, cancers, drugs, and infectious agents.*
pressure ulcer	Skin ulceration caused by prolonged pressure, usually in a person who is bedridden; also known as *decubitus ulcer* or *bedsore* (See Fig. 3–12.) *Pressure ulcers are most commonly found in skin overlying a bony projection, such as the hip, ankle, heel, shoulder, and elbow.*
urticaria ŭr-tĭ-KĀ-rē-ă	Allergic reaction of the skin characterized by eruption of pale red elevated patches that are intensely itchy; also called *wheals* or *hives*
verruca vĕ-ROO-kă	Rounded epidermal growths caused by a virus; also called *wart* *Types of warts include plantar warts, juvenile warts, and venereal warts. Warts may be removed by cryosurgery, electrocautery, or acids; however, they may regrow if the virus remains in the skin.*
vitiligo vĭt-ĭl-Ī-gō	Localized loss of skin pigmentation characterized by milk-white patches; also called *leukoderma* (See Fig. 3–13.)

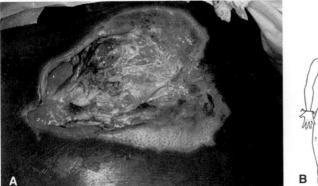 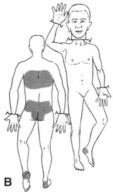

Figure 3-12 Pressure ulcer. (A) Deep pressure ulcer over a bony prominence in a bedridden patient. (B) Common sites of pressure ulcers. From Goldsmith, Lazarus, and Tharp: *Adult and Pediatric Dermatology: A Color Guide to Diagnosis and Treatment.* F. A. Davis, Philadelphia, 1997, p 445, with permission.

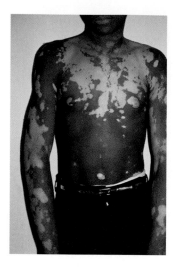

Figure 3-13 Vitiligo. From Goldsmith, Lazarus, and Tharp: *Adult and Pediatric Dermatology: A Color Guide to Diagnosis and Treatment.* F. A. Davis, Philadelphia, 1997, p 121, with permission.

Diagnostic Procedures

biopsy (Bx, bx) BĪ-ŏp-sē	Removal of a small piece of living tissue from an organ or other part of the body for microscopic examination to confirm or establish a diagnosis, estimate prognosis, or follow the course of a disease *Types of biopsy include aspiration biopsy, needle biopsy, punch biopsy, shave biopsy, and frozen section.*
skin test	Method for determining induced sensitivity (allergy) by applying or inoculating a suspected allergen or sensitizer into the skin and determining sensitivity (allergy) to the specific antigen by an inflammatory skin reaction to it *The most commonly used skin tests are the intradermal, patch, and scratch tests. (See Fig. 3–14.)*

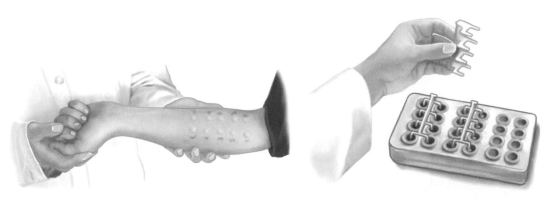

Figure 3-14 Skin tests. (**A**) Intradermal allergy test reactions. (**B**) Scratch (prick) skin test kit for allergy testing.

Medical and Surgical Procedures

cryosurgery krī-ō-SĔR-jĕr-ē	Use of subfreezing temperature, commonly with liquid nitrogen, to destroy abnormal tissue cells, such as unwanted, cancerous, or infected tissue
débridement dā-brēd-MŎN or dĭ-BRĒD-mĕnt	Treatment that involves removal of foreign material and dead or damaged tissue, especially in a wound, and is used to promote healing and prevent infection
excimer laser ĔK-sŭh-mĕr	Aims a high intensity ultraviolet B (UVB) light dose of a very specific wavelength, and a handheld wand allows the energy to be delivered precisely to the affected areas without harming healthy skin around them; also called *exciplex laser*. *Because the laser light never touches the surrounding skin, it reduces the risk of UV radiation exposure. Excimer lasers are used to treat mild-to-moderate psoriasis and require fewer and less vigorous treatments than other light therapies.*
fulguration fŭl-gū-RĀ-shŭn	Tissue destruction by means of a high-frequency electric current; also called *electrodesiccation* *This procedure is used to remove tumors and lesions within and on the body.*
incision and drainage (I&D)	Surgical procedure to release pus or pressure built up under the skin, such as in an abscess, and remove its contents
Mohs surgery MŌZ	Procedure in which layers of cancer-containing skin are progressively excised and examined until only cancer-free tissue remains
skin graft	Surgical procedure to transplant healthy tissue to an injured site *Human, animal, or artificial skin provides a temporary covering or permanent layer of skin over a wound or burn.*
allograft ĂL-ō-grăft	Transplantation of healthy tissue from one person to another person; also called *homograft* *In an allograft, the skin donor is usually a cadaver. This type of skin graft is temporary and used to protect the patient against infection and fluid loss. The allograft is frozen and stored in a skin bank until needed.*
autograft AW-tō-grăft	Transplantation of healthy tissue from one site to another site in the same individual
synthetic sĭn-THĔT-ĭk	Transplantation of artificial skin produced from collagen fibers arranged in a lattice pattern *With a synthetic skin graft, the recipient's body does not reject the synthetic skin (produced artificially), and healing skin grows into it as the graft gradually disintegrates.*
xenograft ZĔN-ō-grăft	Transplantation (dermis only) from a foreign donor (usually a pig) and transferred to a human; also called *heterograft* *A xenograft is used as a temporary graft to protect the patient against infection and fluid loss.*

skin resurfacing	Repair of damaged skin, acne scars, fine or deep wrinkles, or tattoos or improvement of skin tone irregularities using topical chemicals, abrasion, or laser
	In cosmetic surgery, skin resurfacing may involve dermabrasion, chemical peels, cutaneous lasers, and other techniques.
chemical peel	Use of chemicals to remove outer layers of skin to treat acne scarring and general keratoses, as well as cosmetic purposes to remove fine wrinkles on the face; also called *chemabrasion*
cutaneous laser kū-TĀ-nē-ŭs *cutane:* skin -*ous:* pertaining to	Any of several laser treatments employed for cosmetic and plastic surgery *Cutaneous laser includes treatment of pigmented lesions, wrinkles, vascular malformations, and other cosmetic skin surface irregularities.*
dermabrasion DĔRM-ă-brā-zhŭn	Removal of acne scars, nevi, tattoos, or fine wrinkles on the skin through the use of sandpaper, wire brushes, or other abrasive materials on the epidermal layer

PHARMACOLOGY

Drug Category	Action
antibiotics ăn-tĭ-bī-ŎT-ĭks	Kill bacteria that cause skin infections
antifungals ăn-tĭ-FŬNG-găls	Kill fungi that infect the skin
antipruritics ăn-tĭ-proo-RĬT-ĭks	Reduce severe itching
corticosteroids kor-tĭ-kō-STĔR-oyds	Anti-inflammatory agents that treat skin inflammation

Pronunciation Help	Long sound	ā in rāte	ē in rēbirth	ī in īsle	ō in ōver	ū in ūnite
	Short sound	ă in ălone	ĕ in ĕver	ĭ in ĭt	ŏ in nŏt	ŭ in cŭt

ADDITIONAL MEDICAL TERMS REVIEW

Match the medical term(s) below with the definitions in the numbered list.

alopecia	dermabrasion	scabies
biopsy	eczema	tinea
comedo	fulguration	urticaria
cryosurgery	furuncle	verruca
débridement	petechia	vitiligo

1. _____ is a rounded epidermal growth caused by a virus.

2. _____ is localized loss of skin pigmentation characterized by the appearance of milk-white patches.

3. _____ is a fungal skin disease, commonly called *ringworm,* whose name indicates the body part affected.

4. _____ is an abscess that originates in a hair follicle and is also called a *boil.*

5. _____ is a general term for an itchy red rash that may become crusted, thickened, or scaly.

6. _____ is an allergic reaction of the skin characterized by eruption of pale red elevated patches that are intensely itchy and is also called *hives.*

7. _____ refers to excision of a small piece of living tissue from an organ or other part of the body for microscopic examination.

8. _____ refers to use of revolving wire brushes or sandpaper to remove superficial scars on the skin.

9. _____ refers to the procedure in which diseased tissue is destroyed by a high-frequency electric current.

10. _____ refers to the use of liquid nitrogen to destroy or eliminate abnormal tissue cells.

11. _____ refers to removal of foreign material and dead or damaged tissue, especially in a wound.

12. _____ is a contagious skin disease transmitted by the itch mite.

13. _____ is the absence or loss of hair, especially of the head, and is also called *baldness.*

14. _____ is a blackhead.

15. _____ is a minute, hemorrhagic spot on the skin that is a smaller version of ecchymosis.

Competency Verification: Check your answers in Appendix B: Answer Key, page 567. If you are not satisfied with your level of comprehension, review the additional medical terms section and retake the review.

Correct Answers _____ x 6.67 = _____ % Score

PRIMARY AND SECONDARY LESIONS REVIEW

Identify and label the following skin lesions using the terms listed below.

bulla	macule	pustule	vesicle
excoriations	nodule	tumor	wheal
fissure	papule	ulcer	

PRIMARY LESIONS

FLAT LESIONS
Flat, discolored, circumscribed lesions of any size

Flat, pigmented, circumscribed area less than 1 cm in diameter.
Examples: freckle, flat mole, or rash that occurs in rubella.

ELEVATED LESIONS

Solid — *Fluid-filled*

Solid, elevated lesion less than 1 cm in diameter that may be the same color as the skin or pigmented.
Examples: nevus, wart, pimple, ringworm, psoriasis, eczema.

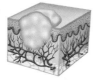

Elevated, circumscribed, fluid-filled lesion less than 0.5 cm in diameter.
Examples: poison ivy, shingles, chickenpox.

Palpable, circumscribed lesion; larger and deeper than a papule (0.6 to 2 cm in diameter); extends into the dermal area.
Examples: intradermal nevus, benign or malignant tumor.

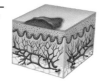

Small, raised, circumscribed lesion that contains pus; usually less than 1 cm in diameter.
Examples: acne, furuncle, pustular psoriasis, scabies.

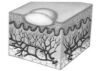

Solid, elevated lesion larger than 2 cm in diameter that extends into the dermal and subcutaneous layers.
Examples: lipoma, steatoma, dermatofibroma, hemangioma.

A vesicle or blister larger than 1 cm in diameter.
Examples: second degree burns, severe poison oak, poison ivy.

Elevated, firm, rounded lesion with localized skin edema (swelling) that varies in size, shape, and color; paler in the center than its surrounding edges; accompanied by itching.
Examples: hives, insect bites, urticaria.

SECONDARY LESIONS

DEPRESSED LESIONS
Depressed lesions caused by loss of skin surface

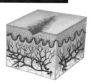

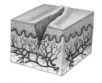

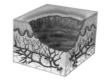

Linear scratch marks or traumatized abrasions of the epidermis.
Examples: scratches, abrasions, chemical or thermal burns.

Small slit or cracklike sore that extends into the dermal layer; could be caused by continuous inflammation and drying.

An open sore or lesion that extends to the dermis and usually heals with scarring.
Examples: pressure sore, basal cell carcinoma.

Competency Verification: Check your answers by referring to Figure 3–11, page 88. Review material that you did not answer correctly.

MEDICAL RECORD ACTIVITIES

Medical reports included in the following activities reflect common real-life clinical scenarios using medical terminology to document patient care.

MEDICAL RECORD ACTIVITY 3-1

COMPOUND NEVUS

Terminology

Terms listed in the table below come from the medical report Compound Nevus that follows. Use a medical dictionary such as Taber's Cyclopedic Medical Dictionary, *the appendices of this book, or other resources to define each term. Then practice the pronunciations aloud for each term.*

Term	Definition
circumscribed SĔR-kŭm-skrībd	
crusting KRŬST-ĭng	
lesion LĒ-zhŭn	
melanoma mĕl-ă-NŌ-mă	
nevus NĒ-vŭs	
trauma TRAW-mă	
vermilion border vĕr-MĬL-yŏn	

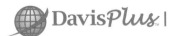 **DavisPlus** | Visit the *Medical Terminology Simplified* online resource center at Davis*Plus* to hear pronunciation and meanings of selected terms from the medical reports sections.

Reading

Practice pronunciation of medical terms by reading the following medical report aloud.

Compound Nevus

A 29-year-old, married white woman was referred for surgical treatment of a nevus of the right lower lip. The patient has had a small nevus located at the vermilion border of her lower lip all of her life, but recently it has enlarged and has become irritated with crusting and bleeding due to local trauma.

The lesion was evaluated initially about 1 month ago during a period of trauma, but it could not be removed at that time because the patient had a prominent upper respiratory infection. Subsequently, there has been healing of the local inflammatory component, and the nevus is clear at this time.

Examination reveals a brownish lesion with a flat, irregular border that is fairly circumscribed, measuring 0.5 cm in the greatest diameter, and located just at the edge of the vermilion border on the right side of the lower lip.

IMPRESSION: Compound nevus, lower lip, rule out melanoma.

Evaluation

Review the medical report above to answer the following questions. Use a medical dictionary such as *Taber's Cyclopedic Medical Dictionary* and other resources if needed.

1. What is a nevus?

   _____

   _____

2. Locate the vermilion border on your lip. Where is it located?

   _____

   _____

3. Was the lesion limited to a certain area?

   _____

   _____

4. In the impression, the pathologist has ruled out melanoma. What does this mean?

   _____

   _____

5. Is melanoma a dangerous condition? If so, explain why.

   _____

   _____

MEDICAL RECORD ACTIVITY 3 - 2

PSORIASIS

Terminology

Terms listed in the table below come from the medical report Psoriasis that follows. Use a medical dictionary such as Taber's Cyclopedic Medical Dictionary, *the appendices of this book, or other resources to define each term. Then practice the pronunciations aloud for each term.*

Term	Definition
Bartholin gland BĂR-tō-lĭn	
diabetes mellitus dī-ă-BĒ-tēz MĔ-lĭ-tŭs	
diaphoresis dī-ă-fō-RĒ-sĭs	
Dx	
enteritis ĕn-tĕr-Ī-tĭs	
erythematous ĕr-ĭ-THĔM-ă-tŭs	
FH	
histiocytoma hĭs-tē-ō-sī-TŌ-mă	
macules MĂK-ūlz	
papules PĂP-ūlz	
PE	
pruritus proo-RĪ-tŭs	

Term	Definition
psoriasis sō-RĪ-ă-sĭs (See Fig. 3–10.)	
sclerosed sklĕ-RŌST	
sinusitis sī-nŭs-Ī-tĭs	
syncope SĬN-kō-pē	
vulgaris vŭl-GĀ-rĭs	

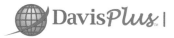 DavisPlus | Visit the *Medical Terminology Simplified* online resource center at Davis*Plus* to hear pronunciation and meanings of terms in this medical report.

Reading

Practice pronunciation of medical terms by reading the following medical report aloud.

Psoriasis

Patient is a 24-year-old white woman who has experienced intermittent psoriasis in various stages of severity since her early teens. Since May, her condition has become more troublesome because of an increase of symptoms after being exposed to the sun. Her past history indicates she had chronic sinusitis of 3 years' duration. Her Bartholin gland was excised in 20XX. She has had pruritus of the scalp and abdominal regions. There is no FH of psoriasis. An uncle has had diabetes mellitus since age 43. Patient has occasional abdominal pains accompanied by diaphoresis and/or syncope. PE showed the patient to have psoriatic involvement of the scalp, external ears, trunk and, to a lesser degree, legs. There are many scattered erythematous (light ruby), thickened plaques covered by thick, yellowish white scales. A few areas on the legs and arms show multiple, sclerosed, brown macules and papules.

DIAGNOSES: 1. Psoriasis vulgaris
2. Multiple histiocytomas
3. Abdominal pain, by history
4. Rule out colitis, regional enteritis

Evaluation

Review the medical report above to answer the following questions. Use a medical dictionary such as Taber's Cyclopedic Medical Dictionary *and other resources if needed.*

1. What causes psoriasis?

   _____

   _____

2. On what parts of the body does psoriasis typically occur?

   _____

   _____

3. How is psoriasis treated?

   _____

   _____

4. What is a histiocytoma?

   _____

   _____

INTEGUMENTARY SYSTEM CHAPTER REVIEW

WORD ELEMENTS SUMMARY

The following table summarizes CFs, suffixes, and prefixes related to the integumentary system.

Word Element	Meaning	Word Element	Meaning
Combining Forms			
adip/o, lip/o, steat/o	fat	**melan/o**	black
cutane/o, derm/o, dermat/o	skin	**myc/o**	fungus
cyt/o	cell	**necr/o**	death, necrosis
cyan/o	blue	**onych/o**	nail
erythr/o, erythemat/o	red	**pil/o, trich/o**	hair
hidr/o, sudor/o	sweat	**scler/o**	hardening; sclera (white of the eye)
hydr/o	water	**squam/o**	scale
ichthy/o	dry, scaly	**xanth/o**	yellow
kerat/o	horny tissue; hard; cornea	**xer/o**	dry
leuk/o	white		
Suffixes			
-al, -ous	pertaining to	**-oma**	tumor
-cele	hernia, swelling	**-osis**	abnormal condition; increase (used primarily with blood cells)
-cyte	cell	**-pathy**	disease
-derma	skin	**-penia**	decrease, deficiency
-emia	blood condition	**-phagia**	swallowing, eating
-esis	condition	**-phoresis**	carrying, transmission
-itis	inflammation	**-plasty**	surgical repair
-logist	specialist in the study of	**-rrhea**	discharge, flow
-logy	study of	**-therapy**	treatment
-malacia	softening	**-tome**	instrument to cut
Prefixes			
auto-	self, own	**hypo-**	under, below; deficient
epi-	above, on	**sub-**	under, below

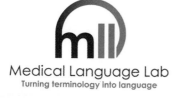

Medical Language Lab
Turning terminology into language

Visit the *Medical Language Lab* at *medicallanguagelab.com*. Use the flash-card activity to reinforce your study of word elements. We recommend you complete the flash-card activity before starting the Word Elements Chapter Review below.

WORD ELEMENTS CHAPTER REVIEW

This review provides a verification of your knowledge of the word elements covered in this chapter. Write the meaning of the word element in the space provided. To reinforce your understanding of the word parts that comprise a medical term, each word element is identified as a prefix (P), word root (WR), combining form (CF), or suffix (S). The first word is completed for you.

Medical Term	Word Elements	Meaning
1. adipocele	*adip/o (CF)*	*fat*
	-cele (S)	*hernia, swelling*
2. anhidrosis		
3. cryotherapy		
4. dermatomycosis		

Continued

Medical Term	Word Elements	Meaning
5. diaphoresis		
6. epidermis		
7. erythrocyte		
8. hidradenitis		
9. hypodermic		

Medical Term	Word Elements	Meaning
10. ichthyosis		
11. keratosis		
12. lipocele		
13. onychomalacia		
14. pyoderma		
15. scleroderma		

Continued

Medical Term	Word Elements	Meaning
16. seborrhea		
17. subcutaneous		
18. trichopathy		
19. xanthoma		
20. xeroderma		

Competency Verification: Check your answers in Appendix B: Answer Key, page 568. If you are not satisfied with your level of comprehension, review the chapter's flash-card activity at *medicallanguagelab.com* and retake the review.

Correct Answers _____ x 5 = _____ % Score

VOCABULARY REVIEW

Match the medical term(s) below with the definitions in the numbered list.

autograft	Kaposi sarcoma	onychomalacia	subcutaneous
diaphoresis	leukemia	onychomycosis	suction lipectomy
ecchymosis	lipocele	papules	trichopathy
erythrocyte	melanoma	pressure ulcer	xanthoma
hirsutism	onychoma	pustule	xeroderma

1. _____ means *beneath the skin.*

2. _____ is a condition in which a person sweats excessively and is also called sudoresis.

3. _____ refers to any disease of the hair.

4. _____ is a transplantation of healthy tissue from one site to another site in the same individual.

5. _____ is a type of malignant skin tumor associated with AIDS.

6. _____ refers to excision of subcutaneous fat tissue by use of a blunt-tipped cannula (tube) and is done for cosmetic reasons.

7. _____ is a fungal infection of the nails.

8. _____ is caused by prolonged pressure against an area of skin from a bed or chair.

9. _____ refers to excessive production of white blood cells and literally means *white blood.*

10. _____ is a black-and-blue mark on the skin, also called a bruise.

11. _____ is a benign tumor of the nail bed.

12. _____ means excessive body hair, especially in women.

13. _____ is an elevated lesion containing pus, as seen in acne, furuncles, and psoriasis.

14. _____ is a medical term for warts, moles, and pimples.

15. _____ is a red blood cell.

16. _____ means excessive dryness of the skin.

17. _____ is a black tumor.

18. _____ refers to a hernia that contains fat or fatty cells.

19. _____ refers to a tumor containing yellow material.

20. _____ is an abnormal softening of the nail or nail bed.

Competency Verification: Check your answers in Appendix B: Answer Key, page 570. If you are not satisfied with your level of comprehension, review the chapter vocabulary and retake the review.

Correct Answers: _____ x 5 = _____ % Score

Respiratory System

OBJECTIVES

Upon completion of this chapter, you will be able to:

- Describe the type of medical treatment the pulmonologist provides.
- Identify respiratory structures by labeling them on anatomical illustrations.
- Describe the primary functions of the respiratory system.
- Describe diseases, conditions, and procedures related to the respiratory system.
- Apply your word-building skills by constructing medical terms related to the respiratory system.
- Describe common abbreviations and symbols related to the respiratory system.
- Recognize, define, pronounce, and spell terms correctly.
- Demonstrate your knowledge of this chapter by successfully completing the frames, reviews, and medical report evaluations.

MEDICAL SPECIALTY

Pulmonology

The medical specialty of **pulmonology,** also called **pulmonary medicine,** is the branch of medicine concerned with the diagnosis and treatment of diseases involving the structures of the lower respiratory tract, including the lungs, their airways and blood vessels, and the chest wall (thoracic cage). Medical doctors who treat respiratory disorders are called **pulmonologists.** Respiratory disorders include but are not limited to asthma, emphysema, chronic bronchitis, lung disease, and pulmonary vascular disease. Pulmonologists also care for patients requiring specialized ventilator support and lung transplantation. In general, they are specialized to diagnose and manage pulmonary disorders and acute and chronic respiratory failure. Diagnosis and management of pulmonary disorders may include pulmonary function tests, arterial blood gas analysis, chest x-rays, and chemical or microbiological tests.

ANATOMY AND PHYSIOLOGY OVERVIEW

The respiratory system consists of the upper and lower respiratory tracts. The upper tract includes the nose, pharynx, larynx, and trachea. The lower tract includes the left and right bronchi, bronchioles, alveoli, and lungs. (See Fig. 4–1.) The main function of the respiratory system is to perform pulmonary ventilation of the body. Respiratory structures, along with the structures of the cardiovascular system, transport oxygen (O_2) and remove carbon dioxide (CO_2), a waste product, from the cells of the body. This process is accomplished by events of respiration, exchanging O_2 and CO_2 between the environmental air and the blood circulating through the lungs. Secondary functions of the respiratory system include warming air as it passes into the body and assisting in the speech function by providing air for the larynx and the vocal cords.

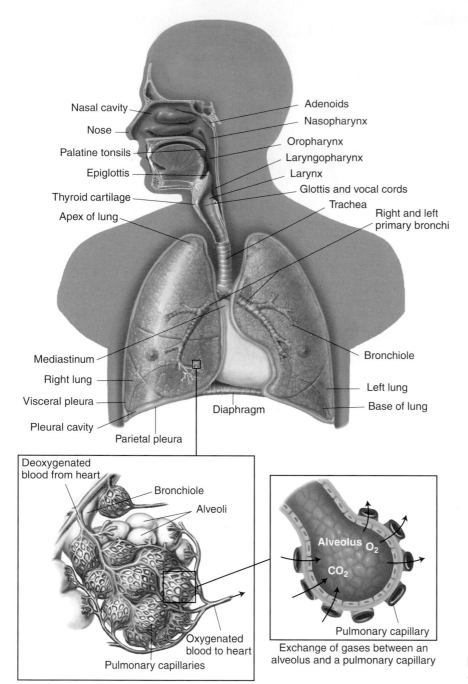

Nasal cavity

Nose

Palatine tonsils

Epiglottis

Thyroid cartilage

Apex of lung

Adenoids

Nasopharynx

Oropharynx

Laryngopharynx

Larynx

Glottis and vocal cords

Trachea

Right and left primary bronchi

Mediastinum

Right lung

Visceral pleura

Pleural cavity

Parietal pleura

Bronchiole

Left lung

Base of lung

Diaphragm

Deoxygenated blood from heart

Bronchiole

Alveoli

Oxygenated blood to heart

Pulmonary capillaries

Alveolus O_2

CO_2

Pulmonary capillary

Exchange of gases between an alveolus and a pulmonary capillary

Figure 4-1 Anterior view of the upper and lower respiratory tracts.

WORD ELEMENTS

This section introduces combining forms (CFs) related to the respiratory system. Included are key suffixes; prefixes are defined in the right-hand column as needed. Review the following table and pronounce each word in the word analysis column aloud before you begin to work the frames.

Word Element	Meaning	Word Analysis
Combining Forms		
Upper Respiratory Tract		
adenoid/o	adenoids	**adenoid**/ectomy (ăd-ĕ-noyd-ĔK-tō-mē): excision of the adenoids 　*-ectomy:* excision, removal
laryng/o	larynx (voice box)	**laryng/o**/scope (lăr-ĬN-gō-skōp): instrument for examining the larynx 　*-scope:* instrument for examining
nas/o	nose	**nas**/al (NĀ-zl): pertaining to the nose 　*-al:* pertaining to
rhin/o		**rhin/o**/rrhea (rī-nō-RĒ-ă): watery discharge from the nose 　*-rrhea:* discharge, flow *Allergies and a cold commonly cause rhinorrhea. The flow of cerebrospinal fluid from the nose after an injury to the head may also cause rhinorrea.*
pharyng/o	pharynx (throat)	**pharyng**/itis (făr-ĭn-JĪ-tĭs): inflammation of the pharynx, usually due to infection 　*-itis:* inflammation
tonsill/o	tonsils	peri/**tonsill**/ar (pĕr-ĭ-TŎN-sĭ-lăr): pertaining to the area surrounding the tonsils *peri-:* around 　*-ar:* pertaining to
trache/o	trachea (windpipe)	**trache/o**/stomy (trā-kē-ŎS-tō-mē): creation of an opening into the trachea 　*-stomy:* forming an opening (mouth) *Tracheostomy is performed to provide and secure an open airway.*
Lower Respiratory Tract		
alveol/o	alveolus (plural, alveoli)	**alveol**/ar (ăl-VĒ-ō-lăr): pertaining to alveoli 　*-ar:* pertaining to
bronchi/o	bronchus (plural, bronchi)	**bronchi**/ectasis (brŏng-kē-ĔK-tă-sĭs): dilation of a bronchus or bronchi 　*-ectasis:* dilation, expansion *Bronchiectasis can be caused by damaging effects of a long-standing infection.*
bronch/o		**bronch/o**/scope (BRŎNG-kō-skōp): curved, flexible tube with a light for visual examination of the bronchi 　*-scope:* instrument for examining *A bronchoscope is used to examine the bronchi or secure a specimen for biopsy or culture. It is also used to aspirate secretions or a foreign body from the respiratory tract.*
bronchiol/o	bronchiole	**bronchiol**/itis (brŏng-kē-ō-LĪ-tĭs): inflammation of the bronchioles 　*-itis:* inflammation
pleur/o	pleura	**pleur**/itic (ploo-RĬT-ĭk): pertaining to pleurisy 　*-itic:* pertaining to
pneum/o	air; lung	**pneum**/ectomy (nū-MĔK-tō-mē): excision of all or part of a lung 　*-ectomy:* excision, removal
pneumon/o		**pneumon**/ia (nū-MŌ-nē-ă): inflammation of one or both lungs, usually due to infection 　*-ia:* condition *Pneumonia is caused primarily by bacteria, viruses, and chemical irritants. Fluid, microorganisms, and white blood cells fill the alveoli and air passages which makes breathing difficult.*

Continued

Word Element	Meaning	Word Analysis
pulmon/o	lung	**pulmon/o/logist** (pŭl-mŏ-NŎL-ŏ-jĭst): physician who specializes in treating pathological conditions of the lungs 　*-logist:* specialist in the study of
thorac/o	chest	**thorac/o/pathy** (thō-răk-ŎP-ă-thē): disease of the thorax or the organs it contains 　*-pathy:* disease

Suffixes

Word Element	Meaning	Word Analysis
-algia	pain	pleur/**algia** (ploo-RĂL-jē-ă): pain in the pleura 　*pleur:* pleura
-dynia		thorac/o/**dynia** (thō-răk-ō-DĬN-ē-ă): pain in the chest 　*thorac/o:* chest
-ectasis	dilation, expansion	atel/**ectasis** (ăt-ĕ-LĔK-tă-sĭs): abnormal condition characterized by the collapse of alveoli 　*atel:* incomplete; imperfect *Atelectasis is characterized by the collapse of alveoli, preventing respiratory exchange of carbon dioxide and oxygen in part of the lungs.*
-osis	abnormal condition; increase (used primarily with blood cells)	*cyan/**osis** (sī-ă-NŌ-sĭs): bluish discoloration of the skin and mucous membranes* 　*cyan:* blue *Cyanosis is caused by a deficiency of oxygen in the blood.*
-osmia	smell	an/**osmia** (ăn-ŎZ-mē-ă): loss or impairment of the sense of smell, which usually occurs as a temporary condition 　*an-:* without, not
-oxia	oxygen	hyp/**oxia** (hī-PŎKS-ē-ă): abnormally low level of oxygen at the cellular level 　*hyp-:* under, below, deficient *In hypoxia, the whole body (generalized) or a portion of the body (tissue hypoxia) is deprived of adequate oxygen.*
-phagia	swallowing, eating	aer/o/**phagia** (ĕr-ō-FĂ-jē-ă): swallowing air 　*aer/o:* air
-pnea	breathing	a/**pnea** (ăp-NĒ-ă): temporary cessation of breathing 　*a-:* without, not *Apnea may be a serious symptom, especially in patients with other potentially life-threatening conditions. Some types of apnea include newborn, cardiac, and sleep.*
-spasm	involuntary contraction, twitching	pharyng/o/**spasm** (făr-ĬN-gō-spăzm): spasm of muscles in the pharynx 　*pharyng/o:* pharynx (throat)
-thorax	chest	py/o/**thorax** (pī-ō-THŌ-răks): accumulation of pus in the thorax 　*py/o:* pus

| **Pronunciation Help** | Long sound
Short sound | ā in rāte
ă in ălone | ē in rēbirth
ĕ in ĕver | ī in īsle
ĭ in ĭt | ō in ōver
ŏ in nŏt | ū in ūnite
ŭ in cŭt |

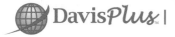 Visit the *Medical Terminology Simplified* online resource center at Davis*Plus* for an audio exercise of the terms in this table. It will help you master pronunciations and meanings of the selected medical terms.

SECTION REVIEW 4-1

For the following medical terms, first write the suffix and its meaning. Then translate the meaning of the remaining elements starting with the first part of the word. The first word is completed for you.

Term	Meaning
1. laryng/o/scope	-scope: instrument for examining; larynx (voice box)
2. py/o/thorax	
3. hyp/oxia	
4. trache/o/stomy	
5. a/pnea	
6. pulmon/o/logist	
7. pneumon/ia	
8. rhin/o/rrhea	
9. an/osmia	
10. pneum/ectomy	

Competency Verification: Check your answers in Appendix B: Answer Key, page 570. If you are not satisfied with your level of comprehension, review the vocabulary and retake the review.

Correct Answers _____ x 10 = _____% Score

RESPIRATORY SYSTEM

Upper Respiratory Tract

nose, stomach	**4–1** External openings of the nose are referred to as nostrils or nares (singular, naris). Nas/o/gastr/ic refers to the nose and stomach. This term is used to describe procedures and devices associated with the nose and the stomach, such as nas/o/gastr/ic feeding and nas/o/gastr/ic suction. When you see the term nas/o/gastr/ic tube, you will know it refers to a device inserted into the _____ and into the _____.
pharynx (throat) FĂR-ĭnks	**4–2** When the term tube is used in association with a medical procedure, it usually refers to a catheter. A catheter is a hollow, flexible tube inserted into a vessel or body cavity. Its purpose is to withdraw or instill fluids into a body cavity or vessel. A pharyng/eal suction catheter is a rigid tube used to suction the pharynx when the physician performs a visual examination or therapeutic procedure of the throat. The CF *pharyng*/o means _____ (_____).

nas/o, rhin/o	**4–3** The CFs for *nose* are _____ / _____ and _____ / _____.
para/nas/al păr-ă-NĀ-săl	**4–4** The prefix *para-* is a directional element that means *near, beside; beyond.* The para/nas/al sinuses are hollow spaces within the skull that open into the nasal cavities. They are lined with ciliated epithelium, which is continuous with the mucosa of the nasal cavities. The term in this frame that means near or beside the nose is _____ / _____ / _____.
rhin/o/plasty RĪ-nō-plăs-tē **rhin/o/tomy** rī-NŎT-ō-mē	**4–5** The CFs *rhin/o* and *nas/o* refer to the nose. As a general rule, *nas/o* is not used to build surgical terms. However, if you are in doubt about which element to use, consult a medical dictionary. Form operative terms that mean *surgical repair of the nose:* _____ / _____ / _____ *incision of the nose:* _____ / _____ / _____
rhin/o/rrhea rī-nō-RĒ-ă	**4–6** Rhin/o/rrhea is a *discharge from the nose.* Sneezing, tearing, and a runny nose are common symptoms of a cold. Build a term that means *discharge from the nose:* _____ / _____ / _____
rhin/o/rrhagia rī-nō-RĂ-jē-ă **rhin/o/rrhea** rī-nō-RĒ-ă	**4–7** Whereas rhin/o/rrhea refers to a runny nose, rhin/o/rrhagia refers to a nosebleed. Profuse bleeding from the nose is charted with the Dx _____ / _____ / _____. A runny discharge from the nose is charted with the Dx _____ / _____ / _____.

![icon] When in doubt about the meaning of a word element, refer to Appendix A: Glossary of Medical Word Elements.

air; lung	**4–8** Air enters the nose and passes through the (1) **nasal cavity,** where fine hairs catch many of the dust particles that we inhale. Label the nasal cavity in Figure 4–2. The CFs *pneum/o* and *pneumon/o* mean _____ ; _____.
aer/o/phagia ĕr-ō-FĀ-jē-ă	**4–9** Swallowing air is not unusual for infants. It can occur as they suck on a nipple to obtain milk, water, or any liquid substance. Doing so commonly causes gaseous discomfort, which is relieved when the infant is burped. Combine *aer/o +-phagia* to form a medical term that means *swallowing air:* _____ / _____ / _____
air	**4–10** The suffix *-therapy* is used in words to mean *treatment.* Aer/o/therapy is the treatment of disease using _____.

Boldface indicates a word root or combining form. Blue indicates a suffix. Pink indicates a prefix.

A

(1) _____ _____

(2) _____ (_____)

(3) _____ (_____)

(4) _____

(6) _____ and _____

_____ _____

(5) _____ (_____)

(7) _____

(8) ____ ____

(11) _____

(12) _____

B

(9) _____

(10) _____ _____

Alveolus O$_2$

CO$_2$

Figure 4-2 Identifying the upper and lower respiratory tracts.

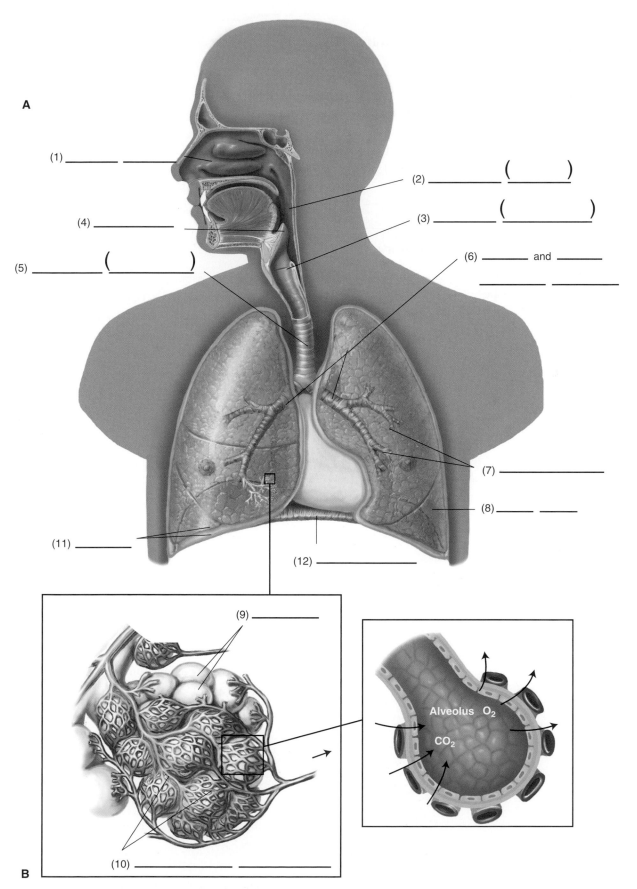

| water | **4-11**   Hydr/o/therapy is the treatment of disease using _____. |

| air, water | **4-12**   Combining air and water to treat a disease or injury is also a form of therapy. Aer/o/hydr/o/therapy is the treatment of disease by using _____ and _____. |

| aer/o/therapy
ĕr-ō-THĔR-ă-pē

hydr/o/therapy
hī-drō-THĔR-ă-pē

aer/o/hydr/o/therapy
ĕr-ō-hī-drō-THĔR-ă-pē | **4-13**   Use *-therapy* to develop words that mean *treatment with*

air: _____ / _____ / _____

water: _____ / _____ / _____

air and water:

_____ / _____ / _____ / _____ / _____ |

| | **4-14**   After passing through the nasal cavity, air reaches the (2) **pharynx (throat)**. Label the pharynx in Figure 4–2. |

| pharyng/o

myc

-osis | **4-15**   From the term pharyng/o/myc/osis, determine the elements that mean

pharynx (throat): _____ / _____

fungus: _____

abnormal condition: _____ |

| pharynx or throat
FĂR-ĭnks | **4-16**   Pharyng/o/myc/osis is a fungal disease of the _____. |

| pharynx
FĂR-ĭnks | **4-17**   The suffix *-plegia* means *paralysis.* Pharyng/o/plegia and pharyng/o/paralysis are terms used to describe muscle paralysis of the _____. |

| cancer
KĂN-sĕr | **4-18**   Smoking, drinking alcohol, and chewing tobacco can cause cancer (CA) of the pharynx. Patients with pharyng/eal CA may require some type of plastic surgery. When you see CA in a medical chart, you will know it is an abbreviation for _____. |

Boldface indicates a word root or combining form. Blue indicates a suffix. Pink indicates a prefix.

pharyng/itis făr-ĭn-JĪ-tĭs **pharyng/o/plasty** făr-ĬN-gō-plăs-tē **pharyng/o/tomy** făr-ĭn-GŎT-ō-mē **pharyng/o/tome** făr-ĬN-gō-tōm **pharyng/o/spasm** făr-ĬN-gō-spăzm	**4–19** Use *pharyng/o* to form medical words that mean *inflammation of the pharynx (throat):* _____ / _____ *surgical repair of the pharynx (throat):* _____ / ____ / _____ *incision of the pharynx (throat):* _____ / ____ / _____ *instrument to incise the pharynx (throat):* _____ / ____ / _____ *involuntary contraction or twitching of the pharynx (throat):* _____ / ____ / _____
pharyng/o/cele făr-ĬN-gō-sēl	**4–20** Use *-cele* to build a word that literally means *hernia or swelling of the pharynx:* _____ / ____ / _____
stricture, pharynx STRĬK-chūr, FĂR-ĭnks	**4–21** Pharyng/o/stenosis is a narrowing, or _____, of the_____.
	4–22 The (3) **larynx (voice box)** is responsible for sound production and makes speech possible. Label the larynx in Figure 4–2.
laryng/o/scope lăr-ĬN-gō-skōp	**4–23** Combine *laryng/o* + *-scope* to form a word that means *instrument to view the larynx:* _____ / ____ / _____
laryng/ectomy lăr-ĭn-JĔK-tō-mē	**4–24** When laryng/eal CA is detected in its early stages, a partial laryng/ectomy may be recommended. For extensive CA of the larynx, the entire larynx is removed. In either case, when excision of the larynx is performed, the surgery is called a _____ / _____.
-stenosis **laryng/o**	**4–25** Laryng/o/stenosis is a narrowing or stricture of the larynx. Determine the elements that mean *narrowing, stricture:* _____ *larynx:* _____ / ____

laryng/itis
lăr-ĭn-JĪ-tĭs

laryng/o/scope
lăr-ĬN-gō-skōp

laryng/o/scopy
lăr-ĭn-GŎS-kō-pē

laryng/o/stenosis
lăr-ĭn-gō-stĕ-NŌ-sĭs

4-26   Form medical words that mean

inflammation of the larynx: _____ / _____

instrument to view or examine the larynx:

_____ / _____ / _____

visual examination of the larynx:

_____ / _____ / _____

narrowing or stricture of the larynx:

_____ / _____ / _____

4-27   A small leaf-shaped cartilage called the (4) **epiglottis** is located in the super/ior portion of the larynx. During swallowing, it closes off the larynx so that foods and liquids are directed into the esophagus. If anything but air passes into the larynx, a cough reflex attempts to expel the material to avoid a serious blockage of breathing. Label the epiglottis in Figure 4–2.

 When defining a medical word, first define the suffix. Second, define the beginning of the word; finally, define the middle of the word. Here is an example of the term

bronch / o / pneumon / itis
(2)   (3)   (1)

SECTION REVIEW 4-2

Using the following table, write the CF, suffix, or prefix that matches its definition in the space provided to the left of the definition. There may be more than one word element that matches a definition.

Combining Forms

aer/o	pharyng/o
hydr/o	rhin/o
laryng/o	trache/o
myc/o	
nas/o	

Suffixes

-cele	-stenosis
-ectasis	-stomy
-phagia	-therapy
-plegia	-tome
-scopy	-tomy

Prefixes

a-
an-
neo-
para-

1. _____ air

2. _____ near, beside; beyond

3. _____ fungus

4. _____ dilation, expansion

5. _____ forming an opening (mouth)

6. _____ incision

7. _____ instrument to cut

8. _____ larynx (voice box)

9. _____ hernia, swelling

10. _____ new

11. _____ nose

12. _____ paralysis

13. _____ pharynx (throat)

14. _____ narrowing, stricture

15. _____ swallowing, eating

16. _____ trachea (windpipe)

17. _____ treatment

18. _____ without, not

19. _____ visual examination

20. _____ water

Competency Verification: Check your answers in Appendix B: Answer Key, page 570. If you are not satisfied with your level of comprehension, go back to Frame 4–1 and rework the frames.

Correct Answers _____ x 5 = _____% Score

Lower Respiratory Tract

bronchi/oles BRŎNG-kē-ōlz	**4–28** Continue to label structures in Figure 4–2, page 113, as you read the following material. The (5) **trachea (windpipe)** is a cylindrical tube composed of smooth muscle embedded with a series of 16 to 20 C-shaped rings of cartilage. The trachea extends downward into the thoracic cavity, where it divides to form the (6) **right and left primary bronchi (singular, bronchus).** Each bronchus enters a lung and continues to subdivide into increasingly finer, smaller branches known as (7) **bronchioles.** The diminutive suffix -ole means *small, minute.* Thus, smaller segments of the bronchus are called _____ / _____.
bronchus BRŎNG-kŭs	**4–29** The continuous branching of bronchi and bronchi/oles from the trachea throughout the lungs resembles an inverted tree. This series of respiratory tubes that branch into progressively narrower tubes as they extend into the lungs is known as the **bronchi/al tree.** Refer to Figure 4–1 to identify the structures of the bronchi/al tree. The singular form of *bronchi* is _____.
cartilage KĂR-tĭ-lĭj	**4–30** The trachea's cartilaginous rings provide necessary rigidity to keep air passage open at all times. The CF *chondr/o* refers to *cartilage.* Chondr/itis is an inflammation of _____.
chondr/o/plasty KŎN-drō-plăs-tē **chondr/o/pathy** kŏn-DRŎP-ă-thē **chondr/oma** kŏn-DRŌ-mă	**4–31** Form medical words that mean *surgical repair of cartilage:* _____ / _____ / _____ *disease of cartilage:* _____ / _____ / _____ *tumor (or tumorlike growth) of cartilage:* _____ / _____
trache/o/stomy trā-kē-ŎS-tō-mē	**4–32** On its way to the lungs, air passes from the larynx to the trachea (windpipe). In a life-threatening situation, when trache/al obstruction causes cessation of breathing, a trache/o/stomy is performed through the neck into the trachea to gain access below the blockage. (See Fig. 4–3.) When an emergency situation warrants creation of an opening (mouth) into the trachea, the procedure performed is a _____ / _____ / _____.
trache/o/malacia trā-kē-ō-mă-LĀ-shē-ă	**4–33** Softening of trache/al cartilage may be caused by pressure of the left pulmonary artery on the trachea. Use *-malacia* to form a word that literally means *softening of the trachea:* _____ / _____ / _____

Boldface indicates a word root or combining form. Blue indicates a suffix. Pink indicates a prefix.

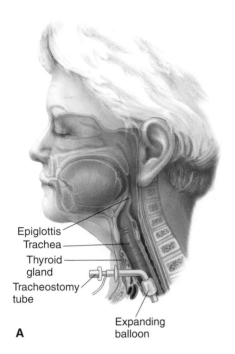

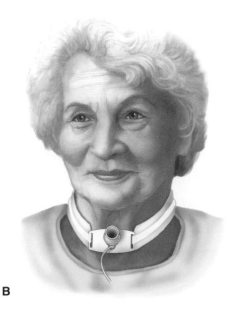

Epiglottis
Trachea
Thyroid gland
Tracheostomy tube

Expanding balloon

A

B

Figure 4-3 Tracheostomy. (**A**) Lateral view with the tracheostomy tube in place. (**B**) Frontal view.

---

trache/o/pathy trā-kē-ŎP-ă-thē	**4-34** Use *trache/o* to develop medical terms that mean *disease of the trachea:* _____ / ____ / _____
trache/o/plasty TRĀ-kē-ō-plăs-tē	*surgical repair of the trachea:* _____ / ____ / _____
trache/o/stenosis trā-kē-ō-stĕn-Ō-sĭs	*narrowing or stricture of the trachea:* _____ / ____ / _____
trache/o/tomy trā-kē-ŎT-ō-mē	*incision of the trachea:* _____ / ____ / _____

---

trachea, larynx TRĀ-kē-ă, LĂR-inks	**4-35** Trache/o/laryng/o/tomy is an incision of the _____ and _____.

4-36 Label the left lung in Figure 4–2 as you continue to read the material in this frame. Then review the position of the trachea to see how it branches into a right and left primary bronchus. Each primary bronchus (plural, bronchi) leads to a separate lung, the right and the (8) **left lung**. Structures of the bronchi and alveoli are part of the lungs, which are the organs of respiration (act of breathing).

---

bronchi BRŎNG-kē	**4-37** Change the singular form of bronchus to its plural form: _____

---

bronch/o/spasm
BRŎNG-kō-spăzm

4–38   Asthmatic patients may experience wheezing caused by bronch/ial spasms. The medical term for this condition is bronchi/o/spasm or

_____ / _____ / _____.

bronchi/ectasis
brŏng-kē-ĔK-tă-sĭs

4–39   Chronic dilation of bronchi is called bronchi/ectasis. Chronic pneumon/ia or flu may result in dilation of bronchi. The medical term for this condition is

_____ / _____.

bronch/itis
brŏng-KĪ-tĭs

bronch/o/spasm
BRŎNG-kō-spăzm

bronch/o/stenosis
brŏng-kō-stĕn-Ō-sĭs

4–40   Use _bronch/o_ to build medical words that mean

inflammation of bronchi: _____ / _____

involuntary contraction or twitching of the bronchus:

_____ / _____ / _____

narrowing or stricture of bronchi:

_____ / _____ / _____

4–41   Structurally, each primary bronchus is similar to that of the trachea, but as they subdivide into finer branches, the amount of cartilage in the walls decreases and finally disappears as it forms bronchi/oles. As cartilage diminishes, a layer of smooth muscle surrounding the tube becomes more prominent. Smooth muscles in the walls of bronchi/oles are designed to constrict or dilate the airways to maintain unobstructed air passages. Bronchi/oles eventually distribute air to the (9) **alveoli** (singular, alveolus), small clusters of grapelike air sacs of the lungs. Each alveolus is surrounded by a network of microscopic (10) **pulmonary capillaries.** Label the alveoli and pulmonary capillaries in Figure 4–2.

erythr/o/cytes
ĕ-RĬTH-rō-sītz

oxygen

carbon dioxide

4–42   The thin walls of the alveoli permit an exchange of gases between the alveolus and the surrounding capillaries. Blood flowing through the capillaries accepts oxygen (O_2) from the alveolus, while depositing carbon dioxide (CO_2) into the alveolus. Erythr/o/cytes in the blood carry O_2 to all parts of the body and CO_2 to the lungs for exhalation.

The medical term for red blood cells is

_____ / _____ / _____.

The abbreviation O_2 means _____.

The abbreviation CO_2 means _____ _____.

micro/scope
MĪ-krō-skōp

4–43   Macro/scopic structures are visible to the naked eye. Micro/scopic structures, such as the alveoli, are visible only through the use of a micro/scope.

Micro/scopic capillaries are visible to the eye through the use of a magnifying instrument called a _____ / _____.

Boldface indicates a word root or combining form. Blue indicates a suffix. Pink indicates a prefix.

alveoli ăl-VĒ-ō-lī	**4–44** If a lung disorder destroys or damages enough alveol/ar sacs, there is less surface area for gas exchange, and breathlessness results. Clusters of air sacs at the end of the bronchi/al tree are called _____ (plural).
O_2 CO_2	**4–45** The abbreviations O_2 and CO_2 are commonly seen in laboratory reports. Whenever you are in doubt about an abbreviation, refer to Appendix E for a list of common abbreviations and symbols. The abbreviation for oxygen is _____. The abbreviation for carbon dioxide is _____.
external respiration **internal respiration**	**4–46** The process of gas exchange between the atmosphere and body cells is called respiration and it occurs in two phases. **External respiration** occurs each time we inhale (breathe in) air. This process results in a gas exchange (O_2 loading and CO_2 unloading) between air-filled chambers of the lungs and the blood in the pulmonary capillaries. **Internal (cellular) respiration** is the exchange of gases (O_2 unloading and CO_2 loading) between the blood and body tissue cells. This process occurs in body tissues when O_2 (carried in blood from the lungs to nourish the body's cells) is exchanged for CO_2. The CO_2 travels in the bloodstream to the lungs and is exhaled through the mouth or nose. You may have to read this frame a few times to understand the process of respiration. Nevertheless, see if you can differentiate between the two types of respiration and identify the symbols for oxygen and carbon dioxide. Gas exchange between the body and the outside environment is called _____ _____. Gas exchange at the cellular level between the blood and body tissue cells is called _____ _____.
inflammation, lung(s) ĭn-flă-MĀ-shŭn	**4–47** The CFs *pneum/o* and *pneumon/o* mean *air; lung.* Pneumon/itis is an _____ of the _____.
air, lung **condition**	**4–48** Pneumon/ia, an acute inflammation and infection of the lungs in which alveoli fill with secretions, is a leading cause of death in the United States. Analyze pneumon/ia by defining the word elements: *pneumon/o,* which means _____ or _____ *-ia,* which means _____ (noun ending)
pneumon/ectomy nū-mōn-ĔK-tō-mē	**4–49** In patients with lung cancer, it may be necessary to remove part or all of the lung. Use *pneumon/o* to form a word that means *excision of a lung:* _____ / _____

pneumon/o/cele nū-MŌN-ō-sēl	**4–50** The suffix *-cele* means *hernia, swelling.* A hernial protrusion of lung tissue may be caused by a partial airway obstruction. Use *pneumon/o* to form a word that means *herniation of the lung:* _____ / _____ / _____
pneumon/osis nū-mōn-Ō-sĭs **pneumon/o/pathy** nū-mō-NŎP-ăth-ē **pneumon/ectomy** nū-mōn-ĔK-tō-mē	**4–51** Use *pneumon/o* to build medical words that mean *abnormal condition of the lungs:* _____ / _____ *disease of the lung:* _____ / _____ / _____ *excision of a lung:* _____ / _____
lung(s)	**4–52** The suffix *-centesis* is used in words to denote a surgical puncture. *Pneum/o/centesis* is a surgical puncture to aspirate the _____.
	4–53 If you are not sure what aspirate means in the previous frame, take a few minutes to use your medical dictionary to define the term. _____ _____
pneumon/o/centesis nū-mō-nō-sĕn-TĒ-sis	**4–54** Lung abscess, an abnormal localized collection of fluid, may be caused by pneumonia. Therapeutic treatment with pneum/o/centesis may be required. Construct another word that means *surgical puncture of a lung:* _____ / _____ / _____
lung(s), air **black** **abnormal condition**	**4–55** Pneumon/o/melan/osis is an abnormal condition of black lung caused by inhalation of black dust (a disease common among coal miners), which is also called *pneumomelanosis* or *pneumoconiosis.* Analyze pneumon/o/melan/osis by defining the word elements: *pneumon/o* means: _____ or _____ *melan/o* means: _____ *-osis* means: _____
oxygen **carbon dioxide**	**4–56** The lungs are divided into five lobes: three lobes in the right lung and two lobes in the left lung. Both lungs supply blood with O_2 inhaled from the environment and dispose of waste CO_2 in the exhaled air. O_2 refers to _____. CO_2 refers to _____ _____.

Boldface indicates a word root or combining form. Blue indicates a suffix. Pink indicates a prefix.

excision or removal ĕk-SĬ-zhŭn	**4-57** Lung CA patients may undergo a lob/ectomy, which is a(n) _____ of a lobe.
lob/o	**4-58** From lob/ar (pertaining to the lobe), construct the CF for *lobe*: _____ / _____
lob/itis lō-BĪ-tĭs **lob/o/tomy** lō-BŎT-ō-mē **lob/ectomy** lō-BĔK-tō-mē	**4-59** Develop medical words that mean *inflammation of a lobe:* _____ / _____ *incision of a lobe:* _____ / _____ / _____ *excision of a lobe:* _____ / _____
	4-60 Each lung is enclosed in a double-folded membrane called the (11) **pleura**. Label the pleura in Figure 4–2.
inflammation ĭn-flă-MĀ-shŭn	**4-61** Pleur/itis is an _____ of the pleura.
pleur/o	**4-62** From pleur/o/dynia, identify the CF for pleura: _____ / _____
pleur/o/dynia, pleur/algia ploo-rō-DĬN-ē-ă, ploo-RĂL-jē-ă	**4-63** Pain in the pleura is known as _____ / _____ / _____ or _____ / _____.
pneumon/o or pneum/o	**4-64** Pleur/o/pneumon/ia is pleurisy complicated with pneumonia. The CF for *air* or *lung* is _____ / _____.
pleur/itis ploo-RĪ-tĭs **pleur/o/cele** PLOO-rō-sēl	**4-65** Form medical words that mean *inflammation of the pleura:* _____ / _____ *hernia or swelling of the pleura:* _____ / _____ / _____
inflammation, pleura PLOO-ră	**4-66** Pleurisy is an inflammation of the pleura. Pleur/itis is also an _____ of the _____.

inflammation, pleura PLOO-ră	**4-67** Whenever you see the word pleur/isy or pleur/itis, you will know it means _____ of the _____.
pleur/o/dynia ploo-rō-DĬN-ē-ă	**4-68** The suffixes *-algia* and *-dynia* refer to *pain*. The pleura commonly becomes inflamed when a person has pneumonia. This condition may cause pleur/algia, which is also called _____ / _____ / _____.
without, not **slow** **bad; painful; difficult** **good, normal** **rapid** **breathing**	**4-69** Prefixes *a-*, *brady-*, *dys-*, *eu-*, and *tachy-* are commonly attached to *-pnea* to describe various types of breathing conditions. Write the meanings of each of the following elements. *a-:* _____, _____ *brady-:* _____ *dys-:* _____; _____; _____ *eu-:* _____, _____ *tachy-:* _____ *-pnea:* _____
a/pnea ĂP-nē-ă	**4-70** A/pnea is a temporary loss of breathing that results in brief or prolonged absence of spontaneous respiration. It is a serious symptom, especially in patients with other potentially life-threatening conditions. Causes include respiratory arrest or respiratory failure. A term that literally means *without breathing* is _____ / _____.
a/pnea ĂP-nē-ă	**4-71** When a/pnea occurs in premature infants, the immature central nervous system (CNS) fails to maintain a consistent respiratory rate. Thus, there are occasional long pauses between periods of regular breathing. An infant whose mother used cocaine during pregnancy is also likely to develop life-threatening a/pnea. When there is temporary cessation of breathing, the event is documented in the medical record as _____ / _____.
CPAP **OSA**	**4-72** Another type of a/pnea, obstructive sleep apnea (OSA), may be due to enlarged tonsils that cause an airway obstruction. Treatment includes the use of a continuous positive airway pressure (CPAP) machine. (See Fig. 4–4.) Provide the abbreviation that means *continuous positive airway pressure:* _____ *obstructive sleep apnea:* _____

Boldface indicates a word root or combining form. Blue indicates a suffix. Pink indicates a prefix.

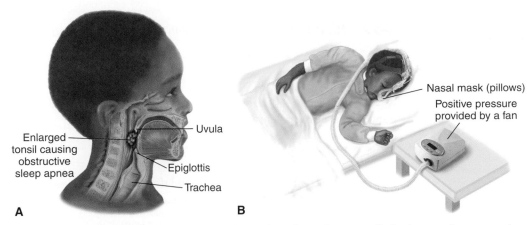

Figure 4-4 Sleep apnea. (A) Airway obstruction caused by enlarged tonsils, eventually leading to obstructive sleep apnea. (B) Continuous positive airway pressure (CPAP) machine.

a/pnea ĂP-nē-ă **dys/pnea** dĭsp-NĒ-ă	**4–73** Because of airway obstruction, OSA patients stop breathing multiple times each night. A/pnea is followed by a gasping breath that commonly awakens the patient and results in sleep deprivation, fatigue, and difficulty concentrating during the day. This condition occurs most commonly in middle-aged, obese men who snore excessively. Build a medical term that means *without or not breathing:* _____ / _____ *painful or difficult breathing:* _____ / _____
dys/pnea dĭsp-NĒ-ă	**4–74** Dys/pnea is normal when due to vigorous work or athletic activity. Dys/pnea can also occur as a result of various disorders of the respiratory system, such as pleurisy. A patient with pleurisy may experience _____ / _____.
eu- **-pnea**	**4–75** Eu/pnea is normal breathing, as distinguished from dys/pnea and a/pnea. From eu/pnea, determine word elements that mean *good, normal:* _____ *breathing:* _____
-pnea **orth/o**	**4–76** Orth/o/pnea is a condition in which there is labored breathing in any posture except in the erect sitting or standing position. Identify word elements in this frame that mean *breathing:* _____ *straight:* _____ / _____

thorac/o/tomy thō-răk-ŎT-ō-mē	**4–77** The CF *thorac/o* means chest. Form a word that means incision of the chest: _____ / _____ / _____
thorac/o/centesis thō-răk-ō-sĕn-TĒ-sĭs	**4–78** To remove fluid from the thorac/ic cavity, a surgeon performs a surgical puncture of the chest. This procedure is called thoracentesis or _____ / _____ / _____. (See Fig. 4–5.)
thoracentesis thō-ră-sĕn-TĒ-sĭs	**4–79** Fluid commonly builds up around the lung(s) in patients with CA or pneumonia. To remove fluid from the thorac/ic cavity, the physician performs the surgical procedure called thorac/o/centesis, also known as _____.
	4–80 The (12) **diaphragm** is a muscular partition that separates the lungs from the abdominal cavity and aids in the process of breathing. The CF *phren/o* refers to the diaphragm. Label the *diaphragm* in Figure 4–2.
phren/o	**4–81** The CF *phren/o* also refers to the mind. When you want to build words that refer to the diaphragm or mind, use the CF _____ / _____.
diaphragm DĪ-ă-frăm	**4–82** Whereas phren/o/logy is the study of the mind, phren/o/ptosis refers to a prolapse or downward displacement of the _____.
phren/o/spasm FRĔN-ō-spăzm	**4–83** Involuntary contraction or twitching of the diaphragm, also known as hiccups, is documented in the medical record as _____ / _____ / _____.

Competency Verification: Check your labeling of Figure 4–2 with Appendix B: Answer Key, page 570.

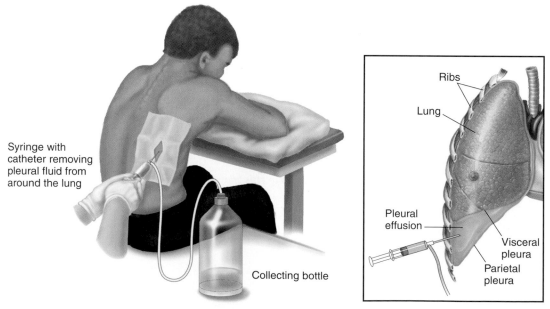

Syringe with catheter removing pleural fluid from around the lung

Collecting bottle

Ribs

Lung

Pleural effusion

Visceral pleura

Parietal pleura

Figure 4-5 Thoracentesis.

Boldface indicates a word root or combining form. Blue indicates a suffix. Pink indicates a prefix.

inspiration or inhalation ĭn-spĭ-RĀ-shŭn, ĭn-hă-LĀ-shŭn **expiration or exhalation** ĕks-pĭ-RĀ-shŭn, ĕks-hă-LĀ-shŭn	**4–84** Identify words in Figure 4–6 that mean *process of breathing air* *into the lungs:* _____ *out of the lungs:* _____
inter/cost/al ĭn-tĕr-KŎS-tăl	**4–85** During inspiration, the diaphragm and the inter/cost/al muscles contract. As their name implies, the muscles between adjacent ribs are known as the _____ / _____ / _____ muscles.
descends **ascends**	**4–86** Examine Figure 4–6A and B and use the term ascends or descends to complete this frame. During inspiration (or inhalation), the diaphragm _____. During expiration (or exhalation), the diaphragm _____.
air	**4–87** Recall that *aer/o* is the CF for _____.
aer/o/phobia ĕr-ō-FŌ-bē-ă	**4–88** Aer/o/phobia is a fear of air, drafts of air, airborne influences, or "bad air" (body odor). The medical word that means fear of air is _____ / _____ / _____.

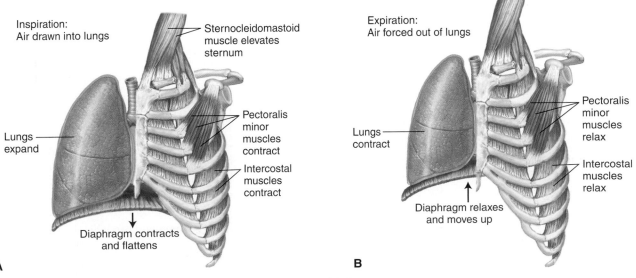

Figure 4-6 Position of the diaphragm during (**A**) inspiration and (**B**) expiration.

hem/o/phobia hē-mō-FŌ-bē-ă	**4–89** Combine **hem/o** and *-phobia* to form a word that means fear of blood: _____ / _____ / _____
muc/o **myc/o**	**4–90** Although the CFs **muc/o** and **myc/o** look similar, they have different meanings. Determine the CF that means *mucus:* _____ / _____ *fungus:* _____ / _____
air, lung **fungus** **abnormal condition**	**4–91** Analyze *pneumon/o/myc/osis* by defining the word elements. *pneumon/o:* _____ or _____ *myc:* _____ *osis:* _____ _____
chronic bronch/itis brŏng-KĪ-tĭs	**4–92** Chronic bronch/itis is an inflammation of the bronchi that persists for a long time. This pulmon/ary disease is commonly caused by cigarette smoking and is characterized by increased production of mucus and obstruction of respiratory passages. Bronch/itis may be of short duration, but when it persists for a long time, it may be a more serious pulmon/ary disease called _____ _____ / _____.
bronchi/al BRŎNG-kē-ăl **bronch/itis** brŏng-KĪ-tĭs	**4–93** Chronic bronch/itis results in expectoration of mucus, sputum, or fluids by coughing or spitting. Use **bronchi/o** to build a term that means *pertaining to the bronchi:* _____ / _____ Use **bronch/o** to build a term that means inflammation of the bronchi: _____ / _____
bronch/o **pneumon** **-ia**	**4–94** Pneumon/ia is lung inflammation caused by bacteria, a virus, or chemical irritants. Some pneumon/ias affect only one lobe of the lung (lobar pneumon/ia). Others, such as bronch/o/pneumon/ia, involve the lungs and bronchi/oles. Identify elements in bronch/o/pneumon/ia that mean *bronchus:* _____ / _____ *air; lung:* _____ *condition:* _____
bronch/o/pneumon/ia brong-kō-nū-MŌ-nē-ă	**4–95** A type of pneumon/ia that involves the lungs and bronchi/oles is called _____ / _____ / _____ / _____.

Boldface indicates a word root or combining form. Blue indicates a suffix. Pink indicates a prefix.

-oles	**4-96** In Frame 4–95, the diminutive element that means *small or minute* is _____.
compromised, immunocompromised ĭm-ū-nō-KŎM-pră-mīzd	**4-97** *Pneumocystis* pneumon/ia (PCP) is closely associated with a compromised immune system, particularly in patients with acquired immunodeficiency syndrome (AIDS). PCP is caused by a fungus that resides in or on the normal flora (potentially path/o/gen/ic organisms that reside in, but are harmless to, healthy individuals). The fungus becomes an aggressive path/o/gen in immunocompromised persons. Identify two terms in this frame that refer to an immune system incapable of resisting path/o/gen/ic organisms: _____ or _____.
PCP **AIDS**	**4-98** Identify the abbreviation for Pneumocystis *pneumon/ia:* _____ *acquired immunodeficiency syndrome:* _____
Pneumocystis pneumonia nū-mō-SĬS-tĭs nū-MŌ-nē-ă	**4-99** A type of pneumonia seen in patients with AIDS is _____ _____.
COPD **asthma, emphys/ema** ĂZ-mă, ĕm-fĭ-SĒ-mă	**4-100** Chronic obstructive pulmonary disease (COPD), a group of respiratory disorders, is characterized by chronic, partial obstruction of the bronchi and lungs. Three major disorders included in COPD are asthma, chronic bronch/itis, and emphys/ema. (See Fig. 4–7.) The abbreviation for *chronic obstructive pulmonary disease* is _____. Three major path/o/logic/al conditions associated with COPD are chronic bronch/itis, _____, and _____ / _____.
bronch/itis brong-KĪ-tĭs	**4-101** Chronic bronch/itis, an inflammation of the mucous membranes lining the bronchial airways, is characterized by increased mucus production resulting in a chronic productive cough. (See Fig. 4–7A.) Cigarette smoking, environmental irritants, allergic response, and infectious agents cause this condition. The medical term that means *inflammation of bronchi* is _____ / _____.
emphys/ema ĕm-fĭ-SĒ-mă	**4-102** The CF *emphys/o* means *to inflate.* The suffix *-ema* means *state of; condition.* Emphys/ema is a chronic disease characterized by overexpansion and destruction of alveoli, and is commonly associated with cigarette smoking. (See Fig. 4–7B.) Destruction of alveoli occurs in the respiratory disease known as _____ / _____.

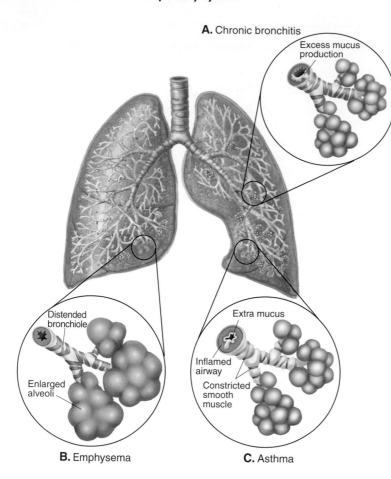

A. Chronic bronchitis

Excess mucus production

Distended bronchiole

Enlarged alveoli

B. Emphysema

Extra mucus

Inflamed airway

Constricted smooth muscle

C. Asthma

Figure 4-7 COPD. **(A)** Chronic bronchitis with inflamed airways and excessive mucus. **(B)** Emphysema with distended bronchioles and alveoli. **(C)** Asthma with narrowed bronchial tubes and swollen mucous membranes.

---

dys/pnea dĭsp-NĒ-ă	**4–103** Asthma is a respiratory condition characterized by recurrent attacks of labored or difficult breathing accompanied by wheezing. (See Fig. 4–7C.) The medical term for painful or difficult breathing is _____ / _____.
metastasize or metastasis mĕ-TĂS-tă-sīz, mĕ-TĂS-tă-sĭs	**4–104** Lung CA, associated with smoking, is the leading cause of cancer-related deaths in men and women in the United States. It usually spreads rapidly and metastasizes to other parts of the body, making it difficult to diagnose and treat in its early stages. When CA spreads to other parts of the body, the medical term used to describe that condition is _____.
tuberculosis tū-bĕr-kū-LŌ-sĭs **tubercles** TŪ-bĕr-klz	**4–105** Tuberculosis (TB), an infectious disease, produces small lesions, or tubercles, in the lungs. If left untreated, it infects the bones and organs of the entire body. An increase in TB is attributed to the increasing prevalence of AIDS. The abbreviation TB refers to _____. The name tuberculosis is derived from small lesions that appear in the lungs called _____.

SECTION REVIEW 4-3

Using the table below, write the CF, suffix, or prefix that matches its definition in the space provided to the left of the definition. There may be more than one word element that matches a definition.

Combining Forms

bronch/o	orth/o
bronchi/o	pleur/o
chondr/o	pneum/o
hem/o	pneumon/o
melan/o	thorac/o
myc/o	

Suffixes

-cele	-scope
-centesis	-spasm
-ectasis	-stenosis
-osis	
-phobia	
-pnea	

Prefixes

a-	tachy-
brady-	
dys-	
eu-	
macro-	
micro-	

1. _____ abnormal condition; increase (used primarily with blood cells)

2. _____ slow

3. _____ bad; painful; difficult

4. _____ black

5. _____ breathing

6. _____ bronchus (plural, bronchi)

7. _____ blood

8. _____ chest

9. _____ dilation, expansion

10. _____ fear

11. _____ fungus

12. _____ good, normal

13. _____ hernia, swelling

14. _____ instrument for examining

15. _____ involuntary contraction, twitching

16. _____ large

17. _____ rapid

18. _____ air; lung

19. _____ pleura

20. _____ small

21. _____ straight

22. _____ narrowing, stricture

23. _____ surgical puncture

24. _____ without, not

25. _____ cartilage

Competency Verification: Check your answers in Appendix B: Answer Key, page 570. If you are not satisfied with your level of comprehension, go back to Frame 4–28 and rework the frames.

Correct Answers _____ x 4 = _____% Score

ABBREVIATIONS

This section introduces respiratory system–related abbreviations and their meanings.

Abbreviation	Meaning	Abbreviation	Meaning
ABGs	arterial blood gases	FVC	forced vital capacity
AIDS	acquired immunodeficiency syndrome	HF	heart failure
ARDS	acute respiratory distress syndrome	MRI	magnetic resonance imaging
CA	cancer; chronological age; cardiac arrest	NMT	nebulized mist treatment
CF	cystic fibrosis	O_2	oxygen
CO_2	carbon dioxide	OSA	obstructive sleep apnea
COPD	chronic obstructive pulmonary disease	PCP	*Pneumocystis* pneumonia; primary care physician
CPAP	continuous positive airway pressure	PE	pulmonary embolism
CT	computed tomography	PFT	pulmonary function test
DPT	diphtheria, pertussis, tetanus	PSG	polysomnography
Dx	diagnosis	SIDS	sudden infant death syndrome
EEG	electroencephalography, electroencephalogram	TB	tuberculosis

ADDITIONAL MEDICAL TERMS

The following terms are additional terms related to the respiratory system. Recognizing and learning these terms will help you understand the connection between common signs, symptoms, and diseases and their diagnoses, as well as the rationale behind methods of medical and surgical treatments selected for a particular disorder.

Diseases and Conditions

acidosis ăs-i-DŌ-sĭs	Excessive acidity of blood due to an accumulation of acids or an excessive loss of bicarbonate *Respiratory acidosis is caused by abnormally high levels of carbon dioxide (CO_2) in the body.*
acute respiratory distress syndrome (ARDS) RĚS-pĭ-ră-tō-rē dĭs-TRĚS SĬN-drōm	Respiratory insufficiency marked by progressive hypoxia *ARDS is due to severe inflammatory damage that causes abnormal permeability of the alveolar-capillary membrane. As a result, the alveoli fill with fluid, which interferes with gas exchange.*
adventitious breath sounds ăd-věn-TĬSH-ŭs	Abnormal breath sounds heard during respiration (breathing in and out) with the use of a stethoscope (auscultation) *Identifying the type of adventitious breath sound is important and assists the physician in determining a diagnosis.*
pleural rub PLOO-răl	Grating sound of the pleural linings rubbing against each other that is heard on auscultation; also called friction rub *A pleural rub helps diagnose pleurisy, pneumonia, and other conditions affecting the lungs. This condition occurs where the pleural layers are inflamed and have lost their lubrication.*
rales RĀLZ	Fine, crackling or bubbling sounds, commonly heard during inspiration when there is fluid in the alveoli; also called *crackles* *Rales are commonly associated with bronchitis, pneumonia, and heart failure (HF). Rales that do not clear after a cough may indicate pulmonary edema or fluid in the alveoli due to HF or acute respiratory distress syndrome (ARDS).*
rhonchi RONG-kē	Snoring, rumbling sounds heard upon auscultation of the chest during respiration *Rhonchi indicate inflammation and congestion of the bronchi caused by inflammation, mucus, or a foreign body that partially obstructs the bronchi.*
stridor STRĪ-dor	High-pitched, musical breathing sound made on inspiration and caused by obstruction in the pharynx or larynx, commonly heard without the use of a stethoscope *Stridor is characteristic of the upper respiratory disorder called croup. It is also caused by an allergic reaction, airway injury, throat abscess, or laryngitis.*
wheezes HWĒZ-ěz	Continuous, high-pitched whistling sounds, usually heard during expiration and caused by narrowing of an airway *Wheezes occur in such conditions as asthma, croup, hay fever, and emphysema.*

anoxia
ăn-ŎK-sē-ă
 	
   an: without, not
  -oxia: oxygen
	Total absence of oxygen (O_2) in body tissues
	
	Anoxia is caused by a lack of O_2 in inhaled air or obstruction that prevents O_2 from reaching the lungs.

atelectasis
ăt-ĕ-LĔK-tă-sĭs
 	
   atel: incomplete;
         imperfect
 -ectasis: dilation,
         expansion
	Collapse of lung tissue, preventing respiratory exchange of oxygen (O_2) and carbon dioxide (CO_2)
	
	Atelectasis can be caused by obstruction of foreign bodies, excessive secretions, or pressure on the lung from a tumor. In fetal atelectasis, the lungs fail to expand normally at birth.

coryza kō-RĪ-ză	Acute inflammation of nasal passages accompanied by profuse nasal discharge; also called a *cold*
croup CROOP	Acute respiratory syndrome that occurs primarily in children and infants and is characterized by laryngeal obstruction and spasm, barking cough, and stridor

cystic fibrosis (CF)
SĬS-tĭk fī-BRŌ-sĭs
 	
   cyst: bladder
     -ic: pertaining to
  fibr: fiber, fibrous tissue
  -osis: abnormal condi-
        tion; increase
        (used primarily
        with blood cells)
	Genetic disease of exocrine glands characterized by excessive secretions of thick mucus that does not drain normally, causing obstruction of passageways (including pancreatic and bile ducts and bronchi)
	
	CF leads to chronic airway obstruction, recurrent respiratory infection, bronchiectasis, and, eventually, respiratory failure.

empyema ĕm-pī-Ē-mă	Pus in a body cavity, especially in the pleural cavity (pyothorax) *Empyema is usually the result of a primary infection in the lungs.*

epiglottitis
ĕp-ĭ-glŏt-Ī-tĭs
 	
  epiglott: epiglottis
     -itis: inflammation
	In the acute form, a severe, life-threatening infection of the epiglottis and surrounding area that occurs most commonly in children between ages 2 and 12 with a sudden onset of fever, dysphagia, inspiratory stridor, and severe respiratory distress
	
	Treatment of epiglottitis involves establishing an open airway for the person to breathe, including a breathing tube (intubation) and moistened (humidified) oxygen. Also, intravenous (IV) therapy with antibiotics will be started immediately to help treat the infection by the bacteria.

epistaxis ĕp-ĭ-STĂK-sĭs	Hemorrhage from the nose; also called *nosebleed*

hypoxemia
hī-pŏks-Ē-mē-ă
  hyp: under, below, deficient
  ox: oxygen
  -emia: blood
	Deficiency of oxygen in blood, usually a sign of respiratory impairment; also called *low blood oxygen*
	
	Blood oxygen can be measured by testing a sample of blood from an artery.

hypoxia
hī-PŎKS-ē-ă
  hyp: under, below, deficient
  ox: oxygen
  -ia: condition
	Deficiency of oxygen in body tissues, usually a sign of respiratory impairment
	
	Generalized hypoxia occurs in healthy people when they ascend to high altitude, where it causes altitude sickness that may lead to potentially fatal complications.

influenza ĭn-floo-ĔN-ză	Acute, contagious respiratory infection characterized by sudden onset of fever, chills, headache, and muscle pain
lung cancer KĂN-sĕr	Pulmonary malignancy commonly attributed to cigarette smoking *Lung cancer comprises various malignant neoplasms that may appear in the trachea, bronchi, or air sacs of the lungs. Survival rates are low in lung cancer due to rapid metastasis and late detection.*
pertussis pĕr-TŬS-ĭs	Acute infectious disease characterized by a cough with a sound like a "whoop"; also called *whooping cough* *Immunization of infants as part of the diphtheria, pertussis, tetanus (DPT) vaccine prevents the spread of pertussis.*

pleural effusion
PLOO-răl ĕ-FŪ-zhŭn
  pleur: pleura
  -al: pertaining to
	Abnormal presence of fluid in the pleural cavity
	
	The fluid may contain blood (hemothorax), serum (hydrothorax), or pus (pyothorax). Treatment includes a surgical puncture of the chest using a hollow-bore needle (thoracentesis, thoracocentesis) to remove excess fluid. (See Fig. 4–5.)

pneumothorax
nū-mō-THŌ-răks
  pneum/o: air; lung
  -thorax: chest
	Collection of air in the pleural cavity, causing the complete or partial collapse of a lung
	
	Pneumothorax can occur with pulmonary disease (emphysema, lung cancer, or tuberculosis) when pulmonary lesions rupture near the pleural surface, allowing communication between an alveolus or bronchus and the pleural cavity. It may also be the result of an open chest wound or a perforation of the chest wall that permits the entrance of air. (See Fig. 4–8.)

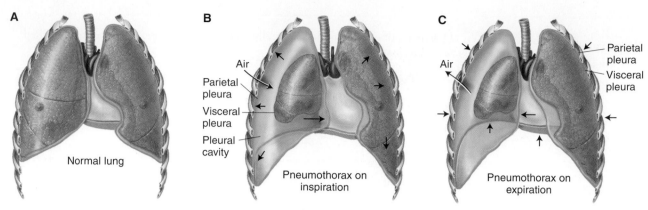

Figure 4-8 Pneumothorax. (**A**) Normal lung. (**B**) Pneumothorax on inspiration in which outside air rushes in due to disruption of chest wall and parietal pleura and the mediastinal contents shift to the side opposite the injury, compressing the uninjured lung. (**C**) Pneumothorax on expiration in which the lung air rushes out due to disruption of the visceral pleura and the mediastinal contents move toward the center.

sudden infant death syndrome (SIDS)	Completely unexpected and unexplained death of an apparently well, or virtually well, infant; also called *crib death* *SIDS is the most common cause of death between the second week and first year of life.*

Diagnostic Procedures

arterial blood gas (ABG) ăr-TĒ-rē-ăl *arteri:* artery *-al:* pertaining to	Measurement of the oxygen (O_2) and carbon dioxide (CO_2) content of arterial blood by various methods *ABG analysis is used to assess the adequacy of ventilation and oxygenation and the acid-base status of the body.*
bronchoscopy brŏng-KŎS-kō-pē *bronch/o:* bronchus (plural, *bronchi*) *-scopy:* visual examination	Visual examination of the interior bronchi using a bronchoscope, a flexible fiber-optic instrument with a light, which can be inserted through the nose or mouth (See Fig. 4–9.) *Bronchoscopy may be performed to remove obstructions, obtain a biopsy specimen, or observe directly for pathological changes.*
computed tomography (CT) cŏm-PŪ-tĕd tō-MŎG-ră-fē *tom/o:* to cut, slice *-graphy:* process of recording	Radiographic study using a narrow beam of x-rays that rotates in a full arc around the patient to acquire multiple views of the body, which a computer interprets to produce cross-sectional images of an internal organ or tissue; also called *computerized axial tomography (CAT) scanning* *In the respiratory system, CT scanning is used to detect lesions in the lungs and thorax, blood clots, and pulmonary embolism. CT scans may be performed with or without a contrast medium.*

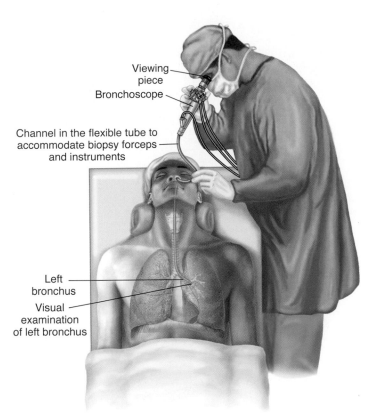

Viewing piece

Bronchoscope

Channel in the flexible tube to accommodate biopsy forceps and instruments

Left bronchus

Visual examination of left bronchus

Figure 4-9 Bronchoscopy of the left bronchus.

magnetic resonance imaging (MRI) mămg-NĚT-ĭc RĚZ-ĕn-ăns ĬM-ĭj-ĭng	Radiographic procedure that uses electromagnetic energy to produce multiplanar, cross-sectional images of the body *In the respiratory system, MRI is used to produce a scan of the chest and lungs. MRI does not require a contrast medium, but it may be used to enhance visualization of internal structures.*
polysomnography (PSG) pŏl-ē-sŏm-NŎG-ră-fē *poly-:* many, much *somn/o:* sleep *-graphy:* process of recording	Test that diagnoses sleep disorders by recording various aspects of sleep, such as eye and muscle movements, respiration, and electroencephalography (EEG) patterns (See Fig. 4–10.)
pulmonary function tests (PFTs) PŬL-mō-nĕ-rē	Group of tests that measure the capacity of the lungs and the volume of air during inhalation and exhalation *PFTs can diagnose lung diseases, measure the severity of lung impairments, and check to see how well treatment for a lung disease is working.*
spirometry spī-RŎM-ĕ-trē *spir/o:* to breathe *-metry:* act of measuring	Common lung function test that measures and records the volume and rate of inhaled and exhaled air and is used to assess pulmonary function by means of a spirometer *Spirometry is most useful when assessing for obstructive lung diseases, especially asthma and chronic pulmonary disease (COPD). (See Fig. 4–11.)*

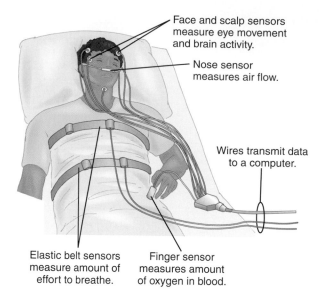

Face and scalp sensors measure eye movement and brain activity.

Nose sensor measures air flow.

Wires transmit data to a computer.

Elastic belt sensors measure amount of effort to breathe.

Finger sensor measures amount of oxygen in blood.

Figure 4-10 Polysomnography.

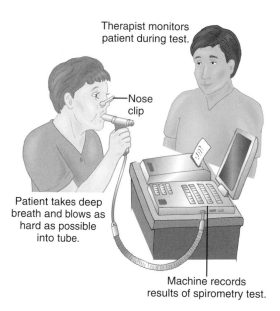

Therapist monitors patient during test.

Nose clip

Patient takes deep breath and blows as hard as possible into tube.

Machine records results of spirometry test.

Figure 4-11 Spirometry.

Medical and Surgical Procedures

endotracheal intubation
ĕn-dŏ- TRĀ-kē-ăl
ĭn-tū-BĀ-shŭn
endo-: in, within
trache-: trachea
(windpipe)
-al: pertaining to

Insertion of an endotracheal tube through the mouth or nose into the trachea (windpipe) just above the bronchi to provide air to patients who are unable to breathe on their own because of airway obstruction or respiratory failure, as well as to administer oxygen, medication, or anesthesia (See Fig. 4–12.)

A lighted laryngoscope is used to hold the airway open and helps visualize the vocal cords before insertion of the endotrachial tube.

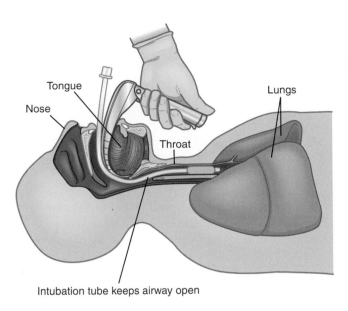

Figure 4-12 Endotracheal intubation.

postural drainage PŎS-chur-ăl	Use of body positioning to assist in removal of secretions from specific lobes of the lung, bronchi, or lung cavities

Pronunciation Help	Long sound	ā in rāte	ē in rēbirth	ī in īsle	ō in ōver	ū in ūnite
	Short sound	ă in ălone	ĕ in ĕver	ĭ in ĭt	ŏ in nŏt	ŭ in cŭt

PHARMACOLOGY

The table below lists common drug categories used to treat urinary disorders, as well as their therapeutic actions.

Drug Category	Action
bronchodilators brŏng-kō-DĪ-lă-tŏrz	Increase airflow by dilating constricted airways through relaxation of the smooth muscles that surround the bronchioles and bronchi *Bronchodilators are used to treat asthma, emphysema, chronic obstructive pulmonary disease (COPD), and exercise-induced bronchospasm. Most bronchodilators provide metered dosages of the medication and may employ a spacer as a reservoir for the medication. (See Fig. 4–13.)*
corticosteroids kor-tĭ-kō-STĔR-oyds	Decrease inflammation in the airways, reducing swelling and mucus production and making breathing easier *Corticosteroids are used to treat chronic lung conditions, such as COPD and asthma.*
nebulized mist treatments (NMTs) NĔB-ū-līzd	Produce a fine spray (nebulizer) to deliver a medication directly into the lungs (See Fig. 4–14.)

Pronunciation Help	Long sound	ā in rāte	ē in rēbirth	ī in īsle	ō in ōver	ū in ūnite
	Short sound	ă in ălone	ĕ in ĕver	ĭ in ĭt	ŏ in nŏt	ŭ in cŭt

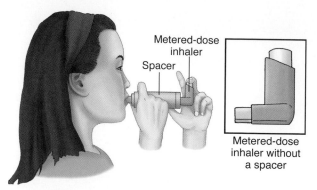

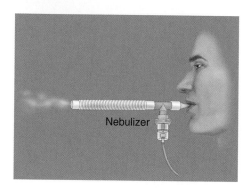

Figure 4-13 Inhaler with spacer.

Figure 4-14 Nebulizer.

ADDITIONAL MEDICAL TERMS REVIEW

Match the medical term(s) below with the definitions in the numbered list.

acidosis	cystic fibrosis	influenza	pneumothorax
ARDS	epiglottitis	lung cancer	rales
atelectasis	epistaxis	MRI	rhonchi
bronchodilators	hypoxemia	pertussis	SIDS
coryza	hypoxia	pleural effusion	stridor

1. _____ is a high-pitched musical breathing sound made on inspiration and caused by obstruction in the pharynx or larynx

2. _____ refers to *nosebleed.*

3. _____ is a contagious respiratory infection characterized by the onset of fever, chills, headache, and muscle pain.

4. _____ is excessive acidity of blood due to an accumulation of acids or excessive loss of bicarbonate.

5. _____ is acute inflammation of nasal passages accompanied by profuse nasal discharge and is also called a cold.

6. _____ is a genetic disorder of exocrine glands characterized by excessive production of mucus, causing severe congestion within the lungs and pancreas.

7. _____ refers to a pulmonary malignancy commonly attributed to cigarette smoking.

8. _____ is an abnormal presence of fluid in the pleural cavity.

9. _____ refers to an accumulation of air in the pleural cavity.

10. _____ is fine, crackling or bubbling sounds, commonly heard during inspiration when there is fluid in the alveoli.

11. _____ are used to dilate bronchial walls to increase airflow.

12. _____ is a form of restrictive lung disease that follows severe infection or trauma in young, previously healthy individuals.

13. _____ uses electromagnetic energy to produce multiplanar cross-sectional images of the body.

14. _____ refers to a collapsed lung.

15. _____ is a severe, life-threatening infection of the epiglottis that occurs most commonly in children.

16. _____ is an acute infectious disease characterized by an explosive cough that is also called whooping cough.

17. _____ is a deficiency of oxygen in the blood.

18. _____ refers to the unexpected, unexplained death of an apparently well, or virtually well, infant.

19. _____ is a deficiency of oxygen in the tissues.

20. _____ refers to abnormal chest sounds resembling snoring that is produced in obstructed airways.

Competency Verification: Check your answers in Appendix B: Answer Key, page 571. If you are not satisfied with your level of comprehension, review the pathological, diagnostic, and therapeutic terms and retake the review.

Correct Answers _____ × 5 = _____ % Score

MEDICAL RECORD ACTIVITIES

Medical reports included in the following activities reflect common real-life clinical scenarios using medical terminology to document patient care.

MEDICAL RECORD ACTIVITY 4-1

UPPER AIRWAY OBSTRUCTION

Terminology

Terms listed in the table below come from the medical report Upper Airway Obstruction that follows. Use a medical dictionary such as Taber's Cyclopedic Medical Dictionary, *the appendices of this book, or other resources to define each term. Then practice reading the pronunciations aloud for each term.*

Term	Definition
anesthesia ăn-ĕs-THĒ-zē-ă	
biopsy BĪ-ŏp-sē	
carcinoma kăr-sĭ-NŌ-mă	
expired	
fascia FĂSH-ē-ă	
hemorrhage HĔM-ĕ-rĭj	
lymph node LĬMF NŌD	
meatus mē-Ā-tŭs	
metastatic mĕt-ă-STĂT-ĭk	

Term	Definition
necropsy NĔK-rŏp-sē	
needle biopsy BĪ-ŏp-sē	
node NŌD	
papillary PĂP-ĭ-lăr-ē	
pneumonia nū-MŌ-nē-ă	
polyp PŎL-ĭp	
snare SNĀR	
submaxillary sŭb-MĂK-sĭ-lăr-ē	

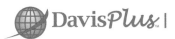 **DavisPlus** | Visit the *Medical Terminology Simplified* online resource center at Davis*Plus* to practice pronunciation and reinforce the meanings of selected terms in this medical report.

Reading

Practice pronunciation of medical terms by reading the following medical report aloud.

Upper Airway Obstruction

A 55-year-old white man was seen 2 years ago because of upper airway obstruction due to large polyps in the right nasal cavity. On examination, a large polypoid mass was observed to fill most of the right nasal cavity. The mass originated in the middle meatus. With the use of a nasal snare, polypectomy was performed to remove several sections. There was a slight hemorrhage. On the next day, a 4 × 3–cm oval soft mass was excised from beneath the left submaxillary region, with the patient under local anesthesia. The mass was just beneath the superficial fascia and appeared to be an enlarged lymph node unconnected with the nasal disease.

The pathological diagnosis of the nasal growth was low-grade papillary carcinoma. The diagnosis of the lymph node was metastatic carcinoma. A chest film was taken that indicated the presence of pulmonary densities attributed to unresolved pneumonia. Also, a needle biopsy of the enlarged liver nodes yielded no results.

After discharge from the hospital, the patient expired at home, and no necropsy was obtained.

Evaluation

Review the medical report above to answer the following questions. Use a medical dictionary such as Taber's Cyclopedic Medical Dictionary *and other resources if needed.*

1. What types of patients are at risk for nasal polyps?

_____

_____

2. When is a polypectomy indicated?

_____

_____

3. Were the patient's nasal polyps cancerous?

_____

_____

4. What contributed to the patient's death?

_____

_____

5. Why was a biopsy of the liver performed?

_____

_____

6. What does "patient expired at home" mean?

_____

_____

MEDICAL RECORD ACTIVITY 4-2

BRONCHOSCOPY

Terminology

Terms listed in the table below come from the medical report Bronchoscopy that follows. Use a medical dictionary such as Taber's Cyclopedic Medical Dictionary, *the appendices of this book, or other resources to define each term. Then practice reading the pronunciations aloud for each term.*

Term	Definition
acid-fast bacilli bă-SĬL-ī	

Term	Definition
bronchopulmonary brŏng-kō-PŬL-mō-nă-rē	
brush biopsies BĬ-ŏp-sēz	
carina kă-RĪ-nă	
culture and sensitivity	
endobronchial ĕn-dō-BRŎNG-kē-ăl	
fluoroscopic FLOR-ō-skŏp-ĭk	
friable FRĬ-ă-bl	
Legionella LĒ-jĭ-nĕl-ă	
lesion LĒ-zhŭn	
mucosal mū-KŌS-ăl	
needle aspiration ăs-pĭ-RĀ-shŭn	

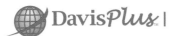 **DavisPlus** | Visit the *Medical Terminology Simplified* online resource center at Davis*Plus* to practice pronunciation and reinforce the meanings of selected terms in this medical report.

Reading

Practice pronunciation of medical terms by reading the following medical report aloud.

Bronchoscopy

The bronchoscope was passed transnasally. The vocal cords, larynx, and trachea were normal. The main carina was sharp. All bronchopulmonary segments were visualized. There was an endobronchial friable mucosal lesion seen in the left lower lobe bronchus, partially occluding the entire left lower lobe bronchus. No other endobronchial lesions or bleeding sites were noted.

Under fluoroscopic control, transbronchial biopsies of this left lower lung area were obtained, as well as transbronchial needle aspiration, bronchial brush biopsies, and bronchial brush washings for cytology evaluation. Sterile brush cultures for culture and sensitivity, acid-fast bacilli, fungus, and *Legionella* were also done.

The patient tolerated the procedure well.

Evaluation

Review the medical record to answer the following questions. Use a medical dictionary such as Taber's Cyclopedic Medical Dictionary *and other resources if needed.*

1. What does "bronchoscope was inserted transnasally" mean?

   _____

   _____

2. What was seen in the left lower bronchus?

   _____

   _____

3. What kinds of biopsies were obtained during the bronchoscopy?

   _____

   _____

4. What type of radiographic procedure was used to enhance visualization to obtain biopsies for cytology evaluation?

   _____

   _____

5. What condition results from the bacterium *Legionella*?

   _____

   _____

RESPIRATORY SYSTEM CHAPTER REVIEW

WORD ELEMENTS SUMMARY

The following table summarizes CFs, suffixes, and prefixes related to the respiratory system.

Word Element	Meaning	Word Element	Meaning
Combining Forms			
acid/o	acid	my/o	muscle
adenoid/o	adenoids	myc/o	fungus
aer/o	air	nas/o, rhin/o	nose
alveol/o	alveolus (plural, *alveoli*)	or/o	mouth
arteri/o	artery	orth/o	straight
atel/o	incomplete, imperfect	ox/o	oxygen
bronch/o, bronchi/o	bronchus (plural, *bronchi*)	pharyng/o	pharynx (throat)
carcin/o	cancer	pleur/o	pleura
chondr/o	cartilage	pneum/o, pneumon/o	air; lung
epiglott/o	epiglottis	pulmon/o	lung
fibr/o	fiber, fibrous tissue	sinus/o	sinus, cavity
hem/o	blood	spir/o	to breathe
hydr/o	water	thorac/o	chest
laryng/o	larynx (voice box)	tom/o	to cut
melan/o	black	tonsill/o	tonsils
muc/o	mucus	trache/o	trachea (windpipe)
Suffixes			
-al, -ic, -ous	pertaining to	-phagia	swallowing, eating
-algia, -dynia	pain	-phobia	fear
-cele	hernia, swelling	-plasm	formation, growth
-centesis	surgical puncture	-plasty	surgical repair
-ectasis	dilation, expansion	-plegia	paralysis
-ectomy	excision, removal	-pnea	breathing
-emia	blood condition	-rrhagia	bursting forth (of)
-graphy	process of recording	-rrhaphy	suture
-ia	condition	-scope	instrument for examining
-ist	specialist	-scopy	visual examination
-logist	specialist in the study of	-spasm	involuntary contraction, twitching
-malacia	softening	-stenosis	narrowing, stricture
-metry	act of measuring	-therapy	treatment

Continued

Word Element	Meaning	Word Element	Meaning
-oma	tumor	-thorax	chest
-osis	abnormal condition; increase (used primarily with blood cells)	-tome	instrument to cut
-pathy	disease	-tomy	incision
Prefixes			
a-, an-	without, not	hyp-, hypo-	under, below, deficient
dys-	bad; painful; difficult	macro-	large
endo-	in, within	micro-	small
epi-	above, upon	neo-	new
eu-	good, normal	peri-	around

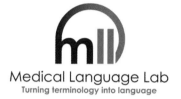

Medical Language Lab
Turning terminology into language

Visit the *Medical Language Lab* at the website *medicallanguagelab.com*. Use the flash-card exercise to reinforce your study of word elements. We recommend you complete the flash-card exercise before starting the Word Elements Chapter Review that follows.

WORD ELEMENTS CHAPTER REVIEW

This review provides a verification of your knowledge of the word elements covered in this chapter. Write the meaning of the word element in the space provided. To reinforce your understanding of the word parts that make up a medical term, identify each word element as a prefix (P), word root (WR), combining form (CF), or suffix (S). The first word is completed for you.

Medical Term	Word Elements	Meaning
1. anoxia	*an- (P)*	*without, not*
	-oxia (S)	*oxygen*
2. apnea		
3. atelectasis		
4. bronchiole		
5. bronchoscopy		

Continued

Medical Term	Word Elements	Meaning
6. cyanosis		
7. endotracheal		
8. epiglottitis		
9. hypoxemia		
10. laryngoscope		

Medical Term	Word Elements	Meaning
11. pleurodynia		
12. pneumectomy		
13. pneumothorax		
14. pulmonologist		
15. polysomnography		
16. pyothorax		

Continued

Medical Term	Word Elements	Meaning
17. rhinorrhea		
18. spirometry		
19. thoracopathy		
20. tracheostomy		

*The *i* in *bronch/i* in the term *bronchiole* is an exception to the rule of using the connecting vowel *o*.

Competency Verification: Check your answers in Appendix B: Answer Key, page 572. If you are not satisfied with your level of comprehension, review the chapter's flash-card exercise at medicallanguagelab.com and retake the review.

Correct Answers _____ x 5 = _____ % Score

VOCABULARY REVIEW

Match the medical terms with the definitions in the numbered list.

aerophagia	atelectasis	diagnosis	pyothorax
anosmia	catheter	pharyngoplegia	rhinoplasty
apnea	chondroma	pleurisy	TB
aspirate	COPD	*Pneumocystis*	thoracentesis
asthma	croup	pneumothorax	tracheostomy

1. _____ refers to presence of pus in the chest.

2. _____ is a surgical puncture of the chest to remove fluid.

3. _____ is a respiratory condition marked by recurrent attacks of difficult or labored breathing accompanied by wheezing.

4. _____ is an acute respiratory syndrome of childhood characterized by laryngeal obstruction and spasm, barking cough, and stridor.

5. _____ is a surgical procedure that creates an opening through the neck into the trachea.

6. _____ refers to the use of scientific methods and medical skill to establish the cause and nature of a person's illness.

7. _____ is a temporary cessation of breathing.

8. _____ refers to swallowing air.

9. _____ refers to using suction to remove fluids from a body cavity.

10. _____ is a cartilaginous tumor.

11. _____ is an abnormal condition characterized by collapse of alveoli.

12. _____ is the loss or impairment of the sense of smell.

13. _____ is paralysis of pharyngeal muscles.

14. _____ is inflammation of the pleura.

15. _____ is a type of pneumonia seen in patients with AIDS and in debilitated children.

16. _____ is a hollow, flexible tube that can be inserted into a vessel or cavity of the body to withdraw or instill fluids.

17. _____ refers to the surgical repair or plastic surgery of the nose.

18. _____ is an infectious disease that produces small lesions or tubercles in the lungs.

19. _____ refers to a group of respiratory disorders characterized by chronic bronchitis, asthma, and emphysema.

20. _____ is the presence of air in the pleural cavity.

Competency Verification: Check your answers in Appendix B: Answer Key, page 573. If you are not satisfied with your level of comprehension, review the chapter vocabulary and retake the review.

Correct Answers _____ x 5 = _____ % Score

Cardiovascular and Lymphatic Systems

OBJECTIVES

Upon completion of this chapter, you will be able to:

- Describe the type of medical treatment the cardiologist, vascular surgeon, and immunologist provide.
- Identify the structures of the cardiovascular and lymphatic systems by labeling them on anatomical illustrations.
- Describe the primary functions of the cardiovascular and lymphatic systems.
- Describe diseases, conditions, and procedures related to the cardiovascular and lymphatic systems.
- Apply your word-building skills by constructing various medical terms related to the cardiovascular and lymphatic systems.
- Describe common abbreviations and symbols related to the cardiovascular and lymphatic systems.
- Recognize, define, pronounce, and spell terms correctly.
- Demonstrate your knowledge of this chapter by successfully completing the frames, reviews, and medical report evaluations.

MEDICAL SPECIALTIES

Cardiology

The medical specialty of **cardiology** encompasses the treatment of heart disease. Generally, three types of cardiology specialists provide medical care: the cardiologist, the pediatric cardiologist, and the cardiothoracic surgeon. The **cardiologist** specializes in treating adults, and the **pediatric cardiologist** specializes in treating infants, children, and teenagers. The cardiologist and pediatric cardiologist provide nonsurgical treatments to detect, prevent, and treat heart and vascular diseases, whereas the **cardiothoracic surgeon** performs surgeries to treat cardiovascular disorders. Some of these critical, lifesaving surgeries include coronary artery bypass, valve replacement or repairs, heart transplants, and repairs of complex heart problems present from birth (congenital heart disease). An **interventional cardiologist** performs other invasive procedures, such as angioplasty, pacemaker insertion, and implantable cardioverter-defibrillator insertion. The physician who further specializes in surgical treatment of blood vessels and vascular disorders is a **vascular surgeon**.

Immunology

Immunology is the medical specialty encompassing the study of the immune system and its functions. The immune system is the body's defense against cancer and foreign invaders, such as bacteria and viruses. The ability to fight off disease and protect the body depends on an adequate functioning immune response. **Immunologists** are physicians who treat autoimmune and immunodeficiency diseases, cancer, or patients who are undergoing bone marrow, organ, or stem cell transplantation.

ANATOMY AND PHYSIOLOGY OVERVIEW

The cardiovascular (CV) system is composed of the heart, which is essentially a muscular pump, and an extensive network of blood vessels. The main purpose of the CV system, also called the circulatory system, is to deliver oxygen, nutrients, and other essential substances to body cells and remove waste products of cellular metabolism. This process is carried out by a complex network of blood vessels that includes arteries, capillaries, and veins—all of which are connected to the heart. A healthy CV system is vital to a person's survival. A CV system that does not provide adequate circulation deprives tissues of oxygen and nutrients and fails to remove waste, resulting in irreversible changes to cells that could be life-threatening.

The lymphatic system is closely linked to the CV system and depends on the pumping action of the heart to circulate its substances throughout the body. The lymphatic system consists of a network of vessels and nodes, and a few specialized organs, including the tonsils, thymus, and spleen. Blood flows from the heart to blood capillaries and back to the heart. Lymph capillaries collect tissue fluid, which is returned to the blood. (See Fig. 5–1.)

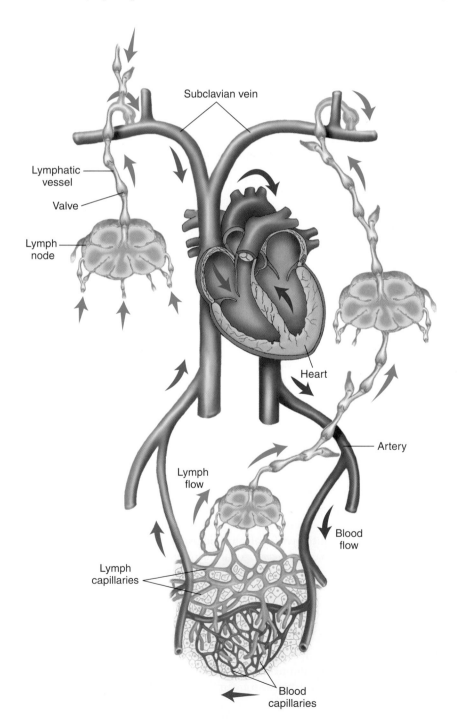

Figure 5-1 Interrelationship of the cardiovascular and lymphatic system, in which the blood flows from the heart to blood capillaries and back to the heart and lymph capillaries to collect tissue fluid, which is returned to the blood (*arrows* indicate the direction of blood and lymph flow).

WORD ELEMENTS

This section introduces combining forms (CFs), suffixes, and prefixes related to the cardiovascular system. Included are key suffixes, prefixes are defined in the right-hand column as needed. Review the following table and pronounce each word in the word analysis column aloud before you begin to work in the frames.

Word Element	Meaning	Word Analysis
Combining Forms		
angi/o	vessel (usually blood or lymph)	**angi/o**/graphy (ăn-jē-ŎG-ră-fē): process of recording blood vessels *-graphy:* process of recording *Angiography is an x-ray visualization of the internal anatomy of the heart and blood vessels after the intravascular introduction of a contrast medium. It is used as a diagnostic aid to visualize blood vessel and heart abnormalities.*
aneurysm/o	widening, widened blood vessel	**aneurysm/o**/rrhaphy (ăn-ū-rĭz-MŌR-ă-fē): suture of a blood vessel *-rrhaphy:* suture *Aneurysmorrhaphy closes the area of dilation and weakness in the wall of an artery. This condition may result from a congenital defect or a damaged vessel wall due to arteriosclerosis.*
aort/o	aorta	**aort/o**/stenosis (ā-or-tō-stĕn-Ō-sĭs): narrowing of the aorta *-stenosis:* narrowing, stricture

arteri/o	artery	**arteri/o**/scler/osis (ăr-tē-rē-ō-sklĕ-RŌ-sĭs): abnormal hardening of arterial walls
		  scler: hardening; sclera (white of eye)
		  -osis: abnormal condition; increase (used primarily with blood cells)
		Arteriosclerosis results in a decreased blood supply, especially to the cerebrum and lower extremities.

arteriol/o	arteriole	**arteriol**/itis (ăr-tēr-ē-ō-LĪ-tĭs): inflammation of an arteriole *-itis:* inflammation
ather/o	fatty plaque	**ather**/oma (ăth-ĕr-Ō-mă): fatty degeneration or thickening of the larger arterial walls, as in atherosclerosis *-oma:* tumor

atri/o	atrium	**atri/o**/ventricul/ar (ā-trē-ō-vĕn-TRĬK-ū-lăr): pertaining to the atrium and the ventricle
		  ventricul: ventricle (of heart or brain)
		  -ar: pertaining to

cardi/o	heart	**cardi/o**/megaly (kăr-dē-ō-MĔG-ă-lē): enlargement of the heart; also called *megalocardia* *-megaly:* enlargement
coron/o		**coron**/ary (KOR-ō-nă-rē): pertaining to the heart *-ary:* pertaining to
phleb/o	vein	**phleb**/itis (flĕb-Ī-tĭs): inflammation of a vein *-itis:* inflammation
ven/o		**ven**/ous (VĒ-nŭs): pertaining to the veins or blood passing through them *-ous:* pertaining to
thromb/o	blood clot	**thromb/o**/lysis (thrŏm-BŎL-ĭ-sĭs): breaking up of a thrombus *-lysis:* separation; destruction; loosening

Continued

Word Element	Meaning	Word Analysis
varic/o	dilated vein	**varic**/ose (VĂR-ĭ-kōs): pertaining to a dilated vein *-ose:* pertaining to; sugar
vas/o	vessel; vas deferens; duct	**vas**/o/spasm (VĂS-ō-spăzm): spasm of a blood vessel *-spasm:* involuntary contraction, twitching
vascul/o	vessel	**vascul**/ar (VĂS-kū-lăr): pertaining to or composed of blood vessels *-ar:* pertaining to

ventricul/o	ventricle (of heart or brain)	intra/**ventricul**/ar (ĭn-tră-věn-TRĬK-ū-lăr): within a ventricle
		   intra: in, within
		   -ar: pertaining to

Suffixes

Word Element	Meaning	Word Analysis
-cardia	heart condition	tachy/**cardia** (tăk-ē-KĂR-dē-ă): rapid heart rate *tachy-:* rapid

-gram	record, writing	electr/o/cardi/o/**gram** (ē-lěk-trō-KĂR-dē-ō-grăm): record of electrical activity of the heart
		   electr/o: electricity
		   cardi/o: heart

-graph	instrument for recording	electr/o/cardi/o/**graph** (ē-lěk-trō-KĂR-dē-ŏ-grăf): instrument for recording electrical activity of the heart
		   electr/o: electricity
		   cardi/o: heart

-graphy	process of recording	electr/o/cardi/o/**graphy** (ē-lěk-trō-kăr-dē-ŎG-ră-fē): process of recording electrical activity of the heart
		   electr/o: electricity
		   cardi/o: heart
		
		Electrocardiography is a noninvasive test that records the electrical activity of the heart during contractions and rest. It is used to diagnose abnormal cardiac rhythm and the presence of heart muscle (myocardial) damage.

-stenosis	narrowing, stricture	arteri/o/**stenosis** (ăr-tē-rē-ō-stě-NŌ-sĭs): narrowing of an artery *arteri/o:* artery *Narrowing of an artery may be caused by fatty plaque buildup, scar tissue, or a blood clot.*

-um	structure, thing	endo/cardi/**um** (ěn-dō-KĂR-dē-ŭm): structure within the heart
		   endo-: in, within
		   cardi: heart

Pronunciation Help	Long sound	ā in rāte	ē in rēbirth	ī in īsle	ō in ōver	ū in ūnite
	Short sound	ă in ălone	ě in ěver	ĭ in ĭt	ŏ in nŏt	ŭ in cŭt

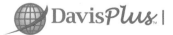

Visit the *Medical Terminology Simplified* online resource center at Davis*Plus* for an audio exercise of the terms in this table. It will help you master pronunciations and meanings of the medical terms.

SECTION REVIEW 5-1

For the following medical terms, first write the suffix and its meaning. Then translate the meaning of the remaining elements starting with the first part of the word. The first word is completed for you.

Term	Meaning
1. endo/cardi/um	-um: structure, thing; in, within; heart
2. cardi/o/megaly	
3. aort/o/stenosis	
4. tachy/cardia	
5. phleb/itis	
6. thromb/o/lysis	
7. vas/o/spasm	
8. ather/oma	
9. electr/o/cardi/o/graphy	
10. atri/o/ventricul/ar	

Competency Verification: Check your answers in Appendix B: Answer Key, page 573. If you are not satisfied with your level of comprehension, review the vocabulary and complete the review again.

Correct Answers _____ x 10 = _____ % Score

CARDIOVASCULAR SYSTEM

Layers of the Heart Wall

5-1   The heart is a four-chambered muscular organ located in the mediastin/um, the area of the chest between the lungs. Its primary purpose is to pump blood through the arteries, veins, and capillaries. The walls of the heart are composed of the (1) **endocardium**, (2) **myocardium**, and (3) **pericardium**. Review the structures of the heart and label its three layers in Figure 5–2.

my/o/cardi/um
mī-ō-KĂR-dē-ŭm

peri/cardi/um
pĕr-ĭ-KĂR-dē-ŭm

5–2   The endo/cardi/um, the inner membranous layer, lines the interior of the heart and the heart valves. The my/o/cardi/um, the middle muscular layer, is composed of a special type of muscle arranged in such a way that the contraction of muscle bundles results in squeezing or wringing of the heart chambers to eject blood from the chambers. The peri/cardi/um, a fibrous sac, surrounds and encloses the entire heart.

When we talk about the muscular layer of the heart, we are referring to the

_____ / _____ / _____ / _____.

When we talk about the fibrous sac that encloses the entire heart, we are referring to

the _____ / _____ / _____.

---

peri/card/itis
pĕr-ĭ-kăr-DĪ-tĭs

peri/cardi/o/centesis
pĕr-ĭ-kăr-dē-ō-sĕn-TĒ-sĭs

5–3   The prefix *peri-* means *around*. Peri/card/itis is an inflammation or infection of the pericardial sac with an accumulation of pericardial fluid. When the fluid presses on the heart and prevents it from beating, the condition is known as cardi/ac tamponade. If necessary, peri/cardi/o/centesis may be performed.

Build medical terms that mean

inflammation around the heart: _____ / _____ / _____

surgical puncture around the heart:

_____ / _____ / _____ / _____

---

peri/cardi/ectomy
pĕr-ĭ-kăr-dē-ĔK-tō-mē

5–4   The surgical procedure that means *excision of all or part of the peri/cardi/um* is

_____ / _____ / _____.

---

peri/cardi/o/rrhaphy
pĕr-ĭ-kăr-dē-OR-ă-fē

5–5   Suturing a wound in the peri/cardi/um is called

_____ / _____ / _____ / _____

---

my/o/cardi/um
mī-ō-KĂR-dē-ŭm

5–6   Cross-striations of cardi/ac muscle provide the mechanics of squeezing blood out of the heart chambers to maintain the flow of blood in one direction. Identify the muscul/ar layer of the heart responsible for this function.

_____ / _____ / _____ / _____

---

endo/cardi/um
ĕn-dō-KĂR-dē-ŭm

peri/cardi/um
pĕr-ĭ-KĂR-dē-ŭm

my/o/cardi/um
mī-ō-KĂR-dē-ŭm

5–7   Review the three layers of the heart by completing the following statements:

The layer that lines the heart and the heart valves is known as the

_____ / _____ / _____.

The fibrous sac surrounding the entire heart and composed of two membranes separated

by fluid is called the _____ / _____ / _____.

The middle specialized muscular layer is called the

_____ / _____ / _____ / _____.

Boldface indicates a word root or combining form. Blue indicates a suffix. Pink indicates a prefix.

(4) _____

(6) _____ _____ _____

(8) _____ _____

(13) _____ _____ _____

(12) _____ _____ _____

(10) _____ _____

(9) _____ _____

(11) _____ _____

(5) _____ _____

Chordae tendineae

(3) _____

(7) _____ _____ _____

(2) _____

(1) _____

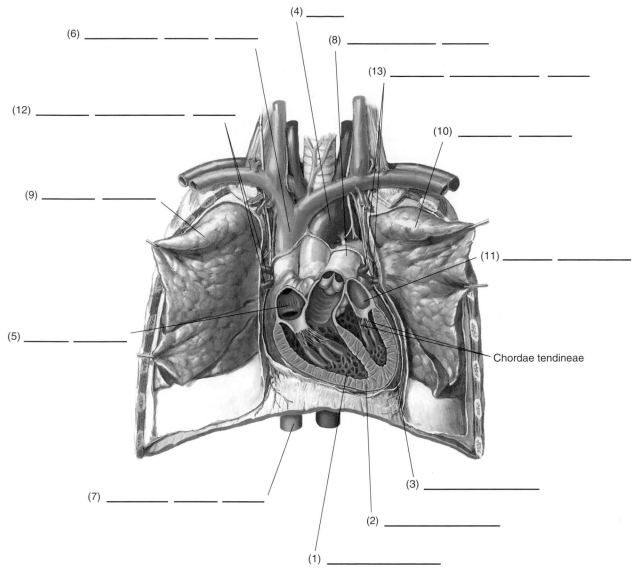

Figure 5-2 Heart structures.

Circulation and Heart Structures

5–8   The circulatory system is commonly divided into the cardiovascular system, which consists of the heart and blood vessels, and the lymphatic system, which consists of lymph vessels, lymph nodes, and lymphoid organs (spleen, thymus, and tonsils). Review Figure 5–1 to see the interrelationship of the cardiovascular system with the lymphatic system.

5–9   Some of the main vessels associated with circulation are illustrated in Figure 5–2. Observe the locations and label the structures as you read the following material. The (4) **aorta,** the largest blood vessel in the body, is the main trunk of systemic circulation. It starts and arches out at the left ventricle. Deoxygenated blood enters the (5) **right atrium** via two large veins, the vena cavae (singular, vena cava). The (6) **superior vena cava** conveys blood from the upper portion of the body (head, arms, and chest); the (7) **inferior vena cava** conveys blood from the lower portion of the body (abdomen, pelvis, and legs).

deoxygenated
dē-ŎK-sĭ-jĕn-ā-tĕd

5–10   Blood in the veins, except for pulmonary veins, has a low oxygen content (deoxygenated) and a relatively high concentration of carbon dioxide. In contrast to the bright red color of the oxygenated blood in the arteries, deoxygenated blood has a dark blue to purplish color.

The term in this frame that means low oxygen content is _____.

5–11   Label Figure 5–2 as you continue to identify and learn about the structures and functions of the circulatory system. The (8) **pulmonary trunk** is the only artery that carries deoxygenated blood. As deoxygenated blood is pumped from the right ventricle, it enters the pulmonary trunk. The pulmonary trunk runs diagonally upward, then divides abruptly to form the branches of the right and left pulmonary arteries. Each branch conveys deoxygenated blood to the lungs. The (9) **right lung** has three lobes; the (10) **left lung** has two lobes. Oxygen-rich blood returns to the heart via four pulmonary veins, which deposit the blood into the (11) **left atrium.** There are two (12) **right pulmonary veins** and two (13) **left pulmonary veins.**

Competency Verification: Check your labeling of Figure 5–2 in Appendix B: Answer Key, page 574.

5–12   Internally, the heart is composed of four chambers. The upper chambers are the (1) **right atrium (RA)** and (2) **left atrium (LA).** The lower chambers are the (3) **right ventricle (RV)** and (4) **left ventricle (LV).** Locate and label the chambers of the heart in Figure 5–3.

atri/al
Ā-trē-ăl

5–13   The CF *atri/o* refers to the atrium. A term that means pertaining to the atrium is _____ / _____.

atrium, left
Ā-trē-ŭm

5–14   The heart consists of two upper chambers, the right _____ and the _____ atrium.

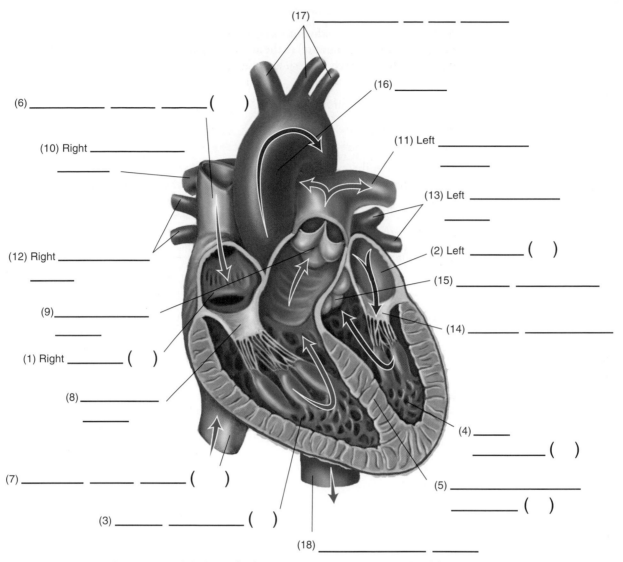

(17) _____ __ ___ _____

(16) _____

(6) _____ _____ _____ ( )

(10) Right _____

_____

(11) Left _____

_____

(12) Right _____

_____

(13) Left _____

_____

(9) _____

_____

(2) Left _____ ( )

(15) _____ _____

(1) Right _____ ( )

(14) _____ _____

(8) _____

_____

(4) _____

_____ ( )

(7) _____ _____ ____ ( )

(5) _____

_____ ( )

(3) _____ _____ ( )

(18) _____ _____

Figure 5-3 Internal structures of the heart (*red arrows* designate oxygen-rich blood flow and *blue arrows* designate oxygen-poor blood flow).

ventricul/o/tomy vĕn-trĭk-ū-LŎT-ō-mē	**5–15** The CF **ventricul**/*o* means *ventricle (of the heart or brain)*. A ventricle is a small cavity, such as the right and left ventricles of the heart or one of the cavities filled with cerebrospinal fluid in the brain. Incisions are sometimes performed into these cavities. An incision of a ventricle is known as a _____ / _____ / _____.
atrium, ventricle Ă-trē-ŭm, VĔN-trĭk-l	**5–16** The term atri/o/ventricul/ar (AV) refers to the atrium and the ventricle. It also pertains to a connecting conduction event between the atria and ventricles. The singular form of atria is _____; the singular form of ventricles is _____.

ventricul/ar
věn-TRĬK-ū-lăr

5-17   Flutter is an a/rrhythm/ia in which there is very rapid but regular rhythm (250 to 300 beats per minute) of the atria or ventricles. The heart chambers do not have time to completely fill with blood before the next contraction. Flutter can progress to fibrillation.

When the flutter occurs in the atrium, it is called an *atri/al flutter*. When the flutter occurs in the ventricle, it is called a _____ / _____ flutter.

---

a/rrhythm/ia
ă-RĬTH-mē-ă

my/o/cardi/um
mī-ō-KĂR-dē-ŭm

5-18   Flutter that progresses to fibrillation (a/rrhythm/ia in which there is a rapid, uncoordinated quivering of the my/o/cardi/um) can affect the atria or the ventricles.

Write the term that means

without rhythm: _____ / _____ / _____

muscular layer of the heart:

_____ / _____ / _____ / _____

RV

LV

5-19   Write the abbreviations for the two lower chambers of the heart:

right ventricle: _____

left ventricle: _____

---

atria
Ā-trē-ă

cardia
KĂR-dē-ă

septa
SĔP-tă

bacteria
băk-Tē-rē-ă

5-20   The rule for forming plural words from singular words that end in *-um* is to drop *-um* and add *-a*. Practice modifying the singular terms below to their plural forms.

Singular	Plural
atrium	_____
cardium	_____
septum	_____
bacterium	_____

5-21   A wall or partition dividing a body space or cavity is known as a septum (plural, septa). Some septa are membranous; others are composed of bone or cartilage. Each is named according to its location in the body. In the heart, there are several septa, one of which is the interventricular septum (IVS), the partition that divides the LV from the RV. Label the (5) **interventricular septum (IVS)** in Figure 5–3.

IVS

IAS

5-22   The ventricles are separated by a thick muscular IVS, whereas the atria are separated by a thinner muscular interatrial septum (IAS).

The abbreviation of the septum situated between the

ventricles is: _____

atria is: _____

Boldface indicates a word root or combining form. Blue indicates a suffix. Pink indicates a prefix.

bacterium băk-TĒ-rē-ŭm **septum** SĔP-tŭm **atrium** Ā-trē-ŭm **cardium** KĂR-dē-ŭm	**5-23** Form singular words from the following plural words. Apply the rule that was covered in Frame 5–20. **Plural** **Singular** bacteria _____ septa _____ atria _____ cardia _____
rapid	**5-24** The prefix *tachy-* is used in words to mean *rapid*. Tachy/cardia is a heart rate that is _____.
rapid eating	**5-25** Tachy/pnea refers to rapid breathing; tachy/phagia refers to rapid swallowing, or _____ _____.
brady/cardia brād-ē-KĂR-dē-ă	**5-26** The prefix *brady-* is used in words to mean *slow*. People with symptoms of brady/cardia commonly have difficulty pumping an adequate supply of blood to the tissues of the body. The medical term that literally means *slow heart* is _____ / _____.
brady/pnea brād-ĭp-NĒ-ă **brady/phagia** brād-ē-FĂ-jē-ă	**5-27** Form medical words that literally mean *slow breathing:* _____ / _____ *slow eating:* _____ / _____
tachy/pnea tăk-ĭp-NĒ-ă **tachy/phagia** tăk-ē-FĂ-jē-ă	**5-28** Construct medical words that mean *rapid breathing:* _____ / _____ *rapid eating:* _____ / _____
RA **LA** **RV** **LV** **IVS**	**5-29** Review the chambers and structures of the heart (see Fig. 5–3) by writing the abbreviation for the *right atrium:* _____ *left atrium:* _____ *right ventricle:* _____ *left ventricle:* _____ *interventricular septum:* _____

Blood Flow Through the Heart

5–30 Although general circulatory information was discussed previously, this section covers in greater detail the specific structures involved in the flow of blood through the heart. The heart's double pump serves two distinct circulations: pulmonary circulation, which is the short loop of blood vessels that runs from the heart to the lungs and back to the heart, and systemic circulation, which routes blood through a long loop to all parts of the body before returning it to the heart.

Continue to label Figure 5–3 as you read the following information. The right atrium receives oxygen-poor blood from all tissues except those of the lungs. The blood from the head and arms is delivered to the RA through the (6) **superior vena cava (SVC)**. The blood from the legs and torso is delivered to the RA through the (7) **inferior vena cava (IVC)**.

---

inferior

superior

5–31 Determine the directional words in Frame 5–30 that mean

below (another structure): _____

above (another structure): _____

---

superior

inferior

5–32 Refer to Figure 5–3 and use the words superior or inferior to complete this frame.

The left atrium is _____ to the left ventricle.

The right ventricle is _____ to the right atrium.

5–33 Blood flows from the right atrium through the (8) **tricuspid valve** and into the right ventricle. The leaflets (cusps) are shaped so that they form a one-way passage, which keeps the blood flowing in only one direction. Label the tricuspid valve in Figure 5–3.

---

tri/cuspid valve

trī-KŬS-pĭd

5–34 The prefix *tri-* means *three*. The valve that has three leaflets, or flaps, is the

_____ / _____ _____ .

---

two

5–35 The prefix *bi-* refers to *two*. A bi/cuspid valve has _____ leaflets, or flaps.

---

three

5–36 In the English language, a bi/cycle has two wheels; a tri/cycle has _____ wheels.

5–37 The ventricles are the pumping chambers of the heart. As the right ventricle contracts to pump oxygen-deficient blood through the (9) **pulmonary valve** into the pulmonary artery, the tri/cuspid valve remains closed, preventing a backflow of blood into the right atrium. When blood passes through the pulmonary trunk, also known as the main *pulmonary artery,* it branches into the (10) **right pulmonary artery** and the (11) **left pulmonary artery**. The pulmonary arteries carry the oxygen-deficient blood to the lungs. Label the structures introduced in this frame in Figure 5–3.

---

artery ĂR-tĕr-ē	**5-38** The CF *arteri/o* refers to an artery. Arteri/al bleeding is bleeding from an _____.
arteries ĂR-tĕr-ēs	**5-39** Arteri/al circulation is movement of blood through the _____.
artery ĂR-tĕr-ē	**5-40** An arteri/al spasm is a spasm of an _____.

5-41 Develop medical words that mean

arteri/o/rrhexis ăr-tē-rē-ō-RĔK-sĭs **arteri/o/rrhaphy** ăr-tē-rē-OR-ă-fē **arteri/o/pathy** ăr-tē-rē-ŎP-ă-thē **arteri/o/spasm** ăr-TĒ-rē-ō-spăzm	*rupture of an artery:* _____ / _____ / _____ *suture of an artery:* _____ / _____ / _____ *disease of an artery:* _____ / _____ / _____ *involuntary contraction or twitching of an artery:* _____ / _____ / _____

stone, artery ĂR-tĕr-ē	**5-42** The suffix *-lith* refers to a *stone,* or *calculus.* An arteri/o/lith, also called an *arteri/al calculus,* is a calculus, or _____, in an _____.

11 **10**	**5-43** The right and left pulmonary arteries leading to the lungs branch and subdivide until they ultimately form capillaries around the alveoli. Carbon dioxide is passed from the blood into the alveoli and expelled out of the lungs. Oxygen inhaled by the lungs is passed from the alveoli into the blood. The left pulmonary artery is identified in Figure 5–3 as number _____. The right pulmonary artery is identified in Figure 5–3 as number _____.

	5-44 Oxygenated blood leaves the lungs and returns to the heart via the (12) **right pulmonary veins** and (13) **left pulmonary veins.** The four pulmonary veins empty into the LA. The LA contracts to force blood through the (14) **mitral valve** into the LV. Label the structures in Figure 5–3.

two	**5-45** The mitral valve, located between the LA and LV, is a bi/cuspid, or bi/leaflet, valve, which means that the number of leaflets or flaps that the mitral valve has is _____.

vein VĀN	**5–46** *Ven/o* is a combining form that means _____.
vein VĀN	**5–47** *Phleb/o* is another CF for *vein*. Phleb/o/tomy is a procedure used to draw blood from a _____.
phleb/o/rrhaphy flĕb-ŎR-ă-fē **phleb/o/rrhexis** flĕb-ō-RĔK-sĭs **phleb/o/stenosis** flĕb-ō-stĕ-NŌ-sĭs	**5–48** Use *phleb/o* to construct words that mean *suture of a vein:* _____ / _____ / _____ *rupture of a vein:* _____ / _____ / _____ *stricture or narrowing of a vein:* _____ / _____ / _____
ven/o/scler/osis vēn-ō-sklĕ-RŌ-sĭs **ven/o/tomy** vē-NŎT-ō-mē **ven/o/spasm** VĒ-nō-spăzm	**5–49** Use *ven/o* to form words that mean *hardening of a vein:* _____ / _____ / _____ / _____ *incision of a vein:* _____ / _____ / _____ *contraction or twitching of a vein:* _____ / _____ / _____
blood	**5–50** *Hemat/o* and *hem/o* mean _____.
hemat/o/logy hē-mă-TŎL-ō-jē **hemat/o/logist** hē-mă-TŎL-ō-jĭst	**5–51** Use *hemat/o* to form words that mean *study of blood:* _____ / _____ / _____ *specialist in the study of blood:* _____ / _____ / _____
lymph vessels	**5–52** The CF *angi/o* means vessel (usually blood or lymph). An angioma is a tumor consisting primarily of blood or _____ _____.
hemangi/oma hē-măn-jē-Ō-mă	**5–53** *Hem/o* and *angi/o* can be combined into a new element that also means *blood vessel*. Use **hemangi/o** (blood vessel) to develop a word that means *tumor of blood vessels:* _____ / _____.
expansion	**5–54** Hemangi/ectasis is a dilation or _____ of a blood vessel.

Boldface indicates a word root or combining form. Blue indicates a suffix. Pink indicates a prefix.

5-55   Label the structures in Figure 5–3 as you continue to learn about the heart. Contractions of the LV send oxygenated blood through the (15) **aortic valve** and into the (16) **aorta.** The three ascending (17) **branches of the aorta** transport blood to the head and arms. The (18) **descending aorta** transports the blood to the legs and torso.

---

aort/o/pathy
ā-ŏr-TŎP-ă-thē

5-56   The aorta is the largest artery of the body and originates at the LV of the heart. The combining form *aort/o* refers to the aorta. Any disease of the aorta is

called _____ / _____ / _____.

---

pulmon/ary
PŬL-mō-nĕ-rē

vascul/ar
VĂS-kū-lăr

cardi/ac
KĂR-dē-ăk

5-57   Aortic stenosis, a narrowing or stricture of the aortic valve, may be due to congenital malformation or fusion of the cusps. The stenosis obstructs the flow of blood from the LV into the aorta, causing decreased cardi/ac output and pulmon/ary vascul/ar congestion. Treatment usually requires surgical repair.

Identify the terms in this frame that mean

pertaining to the lungs: _____ / _____

pertaining to a vessel: _____ / _____

pertaining to the heart: _____ / _____

---

artery, small vein

5-58   The suffixes *-ole* and *-ule* refer to *small, minute.*

An arteri/ole is a small _____; a ven/ule is a

_____ _____.

---

arteries
ĂR-tĕr-ēz

arteri/oles
ăr-TĒ-rē-ōls

5-59   Arteries are large vessels that convey blood away from the heart; they branch into smaller vessels called arteri/oles. The arteri/oles deliver blood to adjoining minute vessels called capillaries. (See Fig. 5–1.)

Large vessels that transport blood away from the heart are called

_____.

Smaller vessels that are formed from arteries are called

_____ / _____.

---

arteri/oles
ăr-TĒ-rē-ōls

5-60   Arteries convey blood to adjacent smaller vessels called

_____ / _____.

---

capillaries
KĂP-ĭ-lă-rēz

5-61   Arteri/oles are thinner than arteries and carry blood to extending minute

vessels called _____.

---

arteri/o/scler/osis
ăr-tē-ō-sklĕ-RŌ-sĭs

5-62   As a person ages, the arteries lose elasticity, thicken, become weakened, and deteriorate. Deterioration of arterial walls is also due to constant high pressure needed to transport blood throughout the body.

The medical term for an *abnormal condition of artery hardening* is

_____ / _____ / _____ / _____.

arteri/o/scler/osis ăr-tē-rē-ō-sklĕ-RŌ-sĭs	**5-63** High blood pressure and high-fat diets contribute greatly to early arteri/o/scler/osis. A healthy diet can decrease the risk for hardening of the arteries, also called _____ / _____ / _____ / _____.
superior vena cava VĒ-nă KĂ-vă **inferior vena cava** VĒ-nă KĂ-vă	**5-64** Capillaries carry blood from arteri/oles to ven/ules. Ven/ules form a collecting system to return oxygen-deficient blood to the heart through two large veins, the SVC and the IVC. Define the following abbreviations SVC: _____ _____ _____ IVC: _____ _____ _____
6, 7	**5-65** In Figure 5–3, the SVC is number _____; the IVC is number _____.
arteri/o/spasm ăr-TĒ-rē-ō-spăzm	**5-66** Combine *arteri/o* and *-spasm* to form a word meaning *arterial spasm:* _____ / _____ / _____.
varic/ose VĂR-ĭ-kōs **competent**	**5-67** Normal veins have competent (healthy) valves whose ven/ous walls are strong enough to withstand the later/al pressure of blood that is exerted upon them. Blood flows through competent valves in one direction, which is toward the heart. In varic/ose veins, also known as *varicosities,* dilation of veins from long periods of pressure prevents complete closure of the valves. (See Fig. 5–4.) Identify the medical term in this frame that means *pertaining to a dilated vein:* _____ / _____ *healthy:* _____
varicosities văr-ĭ-KŎS-ĭ-tēz **incompetent**	**5-68** Incompetent (damaged) valves cause a backflow of blood in the veins, which causes enlarged, twisted superficial veins called varicosities. (See Fig. 5–4.) Identify the terms in this frame that mean *abnormally enlarged, twisted veins:* _____ *damaged:* _____ / _____

Competency Verification: Check your labeling of Figure 5–3 in Appendix B: Answer Key, page 574.

Boldface indicates a word root or combining form. Blue indicates a suffix. Pink indicates a prefix.

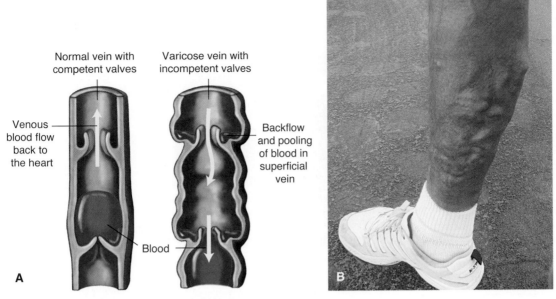

Figure 5-4 Healthy and unhealthy valves and veins. (**A**) Valve function in competent and incompetent valves. (**B**) Varicose veins.

Heart Valves

5-69   Label Figure 5–5 as you read the material about the heart valves and their cusps, also called flaps. Four heart valves maintain the flow of blood in one direction through the heart. The (1) **tricuspid valve** and the (2) **mitral valve** are situated between the upper and lower chambers and are attached to the heart walls by fibrous strands called (3) **chordae tendineae.** The (4) **pulmonary valve** and the (5) **aortic valve** are located at the exits of the ventricles.

Heart valves are composed of thin, fibrous cusps, covered by a smooth membrane called the endocardium, and reinforced by dense connective tissue. The aortic, pulmonary, and tricuspid valves contain (6) **three cusps;** the mitral valve contains (7) **two cusps.** The purpose of the cusps is to open and permit blood to flow through and seal shut to prevent backflow. The opening and closing of the cusps takes place with each heartbeat.

mitral valve
MĪ-trăl

5-70   To classify a heart abnormality, it is important to identify the part of the organ in which the disorder occurs. A mitral valve murmur is caused by an incompetent, or faulty, valve. This type of murmur occurs in the valvular structure of the heart known as the _____ _____.

A

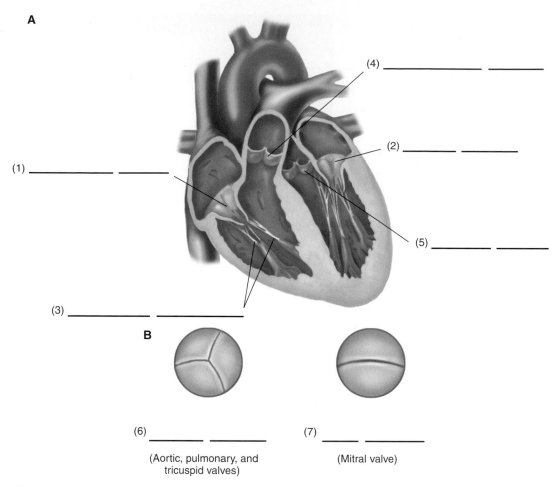

(4) _____ _____

(2) _____ _____

(1) _____ _____

(5) _____ _____

(3) _____ _____

B

(6) _____ _____   (7) _____ _____

(Aortic, pulmonary, and   (Mitral valve)
tricuspid valves)

Figure 5-5 Heart structures with valves and cusps. (**A**) Heart valves. (**B**) Valve cusps.

valve	**5-71** Replacement surgery can be performed to replace a damaged heart valve. When the tri/cuspid valve is damaged, it is replaced at the level of the tri/cuspid _____.

Competency Verification: Check your labeling of Figure 5–5 in Appendix B: Answer Key, page 574.

SECTION REVIEW 5-2

Using the following table, write the CF, suffix, or prefix that matches its definition in the space provided to the left of the definition. There may be more than one word element that matches a definition.

Combining Forms		Suffixes		Prefixes
aort/o	my/o	-ectasis	-rrhaphy	bi-
arteri/o	phleb/o	-ole	-rrhexis	brady-
atri/o	scler/o	-osis	-spasm	epi-
cardi/o	ven/o	-pathy	-stenosis	peri-
hem/o	ventricul/o	-phagia	-ule	tachy-
hemat/o		-pnea		tri-

1. _____ abnormal condition; increase (used primarily with blood cells)

2. _____ above, on

3. _____ aorta

4. _____ around

5. _____ artery

6. _____ atrium

7. _____ blood

8. _____ breathing

9. _____ disease

10. _____ dilation, expansion

11. _____ hardening; sclera (white of the eye)

12. _____ heart

13. _____ involuntary contraction, twitching

14. _____ muscle

15. _____ rapid

16. _____ rupture

17. _____ slow

18. _____ small, minute

19. _____ suture

20. _____ narrowing, stricture

21. _____ swallowing, eating

22. _____ three

23. _____ two

24. _____ vein

25. _____ ventricle (of the heart or brain)

Competency Verification: Check your answers in Appendix B: Answer Key, page 574. If you are not satisfied with your level of comprehension, go back to Frame 5–1 and rework the frames.

Correct Answers _____ × 4 = _____ % Score

Conduction Pathway of the Heart

5-72   Primary responsibility for initiating the heartbeat rests with the (1) **sinoatrial (SA) node**, also known as the pacemaker of the heart. The SA node is a small region of specialized cardiac muscle tissue located on the posterior wall of the (2) **right atrium (RA)**. Label these two structures in Figure 5–6.

SA

RA

5-73   Write the abbreviations for

sinoatrial: _____

right atrium: _____

---

electricity

5-74   The CF *electr/o* refers to electricity. Electric/al and electr/ic both mean

pertaining to _____.

5-75   The electric/al current generated by the heart's pacemaker causes the atri/al walls to contract and forces the flow of blood into the ventricles. The wave of electricity moves to another region of the myo/cardi/um called the (3) **atrioventricular (AV) node**. Label the structure in Figure 5–6 to learn about the conduction pathway of the heart.

---

atri/o/ventricul/ar
ā-trē-ō-věn-TRĬK-ū-lăr

electric/al

atri/al
Ā-trē-ăl

5-76   Identify the words in Frame 5–75 that mean

pertaining to the atrium and ventricles:

_____ / _____ / _____ / _____

pertaining to electricity: _____ / _____

pertaining to the atrium: _____ / _____

AV

SA

5-77   Write the abbreviations for

atri/o/ventricul/ar: _____

sino/atri/al: _____

5-78   The AV node instantaneously transmits impulses to the (4) **bundle of His**, a bundle of specialized fibers that transmits those impulses to the right and left (5) **bundle branches**. Label the structures in Figure 5–6.

5-79   From the right and left bundle branches, impulses travel through the (6) **Purkinje fibers** to the rest of the ventricul/ar my/o/cardi/um and bring about ventricul/ar contraction. Label the Purkinje (pŭr-KĬN-jē) fibers in Figure 5–6.

Boldface indicates a word root or combining form. Blue indicates a suffix. Pink indicates a prefix.

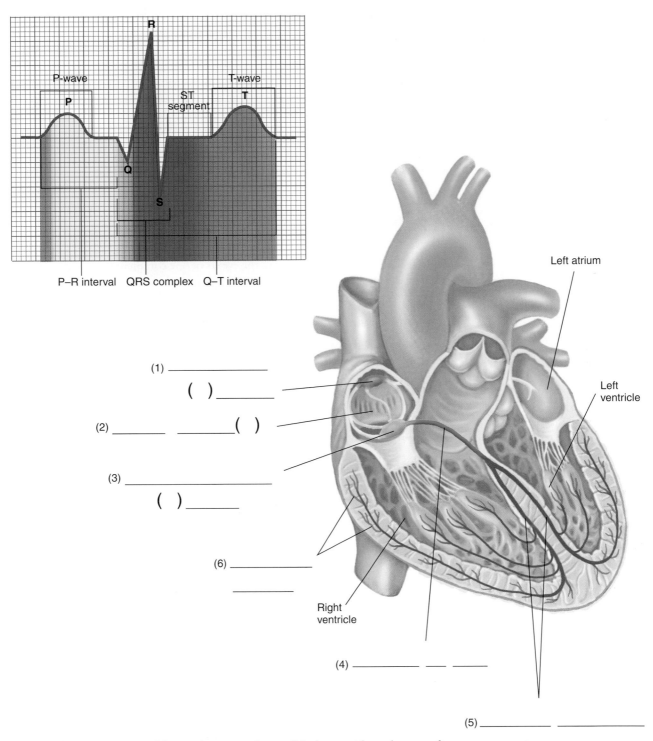

Figure 5-6 Anterior view of the conduction pathway of the heart with an electrocardiogram tracing of one normal heartbeat.

5-80   Use your medical dictionary to define contraction.

_____

_____

_____

_____

Competency Verification: Check your labeling of Figure 5–6 in Appendix B: Answer Key, page 574.

Cardiac Cycle and Heart Sounds

diastole dī-ĂS-tō-lē	**5-81** The cardi/ac cycle refers to the events of one complete heartbeat. Each contraction, or systole, of the heart is followed by a period of relaxation, or diastole. This cycle occurs 60 to 100 times per minute in the normal functioning heart. The normal period of heart contraction is called systole; the normal period of heart relaxation is called _____.
systole SĬS-tō-lē **diastole** dī-ĂS-tō-lē **systole** SĬS-tō-lē	**5-82** When the heart is in the phase of relaxation, it is in diastole. When the heart is in the contraction phase, it is in _____. The pumping action of the heart consists of contraction and relaxation of the myocardial layer of the heart wall. During relaxation (diastole), blood fills the ventricles. The contraction that follows (systole), propels the blood out of the ventricles and into the circulation. Write the medical term relating to the cardi/ac cycle that is in the phase of _relaxation:_ _____ _contraction:_ _____
-graphy **-gram**	**5-83** Recall the suffixes that mean _process of recording:_ _____ _record, writing:_ _____
heart	**5-84** Electr/o/cardi/o/graphy is the process of recording electric/al activity generated by the _____.
record, heart	**5-85** An electr/o/cardi/o/gram is a _____ of electric/al activity generated by the _____. (See Fig. 5–6.)
electr/o/cardi/o/gram ē-lĕk-trō-KĂR-dē-ō-grăm	**5-86** ECG and EKG are abbreviations for electr/o/cardi/o/gram. To evaluate an abnormal cardi/ac rhythm, such as tachy/cardia, an ECG may be helpful. The abbreviations _ECG_ and _EKG_ refer to an _____ / _____ / _____ / _____ / _____.

Boldface indicates a word root or combining form. Blue indicates a suffix. Pink indicates a prefix.

tachy-, brady-	**5-87** The prefix that means rapid is _____ ; the prefix that means slow is _____ .

rapid, slow	**5-88** Tachy/cardia is a heart rate that is _____ ; brady/cardia is a heart rate that is _____ .

> The following summary provides a brief, general interpretation of an ECG. A more comprehensive explanation of ECG abnormalities is beyond the scope of this book. Refer to Figure 5–6 as you read the text that follows.

A normal heart rhythm, or **sinus rhythm,** shows five waves on the ECG strip, which represent electrical changes as they spread through the heart. The waves are known as the **P wave, QRS waves,** and **T wave.**

The **P wave** represents atrial depolarization, conduction of an electrical impulse through the atria. These electrical changes cause atrial contraction. The **QRS waves,** commonly referred to as the *QRS complex,* represent ventricular depolarization, conduction of electrical impulses through the ventricle by way of the bundle of His and the Purkinje fibers. These electrical changes cause ventricular contraction. The **T wave** represents the electrical recovery and relaxation of the ventricles (during diastole).

electr/o/cardi/o/gram ē-lĕk-trō-KĂR-dē-ō-grăm	**5-89** Although the heart itself generates the heartbeat, such factors as hormones, drugs, and nervous system stimulation can also influence the heart rate. To evaluate a patient's heart rate, a physician may order an ECG, an abbreviation for _____ / _____ / _____ / _____ / _____ .

micro/cardia mī-krō-KĂR-dē-ă	**5-90** Micro/cardia, an abnormal smallness of the heart, is a condition that is not usually compatible with a normal life. A person diagnosed with an underdeveloped heart suffers from the condition called _____ / _____ .

enlargement, heart	**5-91** Megal/o/cardia is an enlargement of the heart. Cardi/o/megaly also means _____ of the _____ .

cardi/o/megaly, **megal/o/cardia** kăr-dē-ō-MĔG-ă-lē, mĕg-ă-lō-KĂR-dē-ă	**5-92** In patients with high blood pressure, the heart must work extremely hard. As a result, it enlarges, similar to any other muscle in response to excessive activity or exercise. A patient who develops an enlarged heart has a condition called _____ / _____ / _____ or _____ / _____ / _____ .

	5-93 Use your medical dictionary to define angina pectoris and lumen. _____ _____ _____ _____

-osis **scler** **ather/o**	**5–94** Coronary artery disease (CAD) affects the arteries and may cause various pathological conditions, including a reduced flow of oxygen and nutrients to the myocardium. (See Fig. 5–7.) The most common type of CAD is coronary ather/o/scler/osis. It is now the leading cause of death in the Western world. Identify the word elements in this frame that mean *abnormal condition:* _____ *hardening:* _____ *fatty plaque:* _____ / _____
arteri/o/scler/osis ăr-tē-rē-ō-sklĕ-RŌ-sĭs	**5–95** Arteri/o/scler/osis is a thickening, hardening, and loss of elasticity of arteri/al walls, which results in decreased blood supply. Thus, arteri/o/scler/osis is commonly referred to as *hardening of the arteries.* When the physician diagnoses a hardening of the arteries, the condition is recorded in the medical chart as _____ / _____ / _____ / _____.
ather/o **arteri/o** **scler/o** **my/o** **cardi**	**5–96** Ather/o/scler/osis, the most common form of arteri/o/scler/osis, is characterized by an accumulation of plaque within the arterial wall. This condition results in partial, and eventually total, occlusion. (See Fig. 5–7.) Both conditions develop over a long period and usually occur together. Indicate the word elements used to denote coronary artery disease that mean *fatty plaque:* _____ / _____ *artery:* _____ / _____ *hardening:* _____ / _____ *muscle:* _____ / _____ *heart:* _____

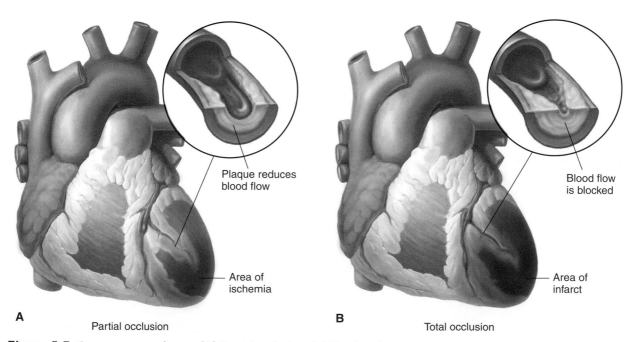

A   Partial occlusion   **B**   Total occlusion

Figure 5-7   Coronary artery disease. (**A**) Partial occlusion. (**B**) Total occlusion.

Boldface indicates a word root or combining form. Blue indicates a suffix. Pink indicates a prefix.

arteri/o/scler/osis
ăr-tē-rē-ō-sklĕ-RŌ-sĭs

ather/o/scler/osis
ăth-ĕr-ō-sklĕ-RŌ-sĭs

5–97   The carotid arteries are a common site of ather/o/scler/osis. When a piece of plaque breaks away from the site, it may travel to the brain, blocking blood flow and causing a stroke. (See Fig. 5–8.)

Build medical words that mean

abnormal condition of arterial hardening:

_____ / _____ / _____ / _____

abnormal condition of fatty plaque hardening:

_____ / _____ / _____ / _____

---

excision or removal

5–98   The CF *necr/o* refers to death or necrosis. *Necr/ectomy* is

_____ of dead tissue.

---

necr/o/phobia
nĕk-rō-FŌ-bē-ă

5–99   Use *-phobia* to form a word that means *fear of death.*

_____ / _____ / _____

---

cardi/ac
KĂR-dē-ăk

necr/osis
nĕ-KRŌ-sĭs

5–100   Necr/osis of the my/o/cardi/um occurs when there is insufficient blood supply to the heart. Eventually, such a condition may result in cardi/ac failure and death of the my/o/cardi/um.

Identify the words in this frame that mean

pertaining to the heart: _____ / _____

abnormal condition of tissue death: _____ / _____

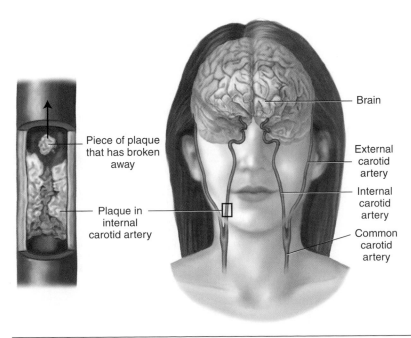

Figure 5-8 Atherosclerosis of the internal carotid artery.

5-101   A my/o/cardi/al infarction (MI), or infarct, is caused by occlusion of one or more coronary arteries. MI is a medical emergency requiring immediate attention. Using your medical dictionary, define infarct.

_____

_____

_____

---

thromb/us
THRŎM-bŭs

5-102   The CF **thromb/o** is used in words to refer to a blood clot; the suffix -us means _condition, structure._

Combine **thromb/o** and -us to form a word that means _condition of a blood clot._

_____ / _____

---

thromb/ectomy
thrŏm-BĚK-tō-mē

5-103   Thromb/osis is a _condition in which a stationary blood clot obstructs a blood vessel at the site of its formation._

The surgical excision of a blood clot is called _____ /

_____.

---

thrombi
THRŎM-bī

anti-

5-104   Anti/coagulants are _agents that prevent or delay blood coagulation_; they are used in the prevention and treatment of a thrombus.

The plural form of _thrombus_ is _____.

The element in this frame that means _against_ is _____.

---

thromb/o/genesis
thrŏm-bō-JĚN-ĕ-sĭs

5-105   Use -genesis to form a word that means _producing or forming a blood clot._

_____ / _____ / _____

---

clot

5-106   If the anti/coagulant does not dissolve the clot, it may be surgically removed. A thromb/ectomy is an excision of a blood _____.

---

anti/coagulant
ăn-tī-kō-ĂG-ū-lănt

5-107   To prevent blood coagulation, the physician uses an agent known as an

_____ / _____.

---

thromb/o/lysis
thrŏm-BŎL-ĭ-sĭs

5-108   Use the surgical suffix -lysis to form a word that means _destruction or dissolving of a thrombus._

_____ / _____ / _____

---

thromb/o/lysis
thrŏm-BŎL-ĭ-sĭs

5-109   The surgical procedure to destroy or remove a clot is thromb/ectomy or

_____ / _____ / _____.

Boldface indicates a word root or combining form. Blue indicates a suffix. Pink indicates a prefix.

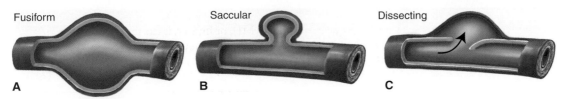

Figure 5-9 Aneurysms. (**A**) Fusiform. (**B**) Saccular. (**C**) Dissecting.

---

aneurysm
ĂN-ū-rĭzm

5-110   An aneurysm is an abnormal dilation of the vessel wall due to a weakness that causes the vessel to balloon and potentially rupture. There are three types of aneurysms: **fusiform**, with a dilation of the entire circumference of the artery; **saccular,** with bulging on only one side of the artery wall; and **dissecting**, with an inner layer tear (dissection) that causes a cavity to form and fill with blood with each heartbeat. (See Fig. 5–9.)

A ballooning out of the wall of the aorta is called an aort/ic

_____.

---

aorta
ā-ŎR-tă

5-111   If a cerebr/al aneurysm ruptures, the hem/o/rrhage occurs in the cerebrum or brain. If an aort/ic aneurysm ruptures, the hem/o/rrhage occurs in the

_____.

---

aort/ic
ā-ŎR-tĭk

hem/o/rrhage
HĔM-ĕ-rĭj

cerebr/al
SĔR-ĕ-brăl

aneurysm
ĂN-ū-rĭzm

5-112   Identify the words in Frame 5–111 that mean

pertaining to the aorta: _____ / _____

bursting forth (of) blood: _____ / _____ / _____

pertaining to the cerebrum: _____ / _____

dilation of a vessel caused by weakness: _____

LYMPHATIC SYSTEM

The lymphatic system consists of lymph, lymph vessels, lymph nodes, and three organs: the tonsils, thymus, and spleen. The lymphatic system has three main functions:

1. It drains excess interstitial fluid from tissue spaces and returns it to circulating blood.
2. It protects the body by defending against foreign or harmful agents, such as bacteria, viruses, and cancerous cells.
3. It absorbs and transports digested fats to venous circulation. These fats are provided by aggregations of lymphatic tissue known as Peyer patches that are present in the lining of the ileum (small intestine).

The fluid (lymph) circulating through the lymphatic system comes from the blood. It contains white blood cells (leukocytes) responsible for immunity, as well as monocytes and lymphocytes. As certain constituents of blood plasma filtrate through tiny capillaries into the spaces between cells, they become interstitial fluid. Most interstitial fluid is absorbed from the interstitial (or intercellular) spaces by thin-walled vessels called lymph capillaries. At this point of absorption, interstitial fluid becomes lymph and is passed through lymphatic tissue called lymph nodes. The nodes are found in clusters in such areas as the neck (cervic/al lymph nodes), under the arm (axill/ary lymph nodes), the pelvis (ili/ac lymph nodes), and the groin (inguin/al lymph nodes). The nodes act as filters against foreign materials. Eventually, lymph reaches large lymph vessels in the upper chest and reenters the bloodstream. (See Fig. 5–1.)

WORD ELEMENTS

This section introduces CFs, suffixes, and prefixes related to the lymphatic system, along with each element's meaning, an example, and additional analysis of key elements in the example. Review the following table and pronounce each word in the word analysis column aloud before you begin to work in the frames.

Word Element	Meaning	Word Analysis
Combining Forms		
aden/o	gland	**aden/o/pathy** (ă-dĕ-NŎP-ă-thē): disease of a gland *-pathy:* disease
agglutin/o	clumping, gluing	**agglutin/ation** (ă-gloo-tĭ-NĀ-shŭn): process of cells clumping together *-ation:* process (of)
immun/o	immune, immunity, safe	**immun/o/gen** (ĭ-MŪ-nō-jĕn): producing immunity *-gen:* forming, producing, origin *An immunogen is a substance capable of producing an immune response.*
lymph/o	lymph	**lymph/o/poiesis** (lĭm-fō-poy-Ē-sĭs): formation of lymphocytes or of lymphoid tissue *-poiesis:* formation, production
lymphaden/o	lymph gland (node)	**lymphaden/itis** (lĭm-făd-ĕn-Ī-tĭs): inflammation of a lymph gland (node) *-itis:* inflammation
lymphangi/o	lymph vessel	**lymphangi/oma** (lĭm-făn-jē-Ō-mă): tumor composed of lymphatic vessels *-oma:* tumor
phag/o	swallowing, eating	**phag/o/cyte** (FĂG-ō-sīt): cell that swallows and eats (cellular debris) *-cyte:* cell *A phagocyte surrounds, engulfs, and digests microorganisms and cellular debris.*
splen/o	spleen	**splen/o/megaly** (splĕ-nō-MĔG-ă-lē): enlargement of the spleen *-megaly:* enlargement
thym/o	thymus gland	**thym/oma** (thī-MŌ-mă): tumor of the thymus gland, usually a benign tumor *-oma:* tumor
Suffix		
-phylaxis	protection	ana/**phylaxis** (ăn-ă-fĭ-LĂK-sĭs): against protection *ana-:* against; up; back *Anaphylaxis is an extreme allergic reaction characterized by a rapid decrease in blood pressure, breathing difficulties, hives, and abdominal cramps.*

Pronunciation Help	Long sound	ā in rāte	ē in rēbirth	ī in īsle	ō in ōver	ū in ūnite
	Short sound	ă in ălone	ĕ in ĕver	ĭ in ĭt	ŏ in nŏt	ŭ in cŭt

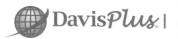

Visit the *Medical Terminology Simplified* online resource center at Davis*Plus* for an audio exercise of the terms in this table. It will help you master pronunciations and meanings of the medical terms.

Boldface indicates a word root or combining form. Blue indicates a suffix. Pink indicates a prefix.

SECTION REVIEW 5-3

For the following medical terms, first write the suffix and its meaning. Then translate the meaning of the remaining elements starting with the first part of the word. The first word is an example that is completed for you.

Term	Meaning
1. agglutin/ation	-ation: process (of); clumping, gluing
2. thym/oma	
3. phag/o/cyte	
4. lymphaden/itis	
5. splen/o/megaly	
6. aden/o/pathy	
7. ana/phylaxis	
8. lymphangi/oma	
9. lymph/o/poiesis	
10. immun/o/gen	

Competency Verification: Check your answers in Appendix B: Answer Key, page 575. If you are not satisfied with your level of comprehension, review the vocabulary and retake the review.

Correct Answers _____ × 10 = _____ % Score

Lymphatic Structures

5-113   Similar to blood capillaries, (1) **lymph capillaries** are thin-walled tubes that carry lymph from the tissue spaces to larger (2) **lymph vessels.** Label these structures in Figure 5–10.

lymph/oma
lĭm-FŌ-mă

lymph/o/cyte
LĬM-fō-sīt

lymph/o/poiesis
lĭm-fō-poy-Ē-sĭs

5-114   Lymph/oma is a malignant tumor of lymph nodes and lymph tissue. Two main kinds of lymphomas are Hodgkin disease and non-Hodgkin lymphoma. These disorders are covered in the diseases section of this chapter.

Use *lymph/o* to build terms that mean

tumor composed of lymph tissue: _____ / _____

cell present in lymph tissue: _____ / _____ / _____

formation or production of lymph:

_____ / _____ / _____

vessels	**5-115** Recall that *angi/o* is used in words to denote a vessel (usually blood or lymph). Angio/card/itis is an inflammation of the heart and blood _____.
lymphangi/o	**5-116** Combine *lymph/o* and *angi/o* to form a new element that means *lymph vessel.* _____ / _____
lymphangi/oma lĭm-făn-jē-Ō-mă	**5-117** Use *lymphangi/o* to form a word that means *tumor composed of lymph vessels.* _____ / _____
angi/o/rrhaphy ăn-jē-OR-ă-fē **angi/o/plasty** ĂN-jē-ō-plăs-tē **angi/o/rrhexis** ăn-jē-ō-RĔK-sĭs	**5-118** Use *angi/o* to develop medical words that mean *suture of a vessel:* _____ / _____ / _____ *surgical repair of a vessel:* _____ / _____ / _____ *rupture of a vessel:* _____ / _____ / _____
chest	**5-119** Similar to veins, lymph vessels contain valves that keep lymph flowing in one direction, toward the thorac/ic cavity. Thorac/ic means *pertaining to the* _____.
	5-120 The (3) **thoracic duct** and the (4) **right lymphatic duct** carry lymph into veins in the upper thoracic region. Label these two ducts in Figure 5–10.
lymph/oid LĬM-foyd	**5-121** Use *-oid* to form a word that means *resembling lymph.* _____ / _____
lymph/o/pathy lĭm-FŎP-ă-thē	**5-122** The word that means any *disease of the lymphat/ic* system is _____ / _____ / _____.
lymph/o/cytes LĬM-fō-sīts	**5-123** Small, round structures called lymph nodes not only produce lymph/o/cytes, but also filter and purify lymph by removing such harmful substances as bacteria and cancerous cells. Lymph cells are known as _____ / _____ / _____.
	5-124 The major lymph node sites are the (5) **cervical nodes**, (6) **axillary nodes**, and (7) **inguinal nodes**. Label the three major lymph node sites in Figure 5–10.

Boldface indicates a word root or combining form. Blue indicates a suffix. Pink indicates a prefix.

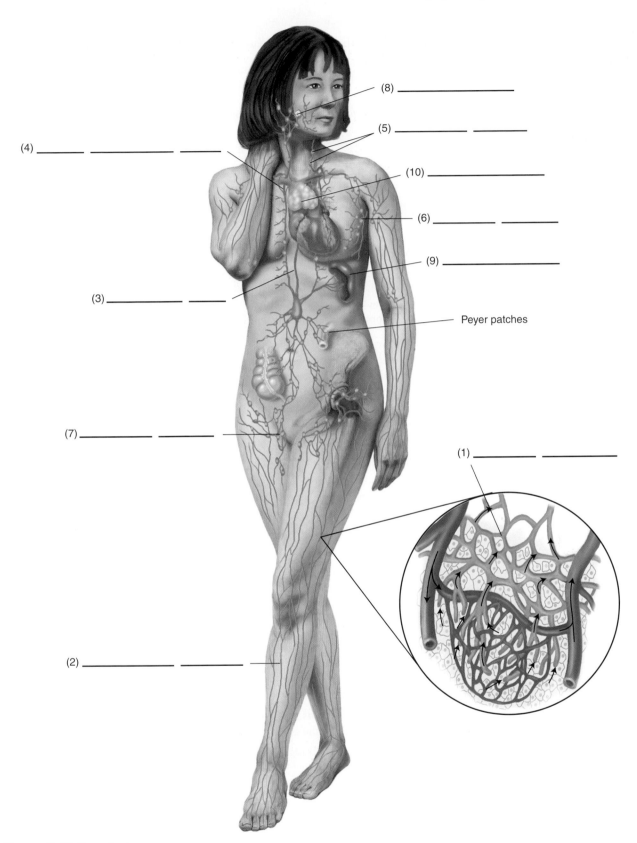

(8) _____

(5) _____ _____

(4) _____ _____ _____

(10) _____

(6) _____ _____

(9) _____

Peyer patches

(3) _____ _____

(7) _____ _____

(1) _____ _____

(2) _____ _____

Figure 5-10 Lymphatic system.

cervic/al SĔR-vĭ-kăl **axill/ary** ĂK-sĭ-lăr-ē **inguin/al** ĬNG-gwĭ-năl	**5-125** Write the name of the lymph node located in the *neck:* _____ / _____ *armpit:* _____ / _____ *groin (depression between the thigh and trunk):* _____ / _____

Tonsil, Spleen, and Thymus

5-126   The (8) **tonsil** is a small mass of lymphoid tissue in the mucous membranes of the pharynx and base of the tongue. Tonsils consist of several masses and are the first line of defense from the external environment. They act as a filter to protect against bacteria and other harmful substances that may enter the body through the nose or mouth. Label the tonsil in Figure 5–10.

5-127   The (9) **spleen** is located in the left upper quadrant (LUQ) of the abdomen and behind the stomach. It is the largest lymphatic organ in the body. Although the spleen is not essential to life, it plays an important role in the immune response by filtering blood in much the same way that lymph nodes filter lymph. Label the spleen in Figure 5–10.

path/o/gen păth-ō-JĔN **hem/o/rrhage** HĔM-ĕ-rĭj **ven/ous** VĒ-nŭs **macro/phage** MĂK-rō-fāj	**5-128** Path/o/gens of all types are filtered from the circulating blood by the macro/phages of the spleen. The spleen also removes and destroys old red blood cells (RBCs) from circulation. The spleen contains ven/ous sinuses that serve as a storage reservoir for blood. In emergencies, such as hem/o/rrhage, the spleen can release blood back into the general circulation. Identify the term in this frame that refers to *micro/organ/ism capable of producing disease:* _____ / _____ / _____ *loss of large amounts of blood in a short period:* _____ / _____ / _____ *pertaining to a vein:* _____ / _____ *phag/o/cyt/ic cell in the spleen:* _____ / _____

5-129   The (10) **thymus**, also an endocrine gland, is a lymphatic organ. It is located near the middle of the chest (mediastinum) just beneath the sternum. Label the thymus in Figure 5–10.

immun/o	**5-130** During fetal life and childhood, the thymus is quite large, but becomes smaller with age as it completes most of its essential work during childhood. The thymus plays an important role in the body's ability to protect itself against disease (immunity), especially during the early years of growth. What CF means *immune, immunity, safe?* _____ / _____

Boldface indicates a word root or combining form. Blue indicates a suffix. Pink indicates a prefix.

T cells	**5–131** The thymus secretes a hormone called thymosin, which stimulates the red bone marrow to produce T lymph/o/cytes, or T cells. T cells are important in the immune process. They originate in the bone marrow but migrate and mature in the thymus. Upon maturation, T cells enter the blood and circulate throughout the body, providing a mechanism of defense against disease because the cells attack and destroy foreign or abnormal cells.
	Specific lymph/o/cytes that attack foreign agents, such as viruses, are known as
	T lympho/cytes or _____.
cyt/o/tox/ic sī-tō-TŎKS-ĭk **CA**	**5–132** Some T cells are called killer T cells or cytotoxic T lymphocytes (CTLs) because they secrete immun/o/logic/ally essential chemical compounds that destroy foreign cells. These killer cells are so named because they are capable of destroying specific cells. The killer cells also play a significant role in the body's resistance to proliferation of cancer (CA) cells.
	Specialized cells that provide surveillance against CA cells are called killer
	T lymph/o/cytes or _____ / _____ / _____ / _____
	T lymph/o/cytes.
	The abbreviation for cancer is _____.
cyt/o/tox/ic T lymph/ **o/cyte** sī-tō-TŎKS-ĭk LĬM-fō-sīt	**5–133** CTLs defend against viral and fung/al infections. They are also responsible for transplant rejection reactions and for immun/o/logic/al surveillance against cancer.
	The abbreviation CTL stands for _____ / _____ / _____ / _____
	_____ _____ / _____ / _____.

Competency Verification: Check your labeling of Figure 5–10 in Appendix B: Answer Key, page 575.

SECTION REVIEW 5-4

Using the following table, write the CF or suffix that matches its definition in the space provided to the left of the definition. There may be more than one word element that matches a definition.

Combining Forms

angi/o	lymph/o
aort/o	my/o
cardi/o	necr/o
cerebr/o	thromb/o
electr/o	
hem/o	

Suffixes

-al	-megaly
-cyte	-pathy
-gram	-plasty
-graphy	-rrhexis
-ic	-stenosis
-lysis	

1. _____ aorta

2. _____ blood

3. _____ blood clot

4. _____ cell

5. _____ cerebrum

6. _____ death, necrosis

7. _____ disease

8. _____ electricity

9. _____ enlargement

10. _____ heart

11. _____ lymph

12. _____ muscle

13. _____ process of recording

14. _____ record, writing

15. _____ pertaining to

16. _____ rupture

17. _____ separation; destruction; loosening

18. _____ narrowing, stricture

19. _____ surgical repair

20. _____ vessel (usually blood or lymph)

Competency Verification: Check your answers in Appendix B: Answer Key, page 575. If you are not satisfied with your level of comprehension, go back to Frame 5–3 and rework the frames.

Correct Answers _____ × 5 = _____ % Score

ABBREVIATIONS

This section introduces cardiovascular and lymphatic systems–related abbreviations and their meanings. Included are abbreviations contained in the medical record activities that follow.

Abbreviation	Meaning	Abbreviation	Meaning
AED	automatic external defibrillator	HTN	hypertension
AICD	automatic implantable cardioverter-defibrillator	IAS	interatrial septum
AIDS	acquired immunodeficiency syndrome	ICD	implantable cardioverter-defibrillator
AV	atrioventricular; arteriovenous	IVC	inferior vena cava
BP	blood pressure	IVS	interventricular
CA	cancer; chronological age; cardiac arrest	LA	left atrium
CAABG	coronary artery bypass graft	LDL	low-density lipoprotein
CAD	coronary artery disease	LUQ	left upper quadrant
CC	cardiac catheterization; chief complaint	LV	left ventricle
CHB	complete heart block	MI	myocardial infarction
CHF	congestive heart failure	MVP	mitral valve prolapse
CV	cardiovascular	PCI	percutaneous coronary intervention
CVA	cerebrovascular accident; costovertebral angle	PTCA	percutaneous transluminal coronary angioplasty
DVT	deep vein thrombosis (also called deep venous thrombosis)	RA	right atrium
EBV	Epstein-Barr virus	RBC	red blood cell
ECG, EKG	electrocardiogram; electrocardiography	RV	right ventricle
ELISA	enzyme-linked immunosorbent assay (test to detect anti-HIV antibodies)	SA	sinoatrial (node)
ELT	endovenous laser ablation; endoluminal laser ablation	SVC	superior vena cava
HDL	high-density lipoprotein	TIA	transient ischemic attack
HF	heart failure	US	ultrasound; ultrasonography
HIV	human immunodeficiency virus	WBC	white blood cell

ADDITIONAL MEDICAL TERMS

The following are additional terms related to the cardiovascular and lymphatic systems. Recognizing and learning these terms will help you understand the connection between common signs, symptoms, and diseases and their diagnoses, as well as the rationale behind methods of treatment selected for a particular disorder.

Diseases and Conditions

Cardiovascular System

angina pectoris ăn-JĪ-nă pĕk-TŌ-rĭs	Mild to severe pain or pressure in the chest caused by ischemia; also called *angina* *Angina pectoris usually results from atherosclerosis of the coronary arteries. It can occur while resting or during exercise and is a warning sign of an impending myocardial infarction (MI).*

arrhythmia
ă-RĬTH-mē-ă
   a-: without, not
rrhythm: rhythm
   -ia: condition
	Irregularity or loss of rhythm of the heartbeat; also called *dysrhythmia*
	
	Arrhythmias occur when the electrical impulses that stem from the conduction system of the heart do not function properly, causing the heart to deviate from the normal heartbeat pattern. Two common types of arrhythmia are flutter and fibrillation.

fibrillation fĭ-brĭl-Ā-shŭn	Arrhythmia of irregular, random contractions of heart fibers *Fibrillation commonly occurs in the atria or ventricles of the heart and is usually described by the part that is contracting abnormally, such as atrial fibrillation or ventricular fibrillation.*
bruit BRWĒ	Abnormal blowing sound heard on auscultation and caused by turbulent blood flow through an artery

deep vein thrombosis (DVT)
DĒP VĀN thrŏm-BŌ-sĭs
   thromb: blood clot
   -osis: abnormal condition; increase (used primarily with blood cells)
	Formation of a blood clot in a deep vein of the body, occurring most commonly in the legs or thighs
	
	Anticoagulants help dissolve clot formations and prevent further clotting. (See Fig. 5–11.)

embolus
ĔM-bō-lŭs
   embol: embolus (plug)
   -us: condition; structure
	Mass of undissolved matter—commonly a blood clot, fatty plaque, or air bubble—that travels through the bloodstream and becomes lodged in a blood vessel
	
	Emboli may be solid, liquid, or gaseous. Occlusion of vessels from an embolus usually results in the development of an infarct.

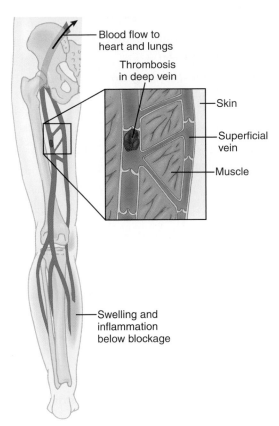

- Blood flow to heart and lungs
- Thrombosis in deep vein
- Skin
- Superficial vein
- Muscle
- Swelling and inflammation below blockage

Figure 5-11 Deep vein thrombosis.

heart block	Interference with normal conduction of electrical impulses that control activity of the heart muscle
	Heart block is usually specified by the location of the block and the type.
first-degree	Atrioventricular (AV) block in which the atrial electrical impulses are delayed by a fraction of a second before being conducted to the ventricles
	First-degree AV block is recognized on ECG by a prolonged PR interval. There is no specific treatment for first-degree AV block, but the condition is monitored because it may precede higher degrees of block.
second-degree	AV block in which occasional electrical impulses from the SA node fail to be conducted to the ventricles
	Because of the dropped beats in second-degree AV block, the QRS complexes are dropped periodically, usually every second, third, or fourth beat.
third-degree	AV block in which electrical impulses from the atria fail to reach the ventricles; also called *complete heart block (CHB)*
	In right- or left-bundle branch block, electrical impulses are unable to travel down the right or left bundle of His. Treatment for second- or third-degree heart block consists of atropine (a drug used to increase heart rate) or pacemaker insertion.

heart failure (HF)	Inability of the heart to circulate blood effectively enough to meet the body's metabolic needs; formerly called *congestive heart failure (CHF)* *Heart failure may result from myocardial infarction, ischemic heart disease, and cardiomyopathy. It may also be caused by the dysfunction of organs other than the heart, especially the lungs, kidneys, and liver.*
hypertension hī-pĕr-TĔN-shŭn *hyper:* excessive, above normal *-tension:* to stretch	Consistently elevated blood pressure (BP) that is higher than 119/79 mm Hg, causing damage to the blood vessels and, ultimately, the heart
ischemia ĭs-KĒ-mē-ă *isch:* to hold back; block *-emia:* blood	Deficiency of blood flow to an organ or tissue due to circulatory obstruction *Some causes of ischemia are arterial embolism, atherosclerosis, thrombosis, and vasoconstriction. (See the ischemic area of an occluded coronary artery in Fig. 5–7.)*
mitral valve prolapse (MVP) MĪ-trăl VĂLV PRŌ-lăps	Condition in which the leaflets of the mitral valve prolapse into the left atrium during systole, resulting in incomplete closure and backflow of blood
myocardial infarction (MI) mī-ō-KĂR-dē-ăl ĭn-FĂRK-shŭn *my/o:* muscle *cardi:* heart *-al:* pertaining to	Necrosis of a portion of cardiac muscle caused by partial or complete occlusion of one or more coronary arteries; also called *heart attack*
patent ductus arteriosus PĂT-ĕnt DŬK-tŭs ăr-tē-rē-Ō-sŭs	Failure of the ductus arteriosus to close after birth, resulting in an abnormal opening between the pulmonary artery and the aorta
Raynaud disease rā-NŌ	Chronic episodes of cyanosis and paleness of the skin, primarily in the fingers or toes, due to intermittent constriction of arterioles in the skin *Episodes may be triggered by cold temperatures or emotional stress. It may also be an indicator of some other, more serious, problem.*

rheumatic heart disease rū-MĂT-ĭk	Streptococcal infection that causes damage to the heart valves and heart muscle, most commonly in children and young adults

Lymphatic System

acquired immunodeficiency syndrome (AIDS) ă-KWĪRD ĭm-ŪN dē-FĬSH-ĕn-sē SĬN-drōm	Deficiency of cellular immunity induced by infection with the human immunodeficiency virus (HIV), characterized by increasing susceptibility to infections, malignancies, and neurological diseases *HIV is transmitted from person to person in cell-rich body fluids (notably blood and semen) through sexual contact, sharing of contaminated needles (as by intravenous drug abusers), or other contact with contaminated blood (as in accidental needle sticks among health-care workers).*
Hodgkin disease HŎJ-kĭn	Malignant disease characterized by painless, progressive enlargement of lymphoid tissue (usually first evident in cervical lymph nodes), splenomegaly, and the presence of unique Reed-Sternberg cells in the lymph nodes
Kaposi sarcoma KĂP-ō-sē săr-KŌ-mă *sarc:* flesh (connective tissue) *-oma:* tumor	Malignancy of connective tissue, including bone, fat, muscle, and fibrous tissue *Kaposi sarcoma is closely associated with AIDS and is commonly fatal because the tumors readily metastasize to various organs.*
mononucleosis mŏn-ō-nū-klē-Ō-sĭs *mono-:* one *nucle:* nucleus *-osis:* abnormal condition; increase (used primarily with blood cells)	Acute infection caused by the Epstein-Barr virus (EBV) and characterized by a sore throat, fever, fatigue, and enlarged lymph nodes
non-Hodgkin lymphoma non-HŎJ-kĭn lĭm-FŌ-mă *lymph:* lymph *-oma:* tumor	Any of a heterogeneous group of malignant tumors involving lymphoid tissue except for Hodgkin disease; previously called lymphosarcoma *These lymphomas include a group of more than 20 different types of lymphomas that occur in older adults and do not show Reed-Sternberg cells.*

| systemic lupus erythe-matosus (SLE)
LŪ-pŭs
ĕr-ĭ-thē-mă-TŌ-sĭs | Chronic inflammatory autoimmune disease characterized by unusual antibodies in the blood that target tissues of the body with a butterfly-shaped rash that appears on the face (See Fig. 5–12.)

There is a sensitivity to sunlight, fatigue, and joint pain. Treatment includes anti-inflammatories, immunosuppressives, and corticosteroids. The rash tends to get worse when exposed to direct sunlight. |

Diagnostic Procedures

Cardiovascular System

| cardiac catheterization (CC)
KĂR-dē-ăk
kăth-ĕ-tĕr-ĭ-ZĀ-shŭn
cardi: heart
-ac: pertaining to | Insertion of a catheter into the heart through a vein or artery, usually of an arm (brachial approach) or leg (femoral approach) to provide evaluation of the heart (See Fig. 5–13.)

During CC, the cardiologist may also inject a contrast medium and take x-rays (angiography). Cardiac catheterization is used mainly in diagnosing and evaluating congenital, rheumatic, and coronary artery lesions, including myocardial infarction. |
| cardiac enzyme studies
KĂR-dē-ăk ĔN-zīm | Tests that measure levels of enzymes and proteins in the blood that increase with an injury to heart muscle, such as from a heart attack

Cardiac enzyme studies help determine whether angina, shortness of breath, or abnormal electrocardiography results indicate a heart attack or imminent heart attack. |

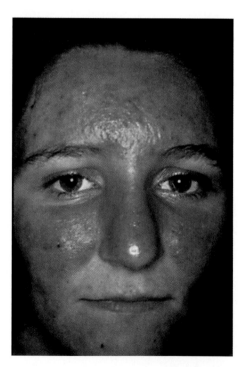

Figure 5-12 Butterfly rash of systemic lupus erythematosus.

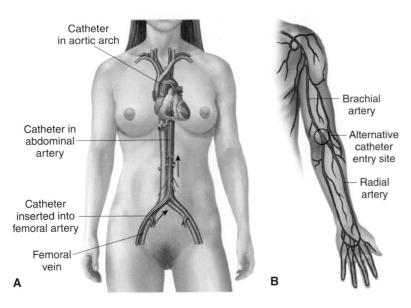

Catheter in aortic arch

Catheter in abdominal artery

Catheter inserted into femoral artery

Femoral vein

Brachial artery

Alternative catheter entry site

Radial artery

A

B

Figure 5-13 Cardiac catheterization. (**A**) Catheter insertion in femoral vein or artery. (**B**) Catheter insertion in brachial or radial artery.

echocardiography ĕk-ō-kăr-dē-ŎG-ră-fē *echo-:* a repeated sound *cardi/o:* heart *-graphy:* process of recording	Use of ultrasound to evaluate the heart and great vessels and diagnose cardiovascular lesions
electrocardiography (ECG, EKG) ē-lĕk-trō-kăr-dē-ŎG-ră-fē *electr/o:* electricity *cardi/o:* heart *-graphy:* process of recording	Creation and study of graphic records (electrocardiograms) produced by electric activity generated by the heart muscle; also called cardiography *A cardiologist analyzes an ECG, which is valuable in diagnosing cases of abnormal heart rhythm and myocardial damage.*
Holter monitor HŌL-ter MŎN-ĭ-tĕr	Device worn by a patient that records prolonged electrocardiograph readings (usually 24 hours) on a portable tape recorder while the patient conducts normal daily activities *Holter monitoring provides a record of cardiac arrhythmia that would not be discovered by means of an ECG of only a few minutes' duration. The patient keeps an activity diary to compare daily events with electrocardiographic tracings. (See Fig. 5–14.)*

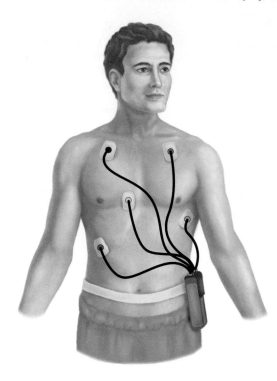

Figure 5-14 Holter monitor.

lipid panel LĬP-ĭd	Panel of blood tests measuring cholesterol components to assess the risk of heart disease *A lipid panel consists of total cholesterol, high-density lipoprotein (HDL), low-density lipoprotein (LDL), and triglycerides.*
stress test	Test in which an ECG is recorded under controlled exercise conditions (typically using a treadmill) to determine the heart's response to physical exertion (stress) *A stress test may show abnormal ECG tracings that do not appear during an ECG taken when the patient is resting.*
nuclear	Stress test that uses a radioisotope to evaluate coronary blood flow *In a nuclear stress test, the radioisotope is injected at the height of exercise. The area not receiving sufficient oxygen is visualized by decreased uptake of the isotope.*
troponin I TRŌ-pō-nĭn	Blood test that measures protein released into the blood by damaged heart muscle (not skeletal muscle) *The troponin I test is a highly sensitive and specific indicator of recent myocardial infarction (MI).*

ultrasonography (US) ŭl-tră-sŏn-ŎG-răf-ē 　*ultra-:* excess, beyond 　*son/o:* sound 　*-graphy:* process of 　　　　recording	Imaging technique in which a small transducer is passed over the skin to transmit high-frequency sound waves (ultrasound) that bounce off body tissues and are then recorded to produce an image of an internal organ or tissue
Doppler DŎP-lĕr	Ultrasonography used to assess blood flow through blood vessels and the heart *Doppler US detects alterations in blood flow caused by plaque or blood clots in arteries and veins. It is used to diagnose deep vein thrombosis (DVT), varicose veins, aneurysms, carotid artery occlusion, and other vessel abnormalities. (See Fig. 5–15.)*

Lymphatic System

bone marrow aspiration biopsy ăs-pĭ-RĀ-shŭn BĪ-ŏp-sē	Removal of living bone marrow tissue, usually taken from the sternum or iliac crest, for microscopic examination *Bone marrow aspiration biopsy evaluates hematopoiesis by revealing the number, shape, and size of red blood cells (RBCs), white blood cells (WBCs), and platelet precursors.*
ELISA	Blood test that detects antibodies in the blood, including screening for an antibody to the AIDS virus; also known as *enzyme-linked immunosorbent assay* *Positive outcome on the ELISA test indicates probable virus exposure and is confirmed with the Western blot test, which is more specific.*
lymphangiography lĭm-făn-jē-ŎG-ră-fē 　*lymph:* lymph 　*angi/o:* vessel (usually 　　　　blood or lymph) 　*-graphy:* process of 　　　　recording	Radiographic examination of lymph glands and lymphatic vessels after an injection of a contrast medium *Lymphangiography is used to show the path of lymph flow as it moves into the chest region.*

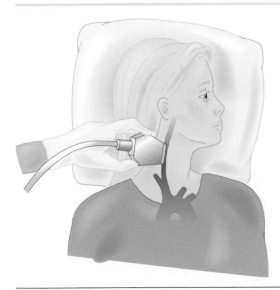

Figure 5-15 Doppler ultrasonography of the carotid artery.

| tissue typing | Technique used to determine the histocompatibility of tissues used in grafts and transplants with the recipient's tissues and cells; also known as histocompatibility testing |

Medical and Surgical Procedures

Cardiovascular System

angioplasty	Endovascular procedure (under x-ray visualization) that widens or opens blocked coronary arteries to restore blood flow to the heart muscle; also called *coronary angioplasty*
	This procedure is used to relieve chest pain caused by reduced blood flow to the heart and minimizes damage to heart muscle caused by a heart attack. A coronary artery stent may also be placed during angioplasty to prevent closure of a coronary artery from an atherosclerotic lesion.
percutaneous transluminal coronary angioplasty (PTCA) pĕr-kū-TĀ-nē-ŭs trăns-LŪ-mĭ-năl KOR-ō-nă-rē ĂN-jē-ō-plăs-tē	Angioplasty in which a balloon catheter is inserted and threaded through the femoral or radial artery into the blocked coronary artery that is narrowed because of atherosclerosis (See Fig. 6–16.)
	Once the catheter is in place, the balloon is inflated and compresses the plaque outward against the wall of the artery. This widens the artery and restores blood flow. Also called percutaneous coronary intervention (PCI).

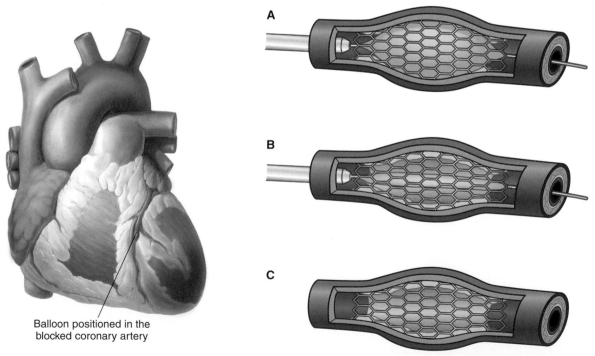

Balloon positioned in the blocked coronary artery

Figure 5-16 PTCA with stent placement. (**A**) Balloon inflated to widen the artery.
(**B**) Deflated balloon. (**C**) Stent remains to hold the artery open when catheter is removed.

cardioversion căr-dē-ō-VĔR-zhŭn *cardi/o:* heart *-version:* turning	Delivery of brief discharges of electricity that pass across the chest to stop a cardiac arrhythmia and restore normal sinus rhythm; also called *defibrillation* *A defibrillator is the electrical device used for cardioversion.*
coronary artery bypass graft (CABG)	Bypass surgery that creates new routes around narrowed or blocked arteries to allow sufficient blood flow to deliver oxygen and nutrients to the heart muscle; also called *coronary artery bypass surgery* (See Fig. 5–17.) *CABG is performed to relieve angina and reduce the risk of death from coronary artery disease. Arteries or veins from elsewhere in the patient's body are grafted to the coronary arteries to bypass atherosclerotic narrowings and improve blood supply to the coronary circulation supplying the myocardium.*
defibrillator dē-FĬB-rĭ-lā-tĕr	Device designed to administer a defibrillating electric shock to restore normal sinus rhythm *There are two types of defibrillators: automatic implantable cardioverter-defibrillators (AICDs) and automatic external defibrillators (AEDs).*
automatic implantable cardioverter-defibrillator (AICD) căr-dē-ō-VĔR-tĕr dē-FĬB-rĭ-lā-tĕr	Surgically implanted defibrillator that automatically detects and corrects potentially fatal arrhythmias, such as ventricular fibrillations; also called *implantable cardioverter-defibrillator (ICD)* (See Fig. 5–18.) *An AICD is implanted, usually in the chest, in a patient who is at high risk for developing a serious arrhythmia. It has leads (wires) that go to the heart, sense its rhythm, and deliver an electrical shock if needed.*
automatic external defibrillator (AED) dē-FĬB-rĭ-lā-tĕr	Portable computerized defibrillator that analyzes the patient's heart rhythm and delivers an electrical shock to stimulate a heart in cardiac arrest *An AED is kept on emergency response vehicles and in public places, such as recreation facilities, and is designed to be used by trained first-responder personnel or lay people.*

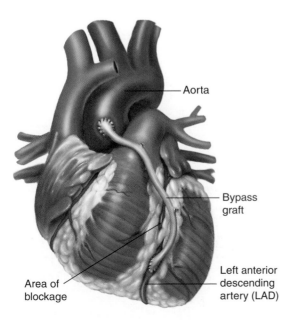

Figure 5-17 Coronary artery bypass graft (CABG).

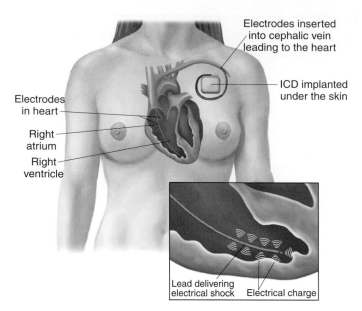

Electrodes inserted into cephalic vein leading to the heart

ICD implanted under the skin

Electrodes in heart

Right atrium

Right ventricle

Lead delivering electrical shock   Electrical charge

Figure 5-18 Automatic implantable cardioverter-defibrillator (AICD).

endarterectomy ĕnd-ăr-tĕr-ĔK-tō-mē *end-:* in, within *arter:* artery *-ectomy:* excision, removal	Surgical removal of the lining of an artery *Endarterectomy is performed on almost any major artery that is diseased or blocked, such as the carotid or femoral artery.*
carotid kă-RŎT-ĭd	Endarterectomy of an occluded carotid artery *Carotid endarterectomy reduces the risk of stroke when it is performed on a patient with moderate or severe stenoses of the artery, with or without a history of transient ischemic attacks (TIAs). (See Fig. 5–19.)*
sclerotherapy sklĕr-ō-THĔR-ă-pē *scler/o:* hardening; sclera (white of the eye) *-therapy:* treatment	Chemical injection into a varicose vein that causes inflammation and formation of fibrous tissue, which closes the vein *When a vein closes, it can no longer fill with blood. In a few weeks the treated varicose vein fades.*
valvuloplasty VĂL-vū-lō-plăs-tē *valvul/o:* valve *-plasty:* surgical repair	Plastic or restorative surgery on a heart valve to correct a prolapse or stenosis *A special type of valvuloplasty, called balloon valvuloplasty, involves insertion of a balloon catheter to open a stenotic heart valve. Inflation of the balloon decreases the constriction.*

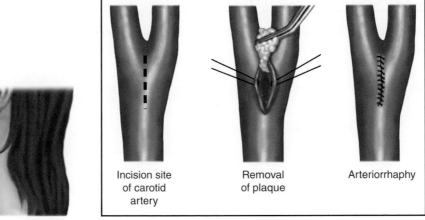

Neck incision

Incision site of carotid artery

Removal of plaque

Arteriorrhaphy

Figure 5-19 Carotid endarterectomy.

Lymphatic System

lymphangiectomy lĭm-făn-jē-ĔK-tō-mē *lymph:* lymph *angi:* vessel (usually blood or lymph) *-ectomy:* excision, removal	Removal of a lymph vessel
bone marrow transplant (BMT) BŌN MĂR-ō	Infusion (transplantation) of healthy bone marrow stem cells to stimulate blood cell production once the diseased bone marrow is destroyed by radiation or chemotherapy drugs *BMT is used to treat patients with leukemia and lymphoma. It can be autologous (from the patient's own bone marrow) or allogenic (from a compatible donor).*

PHARMACOLOGY

The following table lists some common drug categories used to treat cardiovascular and lymph disorders, as well as their therapeutic actions.

Drug Category	Action
Cardiovascular System	
anticoagulants ăn-tĭ-kō-ĂG-ū-lănts	Prevent blood clot formation *Anticoagulants decrease the risk of stroke and deep vein thrombosis and are also used postoperatively to prevent clot formation.*
antiarrhythmics ăn-tē-ă-RĬTH-mĭks	Counteract cardiac arrhythmias (dysrhythmias) by stabilizing the electrical conduction system of the heart
antihypertensives ăn-tē-hī-pĕr-TĔN-sĭvs	Treat hypertension (high blood pressure) *Antihypertensives prevent complications of high blood pressure, such as stroke and myocardial infarctions. There are many classes of antihypertensives that lower blood pressure by different means. Some of the most widely used include beta blockers, diuretics, and angiotensin-converting enzyme (ACE) inhibitors.*
beta blockers	Decrease heart rate and dilate arteries by blocking beta receptors *Beta blockers are used to treat angina, arrhythmias, and hypertension.*
diuretics dī-ū-RĔT-ĭks	Block sodium from being absorbed back into the blood *Diuretics reduce fluid buildup in the body, including fluid in the lungs, a common symptom of heart failure, by increasing secretion of urine. They are commonly prescribed in treating hypertension and heart failure.*
statins STĂ-tĭnz	Lower cholesterol levels in the blood and reduce its production in the liver by blocking the enzyme that produces it
thrombolytics thrŏm-bō-LĬT-ĭks	Dissolve blood clots and help prevent damage to the heart muscle; commonly called *clot busters* *Thrombolytics help manage stroke and may also stop a heart attack that would otherwise be deadly.*
Lymphatic System	
antivirals an-tĭ-VĪ-rălz	Inhibit development of specific viruses *Antivirals are used to treat HIV infection and AIDS.*
immunosuppressants ĭm-ū-nō-sū-PRĔSS-ănts	Suppress the immune response to prevent organ rejection after transplantation or to slow the progression of autoimmune disease

Pronunciation Help	Long sound	ā in rāte	ē in rēbirth	ī in īsle	ō in ōver	ū in ūnite
	Short sound	ă in ălone	ĕ in ĕver	ĭ in ĭt	ŏ in nŏt	ŭ in cŭt

ADDITIONAL MEDICAL TERMS REVIEW

Match the medical term(s) below with the definitions in the numbered list.

AIDS	embolus	ischemia	statins
arrhythmia	fibrillation	lymphadenitis	thrombolytics
atherosclerosis	HF	lymphangiography	tissue typing
bruit	Hodgkin disease	mononucleosis	troponin I
CABG	Holter monitor	Raynaud phenomenon	valvuloplasty
Doppler US	hypertension	rheumatic heart disease	varicose veins
DVT			

1. _____ are swollen, distended veins most commonly seen in the lower legs.

2. _____ is an acute infection caused by Epstein-Barr virus (EBV) and characterized by a sore throat, fever, fatigue, and enlarged lymph nodes.

3. _____ are drugs that dissolve a blood clot.

4. _____ is a mass of undissolved matter present in a blood vessel.

5. _____ is inflammation and enlargement of the lymph nodes.

6. _____ refers to formation of a blood clot in a deep vein of the body.

7. _____ refers to blood pressure that is consistently higher than normal.

8. _____ is irregularity or loss of heart rhythm.

9. _____ are drugs used to lower blood cholesterol levels.

10. _____ is a soft, blowing sound caused by turbulent blood flow.

11. _____ is used to detect blood flow impairment caused by plaque or blood clots in arteries and veins.

12. _____ is a streptococcal infection that causes damage to heart valves and heart muscle.

13. _____ is heart disease caused by an accumulation of fatty substances within the arterial walls.

14. _____ is a small portable device worn on a patient during normal activity to obtain a record of cardiac arrhythmia.

15. _____ is numbness in fingers or toes due to intermittent constriction of arterioles in the skin.

16. _____ is a temporary oxygen deficiency due to an interruption of blood flow to a tissue or organ.

17. _____ refers to malignant solid tumors of the lymphatic system.

18. _____ is a transmissible infection caused by human immunodeficiency virus (HIV).

19. _____ is a condition in which the ability of the heart to pump blood is impaired.

20. _____ means irregular, random contraction of heart fibers.

21. _____ refers to plastic or restorative surgery on a valve, especially a cardiac valve.

22. _____ is a radiographic examination of lymph glands and lymphatic vessels after an injection of a contrast medium.

23. _____ is also known as histocompatibility testing.

24. _____ refers to a blood test that measures protein released into the blood by damaged heart muscle.

25. _____ refers to bypassing one or more blocked coronary arteries to restore blood flow.

Competency Verification: Check your answers in Appendix B: Answer Key, page 575. If you are not satisfied with your level of comprehension, review the additional medical terms and retake the review.

Correct Answers _____ × 4 = _____ % Score

MEDICAL RECORD ACTIVITIES

The following medical reports reflect common, real-life clinical scenarios using medical terminology to document patient care.

MEDICAL RECORD ACTIVITY 5-1

MYOCARDIAL INFARCTION

Terminology

Terms listed in the table below come from the medical report Myocardial Infarction that follows. Use a medical dictionary such as Taber's Cyclopedic Medical Dictionary, *the appendices of this book, or other resources to define each term. Then practice reading the pronunciations aloud for each term.*

Term	Definition
apnea ĂP-nē-ă	
desiccated DĔS-ĭ-kā-tĕd	
dyspnea DĬSP-nē-ă	
fibrillation fĭ-brĭl-Ā-shŭn	
malaise mă-LĀZ	
myocardial infarction mī-ō-KĂR-dē-ăl ĭn-FĂRK-shŭn	

Term	Definition
ST segment–T wave	
syncope SĬN-kō-pē	
tachycardia tăk-ē-KĂR-dē-ă	

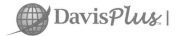 Visit the *Medical Terminology Simplified* online resource center at Davis*Plus* to hear pronunciation and meanings of the selected terms in this medical report listed in the table above.

Reading

Practice pronunciation of medical terms by reading the following medical report aloud.

Myocardial Infarction

A 70-year-old white woman presented to the hospital for evaluation of a syncopal episode. She states that most recently she has experienced generalized malaise, increased shortness of breath while at rest, and dyspnea followed by periods of apnea and syncope.

Her past history includes recurrent episodes of thyroiditis, which led her to have a thyroidectomy 6 years ago while she was under the care of Dr. Knopp. At the time of surgery, the results of her ECG were interpreted as sinus tachycardia with nonspecific ST segment–T wave changes. The tachycardia was attributed to preoperative anxiety and thyroiditis. Postoperatively, under the direction of Dr. Knopp, the patient was treated with a daily dose of 50 mg of desiccated thyroid and has been symptom free until this admission.

On clinical examination, the patient's radial pulse was found to be irregular, and the ECG showed uncontrolled atrial fibrillation with evidence of a recent myocardial infarction.

Evaluation

Review the medical record to answer the following questions. Use a medical dictionary such as Taber's Cyclopedic Medical Dictionary *and other resources if needed.*

   1. What symptoms did the patient experience before admission to the hospital?

      _____

      _____

   2. What was found during clinical examination?

      _____

      _____

   3. What is the danger of atrial fibrillation?

      _____

      _____

4. Did the patient have a prior history of heart problems? If so, describe them.

_____

_____

5. Was the patient's prior heart problem related to her current one?

_____

_____

MEDICAL RECORD ACTIVITY 5-2

CARDIAC CATHETERIZATION

Terminology

Terms listed in the table below come from the medical report Cardiac Catheterization that follows. Use a medical dictionary such as Taber's Cyclopedic Medical Dictionary, _the appendices of this book, or other resources to define each term. Then practice reading the pronunciations aloud for each term._

Term	Definition
angiography ăn-jē-ŎG-ră-fē	
angioplasty ĂN-jē-ō-plăs-tē	
catheter KĂTH-ĕ-tĕr	
heparin HĔP-ă-rĭn	
lidocaine LĪ-dō-kān	
sheath SHĒTH	
ST elevations	
stenosis stĕ-NŌ-sĭs	

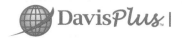

Visit the *Medical Terminology Simplified* online resource center at Davis*Plus* to hear pronunciation and meanings of the selected terms in this medical report listed in the table above.

Reading

Practice pronunciation of medical terms by reading the following medical report aloud.

Cardiac Catheterization

PROCEDURE: Patient was prepared and draped in a sterile fashion and 20 mL of 1% lidocaine was infiltrated into the right groin. A No. 6 French Cordis right femoral arterial sheath was placed and a No. 6 French JL-5 and JR-4 catheter was used to engage the left and right coronary. A No. 6 French pigtail was used for left ventricular angiography. Angioplasty was performed, and further dictation is under the angioplasty report. There were minor irregularities, with a maximal 25% stenosis just after the first diagonal. The remainder of the vessel was free of significant disease.

A 0.014, high-torque, floppy, extra support, exchange-length wire was used to cross the stenosis in the distal right coronary artery. A 3.5 × 20–mm Track Star balloon was inflated in the right coronary artery in the distal portion. The initial stenosis was 50% to 75% with an ulcerated plaque, and the final stenosis was 20% with no significant clot seen in the region. The patient had significant ST elevations in the inferior leads and severe throat tightness and shortness of breath. This would resolve immediately with the inflation of the balloon. The catheters were removed, and the sheath was changed to a No. 8 French Arrow sheath. The patient will be on heparin over the next 12 hours.

IMPRESSION: 1. Two-vessel coronary artery disease with a 75% obtuse marginal and a 75% right coronary artery lesion.
2. Normal left ventricular function.
3. Successful angioplasty to right coronary artery with initial stenosis of 75% and a final stenosis of 20%.

Evaluation

Review the medical record to answer the following questions. Use a medical dictionary such as Taber's Cyclopedic Medical Dictionary *and other resources if needed.*

1. What coronary arteries were under examination?

_____

_____

2. Which surgical procedure was used to clear the stenosis?

_____

3. What symptoms did the patient exhibit before balloon inflation?

_____

_____

4. Why was the patient put on heparin?

_____

_____

CARDIOVASCULAR AND LYMPHATIC SYSTEMS CHAPTER REVIEW

WORD ELEMENTS SUMMARY

The following table summarizes CFs, suffixes, and prefixes related to the cardiovascular and lymphatic systems. Study the word elements and their meanings before completing the Word Elements Chapter Review that follows.

Word Element	Meaning	Word Element	Meaning
Combining Forms			
aden/o	gland	lymph/o	lymph
aneurysm/o	a widening, a widened blood vessel	my/o	muscle
angi/o	vessel (usually blood or lymph)	necr/o	death, necrosis
aort/o	aorta	phleb/o, ven/o	vein
arteri/o	artery	rrhythm/o	rhythm
ather/o	fatty plaque	sarc/o	flesh (connective tissue)
atri/o	atrium	scler/o	hardening; sclera (white of the eye)
cardi/o, coron/o	heart	thromb/o	blood clot
cerebr/o	cerebrum	varic/o	dilated vein
embol/o	embolus (plug)	vas/o	vessel; vas deferens; duct
hem/o	blood	vascul/o	vessel
isch/o	to hold back: block	ventricul/o	ventricle (of the heart or brain)
Suffixes			
-al, -ic, -ary	pertaining to, relating to	-pathy	disease
-cardia	heart condition	-phagia	swallowing, eating
-cyte	cell	-phobia	fear
-ectasis	dilation, expansion	-phylaxis	protection
-ectomy	excision, removal	-plasty	surgical repair
-emia	blood	-pnea	breathing
-genesis	forming, producing, origin	-poiesis	formation, production
-gram	record, writing	-rrhaphy	suture
-graphy	process of recording	-rrhexis	rupture
-ia	condition	-spasm	involuntary contraction, twitching
-lith	stone, calculus	-stenosis	narrowing, stricture
-lysis	separation; destruction; loosening	-tension	to stretch
-malacia	softening	-therapy	treatment
-megaly	enlargement	-tomy	incision
-oid	resembling	-um	structure, thing
-ole, -ule	small, minute	-us	condition, structure

Word Element	Meaning	Word Element	Meaning
-oma	tumor	-version	turning
-osis	abnormal condition; increase (used primarily with blood cells)		
Prefixes			
a-	without, not	epi-	above, upon
anti-	against	micro-	small
bi-	two	peri-	around
brady-	slow	tachy-	rapid
echo-	a repeated sound	trans-	across, through
endo-	in, within	tri-	three

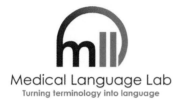

Medical Language Lab
Turning terminology into language

Visit the *Medical Language Lab* at the website *medicallanguagelab.com*. Use the flash-card exercise for this chapter to reinforce your study of word elements. We recommend you complete the flash-card exercise before starting the Word Elements Chapter Review that follows.

WORD ELEMENTS CHAPTER REVIEW

This review provides a verification of your knowledge of the word elements covered in this chapter. Write the meaning of the word element in the space provided. To reinforce your understanding of the word parts that comprise a medical term, identify each word element as a prefix (P), word root (WR), combining form (CF), or suffix (S). The first word is completed for you.

Medical Term	Word Element	Meaning
1. agglutin/ation	*agglutin (WR)*	*clumping, gluing*
	-ation (S)	*process of*
2. ana/phylaxis		
3. aneurysm/o/rrhaphy		
4. a/rrhythm/ia		

Medical Term	Word Element	Meaning
5. arteri/o/scler/osis		
6. ather/oma		
7. atri/o/ventricul/ar		
8. echo/cardi/o/graphy		

Continued

Medical Term	Word Element	Meaning
9. electr/o/cardi/o/gram		
10. embol/us		
11. hem/o/rrhage		
12. hyper/tension		
13. immun/o/gen		
14. isch/emia		

Medical Term	Word Element	Meaning
15. lymph/aden/itis		
16. lymph/angi/oma		
17. phag/o/cyte		
18. phleb/o/stenosis		
19. splen/o/megaly		

Continued

Medical Term	Word Element	Meaning
20. tachy/cardia		
21. thromb/o/genesis		
22. thyroid/ectomy		
23. ultra/son/o/graphy		
24. valv/o/tomy		

Medical Term	Word Element	Meaning
25. varic/ose		

Competency Verification: Check your answers in Appendix B: Answer Key page 576. If you are not satisfied with your level of comprehension, review the chapter's flash-card exercise at *medicallanguagelab.com* and retake the review.

Correct Answers _____ × 4 = _____ % Score

VOCABULARY REVIEW

Match the medical term(s) with the definitions in the numbered list.

agglutination	arteriosclerosis	ECG	pacemaker
anaphylaxis	capillaries	hemangioma	phagocyte
aneurysm	cardiomegaly	malaise	statins
angina pectoris	desiccated	MI	systole
arterioles	diastole	myocardium	tachypnea

1. _____ refers to the muscular layer of the heart.

2. _____ means rapid breathing.

3. _____ is a disease characterized by an abnormal hardening of the arteries.

4. _____ is a cell that engulfs and digests cellular debris.

5. _____ refers to the contraction phase of the heart.

6. _____ refers to the relaxation phase of the heart.

7. _____ is a record of the electrical impulses of the heart.

8. _____ means a vague feeling of bodily discomfort, which may be the first indication of an infection or disease.

9. _____ means dried thoroughly; rendered free from moisture.

10. _____ means enlarged heart.

11. _____ refers to weakness in the vessel wall that balloons and eventually bursts.

12. _____ is severe pain and constriction about the heart caused by an insufficient supply of oxygenated blood to the heart.

13. _____ is necrosis of an area of muscular heart tissue after cessation of blood supply.

14. _____ is a process of cells clumping together.

15. _____ are used to lower cholesterol levels in the blood.

16. _____ is an allergic reaction characterized by a rapid decrease in blood pressure.

17. _____ are the smallest vessels of the circulatory system.

18. _____ is a tumor composed of blood vessels.

19. _____ are small arteries.

20. _____ maintains primary responsibility for initiating the heartbeat.

Competency Verification: Check your answers in Appendix B: Answer Key, page 578. If you are not satisfied with your level of comprehension, review the chapter vocabulary and retake the review.

Correct Answers _____ × 5 = _____ % Score

Digestive System

OBJECTIVES

Upon completion of this chapter, you will be able to:

- Describe the type of medical treatment the gastroenterologist provides.
- Identify digestive structures by labeling them on anatomical illustrations.
- Describe the primary functions of the digestive system.
- Describe diseases, conditions, and procedures related to the digestive system.
- Apply your word-building skills by constructing medical terms related to the digestive system.
- Describe common abbreviations and symbols related to the digestive system.
- Recognize, define, pronounce, and spell terms correctly.
- Demonstrate your knowledge of this chapter by successfully completing the frames, reviews, and medical report evaluations.

MEDICAL SPECIALTY

Gastroenterology

Medical doctors who treat diseases and disorders of the **digestive system,** also called *gastrointestinal (GI) system,* are known as **gastroenterologists.** Various diagnostic procedures are employed to evaluate and treat disorders of the GI system. One of which is a commonly used diagnostic procedure known as **endoscopy.** This procedure involves the use of a flexible lighted instrument to examine the organs of the digestive system and is effectively used to inspect the esophagus, stomach, intestines, and bile ducts. Endoscopy has made it possible to identify various pathological conditions, including cancers, at an early stage. In addition to endoscopy, imaging procedures, blood tests, and tissue biopsies help establish or verify the initial diagnosis.

ANATOMY AND PHYSIOLOGY OVERVIEW

The primary function of the digestive system is to break down food, prepare it for absorption, and eliminate waste substances. The digestive system consists of a digestive tube, called the **GI tract** or **alimentary canal.** It includes the esophagus, stomach, intestines, and several accessory organs: the liver, gallbladder, and pancreas. The GI tract, extending from the oral cavity (mouth) to the anus, varies in size and structure in several distinct regions. It terminates at the anus, where solid wastes are eliminated from the body by means of defecation. (See Fig. 6–1.)

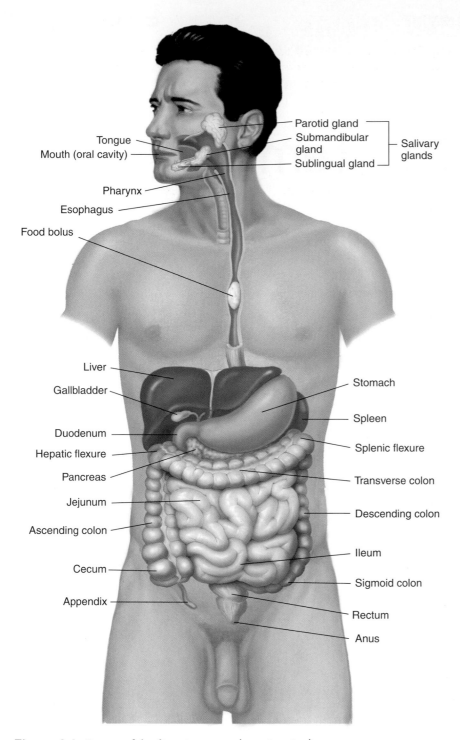

Figure 6-1 Organs of the digestive system (anterior view).

WORD ELEMENTS

This section introduces combining forms (CFs) related to the oral cavity, esophagus, pharynx, and stomach. Included are key suffixes; prefixes are defined in the right-hand column as needed. Review the following table and pronounce each word in the word analysis column aloud before you begin to work the frames.

Word Element	Meaning	Word Analysis
Combining Forms Oral Cavity		

dent/o
 	
odont/o
	teeth	**dent**/ist (DĔN-tĭst): specialist who diagnoses and treats diseases and disorders of the oral cavity (teeth and gums)
		   -ist: specialist
		orth/**odont**/ist (ŏr-thō-DŎN-tĭst): dental specialist in prevention and correction of abnormally positioned or misaligned teeth
		   orth: straight
		    -ist: specialist

gingiv/o	gum(s)	**gingiv**/itis (jĭn-jĭ-VĪ-tĭs): inflammation of the gums *-itis:* inflammation

gloss/o
 	
lingu/o
	tongue	hypo/**gloss**/al (hī-pō-GLŎS-ăl): pertaining to under the tongue
		   hypo-: under, below, deficient
		    -al: pertaining to
		sub/**lingu**/al (sŭb-LĬNG-gwăl): pertaining to under the tongue
		   sub-: under, below
		    -al: pertaining to

or/o
 	
stomat/o
	mouth	**or**/al (OR-ăl): pertaining to the mouth
		   -al: pertaining to
		stomat/o/pathy (stō-mă-TŎP-ă-thē): disease of the mouth
		   -pathy: disease

ptyal/o	saliva	**ptyal**/ism (TĪ-ă-lĭzm): condition of excessive salivation *-ism:* condition
sial/o	saliva, salivary gland	**sial**/o/rrhea (sī-ă-lō-RĒ-ă): excessive flow of saliva; also called *hypersalivation* or *ptyalism* *-rrhea:* discharge, flow
Esophagus, Pharynx, and Stomach		
esophag/o	esophagus	**esophag**/o/scope (ē-SŎF-ă-gō-skōp): instrument for examining the esophagus *-scope:* instrument for examining

pharyng/o	pharynx (throat)	**pharyng**/o/tonsill/itis (fă-rĭng-gō-tŏn-sĭ-LĪ-tĭs): inflammation of the pharynx and tonsils
		   tonsill: tonsils
		    -itis: inflammation

gastr/o	stomach	**gastr**/o/scopy (găs-TRŎS-kō-pē): visual examination of the stomach *-scopy:* visual examination *A gastroscope is a flexible, fiber-optic instrument used to inspect the interior of the stomach.*
pylor/o	pylorus	**pylor**/o/tomy (pī-lor-ŎT-ō-mē): incision of the pylorus (sphincter in the lower portion of the stomach) *-tomy:* incision *Pylorotomy is usually performed to remove an obstruction.*

Continued

Word Element	Meaning	Word Analysis
Suffixes		
-algia	pain	gastr/**algia** (găs-TRĂL-jē-ă): pain in the stomach *gastr:* stomach
-dynia		gastr/o/**dynia** (găs-trō-DĬN-ē-ă): pain in the stomach *gastr/o:* stomach
-emesis	vomiting	hyper/**emesis** (hī-pĕr-ĔM-ĕ-sĭs): excessive vomiting *hyper-:* excessive, above normal
-megaly	enlargement	gastr/o/**megaly** (găs-trō-MĔG-ă-lē): enlargement of the stomach *gastr/o:* stomach
-orexia	appetite	an/**orexia** (ăn-ō-RĔK-sē-ă): loss of appetite *an-:* without, not *Anorexia can result from various conditions, such as adverse effects of medication, as well as other physical or psychological causes.*
-pepsia	digestion	dys/**pepsia** (dĭs-PĔP-sē-ă): difficult or painful digestion; also called *indigestion* *dys-:* bad; painful; difficult *Dyspepsia is a feeling of epigastric discomfort after eating.*
-phagia	swallowing, eating	dys/**phagia** (dĭs-FĀ-jē-ă): difficulty swallowing or eating *dys-:* bad; painful; difficult
-rrhea	discharge, flow	dia/**rrhea** (dī-ă-RĔ-ă): discharge or flow of watery stools from the bowel *dia-:* through, across

Pronunciation Help	Long sound	ā in rāte	ē in rēbirth	ī in īsle	ō in ōver	ū in ūnite
	Short sound	ă in ălone	ĕ in ĕver	ĭ in ĭt	ŏ in nŏt	ŭ in cŭt

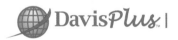

Visit the *Medical Terminology Simplified* online resource center at Davis*Plus* for an audio exercise of the terms in this table. It will help you master pronunciations and meanings of medical terms.

SECTION REVIEW 6-1

For the following medical terms, first write the suffix and its meaning. Then translate the meaning of the remaining elements starting with the first part of the word. The first word is completed for you.

Term	Meaning
1. gingiv/itis	-itis: inflammation; gum(s)
2. dys/pepsia	
3. pylor/o/tomy	
4. dent/ist	
5. esophag/o/scope	
6. gastr/o/scopy	
7. dia/rrhea	
8. hyper/emesis	
9. an/orexia	
10. sub/lingu/al	

Competency Verification: Check your answers in Appendix B: Answer Key, page 578. If you are not satisfied with your level of comprehension, review the word elements tables and retake the review.

Correct Answers _____ × 10 = _____ % Score

UPPER GI TRACT

The upper GI tract consists of the oral cavity, esophagus, pharynx, and stomach.

Oral Cavity

6-1   Label the structures in Figure 6–2 as you read the material in the following frames. Chemical and mechanical processes of digestion begin in the (1) **oral cavity** (mouth) when food is chewed to make it easier to swallow.

---

stomat/o

or/o

6-2   The CFs for the mouth are *or/o* and *stomat/o.*

From stomat/itis, construct the CF for *mouth:* _____ / _____

From or/al, construct the CF for *mouth:* _____ / _____

stomat/itis stō-mă-TĪ-tĭs	**6-3** The suffix *-itis* refers to *inflammation*. It is used in all body systems to describe an inflammation of a particular organ. Use **stomat/o** to form a word that means *inflammation of the mouth*. _____ / _____
pain, mouth **pain, mouth**	**6-4** The suffixes *-dynia* and *-algia* refer to *pain*. Stomat/o/dynia is a _____ in the _____. Stomat/algia is a _____ in the _____.
combining form *or* combining vowel	**6-5** The suffixes *-dynia* and *-algia* are used interchangeably. Because *-algia* begins with a vowel, use a word root to link the suffix. Because *-dynia* begins with a consonant, use a _____ _____ to link the suffix.
stomat/o/dynia, stomat/algia stō-mă-tō-DĬN-ē-ă, stō-mă-TĂL-jē-ă	**6-6** Use **stomat/o** to develop a word that means *pain in the mouth*. _____ / _____ / _____ *or* _____ / _____
	6-7 There are three pairs of salivary glands: the (2) **sublingual gland**, the (3) **submandibular gland**, and the (4) **parotid gland.** The salivary glands, whose primary function is to secrete saliva into the oral cavity, are richly supplied with blood vessels and nerves. Label the salivary glands in Figure 6–2.
sial/o	**6-8** During the chewing process, salivary secretions begin the chemical breakdown of food. The CF **sial/o** means *saliva, salivary glands*. From sial/ic, which means *pertaining to saliva*, construct the CF for *saliva or salivary gland*. _____ / _____
sial/itis sī-ă-LĪ-tĭs	**6-9** Use **sial/o** + *-itis* to form a word that means *inflammation of a salivary gland*. _____ / _____
-rrhea	**6-10** The suffix *-rrhea* is used in words to mean *discharge* or *flow*. From sial/o/rrhea, write the element that means *discharge, flow*. _____

Boldface indicates a word root or combining form. Blue indicates a suffix. Pink indicates a prefix.

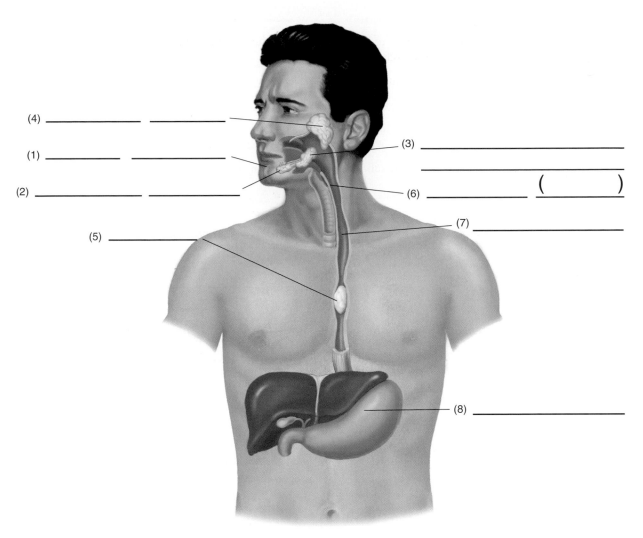

(4) _____ _____

(1) _____ _____

(2) _____ _____

(5) _____

(3) _____

_____

(6) _____ (_____)

(7) _____

(8) _____

Figure 6-2 Upper GI tract.

saliva	**6–11** Sial/o/rrhea, more commonly called ptyal/ism or hyper/salivation, refers to *excessive secretion of saliva.* Analyze sial/o/rrhea by defining the elements:
flow	The CF *sial/o* refers to *salivary glands* or _____.
saliva	The suffix *-rrhea* refers to *discharge* or _____.
condition	The CF *ptyal/o* refers to _____.
	The suffix *-ism* refers to _____.
tongue	**6–12** The CF *lingu/o* means *tongue.* The prefix *sub-* means *under.* Sub/lingu/al means *pertaining to under or below the* _____.
jaw	**6–13** The CF *maxill/o* means *jaw.* Sub/maxill/ary is a directional term that means *under the* _____.

below below above	**6–14** Refer to Figure 6–1 and use the directional terms below or above to complete this frame. The sub/lingu/al gland is located _____ the tongue. The sub/mandibul/ar gland is located _____ the parotid gland. The tongue is located _____ the esophagus.
lingu/o	**6–15** From sub/lingu/al, construct the CF for tongue. _____ / _____
abnormal condition, mouth	**6–16** The suffix *-osis* means *abnormal condition, increase (used primarily with blood cells)*. Stomat/osis literally means _____ _____ of the _____.
myc	**6–17** Stomat/o/myc/osis is an *abnormal condition of a mouth fungus*. From stomat/o/myc/osis, identify the root that means *fungus*. _____
abnormal condition, fungus	**6–18** Myc/osis literally means _____ _____ of a _____.
abnormal condition fungus	**6–19** Whenever you see *-osis* in a word, you will know it means _____ _____ *or increase (used primarily with blood cells)*. Whenever you see *myc/o* in a word, you will know it refers to a _____.
myc/osis mī-KŌS-sĭs	**6–20** Two types of mycoses are athlete's foot and thrush. Change the plural form *mycoses* to its singular form. _____ / _____
-logist	**6–21** The CF *log/o* means *study of*. Combine *log/o* and *-ist* to form a new suffix that means *specialist in study of*. _____

gastr/o/logist găs-TRŎL-ō-jĭst **enter/o/logist** ĕn-tĕr-ŎL-ō-jĭst **gastr/o/enter/o/logist** găs-trō-ĕn-tĕr-ŎL-ō-jĭst	**6-22** Recall that *-logist* means *specialist in the study of.* The gastr/o/logist, enter/o/logist, and gastr/o/enter/o/logist are medical specialists who diagnose and treat digestive disorders. Build medical words that mean *specialist who treats* *stomach disorders:* _____ / _____ / _____ *intestin/al disorders:* _____ / _____ / _____ *stomach and intestin/al disorders:* _____ / _____ / _____ / _____ / _____
gastr/o/logy găs-TRŎL-ō-jē **gastr/o/enter/o/logist** găs-trō-ĕn-tĕr-ŎL-ō-jĭst	**6-23** Use *-logy* or *-logist* to form medical words that mean *study of the stomach:* _____ / _____ / _____ *specialist in the study of stomach and intestines:* _____ / _____ / _____ / _____ / _____
gastr/o/logist găs-TRŎL-ō-jĭst	**6-24** The specialist who diagnoses and treats stomach disorders is a _____ / _____ / _____.
bowel movement **fasting blood sugar** **diagnosis** dī-ăg-NŌ-sĭs **gastr/o/intestin/al** găs-trō-ĭn-TĔS-tĭn-ăl	**6-25** Standardized abbreviations are commonly used in medical reports and insurance claims. Abbreviations are summarized at the end of each chapter and in Appendix E: Abbreviations, page 613. If needed, use one of those references to complete this frame. BM: _____ _____ FBS: _____ _____ _____ Dx: _____ GI: _____ / _____ / _____ / _____
dent/o, odont/o	**6-26** Most of us take our teeth for granted. We do not think about the important mechanical function they perform in the first step of the digestive process—breaking food down into smaller pieces. The CFs for teeth are _____ / _____ and _____ / _____.
teeth, gums, diagnosis dī-ăg-NŌ-sĭs	**6-27** A dent/ist specializes in the prevention, Dx, and treatment of diseases of the teeth and gums. Dentistry is the branch of medicine dealing with the care of the _____ and _____. The abbreviation *Dx* means _____.
pain, tooth **odont/algia** ō-dŏn-TĂL-jē-ă	**6-28** Odont/algia literally means _____ in a _____. A toothache is another word for odont/o/dynia or _____ / _____.

specialist, teeth	**6–29** An orth/odont/ist is a *dent/al specialist who corrects abnormal position and misalignment of the teeth.* *Orth/o* means *straight.* Orth/odont/ist literally means _____ *in* straight _____.
odont **orth** **-ist**	**6–30** From orth/odont/ist, determine the root for *teeth:* _____ root for *straight:* _____ element that means *specialist:* _____
orth/odont/ist ŏr-thō-DŎN-tĭst	**6–31** Being fitted for braces to straighten teeth requires a dent/al specialist known as an _____ / _____ / _____.
specialist **around** **teeth**	**6–32** Another dent/al specialist, the peri/odont/ist, treats abnormal conditions of tissues surrounding the teeth, including the gums and bones. (Use Appendix A: Glossary of Medical Word Elements on page 548 whenever you need help to work the frames.) The suffix *-ist* refers to _____. The prefix *peri-* refers to _____. The root **odont** refers to _____.
gingiv/o	**6–33** Gingiv/itis, a general term for *inflammation of the gums,* is usually caused by accumulation of food particles in crevices between the gums and teeth. From gingiv/itis, construct the CF for gums. _____ / _____
gingiv/itis jĭn-jĭ-VĪ-tĭs	**6–34** Form a word that means *inflammation of the gums.* _____ / _____
inflammation, teeth **inflammation, gums**	**6–35** Primary symptoms of gingiv/itis are bleeding gums. This condition can lead to a more serious disorder, peri/odont/itis. Gingiv/itis is best prevented by correct brushing of teeth and proper gum care. Peri/odont/itis is an _____ *around the* _____. Gingiv/itis means _____ *of the* _____.

Esophagus, Pharynx, and Stomach

6–36   Continue labeling Figure 6–2 as you read the material in this frame. After food is chewed, it is formed into a round, sticky mass called a (5) **bolus.** The bolus is pushed by the tongue into the (6) **pharynx (throat),** where it begins its descent down the (7) **esophagus** to the (8) **stomach.**

Boldface indicates a word root or combining form. Blue indicates a suffix. Pink indicates a prefix.

pharyng/itis **pharyng/o/dynia or pharyng/algia** fă-RĬNG-gō-dĭn-ē-ă, făr-ĭn-GĂL-jē-ă	**6-37** The funnel-shaped pharynx serves as a passageway to the respiratory and GI tracts and provides a resonating chamber for speech sounds. Use the CF **pharyng/o** (throat) to construct words that mean *inflammation of the throat:* _____ / _____ *pain in the throat:* _____ / _____ / _____ or _____ / _____
peristalsis pĕr-ĭ-STĂL-sĭs	**6-38** Food is propelled through the GI tract by coordinated, rhythmic muscle contractions called peristalsis. (See Fig. 6–1.) The bolus is transported to the stomach by involuntary muscle contractions known as _____.
	6-39 Gastr/ic juices in the stomach coupled with mechanical churning turn the bolus into a semiliquid mass called chyme. The chyme slowly leaves the stomach and continues the process of digestion as it enters the first part of the small intestine (duodenum). Review Figure 6–1 to follow the digestive path of the bolus as it enters the duodenum.

Competency Verification: Check your labeling of Figure 6–2 with the answers in Appendix B: Answer Key, page 578.

esophag/eal, **gastr/ic** ē-sŏf-ă-JĒ-ăl, GĂS-trĭk	**6-40** Peptic ulcer disease (PUD) is a condition in which the lining of the esophagus, stomach, or duodenum is eroded, usually from infection with *Helicobacter pylori* bacteria. Ulcers are named by their location: esophag/eal, gastr/ic, or duoden/al. Peptic ulcers that occur in the small intestine are called duoden/al ulcers; peptic ulcers that occur in the esophagus are called _____ / _____ ulcers; peptic ulcers that occur in the stomach are called _____ / _____ ulcers.
muc/oid MŪ-koyd **muc/ous** MŪ-kŭs	**6-41** The erosion in the lining of the esophagus, stomach, and duodenum in PUD can also be due to an increase in the concentration of hydrochloric acid and pepsin. As a result, the damaged mucosa is unable to secrete enough mucus to act as a barrier against the acid, which, combined with hypersecretion of acid, creates a large amount of acid moving into the duodenum. As a result, peptic ulcers occur more commonly in the duodenum. Use **muc/o** to build a term meaning *resembling mucus:* _____ / _____ *pertaining to mucus:* _____ / _____
gastr/itis, peptic ulcer disease găs-TRĪ-tĭs	**6-42** Gastr/ic ulcers may cause severe pain and inflammation of the stomach. A medical term that means *inflammation of the stomach* is _____ / _____. PUD is the abbreviation for _____ _____ _____.
gastr/algia găs-TRĂL-jē-ă	**6-43** Gastr/o/dynia is the medical term for *pain in the stomach*. Another term that means *pain in the stomach* is _____ / _____.

stomach	**6–44** Gastr/o/megaly and megal/o/gastr/ia mean *enlargement of the* _____.
megal/o/gastr/ic mĕg-ă-lō-GĂS-trĭk	**6–45** In megal/o/gastr/ia, the suffix *-ia* is a noun ending that denotes a condition. Use *-ic* to change this word to an adjective. _____ / _____ / _____ / _____
endo/scopy ĕn-DŎS-kō-pē	**6–46** Endo/scopy is a *visual examination of a hollow organ or cavity using a rigid or flexible fiber-optic tube and lighted optical system.* The term in this frame that means *visual examination in or within (an organ)* is _____ / _____.
duoden/o/scopy dū-ŏd-ĕ-NŎS-kō-pē	**6–47** An endo/scope is used to perform endo/scopy. The organ being examined dictates the name of the endoscop/ic procedure. For example, visual examination of the esophagus is known as esophag/o/scopy, of the stomach is gastr/o/scopy, and of the duodenum is duoden/o/scopy. Endo/scopy is performed for bi/opsy, aspirating fluids, and coagulating bleeding areas. A laser can also be passed through the endo/scope for endoscopic surgeries. A camera or video recorder is commonly used during endo/scop/ic procedures to provide a permanent record of the findings. When the physician examines the duodenum, the endoscopic procedure is called _____ / _____ / _____.
esophag/o/scopy ē-sŏf-ă-GŎS-kō-pē	**6–48** Gastr/o/scopy is a *visual examination of the stomach.* Build another term with *-scopy* that means *visual examination of the esophagus.* _____ / _____ / _____.
esophag/o/gastr/o/ **duoden/o/scopy** ĕ-SŎF-ă-gō-găs-trō-dū- ŏd-ĕ-NŎS-kō-pē	**6–49** Upper GI endoscopy, also referred to as EGD, includes visualization of the esophagus, stomach, and duodenum. Use Appendix E, page 615, to define EGD. _____ / _____ / _____ / _____ / _____ / _____ / _____.
gastr/ectomy găs-TRĔK-tō-mē	**6–50** Surgery is the branch of medicine concerned with diseases and trauma requiring an operative procedure. Surgery to remove all or part of the stomach is called _____ / _____.
esophag/o/plasty ē-SŎF-ă-gō-plăs-tē **gastr/o/plasty** GĂS-trō-plăs-tē	**6–51** Form medical words that mean *surgical repair of the* *esophagus:* _____ / _____ / _____ *stomach:* _____ / _____ / _____

Boldface indicates a word root or combining form. Blue indicates a suffix. Pink indicates a prefix.

6-52 Common surgical suffixes that refer to *cutting* are summarized below. Review and use them to complete subsequent frames related to operative procedures.

Surgical Suffix	Meaning
-ectomy	excision, removal
-tome	instrument to cut
-tomy	incision

esophagus
ē-SŎF-ă-gŭs

6-53 Whenever you see a word with the word root (WR) **tom** in it, relate it to an incision. Esophag/o/tomy is an incision through the wall of the

_____.

esophag/o/tome
ē-SŎF-ă-gō-tōm

6-54 When esophag/eal surgery necessitates an incision, the physician will ask for an instrument called an _____ / _____ / _____.

gastr/ectomy
găs-TRĔK-tō-mē

6-55 A surgical procedure to remove all or, more commonly, part of the stomach is called a _____ / _____.

gastr

-ectomy

6-56 Partial or total gastr/ectomy is commonly performed to treat stomach cancer. From gastr/ectomy, identify the element that means

stomach: _____

excision or removal: _____

gastr/ectomy
găs-TRĔK-tō-mē

6-57 A perforated (punctured) stomach ulcer may require a partial

_____ / _____.

stomach

6-58 A gastr/o/tome is an *instrument to cut or incise the* _____.

gastr/o/tome
GĂS-trō-tōm

6-59 When the stomach is incised, the physician uses an instrument called a _____ / _____ / _____.

esophag/us
ē-SŎF-ă-gŭs

6-60 Esophag/o/tomy is an incision of the _____ / _____.

gastr/o/tomy
găs-TRŎT-ō-mē

6-61 Develop a word that means *incision of the stomach.*

_____ / _____ / _____

carcin/oma kăr-sĭ-NŌ-mă	**6-62** Cancer (CA) is a general term used to indicate various types of malignant neoplasms. Most cancers invade surrounding tissues and metastasize (spread) to other sites in the body. The CF for *cancer* is **carcin/o.** Combine **carcin/o** + -*oma* to build a word that means *cancerous tumor.* _____ / _____
cancer	**6-63** CA, especially sarc/oma, can recur even though the tumor is excised. Ultimately, it may cause death. Whenever you see CA in a medical report, you will know it means _____.
-ous	**6-64** Cancer/ous means *pertaining to cancer.* Identify the adjective element that means *pertaining to.* _____
cancerous *or* **malignant**	**6-65** A carcin/oma is a tumor that is _____.
cancer **tumor**	**6-66** The largest group of carcin/omas are solid tumors derived from epithelial tissue, which is the tissue that lines the surfaces of the body. It includes the skin and the tissues that line the internal organs, including the digestive organs. Analyze carcin/oma by defining the elements *carcin:* _____ *-oma:* _____
gastr/itis găs-TRĪ-tĭs **epi/gastr/ic** ĕp-ĭ-GĂS-trĭk	**6-67** *Epi-* means *above, upon.* Epi/gastr/ic pain may result from an acute form of gastr/itis. Identify words in this frame that mean *inflammation of the stomach:* _____ / _____ *pertaining to above or upon the stomach:* _____ / _____ / _____
hyper/emesis hī-pĕr-ĔM-ĕ-sĭs	**6-68** Emesis is a term that means *vomiting;* however, it may also be used as a suffix. A symptomatic term that means *excessive vomiting* is *hyper* / _____.
hyper- **-emesis**	**6-69** Hyper/emesis is characterized by excessive vomiting. Unless treated, it can lead to malnutrition. Determine elements in this frame that mean *excessive, above normal:* _____ *vomiting:* _____

Boldface indicates a word root or combining form. Blue indicates a suffix. Pink indicates a prefix.

hemat/emesis hĕm-ăt-ĔM-ĕ-sĭs	**6-70** *Hemat/o* refers to *blood*. A patient with acute gastr/itis or a peptic ulcer may vomit blood. Build a word that means *vomiting blood*. _____ / _____
hemat/emesis hĕm-ăt-ĔM-ĕ-sĭs	**6-71** Bleeding in the stomach may be due to a gastr/ic ulcer and may cause vomiting of blood. A Dx of vomiting blood is entered in the medical record as _____ / _____.
epi/gastr/ic ĕp-ĭ-GĂS-trĭk	**6-72** A common symptom of gastr/ic disease is pain. When pain occurs in the region above the stomach, it is called epi/gastr/ic pain. Form a word that means *pertaining to above or on the stomach*. _____ / _____ / _____
-pepsia **dys-**	**6-73** Dys/pepsia literally means *painful or difficult digestion* and is a form of gastric indigestion. It is not a disease in itself but may be a symptom of disease. Determine word elements in this frame that mean *digestion:* _____ *bad, painful, difficult:* _____
dys/pepsia dĭs-PĔP-sē-ă	**6-74** Over-the-counter antacids (agents that neutralize acidity) usually provide prompt relief of pain from _____ / _____.
dys/phagia dĭs-FĀ-jē-ă **bad, painful, difficult** **swallowing, eating**	**6-75** The suffix *-phagia* means *swallowing, eating*. Use *dys-* and *-phagia* to form a word that means *difficult or painful swallowing*. _____ / _____ Analyze dys/phagia by defining its elements: *dys-:* _____, _____, _____ *-phagia:* _____, _____
aer/o	**6-76** Swallowing air, usually followed by belching and gastric distention, is a condition known as aer/o/phagia. The CF for *air* is _____ / _____.
aer/o/phagia ĕr-ō-FĀ-jē-ă	**6-77** Infants have a tendency to swallow air as they suck milk from a bottle, a condition charted as _____ / _____ / _____.

SECTION REVIEW 6-2

Using the following table, write the combining form, suffix, or prefix that matches its definition in the space provided to the left of the definition. There may be more than one word element that matches a definition.

Combining Forms		Suffixes		Prefixes
dent/o	or/o	-al	-orexia	an-
gastr/o	orth/o	-ary	-pepsia	dia-
gingiv/o	pylor/o	-algia	-phagia	dys-
gloss/o	sial/o	-dynia	-rrhea	hyper-
lingu/o	stomat/o	-ic	-scope	hypo-
myc/o		-ist	-tomy	peri-
odont/o		-oma		

1. _____ tumor

2. _____ pertaining to

3. _____ around

4. _____ under, below, deficient

5. _____ discharge, flow

6. _____ fungus

7. _____ gum(s)

8. _____ pylorus

9. _____ bad; painful; difficult

10. _____ excessive, above normal

11. _____ saliva, salivary gland

12. _____ stomach

13. _____ specialist

14. _____ straight

15. _____ teeth

16. _____ through, across

17. _____ tongue

18. _____ instrument for examining

19. _____ incision

20. _____ appetite

21. _____ mouth

22. _____ pain

23. _____ swallowing, eating

24. _____ without, not

25. _____ digestion

Competency Verification: Check your answers in Appendix B: Answer Key, page 578. If you are not satisfied with your level of comprehension, go back to Frame 6–1 and rework the frames.

Correct Answers _____ × 4 = _____ % Score

WORD ELEMENTS

This section introduces CFs related to the small intestine and colon. Key suffixes are defined in the right-hand column as needed. Review the following table, and pronounce each word in the word analysis column aloud before you begin to work the frames.

Word Element	Meaning	Word Analysis
Combining Forms **Small Intestine**		
duoden/o	duodenum (first part of the small intestine)	**duoden/o/scopy** (dū-ŏd-ĕ-NŎS-kō-pē): visual examination of the duodenum *-scopy:* visual examination
enter/o	intestine (usually the small intestine)	**enter/o/pathy** (ĕn-tĕr-ŎP-ă-thē): any intestinal disease *-pathy:* disease
jejun/o	jejunum (second part of the small intestine)	**jejun/o/rrhaphy** (jĕ-joo-NOR-ă-fē): suture of the jejunum *-rrhaphy:* suture
ile/o	ileum (third part of the small intestine)	**ile/o/stomy** (ĭl-ē-ŎS-tō-mē): incision of the ileum (ileotomy) and creation of a permanent opening *-stomy**: forming an opening (mouth) *Ileostomy is performed following a total colectomy. The ileum is pulled out through the abdominal wall. The edges of the wall of the colon are rolled to make a mouth (stoma) that is then sutured to the abdominal wall. The patient wears a plastic pouch on the abdomen to collect feces.*
Large Intestine		
append/o	appendix	**append/ectomy** (ăp-ĕn-DĔK-tō-mē): removal of the appendix *-ectomy:* excision, removal *Appendectomy is performed to remove a diseased appendix that is in danger of rupturing.*
appendic/o		**appendic/itis** (ă-pĕn-dĭ-SĪ-tĭs): inflammation of the appendix *-itis:* inflammation
col/o	colon	**col/o/stomy** (kō-LŎS-tō-mē): creation of an opening between the colon and the abdominal wall *-stomy**: forming an opening (mouth) *A colostomy creates a place for fecal matter to exit the body other than through the anus. It may be temporary or permanent.*
colon/o		**colon/o/scopy** (kō-lŏn-ŎS-kō-pē): visual examination of the inner surface of the colon using a long, flexible endoscope *-scopy:* visual examination
proct/o	anus, rectum	**proct/o/logist** (prŏk-TŎL-ō-jĭst): physician who specializes in treating disorders of the colon, rectum, and anus *-logist:* specialist in the study of
rect/o	rectum	**rect/o/cele** (RĔK-tō-sēl): herniation or protrusion of the rectum; also called *proctocele* *-cele:* hernia, swelling
sigmoid/o	sigmoid colon	**sigmoid/o/tomy** (sĭg-moyd-ŎT-ō-mē): incision of the sigmoid colon *-tomy:* incision

Pronunciation Help						
	Long sound	ā in rāte	ē in rēbirth	ī in īsle	ō in ōver	ū in ūnite
	Short sound	ă in ălone	ĕ in ĕver	ĭ in ĭt	ŏ in nŏt	ŭ in cŭt

*When the suffix *-stomy* is used with a combining form that denotes an organ, it refers to a surgical opening to the outside of the body.

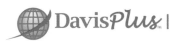 DavisPlus | Visit the *Medical Terminology Simplified* online resource center at Davis*Plus* for an audio exercise of the terms in this table. It will help you master pronunciations and meanings of medical terms.

SECTION REVIEW 6-3

For the following medical terms, first write the suffix and its meaning. Then translate the meaning of the remaining elements, starting with the first part of the word. The first word is completed for you.

Term	Meaning
1. duoden/o/scopy	-scopy: visual examination; duodenum (first part of the small intestine)
2. appendic/itis	
3. enter/o/pathy	
4. col/o/stomy	
5. rect/o/cele	
6. sigmoid/o/tomy	
7. proct/o/logist	
8. jejun/o/rrhaphy	
9. append/ectomy	
10. ile/o/stomy	

Competency Verification: Check your answers in Appendix B: Answer Key, page 579. If you are not satisfied with your level of comprehension, study the word elements tables and retake the review.

Correct Answers _____ × 10 = _____ % Score

LOWER GI TRACT

The lower GI tract consists of the small and large intestine, as well as the anus and rectum.

Small and Large Intestine

6–78 The small intestine is a continuation of the GI tract. It is where digestion of food is completed as nutrients are absorbed into the bloodstream through tiny, fingerlike projections called villi. Any unabsorbed material is passed on to the large intestine to be excreted from the body. There are three parts of the small intestine: the (1) **duodenum,** the (2) **jejunum,** and the (3) **ileum.** Label these parts in Figure 6–3.

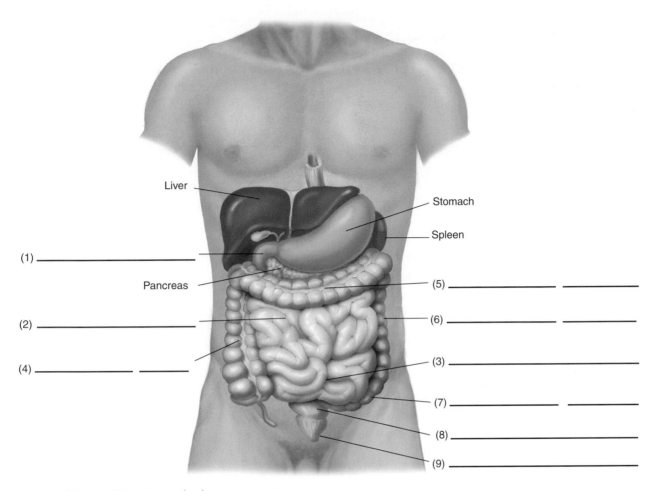

Liver
Stomach
Spleen
(1) _____
Pancreas
(5) _____ _____
(2) _____
(6) _____ _____
(4) _____ _____
(3) _____
(7) _____ _____
(8) _____
(9) _____

Figure 6-3 Small intestine and colon.

duodenum dū-ŎD-ĕ-nŭm **jejunum** jĕ-JŪ-nŭm **ileum** ĬL-ē-ŭm	**6–79** Here is a review of the small intestine. The CF *duoden/o* refers to the first part of the small intestine, called the _____. The CF *jejun/o* refers to the second part of the small intestine, called the _____. The CF *ile/o* refers to the third part of the small intestine, called the _____.
duoden/ectomy dū-ŏd-ĕ-NĔK-tō-mē **jejun/ectomy** jē-jū-NĔK-tō-mē **ile/ectomy** ĭl-ē-ĔK-tō-mē	**6–80** Duoden/ectomy, jejun/ectomy, and ile/ectomy are total or partial excisions of different sections of the small intestine. Build a word that means *excision of the* *duodenum:* _____ / _____ *jejunum:* _____ / _____ *ileum:* _____ / _____

duodenum, duoden/o dū-ŎD-ĕ-nŭm **jejunum, jejun/o** jĕ-JŪ-nŭm **ileum, ile/o** ĬL-ē-ŭm	**6–81** Name the three parts of the small intestine and their CFs. **Part** **Combining Form** 1. _____ _____ / ____ 2. _____ _____ / ____ 3. _____ _____ / ____
duodenum dū-ŎD-ĕ-nŭm	**6–82** Duoden/o/stomy is performed to form an opening (mouth) into the _____.
stomy	**6–83** Identify the element in Frame 6–82 that means *forming an opening* *(mouth):* _____.
opening, jejunum jē-JŪ-nŭm	**6–84** Jejun/o/stomy is a surgical procedure that means *forming an* _____ *into the* _____.
opening, ileum ĬL-ē-ŭm	**6–85** When the colon is removed because of colon CA, an ile/o/stomy is performed. The patient must wear an ile/o/stomy bag to collect fecal material from the ile/um. The surgical procedure *ile/o/stomy* means *forming an* _____ *into the* _____.
-stomy	**6–86** The medical term stoma refers to an *opening shaped like a mouth*. The suffix that means *forming an opening (mouth)* is _____.
-tomy **jejun/o/tomy** jĕ-jū-NŎT-ō-mē	**6–87** For patients who cannot eat by mouth, a jejun/al (pertaining to the jejunum) feeding tube is commonly placed through a jejun/o/tomy incision. The surgical suffix that means *incision* is _____. An *incision of the jejunum* is called _____ / _____ / _____.
duoden/o/tomy dū-ŏd-ĕ-NŎT-ō-mē	**6–88** *Incision of the duodenum* is called _____ / _____ / _____.
ile/o/tomy ĭl-ē-ŎT-ō-mē	**6–89** *Incision of the ileum* is called _____ / _____ / _____.

Boldface indicates a word root or combining form. Blue indicates a suffix. Pink indicates a prefix.

ileum ĬL-ē-ŭm **suture**	**6–90** The suffix *-rrhaphy* refers to *suture (sew)*. Ile/o/rrhaphy is performed to surgically repair the ile/um. Analyze ile/o/rrhaphy by defining its elements. *ile/o:* _____ *-rrhaphy:* _____
duoden/ectomy dū-ŏd-ĕ-NĔK-tō-mē **duoden/o/rrhaphy** dū-ŏ-dĕ-NOR-ă-fē	**6–91** In a bleeding duoden/al ulcer, a suture over the bleeding portion can prevent performing duoden/ectomy. Develop surgical words that mean *excision of the duodenum:* _____ / _____ *suture of the duodenum:* _____ / _____ / _____
jejun/o/rrhaphy jĕ-joo-NOR-ă-fē **ile/o/rrhaphy** ĭl-ē-OR-ă-fē	**6–92** Form surgical words that mean *suture of the* *jejunum:* _____ / _____ / _____ *ileum:* _____ / _____ / _____
stomach, duodenum dū-ŎD-ĕ-nŭm	**6–93** Gastr/o/duoden/o/stomy is the *formation of an opening between the* _____ *and* _____.
stomach, ileum ĬL-ē-ŭm	**6–94** Gastr/o/ile/o/stomy is the *formation of an opening between the* _____ *and* _____.
stomach, small intestine	**6–95** Anastomosis (connection between two vessels, bowel segments, or ducts) is performed to provide a connection from one structure to another. Gastr/o/enter/o/anastomosis is a *surgical connection between the* _____ *and* _____ _____.
gastr/o/enter/o/ anastomosis, gastr/o/ enter/o/stomy găs-trō-ĕn-tĕr-ō-ă-năs-tō- MŌ-sĭs, găs-trō-ĕn-tĕr- ŎS-tō-mē	**6–96** Gastr/o/enter/o/anastomosis, also called *gastr/o/enter/o/stomy,* may be performed when there is a malignant or benign gastr/o/duoden/al disease. Identify terms in this frame that mean *creation of a passage between the stomach and some part of the small intestine.* _____ / _____ / _____ / _____ / _____ *and* _____ / _____ / _____ / _____ / _____
-stomy	**6–97** Another type of anastomosis, gastr/o/duoden/o/stomy, is a procedure in which the lower part of the stomach is excised and the remainder is anastomosed to the duodenum. The element in this frame that means *forming an opening (mouth)* is _____.

ileum ĬL-ē-ŭm	**6–98** Most absorption of food takes place in the third part of the small intestine, which is the _____.
inflammation, ileum ĬL-ē-ŭm	**6–99** Crohn disease, a chronic inflammation of the ile/um, may affect any part of the intestinal tract. This disease is distinguished from closely related bowel disorders by its inflammatory pattern; it is also called *regional ile/itis*. Ile/itis is an _____ *of the* _____.
enter/o	**6–100** Enter/al means pertaining to the intestine (usually the small intestine). From enter/al, construct the CF for *intestine*. _____ / _____
enter/ectomy ĕn-tĕr-ĔK-tō-mē **enter/o/rrhaphy** ĕn-tĕr-OR-ă-fē	**6–101** Build medical terms that mean *excision of intestine (usually small):* _____ / _____ *suture of intestine (such as an intestinal wound):* _____ / _____ / _____
inflammation, intestine	**6–102** Enter/itis is an _____ *of the* _____ *(usually small).*
	6–103 Continue labeling Figure 6–3 as you read the following: The large intestine, also called the colon, extends from the ileum of the small intestine to the anus. The colon consists of four segments: (4) **ascending colon,** (5) **transverse colon,** (6) **descending colon,** and (7) **sigmoid colon.**
col/ectomy kō-LĔK-tō-mē **col/itis** kō-LĪ-tĭs **col/o/tomy** kō-LŎT-ō-mē	**6–104** The CF *col/o* refers to the *colon*. Form medical words that mean *excision of the colon:* _____ / _____ *inflammation of the colon:* _____ / _____ *incision of the colon:* _____ / _____ / _____
col/o/stomy kō-LŎS-tō-mē **col/o/rrhaphy** kō-LOR-ă-fē	**6–105** Col/o/stomy is the surgical creation of an opening into the colon (through the surface of the abdomen). It may be temporary or permanent and may be performed as treatment for CA or diverticul/itis. Col/o/stomy allows elimination of feces into a bag attached to the skin. (See Fig. 6–4.) Build medical terms that mean *forming an opening (mouth) into the colon:* _____ / _____ / _____ *suture of the colon:* _____ / _____ / _____

Boldface indicates a word root or combining form. Blue indicates a suffix. Pink indicates a prefix.

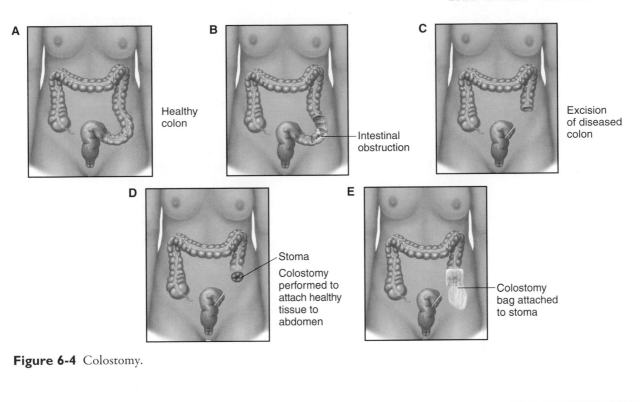

A   Healthy colon

B   Intestinal obstruction

C   Excision of diseased colon

D   Stoma
Colostomy performed to attach healthy tissue to abdomen

E   Colostomy bag attached to stoma

Figure 6-4 Colostomy.

6–106   Absorption of water by the colon changes intestin/al contents from a fluid to a more solid consistency known as feces or stool. Use your medical dictionary to define feces.

_____

_____

---

peristalsis
pĕr-ĭ-STĂL-sĭs

6–107   Recall that the muscular contractions that propel a bolus through the digestive system are known as peristalsis. These muscular contractions also move feces through the colon during the process of defecation.

Elimination of waste products from the colon is possible because of the wavelike

contractions known as _____.

---

liver

spleen

6–108   The ascending colon is located superior to the cecum. (See Fig. 6–1.) It curves horizontally at the hepatic flexure and descends at the splenic flexure.

Name the organ that is in close proximity to the

hepat/ic flexure: _____

splen/ic flexure: _____

6–109   The sigmoid colon is S-shaped and extends from the descending colon into the (8) **rectum.** The rectum terminates in the lower opening of the gastrointestinal tract, the (9) **anus.** Label Figure 6–3 to identify and locate the rectum and anus.

---

sigmoid/o	**6–110** Sigmoid/ectomy, an excision of all or part of the sigmoid colon, is most commonly performed to remove a malignant tumor. A large percentage of lower bowel cancers occur in the sigmoid colon. From sigmoid/ectomy, construct the CF for sigmoid colon. _____ / _____
sigmoid/itis sĭg-moyd-Ī-tĭs	**6–111** Form a term that means *inflammation of the sigmoid colon.* _____ / _____

Competency Verification: Check your labeling of Figure 6–3 with the answers in Appendix B: Answer Key, page 579.

Rectum and Anus

inflammation, rectum RĔK-tŭm	**6–112** The CF *rect/o* refers to the rectum. Rect/itis is a(n) _____ *of the* _____.
inflammation, rectum, colon RĔK-tŭm, KŌ-lŏn	**6–113** Rect/o/col/itis is a(n) _____ *of the* _____ *and* _____.
pain	**6–114** Proct/algia refers to a neur/o/logic/al *pain in or around the anus or lower rectum,* which is also called rect/algia. Whenever you see *-algia* in a term, you will know it means _____.
surgical repair, rectum RĔK-tŭm	**6–115** Rect/o/plasty is a _____ _____ *of* *the* _____.
pertaining to, rectum RĔK-tŭm	**6–116** Rect/o/vagin/al means _____ _____ *the* _____ *and vagina.*
through, across **discharge, flow**	**6–117** *Dia-* is a prefix that means through, across. Dia/rrhea refers to frequent passage of watery bowel movements. Analyze dia/rrhea by defining the elements. dia-: _____, _____ -rrhea: _____, _____
dia/rrhea dī-ă-RĒ-ă	**6–118** A patient with an irritable bowel (IB) may experience frequent passage of watery bowel movements or have symptoms of a condition called _____ / _____.

Boldface indicates a word root or combining form. Blue indicates a suffix. Pink indicates a prefix.

stenosis stĕ-NŌ-sĭs	**6-119** Stenosis refers to a narrowing or stricture of a passageway or orifice. This condition may result in an obstruction. Stenosis may also be used as a suffix. A narrowing or stricture of the pylorus is called *pyloric* _____.
rect/o **-stenosis**	**6-120** Rect/o/stenosis is a *narrowing or stricture of the rectum.* Determine elements in this frame that mean *rectum:* _____ / _____ *narrowing, stricture:* _____
proct/itis prŏk-TĪ-tĭs	**6-121** The CF *proct/o* refers to the *anus and rectum.* Locate the anus and rectum in Figure 6–1. Inflammation of the anus and rectum is known as _____ / _____.
rectum RĔK-tŭm **rectum, anus** RĔK-tŭm, Ā-nŭs	**6-122** The word spasm refers to an *involuntary contraction or twitching.* It is also used in medical words as a suffix. Rect/o/spasm is an involuntary contraction of the _____. Proct/o/spasm is an involuntary contraction of the _____ *and* _____.
path/o/log/ical păth-ō-LŎJ-ĭ-kăl	**6-123** Endo/scopy is an important tool in establishing or confirming a Dx or detecting a path/o/log/ical condition. A video recorder is commonly used during an endo/scop/ic procedure to guide the endo/scope and document abnormalities. Determine the word in this frame that means *study of disease.* _____ / _____ / _____ / _____
colon/o/scopy kō-lŏn-ŎS-kō-pē **proct/o/scopy** prŏk-TŎS-kō-pē	**6-124** The organ being examined dictates the name of the endoscopic procedure. Visual examination of the colon is called col/o/scopy or _____ / _____ / _____. Visual examination of the anus and rectum is called _____ / _____ / _____.
sigmoid colon SĬG-moyd KŌ-lŏn **visual examination**	**6-125** A colonoscopy involves examination of the entire length of the colon; a sigmoidoscopy involves examination of only the lower third of the colon. (See Fig. 6–5.) Sigmoid/o/scopy is used to screen for colon cancer. The American Cancer Society recommends a first sigmoid/o/scopy after age 50. It is done sooner if there is a family history (FH) of colon cancer. Analyze sigmoid/o/scopy by defining its elements. The CF *sigmoid/o* means _____ _____. The suffix *-scopy* means _____ _____.

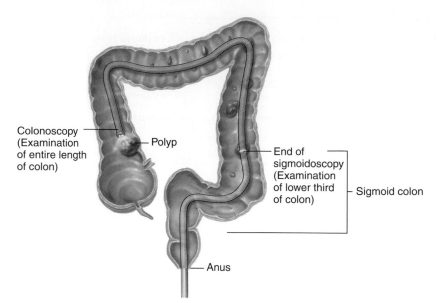

Colonoscopy
(Examination
of entire length
of colon)

Polyp

End of
sigmoidoscopy
(Examination
of lower third
of colon)

Sigmoid colon

Anus

Figure 6-5 Sigmoidoscopy and colonoscopy.

---

sigmoid/o/scopy
sĭg-moy-DŎS-kō-pē

6-126 To examine an abnormality in the colon, the physician performs a visual examination of the sigmoid colon called a _____ / _____ / _____.

---

sigmoid/o/scope
sĭg-MOY-dō-skōp

6-127 A sigmoid/o/scope, a flexible fiber-optic tube that permits transmission of light to visualize images around curves and corners, is placed through the anus to assess the gastro/intestin/al tract.

To examine the colon, the physician uses a flexible fiber-optic instrument called a

_____ / _____ / _____.

---

sigmoid/ectomy
sĭg-moyd-ĔK-tō-mē

carcin/oma
kăr-sĭ-NŌ-mă

6-128 The sigmoid colon is S-shaped and is the last part of the colon. (See Fig. 6–5.) Sigmoid/ectomy is most commonly performed for carcin/oma of the sigmoid colon.

Identify words in this frame that mean

excision of the sigmoid colon: _____ / _____

cancerous tumor: _____ / _____

---

examination, colon
KŌ-lŏn

6-129 A col/o/scopy is commonly referred to as a colon/o/scopy. Both terms mean *visual* _____ *of the* _____.

---

colon/itis
kō-lŏn-Ī-tĭs

colon/o/scope
kō-LŎN-ō-skōp

colon/o/scopy
kō-lŏn-ŎS-kō-pē

6-130 Use *colon/o* to form medical words that mean

inflammation of the colon: _____ / _____

instrument to examine the colon: _____ / _____ / _____

visual examination of the colon: _____ / _____ / _____

Boldface indicates a word root or combining form. Blue indicates a suffix. Pink indicates a prefix.

SECTION REVIEW 6-4

Using the following table, write the CF or suffix that matches its definition in the space provided to the left of the definition. There may be more than one word element that matches a definition.

Combining Forms

col/o	jejun/o
colon/o	proct/o
duoden/o	rect/o
enter/o	sigmoid/o
ile/o	

Suffixes

-rrhaphy	-tome
-scopy	-tomy
-spasm	
-stenosis	
-stomy	

1. _____ intestine (usually small intestine)

2. _____ instrument to cut

3. _____ rectum

4. _____ involuntary contraction, twitching

5. _____ ileum (third part of the small intestine)

6. _____ visual examination

7. _____ jejunum (second part of the small intestine)

8. _____ colon

9. _____ duodenum (first part of the small intestine)

10. _____ forming an opening (mouth)

11. _____ anus, rectum

12. _____ narrowing, stricture

13. _____ suture

14. _____ incision

15. _____ sigmoid colon

Competency Verification: Check your answers in Appendix B: Answer Key, page 579. If you are not satisfied with your level of comprehension, go back to Frame 6–78 and rework the frames.

Correct Answers _____ × 6.67 = _____ % Score

WORD ELEMENTS

This section introduces CFs related to the accessory organs of digestion. Included are key suffixes; prefixes are defined in the right-hand column as needed. Review the following table and pronounce each word in the word analysis column aloud before you begin to work the frames.

Word Elements	Meaning	Word Analysis
Combining Forms		
cholangi/o	bile vessel	**cholangi**/ole (kō-LĂN-jē-ōl): small terminal portion of the bile duct *-ole:* small, minute
chol/e*	bile, gall	**chol**/e/lith (kō-lē-LĬTH): gallstone *-lith:* stone, calculus
cholecyst/o	gallbladder	**cholecyst**/ectomy (kō-lē-sĭs-TĔK-tō-mē): removal of the gallbladder by laparoscopic or open surgery *-ectomy:* excision, removal *Cholecystectomy can be performed by open surgery or laparoscopically (placing a tube into the abdomen).*
choledoch/o	bile duct	**choledoch**/o/tomy (kō-lĕd-ō-KŎT-ō-mē): incision of the common bile duct *-tomy:* incision
hepat/o	liver	**hepat**/itis (hĕp-ă-TĪ-tĭs): inflammation of the liver *-itis:* inflammation
pancreat/o	pancreas	**pancreat**/itis (păn-krē-ă-TĪ-tĭs): inflammation or infection of the pancreas *-itis:* inflammation
Suffixes		
-iasis	abnormal condition (produced by something specified)	chol/e/lith/**iasis** (kō-lē-lĭ-THĪ-ă-sĭs): presence or formation of gallstones *chol/e:* bile, gall *lith/o:* stone, calculus
-megaly	enlargement	hepat/o/**megaly** (hĕp-ă-tō-MĔG-ă-lē): enlargement of the liver *hepat/o:* liver *Hepatomegaly may be caused by infection; fatty infiltration, as in alcoholism; biliary obstruction; or malignancy.*
-prandial	meal	post/**prandial** (pōst-PRĂN-dē-ăl): following a meal *post-:* after, behind

Pronunciation Help	Long sound	ā in rāte	ē in rēbirth	ī in īsle	ō in ōver	ū in ūnite
	Short sound	ă in ălone	ĕ in ĕver	ĭ in ĭt	ŏ in nŏt	ŭ in cŭt

*Using the combining vowel e instead of o is an exception to the rule.

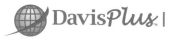

Visit the *Medical Terminology Simplified* online resource center at Davis*Plus* for an audio exercise of the terms in this table. It will help you master pronunciations and meanings of medical terms.

SECTION REVIEW 6-5

For the following medical terms, first write the suffix and its meaning. Then translate the meaning of the remaining elements starting with the first part of the word. The first word is completed for you.

Term	Meaning
1. hepat/itis	-itis: inflammation; liver
2. hepat/o/megaly	
3. chol/e/lith	
4. cholangi/ole	
5. cholecyst/ectomy	
6. post/prandial	
7. chol/e/lith/iasis	
8. choledoch/o/tomy	
9. pancreat/o/lith	
10. pancreat/itis	

Competency Verification: Check your answers in Appendix B: Answer Key, page 579. If you are not satisfied with your level of comprehension, go back to the word elements tables and retake the review.

Correct Answers _____ × 10 = _____ % Score

ACCESSORY ORGANS OF DIGESTION

The accessory organs of digestion include the liver, gallbladder, and pancreas.

liver, gallbladder, pancreas	**6-131** Label Figure 6–6 as you learn about the accessory organs of digestion. Even though food does not pass through the (1) **liver,** (2) **gallbladder,** and (3) **pancreas,** these organs play a vital role in proper digestion and absorption of nutrients. The gallbladder serves as a storage site for bile, which is produced by the liver. When bile is needed for digestion, the gallbladder releases it through ducts into the (4) **duodenum** through the (5) **common bile duct.** The three accessory organs of digestion are the _____, _____, and _____.
hepat/o **cholecyst/o** **pancreat/o**	**6-132** Construct CFs for *liver:* _____ / _____ *gallbladder:* _____ / _____ *pancreas:* _____ / _____

Liver

hepat/itis hĕp-ă-TĪ-tĭs	**6-133** Hepat/itis, an inflammatory condition of the liver, may be caused by bacteri/al or viral infection, parasitic infestation, alcohol, drugs, toxins, or transfusion of incompatible blood. It may be mild and brief or severe and life-threatening. When a person has inflammation of the liver caused by a virus, the Dx is most likely _____ / _____.
hepat/o/megaly hĕp-ă-tō-MĔG-ă-lē	**6-134** Hepat/itis may be characterized by an enlarged liver. The medical term for an enlarged liver is _____ / _____ / _____.
hepat/oma hĕp-ă-TŌ-mă	**6-135** Hepat/o/megaly may be a symptom of a malignant tumor of the liver called hepat/oma. The tumor occurs most commonly in association with hepat/itis or liver cirrh/osis. The Dx of a liver tumor is charted as _____ / _____.
hepat/itis hĕp-ă-TĪ-tĭs	**6-136** **Hepatitis B**, the most common infectious hepatitis seen in hospitals, is transferred by blood and body secretions. As a preventive measure, hospital personnel are usually required to be vaccinated. The medical term for *inflammation of the liver* is _____ / _____.
hepat/o/dynia, **hepat/algia** hĕp-ă-tō-DĬN-ē-ă, hĕp-ă-TĂL-jē-ă **hepat/o/rrhaphy** hĕp-ă-TŌR-ă-fē **hepat/ectomy** hĕp-ă-TĔK-tō-mē	**6-137** Form medical words that mean *pain in the liver:* _____ / _____ / _____ *or* _____ / _____ *suture of the liver:* _____ / _____ / _____ *excision of (a portion of) the liver:* _____ / _____
hepat/o/cyte HĔP-ă-tō-sīt	**6-138** Combine **hepat/o** and *-cyte* to form a word that means *liver cell.* _____ / _____ / _____

6-139 Identify and label the following structures in Figure 6–6 as you read about the accessory organs of digestion. Bile is released from the gallbladder and also drained directly from the liver through the (6) **right hepatic duct** and the (7) **left hepatic duct.** These two ducts eventually form the (8) **hepatic duct.** The (9) **cystic duct** merges with the hepatic duct to form the common bile duct and the (10) **pancreatic duct.** These ducts carry their digestive juices into the duodenum.

Boldface indicates a word root or combining form. Blue indicates a suffix. Pink indicates a prefix.

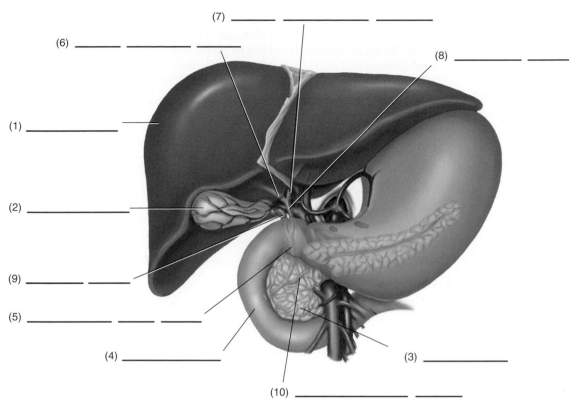

(7) _____ _____ _____

(6) _____ _____ _____

(8) _____ _____

(1) _____

(2) _____

(9) _____ _____

(5) _____ _____ _____

(4) _____

(3) _____

(10) _____ _____

Figure 6-6 Liver, gallbladder, pancreas, and duodenum with associated ducts and blood vessels.

---

hepat/ic hĕ-PĂT-ĭk **cyst/ic** SĬS-tĭk **pancreat/ic** păn-krē-ĂT-ĭk	**6–140** Use *-ic* to form medical words that mean *pertaining to the* *liver:* _____ / _____ *bladder:* _____ / _____ *pancreas:* _____ / _____

---

hepat/ic, cyst/ic, **pancreat/ic** hĕ-PĂT-ĭk, SĬS-tĭk, păn-krē-ĂT-ĭk	**6–141** Refer to Frame 6–140 to write the names of the ducts responsible for transporting digestive juices. _____ / _____ duct, _____ / _____ duct, _____ / _____ duct, and common bile duct

---

Competency Verification: Check your labeling of Figure 6–6 in Appendix B: Answer Key, page 580.

Gallbladder

vomiting	**6–142** The CF *chol/e* means *bile, gall.* Chol/emesis means _____ bile.

cholecyst/o	**6-143** Bile, also called *gall,* is a yellow-green bitter secretion produced by the liver and stored in the gallbladder. It receives its color from the presence of bile pigments such as bilirubin. Bile passes from the gallbladder through the common bile duct into the small intestine. Bile emulsifies (breaks down) fats and prepares them for further digestion and absorption in the small intestine. Combine *chol/e* and *cyst/o* to develop the CF _____ / _____.
gallbladder	**6-144** Cholecyst/itis is an *inflammation of the* _____.
o	**6-145** The vowel *e* in *chol/e* is an exception to the rule of using an _____ as a connecting vowel.
bile, gall **vomiting**	**6-146** When a patient vomits bile, the condition is called chol/emesis. Analyze chol/emesis by defining the elements. The CF *chol/e* refers to _____ or _____. The suffix *-emesis* refers to _____.
liver	**6-147** The suffix *-lith* is used in words to mean *stone,* or *calculus.* A hepat/o/lith is a *stone, or calculus, in the* _____.
pancreat/o/lith păn-krē-ĂT-ō-lĭth **cholecyst/o/lith** kō-lē-SĬS-tō-lĭth **hepat/o/lith** hĕp-Ă-tō-lĭth	**6-148** Form medical words that mean *stone, or calculus, in the* *pancreas:* _____ / _____ / _____ *gallbladder:* _____ / _____ / _____ *liver:* _____ / _____ / _____
chol/e	**6-149** Chol/e/liths are gallstones; chol/e/lith/iasis is an abnormal condition of gallstones. Unless the gallstones obstruct a biliary duct, the condition may remain asymptomatic. Exact causes of gallstones are unknown; however, they occur more commonly in women, elderly people, and obese persons. Figure 6–7 illustrates sites of gallstones. From chol/e/lith, determine the CF that means *bile, gall.* _____ / _____
chol/e/lith kō-lē-LĬTH	**6-150** The most common type of gallstone contains cholesterol. These calculi are formed in the gallbladder or bile ducts. The medical name for gallstone is _____ / _____ / _____.

jaund/o **hyper-** **-emia**	**6-151** Jaund/ice, a yellowish discoloration of the skin and whites of the eyes (sclerae) due to abnormally high levels of bilirubin in the blood (hyper/bilirubin/emia). This condition is usually a sign of liver dysfunction or obstruction of the bile ducts. The CF for *yellow* is: _____ / _____ The prefix for *excessive, above normal* is: _____ The suffix for *blood* is: _____
right upper quadrant	**6-152** Calculi that form in the gallbladder or bile ducts may cause jaund/ice, RUQ pain, obstruction, and inflammation of the gallbladder. RUQ means _____ _____ _____.
cholangi/oma kō-lăn-jē-Ō-mă	**6-153** A bil/i/ary duct, also called a *bile duct,* may become inflamed from a chol/e/lith. The CF *cholangi/o* refers to a bile vessel. A tumor of the bile vessel is called _____ / _____.
cholangi/o/graphy kō-lăn-jē-ŎG-ră-fē	**6-154** The Dx of cholang/itis is determined by ultrasound evaluation and cholangi/o/graphy. The radiographic procedure in this frame for outlining the major bile vessel is _____ / _____ / _____.
bile duct	**6-155** The CF *choledoch/o* means *bile duct.* A choledoch/o/lith is a *stone in the* _____ _____.
choledoch/o	**6-156** Choledoch/o/lith/iasis refers to the *formation of a stone in the common bile duct,* as illustrated in Figure 6–7. The CF for bile duct is _____ / _____.
choledoch/itis kō-lĕ-dō-KĪ-tĭs **choledoch/o/rrhaphy** kō-lĕd-ō-KŎR-ă-fē **choledoch/o/plasty** kō-LĔD-ō-kō-plăs-tē	**6-157** Use *choledoch/o* (bile duct) to develop medical words that mean *inflammation of the bile duct:* _____ / _____ *suture of the bile duct:* _____ / _____ / _____ *surgical repair of the bile duct:* _____ / _____ / _____
choledoch/o/lith kō-LĔD-ō-kō-lĭth **choledoch/o/rrhaphy** kō-lĕd-ō-KŎR-ă-fē **choledoch/o/tomy** kō-lĕd-ō-KŎT-ō-mē	**6-158** When a stone is trapped in the common bile duct, the duct may require an incision to remove the stone. Once the stone is removed, the duct is sutured. Form medical words that mean *stone in the bile duct:* _____ / _____ / _____ *suture of the bile duct:* _____ / _____ / _____ *incision of the bile duct:* _____ / _____ / _____

gallbladder	**6-159** Locate the gallbladder, also known as *cholecyst*, in Figure 6–6. This pouchlike structure stores bile, which is produced by the liver. Cholecyst is the medical name for _____.
cholecyst/itis kō-lē-sĭs-TĬ-tĭs	**6-160** Inflammation of the gallbladder may be caused by the presence of gallstones. The Dx *inflammation of the gallbladder* is charted as _____ / _____.
gallstone	**6-161** A chole/lith is a _____.
stone, calculus KĂL-kū-lŭs	**6-162** The pancreat/ic duct transports pancreatic juices to the duodenum to help the digestive process. A pancreat/o/lith is a _____, *or* _____, *within the pancreas.*
stone, calculus KĂL-kū-lŭs	**6-163** The suffixes *-osis* and *-iasis* are used to indicate an abnormal or diseased condition. The difference between the two is that *-osis* is used to denote a disorder but does not indicate the specific cause of the abnormality. In contrast, *-iasis* is attached to a word root to identify an abnormal condition produced by something that is specified.* For example, lith/iasis is an abnormal condition produced by a _____, *or* _____.
liver	**6-164** Hepat/osis is an *abnormal or diseased condition of the* _____. The cause of the abnormality is not specified and could be the result of any number of liver diseases.
lith/iasis lĭth-Ī-ă-sĭs **pancreat/o/lith/iasis** păn-krē-ă-tō-lĭ-THĪ-ă-sĭs	**6-165** When forming a word that means *abnormal condition of stones, or calculi,* use *-iasis* because the abnormal condition is produced by something specified.* In this case, it is produced by the stones. Use *-iasis* to construct medical words that mean *abnormal condition of stones:* _____ / _____ *pancreat/ic stones:* _____ / _____ / _____ / _____
chol/e/lith/iasis kō-lē-lĭ-THĪ-ă-sĭs	**6-166** Chol/e/lith/iasis is common in obese women over age 40. (See Fig. 6–7.) A patient with a Dx of an *abnormal or diseased condition of gallstones* suffers from _____ / _____ / _____ / _____.

 In some instances, you will find that *-osis* and *-iasis* are interchangeable. Whenever you are in doubt about which suffix to use, refer to your medical dictionary.

---

*There are a few exceptions to this rule.

Boldface indicates a word root or combining form. Blue indicates a suffix. Pink indicates a prefix.

inflammation **gallbladder**	**6-167** Acute cholecyst/itis commonly leads to infection of the gallbladder and duct. Analyze cholecyst/itis by defining the elements. The suffix *-itis* refers to _____. The CF *cholecyst/o* refers to the _____.
cholecyst/itis kō-lē-sĭs-TĪ-tĭs **cholecyst/o/dynia,** **cholecyst/algia** kō-lē-sĭs-tō-DĬN-ē-ă, kō-lē-sĭs-TĂL-jē-ă **cholecyst/o/lith/iasis** kŏ-lē-sĭs-tō-lĭ-THĪ-ă-sĭs	**6-168** Cholecyst/itis is an inflammation of the gallbadder, usually caused by obstruction of gallstones in the bil/i/ary ducts. The disease is marked by pain in the RUQ of the abdomen. Usually, pain develops shortly after a meal and radiates to the shoulder and back. Use *cholecyst/o* to form medical words that mean *inflammation of the gallbladder:* _____ / _____ *pain in the gallbladder:* _____ / _____ / _____ *or* _____ / _____ *abnormal condition of gallbladder stone(s):* _____ / _____ / _____ / _____
cholecyst/ectomy kō-lē-sĭs-TĔK-tō-mē **bil/i/ary*** BĬL-ē-ār-ē **lapar/o/scop/ic** lăp-ă-rō-SKŎP-ĭk	**6-169** Chol/e/cyst/ectomy is performed by lapar/o/scop/ic or open surgery. If bile ducts are obstructed, a classic "gallbladder attack," more properly referred to as bili/ary colic, this results in pain in the RUQ. Nausea and vomiting may accompany the attack. Form medical terms that mean *excision of the gallbladder:* _____ / _____ *pertaining to bile or gall:* _____ / _____ / _____ *pertaining to visual examination of the abdomen:* _____ / _____ / _____ / _____

Pancreas

pancreat/ectomy păn-krē-ă-TĔK-tō-mē	**6-170** Because of its critical function of producing insulin and digestive enzymes, a complete excision of the pancreas is not usually performed. When excision of the pancreas is indicated, the surgeon performs a _____ / _____.
pancreat/ectomy păn-krē-ă-TĔK-tō-mē	**6-171** Pancreat/ic CA is an extremely lethal disease. Surgery is performed for relief, but it is not a cure for the CA. When part or all of the pancreas is removed, the surgeon performs a _____ / _____.
cholecyst/ectomy kō-lē-sĭs-TĔK-tō-mē	**6-172** Because the gallbladder performs no function except storage, it is not essential for life. When the gallbladder is excised, the surgical procedure is called _____ / _____.

---

*Using the combining vowel *i* instead of *o* is an exception to the rule.

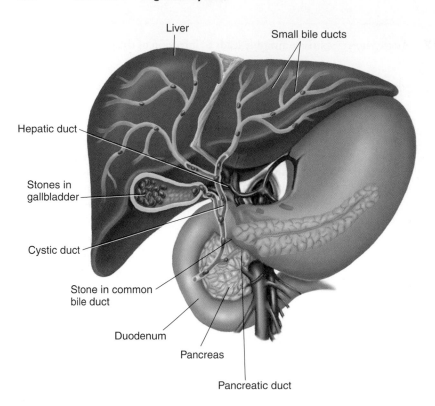

Liver

Small bile ducts

Hepatic duct

Stones in gallbladder

Cystic duct

Stone in common bile duct

Duodenum

Pancreas

Pancreatic duct

Figure 6-7 Cholelithiasis and choledocholithiasis.

---

esophag/o/plasty
ē-SŎF-ă-gō-plăs-tē

choledoch/o/plasty
kō-LĔD-ō-kō-plăs-tē

6-173   Plastic surgery is the specialty for restoration, repair, or reconstruction of body structures.

Develop operative terms that mean *surgical repair of the*

esophagus: _____ / _____ / _____

bile duct: _____ / _____ / _____

---

therm/o/meter
thĕr-MŎM-ĕ-tĕr

6-174   A therm/o/meter is an instrument for measuring degrees of heat or cold. Normal temperature taken orally ranges from about 97.6°F to 99.6°F. Infection, malignancy, severe trauma, and drugs may cause fever. However, other conditions may also cause an elevated temperature.

The CF *therm/o* refers to heat. The instrument used to determine body temperature

is called a _____ / _____ / _____ .

---

poison

6-175   Poison is any substance taken into the body by ingestion, inhalation, injection, or absorption that interferes with normal physiological function. Common elements used to refer to poison are ***tox/o, toxic/o,*** and *-toxic.* Whenever you see any of these elements in

a word, you will know that the element refers to _____ .

---

toxic/o/logy
tŏks-ĭ-KŎL-ō-jē

6-176   Virtually any substance can be poisonous if consumed in sufficient quantity. The term poison usually implies an excessive degree of a tox/ic dosage, rather than a specific group of substances. Aspirin is not usually thought of as a poison, but overdoses of this drug can result in the accidental death of a child.

Form a word that means *study of poisons.*

_____ / _____ / _____

Boldface indicates a word root or combining form. Blue indicates a suffix. Pink indicates a prefix.

abnormal condition, poison **toxic/o, tox/o**	**6-177** Toxic/osis literally means _____ _____ of _____. The CF for *poison* is _____ / _____ or _____ / _____.
toxic/o/logy tŏks-ĭ-KŎL-ō-jē	**6-178** Substances that impair health or destroy life when ingested, inhaled, or absorbed by the body in relatively small amounts are considered tox/ic substances. Identifying the tox/ic substance is critical to expeditious treatment. Scientific study of poisons is known as _____ / _____ / _____.
ultra/son/o/graphy ūl-tră-sŏn-ŎG-ră-fē	**6-179** The suffix -*gram* is used in words to mean *record, writing*. The suffix -*graphy* is used in words to mean *process of recording*. Ultra/son/o/graphy (US) is the *process of imaging deep structures of the body by recording reflection of high-frequency sound waves (ultrasound) and displaying the reflected echoes on a monitor.* US is also called ultrasound and echo. When confirmation of a suspected disease or tumor is needed, the physician may order the radi/o/graph/ic imaging procedure called ultrasound, also known as _____ / _____ / _____ / _____ (US).
adjective **noun** **noun** **noun** **adjective**	**6-180** Adjective and noun suffixes are attached to roots to indicate a part of speech. Some adjective suffixes that mean pertaining to (such as -*ile, -ior,* and -*ous*) were previously introduced. Noun suffixes that mean condition (such as -*ia, -ism,* and -*ist*) were also introduced. Identify the part of speech for the following terms. The first one is completed for you. pen/ile *adjective* _____ cutane/ous _____ gastr/o/log/ist _____ thyroid/ism _____ pneumon/ia _____ poster/ior _____
gastr/o/megaly găs-trō-MĔG-ă-lē	**6-181** Use -*megaly* to build a word that means *enlargement of the stomach*. _____ / _____ / _____
hepat/o/megaly hĕp-ă-tō-MĔG-ă-lē	**6-182** Hepat/o/megaly may be caused by hepat/itis or another condition, such as bil/i/ary obstruction, malignancy, or fatty infiltration caused by alcoholism. The term used in the Dx of an *enlargement of the liver* is _____ / _____ / _____.

SECTION REVIEW 6-6

Using the following table, write the combining form or suffix that matches its definition in the space provided to the left of the definition. There may be more than one word element that matches a definition.

Combining Forms

chol/e	pancreat/o
cholecyst/o	therm/o
choledoch/o	toxic/o
cyst/o	tox/o
hepat/o	

Suffixes

-algia	-graphy	-plasty
-dynia	-iasis	-rrhaphy
-ectomy	-lith	-stomy
-emesis	-megaly	-toxic
-gram	-oma	

1. _____ tumor

2. _____ abnormal condition (produced by something specified)

3. _____ bile duct

4. _____ bile, gall

5. _____ bladder

6. _____ enlargement

7. _____ excision, removal

8. _____ forming an opening (mouth)

9. _____ gallbladder

10. _____ heat

11. _____ liver

12. _____ pain

13. _____ pancreas

14. _____ poison

15. _____ process of recording

16. _____ record, writing

17. _____ stone, calculus

18. _____ surgical repair

19. _____ suture

20. _____ vomiting

Competency Verification: Check your answers in Appendix B: Answer Key, page 580. If you are not satisfied with your level of comprehension, go back to Frame 6–131 and rework the frames.

Correct Answers _____ × 5 = _____ % Score

ABBREVIATIONS

This section introduces digestive system–related abbreviations and their meanings. Included are abbreviations contained in the medical record activities that follow.

Abbreviation	Meaning	Abbreviation	Meaning
BM	bowel movement	GI	gastrointestinal
BMI	body mass index	IBD	inflammatory bowel disease
CA	cancer; chronological age; cardiac arrest	IBS	irritable bowel syndrome
CT	computed tomography	IV	intravenous
Dx	diagnosis	LES	lower esophageal sphincter
EGD	esophagogastroduodenoscopy	MRI	magnetic resonance imaging
ERCP	endoscopic retrograde cholangiopancreatography	NG	nasogastric
ESWL	extracorporeal shock-wave lithotripsy	RGB	Roux-en-Y gastric bypass
FBS	fasting blood sugar	RUQ	right upper quadrant
GERD	gastroesophageal reflux disease	US	ultrasound; ultrasonography

ADDITIONAL MEDICAL TERMS

The following are additional medical terms related to the digestive system. Recognizing and learning these terms will help you understand the connection between a pathological condition, its diagnosis, and the rationale behind the method of treatment selected for a particular disorder.

Diseases and Conditions

appendicitis
ă-pĕn-dĭ-SĪ-tĭs
  appendic: appendix
    -itis: inflammation

Inflammation of the appendix, which is usually acute and caused by blockage of the appendix followed by infection

Treatment for acute appendicitis is appendectomy within 48 hours of the first symptom. When left untreated, appendicitis rapidly leads to perforation and peritonitis as fecal matter is released into the peritoneal cavity. (See Fig. 6–8.)

---

ascites
ă-SĪ-tēz

Abnormal accumulation of serous fluid in the peritoneal cavity

Ascites may be a symptom of inflammatory disorders in the abdomen, venous hypertension caused by liver disease, or heart failure (HF). (See Fig. 6–9.)

---

borborygmus
bŏr-bō-RĬG-mŭs

Gurgling or rumbling sound heard over the large intestine caused by gas moving through the intestines

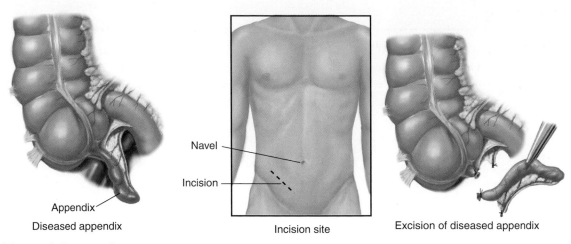

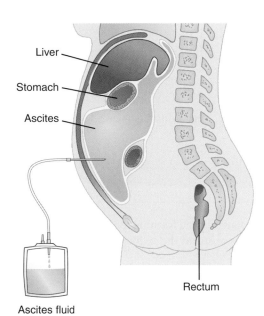

Diseased appendix

Incision site

Excision of diseased appendix

Figure 6-8 Appendectomy.

Ascites fluid

Figure 6-9 Ascites with removal of fluid from the abdominal cavity using a catheter.

cirrhosis
sĭ-RŌ-sĭs
   cirrh: yellow
   -osis: abnormal condition; increase (used primarily with blood cells)
	Chronic liver disease characterized by destruction of liver cells that eventually leads to ineffective liver function and jaundice
	
	Cirrhosis is most commonly caused by chronic alcoholism. It may also be caused by hepatitis, toxins, infectious agents, and circulatory disorders.

celiac disease SĒ-lē-ăk	Disorder that damages the lining of the small intestine in response to gluten (protein found in barley, oats, and wheat) ingestion, which results in malabsorption of nutrients *Treatment for celiac disease consists of the adoption of a gluten-free diet. Patients generally recover by adhering to strict gluten-free dietary guidelines.*

diverticular disease dī-věr-TĬK-ū-lăr	Condition in which bulging pouches (diverticula) in the gastrointestinal (GI) tract push the mucosal lining through the surrounding muscle *When feces become trapped inside a diverticular sac, it causes inflammation, infection, abdominal pain, and fever, a condition known as diverticulitis. (See Fig. 6–10).*

dysentery
DĬS-ĕn-tĕr-ē
   dys-: bad; painful;
        difficult
   enter: intestine (usually
        small intestine)
   -y: condition;
       process
	Inflammation of the intestine, especially of the colon, which may be caused by chemical irritants, bacteria, protozoa, or parasites
	
	Dysentery is common in underdeveloped areas of the world and in times of disaster and social disorganization when sanitary living conditions, clean food, and safe water are not available. It is characterized by diarrhea, colitis, and abdominal cramps.

fistula FĬS-tū-lă	Abnormal passage from one organ to another or from a hollow organ to the surface *An anal fistula is located near the anus and may open into the rectum.*

gastroesophageal reflux disease (GERD)
găs-trō-ē-sŏf-ă-JĒ-ăl
RĒ-flŭks dĭ-ZĒZ
   gastr/o: stomach
   esophag: esophagus
     -eal: pertaining to
	Backflow (reflux) of gastric contents into the esophagus due to malfunction of the lower esophageal sphincter (LES)
	
	Symptoms of GERD include heartburn (burning sensation caused by regurgitation of hydrochloric acid from the stomach to the esophagus), belching, and regurgitation of food. Treatment includes elevating the head of the bed while sleeping, avoiding alcohol and foods that stimulate acid secretion, and administering drugs to decrease production of acid.

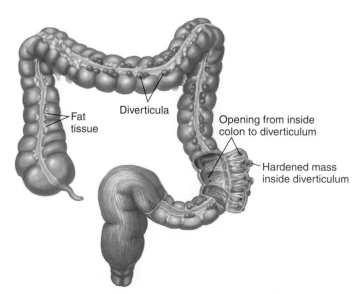

Figure 6-10 Diverticular disease.

hematochezia hĕm-ă-tō-KĒ-zē-ă	Passage of stools containing bright red blood
hemorrhoid HĔM-ō-royd	Mass of enlarged, twisted varicose veins in the mucous membrane inside (internal) or just outside (external) the rectum; also known as *piles*
hernia HĔR-nē-ă	Protrusion or projection of an organ or a part of an organ through the wall of the cavity that normally contains it (See Fig. 6–11.)
inflammatory bowel disease (IBD) ĭn-FLĂM-ă-tŏr-ē BŎWL	Ulceration of the colon mucosa *Crohn disease and ulcerative colitis are forms of IBD.*
Crohn disease KRŌN	Chronic IBD that usually affects the ileum but may affect any portion of the intestinal tract *Crohn disease is distinguished from closely related bowel disorders by its inflammatory pattern, which tends to be patchy or segmented; also called regional colitis.*

ulcerative colitis
   ŬL-sĕr-ā-tĭv kō-LĪ-tĭs
      col: colon
      -itis: inflammation
	Chronic IBD of the colon characterized by episodes of diarrhea, rectal bleeding, and pain

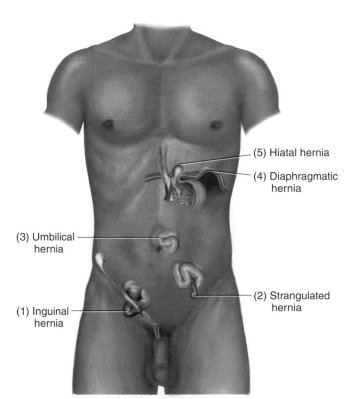

(5) Hiatal hernia

(4) Diaphragmatic hernia

(3) Umbilical hernia

(1) Inguinal hernia

(2) Strangulated hernia

Figure 6-11 Common locations of hernias.

irritable bowel syndrome (IBS) ĬR-ĭ-tă-bl BŎWL SĬN-drōm	Condition characterized by gastrointestinal signs and symptoms, including constipation, diarrhea, gas, and bloating, all in the absence of organic pathology; also called spastic colon *Contributing factors of IBS include stress and tension. Treatment consists of dietary modifications, such as avoiding irritating foods or adding a high-fiber diet and laxatives if constipation is a symptom. It also includes antidiarrheal and antispasmodic drugs, as well as alleviating anxiety and stress.*
obesity **morbid obesity**	Condition in which a person accumulates an amount of fat that exceeds the body's skeletal and physical standards, usually an increase of 20 percent or more above ideal body weight More severe obesity in which a person has a body mass index (BMI) of 40 or greater, which is generally 100 or more pounds over ideal body weight *Morbid obesity is a disease with serious medical, psychological, and social ramifications.*
pancreatitis păn-krē-ă-TĪ-tĭs *pancreat:* pancreas *-itis:* inflammation	Inflammation or infection of the pancreas that occurs when pancreatic enzymes that digest food are activated in the pancreas instead of the duodenum and attack pancreatic tissue, causing damage to the gland *Pancreatitis is caused by chronic alcoholism, gallstones, drug toxicity, infections, and metabolic disorders. Treatment includes administration of pancreatic enzymes, medications to relieve epigastric pain, intravenous fluids, subtotal pancreatectomy, or choledocholithotomy to remove a gallstone.*
peritonitis pĕr-ĭ-tō-NĪ-tĭs	Bacterial or fungal infection of the peritoneum that can result from any rupture (perforation) in the abdomen or as a complication of other medical conditions *Peritonitis requires prompt medical attention. Treatment involves antibiotics and, in some cases, surgery. If left untreated, peritonitis can lead to severe, potentially life-threatening infection throughout the body.*
polyp PŎL-ĭp	Small, stalklike growth that resembles a mushroom and protrudes upward or outward from a mucous membrane surface *Polyps detected during colonoscopy are excised (polypectomy) and sent to the laboratory for microscopic tissue examination (biopsy). This test is used to screen for cancerous or abnormal cells. (See Fig. 6–12.)*

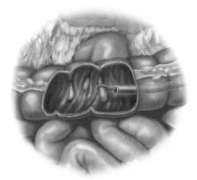

Figure 6-12 Polypectomy.

volvulus VŎL-vū-lŭs	Twisting of the bowel on itself, causing obstruction *Volvulus usually requires surgery to untwist the loop of bowel.*

Diagnostic Procedures

barium enema (BE) BĂ-rē-ŭm ĔN-ĕ-mă	Radiographic examination of the rectum and colon after administration of barium (radiopaque contrast medium) into the rectum; also called *lower GI series (See Fig. 6–13.)* *BE is used for diagnosis of obstructions, tumors, and other abnormalities of the colon.*
barium swallow BĂ-rē-ŭm	Radiographic examination of the esophagus, stomach, and small intestine after oral administration of barium (radiopaque contrast medium); also called *upper GI series* *Barium swallow is commonly performed in patients experiencing dysphagia. Structural abnormalities of the esophagus, stomach, and small intestine may also be diagnosed using this technique.*
computed tomography (CT) kŏm-PŪ-tĕd tō-MŎG-ră-fē *tom/o:* to cut *-graphy:* process of recording	Tomography in which a narrow beam of x-rays rotates in a full arc around the patient to acquire multiple views of the body, which a computer interprets to produce cross-sectional images of an internal organ or tissue; also called *computerized axial tomography (CAT)* *CT scans are used to view the gallbladder, liver, bile ducts, and pancreas and diagnose tumors, cysts, inflammation, abscesses, perforation, bleeding, and obstructions. A contrast material may be used to enhance the structures.*

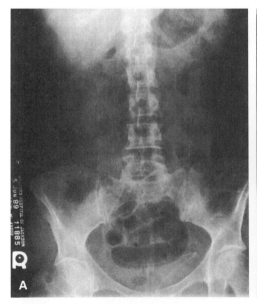 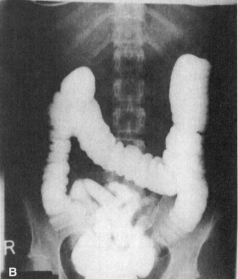

Figure 6-13 Barium enema done poorly (**A**) and correctly (**B**).

endoscopy ĕn-DŎS-kō-pē *endo-:* in, within *-scopy:* visual examination	Visual examination of a cavity or canal using a specialized lighted instrument called an *endoscope* *The organ, cavity, or canal being examined dictates the name of the endoscopic procedure. A camera and video recorder are commonly used during the procedure to provide a permanent record.*
upper GI	Endoscopy of the esophagus (esophagoscopy), stomach (gastroscopy), and duodenum (duodenoscopy) *Endoscopy of the upper GI tract is performed to identify tumors, esophagitis, gastroesophageal varices, peptic ulcers, and the source of upper GI bleeding. It is also used to confirm the presence and extent of varices in the lower esophagus and stomach in patients with liver disease.*
lower GI	Endoscopy of the colon (colonoscopy), sigmoid colon (sigmoidoscopy), and rectum and anal canal (proctoscopy) *Endoscopy of the lower GI tract is used to identify pathological conditions in the colon. It may also be used to remove polyps. When polyps are discovered in the colon, they are removed and tested for cancer.*
magnetic resonance imaging (MRI) măg-NĔT-ĭc RĔZ-ĕn-ăns ĬM-ĭj-ĭng	Radiographic technique that uses electromagnetic energy to produce multiplanar cross-sectional images of the body *In the digestive system, MRI is particularly useful in detecting abdominal masses and viewing images of abdominal structures.*
stool guaiac GWĪ-ăk	Laboratory test performed on feces to detect the presence of blood in the stool (bowel movement) that is not apparent on visual inspection; also called *Hemoccult test*
ultrasonography (US) ŭl-tră-sŏn-ŎG-ră-fē *ultra-:* excess, beyond *son/o:* sound *-graphy:* process of recording	Radiographic procedure in which a small transducer passed over the skin transmits high-frequency sound waves (ultrasound) that bounce off body tissues and are then recorded to produce an image of an internal organ or tissue *Ultrasound is used to view the liver, gallbladder, bile ducts, and pancreas, among other structures. It is also used to diagnose digestive disorders, locate cysts and tumors, and guide insertion of instruments during surgical procedures.*

Medical and Surgical Procedures

bariatric surgery
BĂR-ē-ă-trĭk

Group of procedures that treat morbid obesity

Commonly employed bariatric surgeries include vertical banded gastroplasty and Roux-en-Y gastric bypass. (See Fig. 6–14.)

  vertical banded gastroplasty
  găs-trō-PLĂS-tē
   gastr/o: stomach
   -plasty: surgical repair

Bariatric surgery in which the upper stomach near the esophagus is stapled vertically to reduce it to a small pouch and a band is inserted that restricts and delays food from leaving the pouch, causing a feeling of fullness (See Fig. 6–14A.)

  Roux-en-Y gastric bypass (RGB)
  rū-ĕn-WĪ GĂS-trĭk

Bariatric surgery in which the stomach is first stapled to decrease it to a small pouch and then the jejunum is shortened and connected to the small stomach pouch, causing the base of the duodenum leading from the nonfunctioning portion of the stomach to form a Y configuration, which decreases the pathway of food through the intestine, thus reducing absorption of calories and fats

RGB is performed laparoscopically using instruments inserted through small incisions in the abdomen. When laparoscopy is not possible, gastric bypass can be performed as an open procedure (laparotomy) and involves a large incision in the middle of the abdomen. RGB is the most commonly performed weight loss surgery today. (See Fig. 6–14B.)

lithotripsy
LĬTH-ō-trĭp-sē
 lith/o: stone, calculus
 -tripsy: crushing

Procedure for eliminating a stone within the gallbladder or urinary system by crushing the stone surgically or using a noninvasive method, such as ultrasonic shock waves, to shatter it

The crushed fragments may be expelled or washed out.

  extracorporeal shock-wave lithotripsy (ESWL)
  ĕks-tră-kor-POR-ē-ăl
  LĬTH-ō-trĭp-sē
   extra-: outside
   corpor: body
    -eal: pertaining to
   lith/o: stone, calculus
   -tripsy: crushing

Use of shock waves as a noninvasive method to destroy stones in the gallbladder and biliary ducts

In ESWL, ultrasound is used to locate the stone or stones and monitor their destruction. The patient usually undergoes a course of oral dissolution drugs to ensure complete removal of all stones and stone fragments.

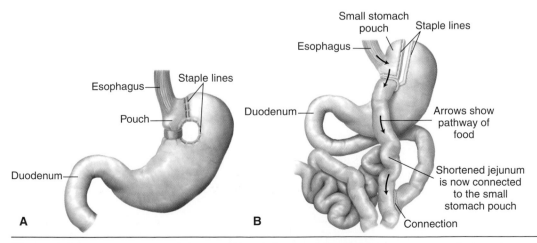

Figure 6-14 Bariatric surgery. (**A**) Vertical banded gastroplasty. (**B**) Roux-en-Y gastric bypass.

nasogastric (NG) intubation nā-zō-GĂS-trĭk ĭn-tū-BĀ-shŭn *nas/o:* nose *gastr:* stomach *-ic:* pertaining to	Insertion of a nasogastric tube through the nose into the stomach *Nasogastric intubation is used to relieve gastric distention by removing gas, gastric secretions, or food. It is also used to instill medication, food, or fluids or obtain a specimen for laboratory analysis.*

PHARMACOLOGY

The following table lists common drug categories used to treat gastrointestinal disorders, as well as their therapeutic actions.

Drug Category	Action
antacids ănt-ĂS-ĭds	Neutralize acids in the stomach
antidiarrheals ăn-tĭ-dī-ă-RĒ-ăls	Control loose stools and relieve diarrhea by absorbing excess water in the bowel or slowing peristalsis in the intestinal tract
antiemetics ăn-tĭ-ē-MĔT-ĭks	Control nausea and vomiting by blocking nerve impulses to the vomiting center of the brain
laxatives LĂK-să-tĭvz	Relieve constipation and facilitate passage of feces through the lower GI tract

Pronunciation Help	Long sound Short sound	ā in rāte ă in ălone	ē in rēbirth ĕ in ĕver	ī in īsle ĭ in ĭt	ō in ōver ŏ in nŏt	ū in ūnite ŭ in cŭt

ADDITIONAL MEDICAL TERMS REVIEW

Match the medical term(s) below with the definitions in the numbered list.

ascites	cirrhosis	hematochezia	IBS	NG intubation
barium enema	Crohn disease	Hemoccult	jaundice	polyp
barium swallow	fistula	IBD	lithotripsy	volvulus

1. _____ is a test performed on feces that detects the presence of blood that is not apparent on visual inspection and is also called *stool guaiac*.

2. _____ refers to the insertion of a tube through the nose into the stomach for therapeutic and diagnostic purposes.

3. _____ is a small benign growth that projects from a mucous membrane.

4. _____ is an abnormal accumulation of serous fluid in the peritoneal cavity.

5. _____ refers to chronic inflammatory bowel disease, which usually affects the ileum.

6. _____ refers to surgically crushing a stone.

7. _____ is an abnormal, tubelike passage from one organ to another or from one organ to the surface.

8. _____ is a yellow discoloration of the skin caused by hyperbilirubinemia.

9. _____ is a radiographic examination of the rectum and colon after administration of barium sulfate.

10. _____ refers to ulceration of the mucosa of the colon, as seen in Crohn disease.

11. _____ refers to passage of stools containing red blood.

12. _____ means twisting of the bowel on itself, causing obstruction.

13. _____ refers to a chronic liver disease characterized pathologically by destruction of liver cells and jaundice.

14. _____ is a radiographic examination of the esophagus, stomach, and small intestine after oral administration of barium sulfate.

15. _____ is a condition characterized by constipation, diarrhea, gas, and bloating without organic pathology and is also called *spastic colon*.

Competency Verification: Check your answers in Appendix B: Answer Key, page 580. If you are not satisfied with your level of comprehension, review the pathological, diagnostic, and therapeutic terms and retake the review.

Correct Answers _____ × 6.67 = _____ % Score

MEDICAL RECORD ACTIVITIES

Medical reports included in the following activities reflect common, real-life clinical scenarios to show how medical terminology is used to document patient care.

MEDICAL RECORD ACTIVITY 6-1

RECTAL BLEEDING

Terminology

Terms listed in the table below come from the medical report Rectal Bleeding that follows. Use a medical dictionary such as Taber's Cyclopedic Medical Dictionary, *the appendices of this book, or other resources to define each term. Then practice reading the pronunciations aloud for each term.*

Term	Definition
angulation ăng-ū-LĂ-shŭn	
anorectal ā-nō-RĔK-tăl	
carcinoma kăr-sĭ-NŌ-mă	
diverticulum dī-věr-TĬK-ū-lŭm	
dysphagia dĭs-FĀ-jē-ă	
emesis ĔM-ĕ-sĭs	
enteritis ĕn-tĕr-Ī-tĭs	
hematemesis hĕm-ăt-ĔM-ĕ-sĭs	

Continued

Term	Definition
ileostomy ĭl-ē-ŎS-tō-mē	
postprandial pōst-PRĂN-dē-ăl	

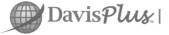 **DavisPlus** | Visit the *Medical Terminology Simplified* online resource center at Davis*Plus* to hear pronunciation and meanings of selected terms in this medical report.

Reading

Practice pronunciation of medical terms by reading the following medical report aloud.

Rectal Bleeding

This 50-year-old white man has lost approximately 40 pounds since his last examination. The patient says he has had no dysphagia or postprandial distress, and there is no report of diarrhea, nausea, emesis, hematemesis, or constipation. The patient has had a history of regional enteritis, appendicitis, and colonic bleeding.

The regional enteritis resulted in an ileostomy with appendectomy about 6 months ago. On 5/30/xx, a sigmoidoscopy using a 10-cm scope showed no evidence of bleeding at the anorectal area. A 35-cm scope was then inserted to a level of 13 cm. At this point, angulation prevented further passage of the scope. No abnormalities had been encountered, but there was dark blood noted at that level.

My impression is that the rectal bleeding could be due to a polyp, bleeding diverticulum, or rectal carcinoma.

Evaluation

Review the medical report above to answer the following questions. Use a medical dictionary such as Taber's Cyclopedic Medical Dictionary *and other resources if needed.*

1. What is the patient's symptom that made him seek medical help?

   _____

   _____

2. What surgical procedures were performed on the patient for regional enteritis?

   _____

   _____

3. What abnormality was found with the sigmoidoscopy?

   _____

   _____

4. What is causing the rectal bleeding?

   _____

   _____

5. Write the plural form of *diverticulum*.

_____

_____

MEDICAL RECORD ACTIVITY 6-2

CARCINOSARCOMA OF THE ESOPHAGUS

Terminology

Terms listed in the table below come from the medical report Carcinosarcoma of the Esophagus that follows. Use a medical dictionary such as Taber's Cyclopedic Medical Dictionary, *the appendices of this book, or other resources to define each term. Then practice reading the pronunciations aloud for each term.*

Term	Definition
aortic arch ā-OR-tĭk	
carcinosarcoma kăr-sĭ-nō-săr-KŌ-mă	
esophagoscopy ē-sŏf-ă-GŎS-kō-pē	
friable FRĪ-ă-bl	
intraluminal ĭn-tră-LŪ-mĭ-năl	
malignant mă-LĬG-nănt	
mediastinal mē-dē-ăs-TĪ-năl	
OR	
polypoid PŎL-ē-poyd	
reanastomosis rē-ăn-ăs-tō-MŌ-sĭs	

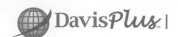 | Visit the *Medical Terminology Simplified* online resource center at Davis*Plus* to hear pronunciation and meanings of selected terms in this medical report.

Reading

Practice pronunciation of medical terms by reading the following medical report aloud.

Carcinosarcoma of the Esophagus

ADMITTING DIAGNOSIS: Carcinosarcoma of the esophagus.

DISCHARGE DIAGNOSIS: Carcinosarcoma of the esophagus.

HISTORY OF PRESENT ILLNESS: Patient had been complaining of dysphagia over the last 4 months with a worsening recently in symptoms.

SURGERY: Esophagoscopy was performed, and a small, friable biopsy specimen was obtained. Pathology tests confirmed it to be malignant. A barium x-ray study revealed polypoid, intraluminal, esophageal obstruction. Surgical findings revealed an infiltrating tumor of the middle third of the esophagus with intraluminal, friable, polypoid masses, each 3 cm in diameter. A resection of the esophagus was performed with reanastomosis of the stomach at the aortic arch. An adjacent mediastinal lymph node was excised. There were no complications during the procedure. Patient left the OR in stable condition.

Evaluation

Review the medical report above to answer the following questions. Use a medical dictionary such as Taber's Cyclopedic Medical Dictionary *and other resources if needed.*

1. What surgery was performed on this patient?

   _____

   _____

2. What diagnostic testing confirmed malignancy?

   _____

   _____

3. Where was the carcinosarcoma located?

   _____

   _____

4. Why was the adjacent lymph node excised?

   _____

   _____

DIGESTIVE SYSTEM CHAPTER REVIEW

WORD ELEMENTS SUMMARY

The following table summarizes CFs, suffixes, and prefixes related to the digestive system. Study the word elements and their meanings before completing the Word Elements Chapter Review that follows.

Word Element	Meaning	Word Element	Meaning
Combining Forms			
appendic/o	appendix	ile/o	ileum (third part of the small intestine)
carcin/o	cancer	jejun/o	jejunum (second part of the small intestine)
chol/e	bile, gall	lith/o	stone, calculus
cholecyst/o	gallbladder	myc/o	fungus
choledoch/o	bile duct	nas/o	nose
cirrh/o, jaund/o	yellow	or/o, stomat/o	mouth
col/o, colon/o	colon	orth/o	straight
corpor/o	body	pancreat/o	pancreas
dent/o, odont/o	teeth	peritone/o	peritoneum
duoden/o	duodenum (first part of the small intestine)	polyp/o	small growth
enter/o	intestine (usually the small intestine)	proct/o	anus, rectum
esophag/o	esophagus	ptyal/o, sial/o	saliva, salivary gland
gastr/o	stomach	rect/o	rectum
gingiv/o	gum(s)	sigmoid/o	sigmoid colon
gloss/o, lingu/o	tongue	son/o	sound
hemat/o, hem/o	blood	tom/o	to cut
hepat/o	liver	tox/o, toxic/o	poison
Suffixes			
-algia, -dynia	pain	-phagia	swallowing, eating
-ectomy	excision, removal	-plasty	surgical repair
-emesis	vomiting	-rrhaphy	suture
-gram	record, writing	-rrhea	discharge, flow
-graphy	process of recording	-scope	instrument for examining
-iasis	abnormal condition (produced by something specified)	-scopy	visual examination
-itis	inflammation	-spasm	involuntary contraction, twitching
-lith	stone, calculus	-stenosis	narrowing, stricture

Continued

Word Element	Meaning	Word Element	Meaning
-logist	specialist in the study of	-stomy	forming an opening (mouth)
-megaly	enlargement	-tome	instrument to cut
-oma	tumor	-tomy	incision
-osis	abnormal condition; increase (used primarily with blood cells)	-tripsy	crushing
-pepsia	digestion		
Prefixes			
dia-	through, across	hyper-	excessive, above normal
dys-	bad; painful; difficult	hypo-	under, below, deficient
endo-	in, within	peri-	around
epi-	above, upon	sub-	under, below
extra-	outside	ultra-	excess, beyond

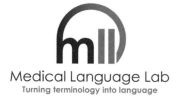

Medical Language Lab
Turning terminology into language

Visit the *Medical Language Lab* at *medicallanguagelab.com.* Use the flash-card–word elements exercise to reinforce your study of word elements. We recommend you complete the flash-card activity before starting the Word Elements Chapter Review that follows.

WORD ELEMENTS CHAPTER REVIEW

This review provides a verification of your knowledge of the word elements covered in this chapter. Write the meaning of the word element in the space provided. To reinforce your understanding of the word parts that comprise a medical term, identify each word element as a prefix (P), word root (WR), combining form (CF), or suffix (S). The first word is completed for you.

Medical Term	Word Element	Meaning
1. anorexia	an- (P)	without, not
	-orexia (S)	appetite
2. appendicitis		
3. cholangiography		
4. cholecystectomy		
5. choledochotomy		

Continued

Medical Term	Word Element	Meaning
6. cirrhosis		
7. colonoscopy		
8. colostomy		
9. duodenorrhaphy		
10. enteropathy		
11. gastroenterologist		

Medical Term	Word Element	Meaning
12. gingivitis		
13. hematemesis		
14. hepatomegaly		
15. ileostomy		
16. jejunorrhaphy		
17. lithotripsy		

Continued

Medical Term	Word Element	Meaning
18. pancreatolysis		
19. peritonitis		
20. postprandial		
21. proctologist		
22. rectostenosis		
23. sigmoidotomy		

Medical Term	Word Element	Meaning
24. sublingual		
25. toxicology		

Competency Verification: Check your answers in Appendix B: Answer Key, page 581. If you are not satisfied with your level of comprehension, review the chapter's flash-card exercise at *medicallanguagelab.com* and retake the review.

Correct Answers _____ × 4 = _____ % Score

VOCABULARY REVIEW

Match the medical word(s) below with the definitions in the numbered list.

anastomosis   cholelithiasis   gastroscopy   peritonitis
antiemetics   duodenotomy   GERD   rectoplasty
bariatric   dyspepsia   hematemesis   sigmoidotomy
celiac disease   dysphagia   hepatomegaly   stomatalgia
cholecystectomy   friable   ileostomy   ultrasound

1. _____ refers to visual examination of the stomach.

2. _____ means bad, painful, difficult digestion.

3. _____ means vomiting blood.

4. _____ refers to high-frequency sound waves that produce internal images of the body.

5. _____ controls nausea and vomiting by blocking nerve impulses to the vomiting center of the brain.

6. _____ damages the lining of the small intestine in response to gluten and results in mal-absorption of nutrients

7. _____ means pain in the mouth.

8. _____ is an incision of the duodenum.

9. _____ means enlargement of the liver.

10. _____ refers to painful swallowing.

11. _____ means removal of the gallbladder.

12. _____ is a surgical connection between two vessels.

13. _____ is an incision of the sigmoid colon.

14. _____ refers to surgical repair of the rectum.

15. _____ is a reflux of gastric contents into the esophagus with heartburn.

16. _____ refers to formation of an opening (mouth) into the ileum.

17. _____ refers to the presence or formation of gallstones.

18. _____ means easily broken or pulverized.

19. _____ is an infection of the lining of the abdomen.

20. _____ is surgery that treats morbid obesity by altering digestive structures to limit food intake.

Competency Verification: Check your answers in Appendix B: Answer Key, page 582. If you are not satisfied with your level of comprehension, review the chapter vocabulary and retake the review.

Correct Answers _____ × 5 = _____ % Score

Urinary System

OBJECTIVES

Upon completion of this chapter, you will be able to:

• Describe the type of medical treatment urologists and nephrologists provide.

• Identify urinary structures by labeling them on anatomical illustrations.

• Describe the primary functions of the urinary system.

• Describe diseases, conditions, and procedures related to the urinary system.

• Apply your word-building skills by constructing medical terms related to the urinary system.

• Describe common abbreviations and symbols related to the urinary system.

• Recognize, define, pronounce, and spell terms correctly.

• Demonstrate your knowledge of this chapter by successfully completing the frames, reviews, and medical report evaluations.

MEDICAL SPECIALTIES

Urology

Physicians who specialize in diagnosis and treatment of disorders of the female and the male urinary systems are called **urologists.** Because some urinary structures in the male perform a dual role (both urinary functions and reproductive functions), the urologist also treats male reproductive disorders. These male disorders include but are not limited to treatment of bladder cancer, infertility, and sexual dysfunctions. Generally, the urologist performs surgery, and treats urination problems, such as difficulty holding urine (incontinence) or obstruction or urinary flow due to tumors or stones in the urinary organs. Also, they manage male reproductive disorders, such as impotence (erectile dysfunction). Other types of urologists include, the **urogynecologist** who specializes in treating urinary problems involving the female reproductive system, and the **pediatric urologist** who specializes in diagnosing and treating urinary problems in children.

Nephrology

The medical specialty of **nephrology** is a subspecialty of internal medicine. **Nephrologists** provide diagnostic evaluation and ongoing care of patients with medical disorders related to the kidneys. These include but are not limited to chronic kidney disease, diabetic kidney disease, complicated hypertension, inherited renal disease, such as polycystic kidney disease, kidney stone prevention, pre- and post-kidney transplantation, and excess fluid accumulation, and problems with electrolyte and mineral metabolism. They also supervise the provision of dialysis services to individuals whose kidneys have deteriorated to the point that their lives would be in jeopardy without renal replacement therapy, a problem commonly known as end-stage renal disease (ESRD).

ANATOMY AND PHYSIOLOGY OVERVIEW

The urinary system is composed of the kidneys, ureters, bladder, and urethra. Its purpose is to regulate the volume and composition of fluids in the body and remove waste substances and excess fluid from the blood. Waste substances are filtered from the blood by the kidneys and excreted in the urine, which exits via the ureters into the urinary bladder. Urine is stored in the bladder until the urge to urinate occurs, at which point the muscles at the bladder outlet relax, allowing the urine to be expelled through the urethra. Review Figure 7–1 to identify the location of urinary structures within the body.

The kidneys perform the major work of the urinary system. The other parts of the system are mainly passageways and storage areas. Functions of the kidneys include regulating the amount of water in the body and keeping body fluids at a constant concentration and acid-base level. They achieve these functions by filtering blood and excreting waste substances and excess water as urine. Other essential substances are reabsorbed into the bloodstream by the process called **reabsorption.**

The filtering–reabsorption process is necessary to maintain the balance of substances required for a relatively stable internal body environment. This stable internal environment, known as **homeostasis,** is necessary for the cells of the body to survive and carry out their functions effectively. If the kidneys fail, waste substances cannot be eliminated from the body. Thus, the substances accumulate in the blood to toxic levels and the cells can no longer function. Death ultimately results unless impurities are filtered out of the blood by means of an artificial kidney known as **kidney dialysis** or the nonfunctioning kidneys are replaced with a healthy kidney through kidney transplantation.

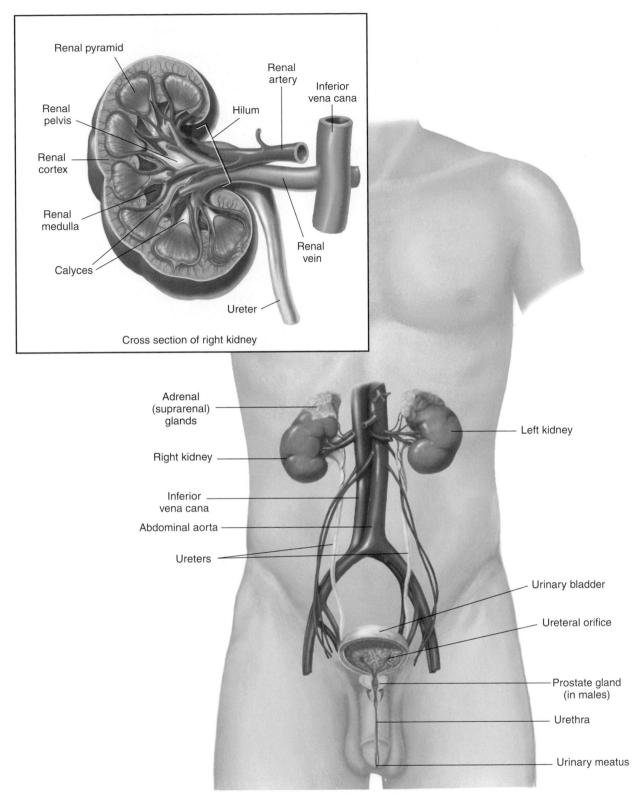

Cross section of right kidney

Figure 7-1 Urinary system with a cross section of the right kidney showing internal structures.

WORD ELEMENTS

This section introduces combining forms (CFs) related to the urinary system. Included are key suffixes; prefixes are defined in the right-hand column as needed. Review the following table, and pronounce each word in the word analysis column aloud before you begin to work in the frames.

Word Element	Meaning	Word Analysis
Combining Forms		
cyst/o	bladder	**cyst/o**/scopy (sĭs-TŎS-kō-pē): visual examination of the urinary tract using a cystoscope inserted through the urethra *-scopy*: visual examination *Cystoscopy helps diagnose urinary tract disorders, obtain tissue and urine samples, excise tumors, or inject a contrast medium into the bladder.*
vesic/o		**vesic/o**/cele (VĔS-ĭ-kō-sēl): hernial protrusion of the urinary bladder; also called *cystocele* *-cele*: hernia, swelling
glomerul/o	glomerulus	**glomerul**/ar (glō-MĔR-ū-lăr): pertaining to the glomerulus *-ar*: pertaining to *The glomerulus is a cluster of capillaries forming the structural and functional unit of the kidney known as the nephron. Glomerular capillaries filter fluid, the first step in urine formation.*
meat/o	opening, meatus	**meat**/us (mē-Ā-tŭs): opening or tunnel through any part of the body, such as the external opening of the urethra *-us*: condition, structure
nephr/o	kidney	**nephr**/oma (nĕ-FRŌ-mă): tumor of the kidney *oma:* tumor
ren/o		**ren**/al (RĒ-năl): pertaining to the kidney *-al:* pertaining to
pyel/o	renal pelvis	**pyel/o**/plasty (PĪ-ĕ-lō-plăs-tē): surgical repair of the renal pelvis *-plasty*: surgical repair
ur/o	urine, urinary tract	**ur**/emia (ū-RĒ-mē-ă): excessive urea and other nitrogenous waste products in the blood; also called *azotemia* *-emia:* blood condition *Healthy kidneys excrete waste products normally. Uremia occurs in renal failure.*
urin/o		**urin**/ary (Ū-rĭ-nār-ē): pertaining to urine or the formation of urine or the urinary tract *-ary*: pertaining to
ureter/o	ureter	**ureter/o**/stenosis (ū-rē-tĕr-ō-stĕ-NŌ-sĭs): narrowing or stricture of a ureter *-stenosis:* narrowing, stricture
urethr/o	urethra	**urethr/o**/cele (ū-RĒ-thrō-sēl): hernial protrusion of the urethra *-cele*: hernia, swelling *Urethrocele may be congenital or acquired and secondary to obesity, childbirth, and poor muscle tone.*

Word Element	Meaning	Word Analysis
Suffixes		
-emia	blood condition	azot/**emia** (ăz-ō-TĒ-mē-ă): excessive amounts of nitrogenous compounds in the blood *azot*: nitrogenous compounds *Azotemia is a toxic condition caused by the kidneys' failure to remove urea from the blood.*
-iasis	abnormal condition (produced by something specified)	lith/**iasis** (lĭth-Ī-ă-sĭs): abnormal condition of stones or calculi *lith*: stone, calculus *The calculi occur most commonly in the kidney, lower urinary tract, and gallbladder.*
-lysis	separation; destruction; loosening	dia/**lysis** (dī-ĂL-ĭ-sĭs): process of removing toxic wastes from the blood when the kidneys are unable to do so *dia-*: through, across
-pathy	disease	nephr/o/**pathy** (nĕ-FRŎP-ă-thē): disease of the kidneys *nephr*: kidney
-pexy	fixation (of an organ)	nephr/o/**pexy** (NĔF-rō-pĕks-ē): surgical procedure to affix a displaced kidney *nephr/o*: kidney
-ptosis	prolapse, downward displacement	nephr/o/**ptosis** (nĕf-rŏp-TŌ-sĭs): downward displacement or dropping of a kidney *nephr/o*: kidney
-tripsy	crushing	lith/o/**tripsy** (LĬTH-ō-trĭp-sē): crushing of a stone *lith/o*: stone, calculus *Lithotripsy is a surgical procedure that employs sound waves to crush a stone in the kidney, ureter, bladder, or gallbladder. The fragments may then be expelled or washed out.*
-uria	urine	poly/**uria** (pŏl-ē-Ū-rē-ă): excessive urination *poly-*: many, much

Pronunciation Help	Long sound	ā in rāte	ē in rēbirth	ī in īsle	ō in ōver	ū in ūnite
	Short sound	ă in ălone	ĕ in ĕver	ĭ in ĭt	ŏ in nŏt	ŭ in cŭt

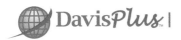

Visit the *Medical Terminology Simplified* online resource center at Davis*Plus* for an audio exercise of the terms in this table. It will help you master pronunciations and meanings of medical terms.

SECTION REVIEW 7-1

For the following medical terms, first write the suffix and its meaning. Then translate the meaning of the remaining elements starting with the first part of the word. The first word is completed for you.

Term

Meaning

1. glomerul/o/scler/osis

   -osis: abnormal condition, increase (used primarily with blood cells);

   glomerulus; hardening, sclera (white of the eye)

2. cyst/o/scopy

3. poly/uria

4. lith/o/tripsy

5. dia/lysis

6. ureter/o/stenosis

7. meat/us

8. ur/emia

9. nephr/oma

10. azot/emia

Competency Verification: Check your answers in Appendix B: Answer Key, page 582. If you are not satisfied with your level of comprehension, review the vocabulary and retake the review.

Correct Answers _____ × 10 = _____ % Score

MACROSCOPIC STRUCTURES

The macroscopic structures that make up the urinary system include two kidneys, two ureters, a bladder, and a urethra.

Kidneys

7-1   Label urinary structures in Figure 7–2 as you read the following material.

The urinary system is composed of a (1) **right kidney** and a **left kidney**. These are the primary structural units responsible for urine formation. Each kidney is composed of an outer layer, called the (2) **renal cortex,** and an inner region, called the (3) **renal medulla.** Blood enters the kidneys through the (4) **renal artery** and leaves through the (5) **renal vein.** Inside the kidney, the renal artery branches into smaller arteries called arterioles that lead into microscopic filtering units called nephrons. Each (6) **nephron** is designed to filter urea and other waste products effectively from the blood.

Boldface indicates a word root or combining form. Blue indicates a suffix. Pink indicates a prefix.

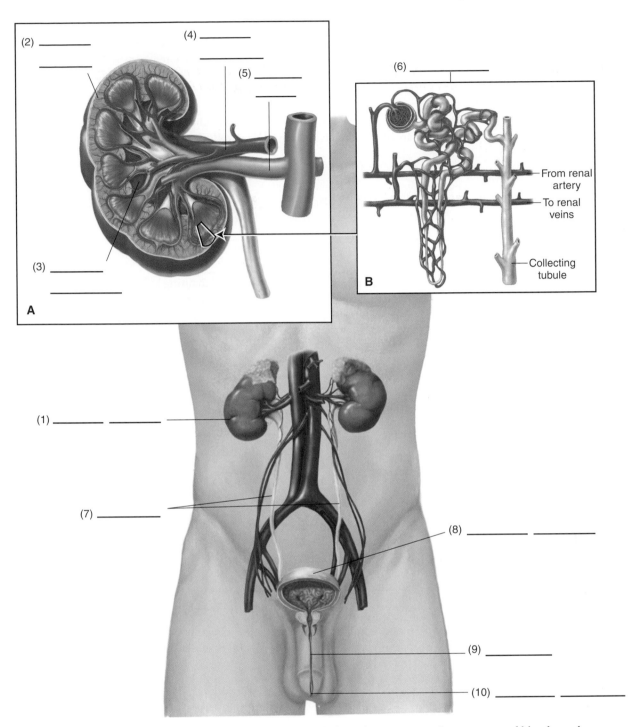

(2) _____

(4) _____

(5) _____

(6) _____

From renal artery

To renal veins

Collecting tubule

(3) _____

_____

A

B

(1) _____ _____

(7) _____

(8) _____ _____

(9) _____

(10) _____ _____

Figure 7-2 Urinary system. (**A**) Cross section of the right kidney showing internal structures and blood vessels. (**B**) Single nephron with a collecting duct and associated blood vessels.

kidney(s)	**7-2** The CFs *nephr/o* and *ren/o* refer to the kidneys. Whenever you see terms such as nephr/itis and ren/al, you will know they refer to the _____.
kidney(s)	**7-3** The term ren/al is commonly used as an adjective to modify a noun. Some examples are ren/al dialysis and ren/al biopsy. Both of these terms mean *pertaining to the* _____.
nephr/ectomy ně-FRĔK-tō-mē	**7-4** A diseased kidney, or renal cancer, may necessitate its removal. Use *nephr/o* to form a word that means *excision of a kidney*. _____ / _____
nephr/o/megaly něf-rō-MĔG-ă-lē	**7-5** When nephr/ectomy is performed, the remaining kidney most likely will become enlarged. Build a word that means *enlargement of a kidney*. _____ / _____ / _____

> If you had difficulty deciding whether to use **nephr/o** or **ren/o** in the previous frames, refer to your medical dictionary. Until you master the language of medicine, the dictionary will help you identify commonly used terms in medicine.

lith/iasis lĭth-Ī-ă-sĭs	**7-6** The suffix *-iasis* is used to describe an abnormal condition (produced by something specified). An abnormal condition of stones is called _____ / _____.
nephr/o/lith NĔF-rō-lĭth **nephr/o/lith/iasis** něf-rō-lĭth-Ī-ă-sĭs	**7-7** Use *nephr/o* to construct a medical word that means *stone (in the) kidney:* _____ / _____ / _____ *abnormal condition of kidney stone(s):* _____ / _____ / _____ / _____
nephr/algia ně-FRĂL-jē-ă **nephr/itis** něf-RĪ-tĭs	**7-8** Formation of a kidney stone, or ren/al calculus, can vary in size from micro/scop/ic (commonly referred to as sand or gravel) to a stone large enough to block the ureter or fill the ren/al pelvis. The stone commonly causes nephr/itis and nephr/algia. (See Fig. 7–3.) Use *nephr/o* to build a word that means *pain in the kidney:* _____ / _____ *inflammation of the kidney:* _____ / _____
stone	**7-9** Nephr/o/lith and ren/al calculus mean the patient suffers from a kidney _____.

Boldface indicates a word root or combining form. Blue indicates a suffix. Pink indicates a prefix.

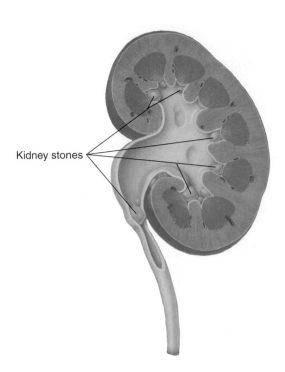

Kidney stones

Figure 7-3 Kidney stones shown in the calyces and ureter.

lith/ectomy lĭ-THĔK-tō-mē **lith/o/tripsy** LĬTH-ō-trĭp-sē	**7–10** Nephr/o/lith/iasis occurs when salts in the urine precipitate (settle out of solution and grow in size). Elimination of the stone(s) may occur spontaneously, but crushing the stone(s) by means of lith/o/tripsy may sometimes be necessary. Build medical terms that mean *excision of a stone:* _____ / _____ *crushing a stone:* _____ / _____ / _____
US **ESWL**	**7–11** Extracorporeal shock-wave lithotripsy (ESWL) is a surgical procedure used to treat ren/al calculi. Powerful ultrasound (US) vibrations break up and destroy calculi in the urinary tract. (See Fig. 7–4.) The calculi and their fragments are removed during urination and by administration of an oral dissolution drug. Identify the following abbreviations: *ultrasound:* _____ *extracorporeal shock-wave lithotripsy:* _____

7–12 Surgical suffixes *-ectomy, -tomy,* and *-tome* are commonly confusing to beginning medical terminology students. To reinforce your understanding of their meanings, review them in the following chart.

Surgical Suffix	**Meaning**
-ectomy	excision, removal
-tomy	incision
-tome	instrument to cut

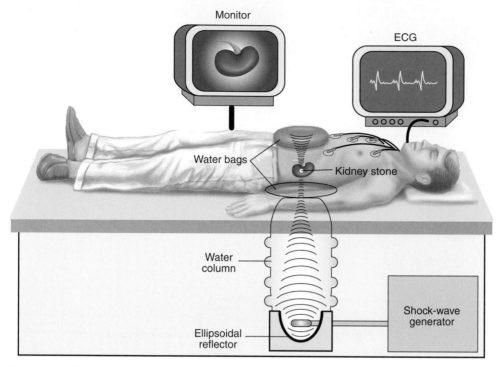

Figure 7-4 Extracorporeal shock-wave lithotripsy.

incision, stone *or* **calculus**	**7-13** Stones trapped in the kidney or ureter may be removed surgically. Nephr/o/lith/o/tomy is an _____ to remove a ren/al _____ .
ren/al RĒ-năl **sten/osis** stĕ-NŌ-sĭs **glomerul/o/nephr/itis** glō-mĕr-ū-lō-nĕ-FRĪ-tĭs **hyper/tension** hī-pĕr-TĔN-shŭn	**7-14** Ren/al hyper/tension produced by kidney disease is the most common type of hyper/tension caused by glomerul/o/nephr/itis or ren/al artery sten/osis. Identify terms in this frame that mean *pertaining to the kidney(s):* _____ / _____ *narrowing, stricture:* _____ / _____ *inflammation of the glomerulus of the kidney:* _____ / ____ / _____ / _____ *high blood pressure:* _____ / _____
protein/uria prō-tēn-Ū-rē-ă	**7-15** Nephr/o/tic syndrome, a group of symptoms characterized by chronic loss of protein in the urine (protein/uria), leads to depletion of body protein, especially albumin. Normally, albumin and other serum proteins maintain fluid within the vascular space. When levels of these proteins are low, fluid leaks from blood vessels into tissues, resulting in edema. The syndrome may also occur as a result of other disease processes. A chronic loss of protein in the urine is called _____ / _____ .

Boldface indicates a word root or combining form. Blue indicates a suffix. Pink indicates a prefix.

swelling	**7-16** Although many disorders manifest fluid retention (excess fluid in tissues), a characteristic of nephr/o/tic syndrome is edema (swelling), especially around the ankles, feet, and eyes. The term edema indicates a _____.
edema ĕ-DĒ-mă	**7-17** When body tissues contain excessive amounts of fluid that cause swelling, the nurse charts this condition as _____.
diuretic dī-ū-RĔT-ĭc	**7-18** Diuretics are drugs prescribed to control edema and stimulate the flow of urine. Edema around the ankles and feet may also be due to a diet high in sodium. When this condition occurs, the physician may recommend a low-sodium diet and prescribe a drug known as a _____.
supra- **ren** **-al**	**7-19** Supra/ren/al is a directional term that means *above the kidney*. Identify elements in this frame that mean *above, excessive, superior:* _____ *kidney:* _____ *pertaining to:* _____
scler/o	**7-20** The CF *scler/o* is used in words to indicate hardening of a body part. It also refers to the sclera (white of the eye). To indicate a hardening, use the CF _____ / _____.
hardening	**7-21** Scler/osis is an abnormal condition of _____.
nephr/osis nĕf-RŌ-sĭs **nephr/o/scler/osis** nĕf-rō-sklĕ-RŌ-sĭs **nephr/o/lith** NĔF-rō-lĭth **nephr/o/lith/iasis** nĕf-rō-lĭth-Ī-ă-sĭs	**7-22** Hyper/tension damages kidneys by causing scler/o/tic changes, such as arteri/o/scler/osis with thickening and hardening of ren/al blood vessels (nephr/o/scler/osis). Recall that *-iasis* is used to denote an abnormal condition (produced by something specified). Use *nephr/o* to form medical words that mean *abnormal condition of a kidney:* _____ / _____ *abnormal condition of kidney hardening:* _____ / _____ / _____ / _____ *calculus in a kidney:* _____ / _____ / _____ *abnormal condition of kidney stone(s):* _____ / _____ / _____ / _____

nephr/ectomy nĕ-FRĔK-tō-mē	**7-23** Many kidney disorders can be treated surgically. Learn these procedures by building surgical terms with ***nephr/o*** that mean
nephr/o/rrhaphy nĕf-ROR-ă-fē	*excision of a kidney:* _____ / _____
nephr/o/tomy nĕ-FRŎT-ō-mē	*suture of a kidney:* _____ / _____ / _____ *incision of the kidney:* _____ / _____ / _____
nephr/o/lith/o/tomy nĕf-rō-lĭth-ŎT-ō-mē	*incision (to remove a) kidney stone:* _____ / _____ / _____ / _____ / _____

nephr/o/ptosis nĕf-rŏp-TŌ-sĭs	**7-24** A kidney may prolapse from its normal position because of a birth defect or injury. The downward displacement may occur because the kidney supports are weakened due to a sudden strain or blow. This condition is called nephr/o/ptosis, or floating kidney. A prolapsed kidney is charted in a medical record as _____ / _____ / _____.

-ptosis **nephr/o**	**7-25** Determine the element in nephr/o/ptosis that means *prolapse, downward displacement:* _____ *kidney:* _____ / _____

nephr/o/ptosis nĕf-rŏp-TŌ-sĭs	**7-26** Downward displacement of a kidney that results from a congenital defect or an injury is called _____ / _____ / _____.

nephr/o/pexy NĔF-rō-pĕks-ē	**7-27** Nephr/o/ptosis can be treated surgically. Use *-pexy* to build a surgical term that means *fixation of the kidney:* _____ / _____ / _____.

Boldface indicates a word root or combining form. Blue indicates a suffix. Pink indicates a prefix.

SECTION REVIEW 7-2

Using the following table, write the combining form, suffix, or prefix that matches its definition in the space provided to the left of the definition. There may be more than one word element that matches a definition.

Combining Forms	Suffixes		Prefixes
lith/o	-iasis	-ptosis	dia-
nephr/o	-megaly	-rrhaphy	poly-
ren/o	-osis	-tome	supra-
scler/o	-pathy	-tomy	
	-pexy		

1. _____ abnormal condition; increase (used primarily with blood cells)

2. _____ abnormal condition (produced by something specified)

3. _____ above; excessive; superior

4. _____ disease

5. _____ enlargement

6. _____ through, across

7. _____ fixation (of an organ)

8. _____ hardening; sclera (white of the eye)

9. _____ instrument to cut

10. _____ incision

11. _____ kidney

12. _____ prolapse, downward displacement

13. _____ stone, calculus

14. _____ suture

15. _____ many, much

Competency Verification: Check your answers in Appendix B: Answer Key, page 583. If you are not satisfied with your level of comprehension, go back to Frame 7–1 and rework the frames.

Correct Answers _____ × 6.67 = _____ % Score

Ureters, Bladder, and Urethra

7-28   The ureters, bladder, and urethra are mainly passageways for transportation, storage, and elimination of urine. Within both kidneys, the renal pelvis narrows to form two muscular tubes called the (7) **ureters.**

Label the ureters in Figure 7–2.

7-29   The contraction of ureteral muscles pushes urine away from the kidneys. It is temporarily stored in the (8) **urinary bladder** until it is expelled from the body through the (9) **urethra** and (10) **urinary meatus** during the process of urination (micturition).

Label Figure 7–2 to locate the urinary structures.

cyst/itis sĭs-TĪ-tĭs **cyst/o/lith/iasis** sĭs-tō-lĭ-THĪ-ă-sĭs **cyst/o/lith/o/tomy** sĭs-tō-lĭth-ŎT-ō-mē	**7–30** The CFs *cyst/o* and *vesic/o* are used in words to refer to the bladder. Use *cyst/o* to form words that mean *inflammation of the bladder:* _____ / _____ *abnormal condition of a bladder stone:* _____ / _____ / _____ / _____ *incision of the bladder to remove a stone:* _____ / _____ / _____ / _____ / _____

Competency Verification: Check your labeling of Figure 7–2 in Appendix B: Answer Key, page 583.

py/uria pī-Ū-rē-ă **dys/uria** dĭs-Ū-rē-ă **bacteri/uria** băk-tē-rē-Ū-rē-ă **cyst/itis** sĭs-TĪ-tĭs	**7–31** Cyst/itis is more common in women, due to their shorter urethra and the closeness of the urethr/al orifice to the anus. Symptoms of cyst/itis include dys/uria, urgency, and urinary frequency. Urinalysis reveals bacteri/uria and py/uria. Identify the words in this frame that mean *pus in urine:* _____ / _____ *painful urination:* _____ / _____ *bacteria in urine:* _____ / _____ *inflammation of the bladder:* _____ / _____

suture SŪ-chūr	**7–32** The surgical suffix *-rrhaphy* is used in words to mean _____.

ureter/o/rrhaphy ū-rē-tĕr-OR-ră-fē **cyst/o/rrhaphy** sĭs-TOR-ă-fē	**7–33** Construct surgical words that mean *suture of the ureter:* _____ / _____ / _____ *suture of the bladder:* _____ / _____ / _____

bladder, intestine	**7–34** Vesic/o/enter/ic means *pertaining to the* _____ *and* _____.

Boldface indicates a word root or combining form. Blue indicates a suffix. Pink indicates a prefix.

bladder

hernia, swelling

rectum
RĔK-tŭm

7–35 A hernia is a protrusion of an anatomical structure through the wall that normally contains it. Hernias may develop in several parts of the body. Examples of hernias are cyst/o/cele and rect/o/cele. (See Fig. 7–5.)

A cyst/o/cele is a herniation of part of the urin/ary bladder through the vagin/al wall caused by weakened pelv/ic muscles. A rect/o/cele is a herniation of a portion of the rectum toward the vagina through weakened vagin/al muscles.

Define the following word elements in this frame:

cyst/o: _____

-cele: _____, _____

rect/o: _____

cyst/o/cele
SĬS-tō-sēl

7–36 Cyst/o/cele develops over years as vaginal muscles weaken and can no longer support the weight of urine in the urinary bladder. This condition usually occurs after a woman has delivered several infants. It also occurs in elderly people because of weakened pelvic muscles resulting from the aging process.

When the physician diagnoses *herniation of the bladder,* you know the Dx will be

charted as a _____ / _____ / _____.

rect/o/cele
RĔK-tō-sēl

7–37 Can you determine the Dx of a patient with a *herniation of the rectum into the vagina*?

_____ / _____ / _____

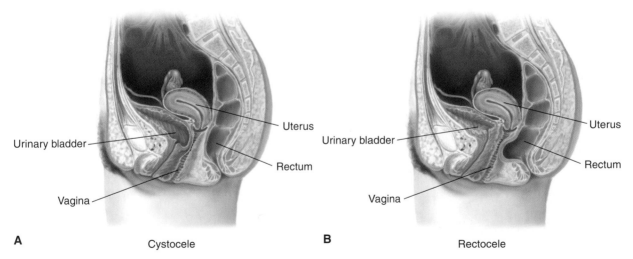

A   Cystocele   B   Rectocele

Figure 7-5 Herniations. (**A**) Cystocele. (**B**) Rectocele.

cyst/o/scope
SĬST-ō-skōp

**cyst/o/scopy,
cyst/o/urethr/o/scopy**
sĭs-TŎS-kō-pē, SĬS-tō-ū-
rē-THRŎS-kō-pē

7–38   Cyst/o/scopy, also called cyst/o/urethr/o/scopy, is a procedure that uses a rigid or flexible cyst/o/scope inserted into the urinary meatus and through the urethra to examine the urinary bladder. (See Fig. 7–6.)

The endo/scope used to perform cyst/o/scopy is called a

_____ / _____ / _____.

The cyst/o/scope is used to perform the diagnostic procedure called

_____ / _____ / _____ or

_____ / _____ / _____ / _____ / _____.

cyst/o/scope
SĬST-ō-skōp

7–39   The cyst/o/scope has an optical lighting system and special lenses and mirrors. It also contains a hollow channel for inserting operative devices to obtain biopsy specimens and remove growths and small stones. A video attachment can be used to create a permanent visual record.

To excise polyps from the bladder, the ur/o/logist uses the special instrument called a

_____ / _____ / _____.

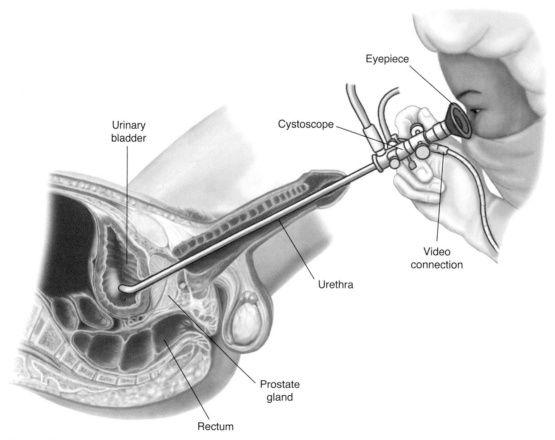

Urinary bladder

Eyepiece

Cystoscope

Video connection

Urethra

Prostate gland

Rectum

Figure 7-6 Cystoscopy of the urinary bladder via the urethra using a cystoscope.

Boldface indicates a word root or combining form. Blue indicates a suffix. Pink indicates a prefix.

cyst/o -scope radi/o -graphy	**7–40** In addition to inserting operative devices through a cyst/o/scope, the physician may place catheters through the cyst/o/scope to obtain urine samples and inject a contrast medium into the bladder during radi/o/graphy. Determine elements in this frame that mean *bladder:* _____ / _____ *instrument for examining:* _____ *radiation, x-ray; radius (lower arm bone on thumb side):* _____ / _____ *process of recording:* _____
urethr/o	**7–41** The urethra differs in men and women. In men, it serves a dual purpose of conveying sperm and discharging urine from the bladder. The female urethra performs only the latter function. Regardless of the sex, the CF for urethra is _____ / _____.
urethr/itis ū-rē-THRĪ-tĭs urethr/ectomy ū-rē-THRĔK-tō-mē urethr/o/pexy ū-RĒ-thrō-pĕks-ē urethr/o/plasty ū-RĒ-thrō-plăs-tē	**7–42** Form medical words that mean *inflammation of the urethra:* _____ / _____ *excision of the urethra:* _____ / _____ *surgical fixation of the urethra:* _____ / ____ / _____ *surgical repair of the urethra:* _____ / ____ / _____
pain, urethra ū-RĒ-thră	**7–43** Urethr/algia and urethr/o/dynia refer to _____ in the _____.
urethr/algia ū-rē-THRĂL-jē-ă	**7–44** In addition to urethr/o/dynia, construct a word that means *pain in the* *urethra:* _____ / _____
cyst/itis sĭs-TĪ-tĭs urethr/itis ū-rē-THRĪ-tĭs	**7–45** Build words that mean *inflammation of the bladder:* _____ / _____ *inflammation of the urethra:* _____ / _____
urinary tract infections	**7–46** Urinary tract infections (UTIs) account for most office visits by patients experiencing urinary tract problems. What does the abbreviation UTIs stand for? _____ _____ _____

urethr/al ū-RĒ-thrăl **lumen** LŪ-měn **dys/uria** dĭs-Ū-rē-ă	**7–47** Urethr/al stricture is a condition of narrowing of the lumen (tubular space within a structure). It is usually caused by infection, cancer, or scar tissue. Dys/uria is the primary symptom due to increased strain caused by difficulty urinating. Identify the terms in this frame that mean *pertaining to the urethra:* _____ / _____ *tubular space within a structure:* _____ *painful urination:* _____ / _____
urethr/o/plasty ū-RĒ-thrō-plăs-tē **sten/osis** stĕ-NŌ-sĭs **dys/uria** dĭs-Ū-rē-ă	**7–48** Urethr/al stricture, also called urethr/al sten/osis, is treated with the surgical procedure called urethr/o/plasty. This procedure is used to relieve dys/uria and recurrent UTIs by restoring unobstructed urine flow. Identify the terms in this frame that mean *surgical repair of the urethra:* _____ / _____ / _____ *abnormal condition of narrowing or stricture:* _____ / _____ *painful urination:* _____ / _____
urethra, rectum ū-RĒ-thră, RĔK-tŭm	**7–49** Urethr/o/rect/al means *pertaining to the* _____ *and* _____.
urethr/o/scope ū-RĒ-thrō-skōp **urethr/o/scopy** ū-rē-THRŎS-kō-pē	**7–50** Form diagnostic terms that mean *instrument for examining the urethra:* _____ / _____ / _____ *visual examination of the urethra:* _____ / _____ / _____
urethr/o/cyst/itis ū-rē-thrō-sĭs-TĪ-tĭs	**7–51** Construct a medical word that means *inflammation of urethra and bladder:* _____ / _____ / _____ / _____
cyst/o/urethr/o/scope sĭs-tō-ū-RĒ-thrō-skōp	**7–52** Cyst/o/urethr/o/scopy is a visual examination of the urethra and bladder. The instrument used to perform a cyst/o/urethr/o/scopy is a _____ / _____ / _____ / _____ / _____.
meat/o/tomy mē-ă-TŎT-ō-mē **meat/o/rrhaphy** MĒ-ă-TŎR-ăf-ē	**7–53** The CF *meat/o* means *opening, meatus.* The urinary meatus is the external opening of the urethra, located at the tip of the penis in males and anterior to the vagina in females. The urinary meatus is where urine is discharged from the body. Use *meat/o* to construct medical words that mean *incision of the meatus:* _____ / _____ / _____ *suture of the meatus:* _____ / _____ / _____

Boldface indicates a word root or combining form. Blue indicates a suffix. Pink indicates a prefix.

-ia	**7–54** Identify the element in *-algia, -dynia, -pepsia,* and *-phagia* that means *condition:* _____.
malignant mă-LĬG-nănt **benign** bĕ-NĪN	**7–55** Malignant tumors are cancerous; benign tumors are noncancerous. Use *malignant* or *benign* to complete the following statements. Cancerous tumors are _____ tumors. Noncancerous tumors are _____ tumors.
noncancerous	**7–56** Benign tumors do not invade surrounding tissue and are contained within a capsule. They become harmful only when they start placing pressure on adjacent structures. For example, a benign tumor of the uterus may place pressure on the urinary bladder and cause frequent urination. Benign tumors are (cancerous, noncancerous) _____ growths.
cancerous	**7–57** Malignant tumors spread rapidly and are invasive and life-threatening. Malignant tumors are (cancerous, noncancerous) _____.
pain, gland	**7–58** The CF *aden/o* is used in words to denote a gland. Aden/o/dynia is _____ in a _____.
gland **cancer** **tumor**	**7–59** Urin/ary tract tumors may be benign or malignant. The most common malignant ren/al tumor is an aden/o/carcin/oma. Define these elements: *aden/o:* _____ *carcin/o:* _____ *-oma:* _____
aden/oma ăd-ĕ-NŌ-mă **aden/o/carcin/oma** ăd-ĕ-nō-kăr-sĭn-Ō-mă	**7–60** An aden/oma is a benign glandular tumor composed of tissue from which it is developing; an aden/o/carcin/oma is a malignant glandular tumor. Determine words in this frame that mean *benign glandular tumor:* _____ / _____ *malignant glandular tumor:* _____ / _____ / _____ / _____

SECTION REVIEW 7-3

Using the following table, write the CF or suffix that matches its definition in the space provided to the left of the definition. There may be more than one word element that matches a definition.

Combining Forms

aden/o	ureter/o
carcin/o	urethr/o
cyst/o	vesic/o
enter/o	
pyel/o	
rect/o	

Suffixes

-ectomy	-oma
-ectasis	-pathy
-iasis	-plasty
-itis	-rrhaphy
-lith	-scope
-megaly	-tomy

1. _____ abnormal condition (produced by something specified)

2. _____ bladder

3. _____ cancer

4. _____ disease

5. _____ enlargement

6. _____ excision, removal

7. _____ dilation, expansion

8. _____ gland

9. _____ incision

10. _____ inflammation

11. _____ instrument for examining

12. _____ intestine (usually small intestine)

13. _____ renal pelvis

14. _____ rectum

15. _____ stone, calculus

16. _____ surgical repair

17. _____ suture

18. _____ tumor

19. _____ ureter

20. _____ urethra

Competency Verification: Check your answers in Appendix B: Answer Key, page 583. If you are not satisfied with your level of comprehension, go back to Frame 7–28 and rework the frames.

Correct Answers _____ × 5 = _____ % Score

MICROSCOPIC STRUCTURES

The **nephron** is the functional unit of the kidney. It is the structure that produces urine in the process of removing wastes and excess substances from the blood. Each nephron contains a glomerulus and a renal tubule.

Boldface indicates a word root or combining form. Blue indicates a suffix. Pink indicates a prefix.

7–61   Microscopic examination of the kidney reveals about one million nephrons, all of which play a vital role in the maintenance of normal fluid balance (homeostasis) in the body. The nephrons are located within the outer layer of the kidney, called the (1) **renal cortex**, and the inner region, called the (2) **renal medulla.**

The first part of the nephron, the (3) **glomerular capsule**, also called **Bowman capsule,** surrounds a tiny ball of coiled intertwining capillaries known as the (4) **glomerulus.** In the first step of urine production, water, salts, sugar, urea, and other nitrogenous waste products are filtered across the wall of glomerular capillaries and into the glomerular capsule. This waste-containing fluid is known as **renal filtrate.**

Label the structures in Figure 7–7.

7–62   The collection of filtrate in the glomerular capsule flows into the long, twisted tube called the (5) **renal tubule,** where **reabsorption** of nutrients continues. The reabsorption process ensures that the body retains essential substances, such as glucose, water, and salts. On the other hand, waste products of metabolism become toxic if allowed to accumulate in the body. Thus, acids, drugs, and other wastes leave the body in the urine. This final process of urine formation occurs in the (6) **collecting tubule** that conveys the newly formed urine to the renal pelvis, which narrows into the ureter. The urine flows through the ureters into the bladder for temporary storage. The bladder eventually expels the urine through the urethra during the process of **urination.**

Label the structures of the nephron in Figure 7–7.

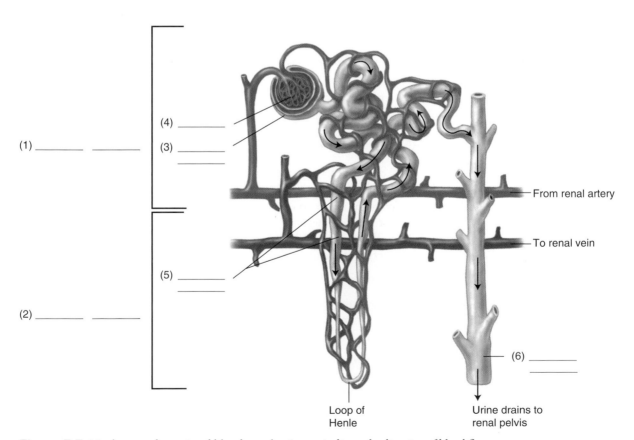

From renal artery

To renal vein

Loop of Henle

Urine drains to renal pelvis

Figure 7-7 Nephron and associated blood vessels. *Arrows indicate the direction of blood flow and flow of renal filtrate.*

hyper/tension hī-pĕr-TĔN-shŭn	**7-63** Glomerul/o/nephr/itis is an inflammatory disease of the kidney that primarily involves the glomerulus. It is characterized by hyper/tension, olig/uria, electrolyte imbalances, and edema. The CF *olig/o* means *scanty*.
olig/uria ŏl-ĭg-Ū-rē-ă	Identify terms in this frame that mean
	high blood pressure: _____ / _____
edema ĕ-DĒ-mă	*diminished capacity to pass urine:* _____ / _____
	swelling (of a body part): _____
glomerul/o/nephr/itis glō-mĕr-ū-lō-nĕ-FRĪ-tĭs	*inflammation of the glomerulus and kidney:*
	_____ / _____ / _____ / _____

glomerul/itis glō-mĕr-ū-LĪ-tĭs	**7-64** Use *glomerul/o* to form medical words that mean
	inflammation of a glomerulus: _____ / _____
glomerul/o/pathy glō-mĕr-ū-LŎP-ă-thē	*disease of a glomerulus:* _____ / _____ / _____

glomerulus *or* glomeruli, hardening glō-MĔR-ū-lŭs, glō-MĔR-ū-lī	**7-65** Glomerul/o/scler/osis literally means *an abnormal condition* of the _____ _____.

Competency Verification: Check your labeling of Figure 7–7 with Appendix B: Answer Key, page 583.

pyel/o/pathy pī-ĕ-LŎP-ă-thē	**7-66** The CF *pyel/o* refers to the renal pelvis, a funnel-shaped chamber that collects urine from the kidney before flowing into the ureter. Use the CF *pyel/o* to construct the word that means *any disease of the renal pelvis:* _____ / _____ / _____

KUB	**7-67** To determine urinary tract abnormalities, such as tumors, swollen kidneys, and calculi, the physician may order a radi/o/graph/ic examination called KUB (kidney, ureter, bladder). The radi/o/graph identifies location, size, shape, and malformation of the kidneys, ureters, and bladder. Stones and calcified areas may also be detected. The diagnostic test of the kidneys, ureters, and bladder is charted with the abbreviation _____.

IVP	**7-68** Intra/ven/ous pyel/o/graphy (IVP) provides multiple radi/o/graph/ic images of the ren/al pelvis and urin/ary tract after injection of a contrast medium. IVP provides detailed information about the structure and function of the kidneys, ureters, bladder, and urethra. To confirm a diagnosis (Dx) of ren/al calculi or other urin/ary disorders, a radi/o/graph involving IV injection of a contrast dye may be ordered. The abbreviation for this type of radiograph is _____.

Boldface indicates a word root or combining form. Blue indicates a suffix. Pink indicates a prefix.

intra/ven/ous ĭn-tră-VĒ-nŭs **pyel/o/gram** PĪ-ĕ-lō-grăm **nephr/o/liths** NĔF-rō-lĭths **ureter/o/liths** ū-RĒ-tĕr-ō-lĭths	**7–69** An intra/ven/ous pyel/o/gram (IVP) provides visualization of urinary structures. It is used to assess the urinary tract and identify nephr/o/liths and ureter/o/liths. Determine words in this frame that mean *within a vein:* _____ / _____ / _____ *record (x-ray) of the renal pelvis:* _____ / ___ / _____ *stones in the kidney:* _____ / ___ / _____ *stones in the ureter:* _____ / ___ / _____
intra/ven/ous pyel/o/graphy (IVP) ĭn-tră-VĒ-nŭs pī-ĕ-LŎG-ră-fē **retro/grade pyel/o/graphy (RP)** RĔT-rō-grād pī-ĕ-LŎG-ră-fē	**7–70** The prefix *retro-* means *backward, behind.* The suffix *-grade* means *to go.* The term retro/grade is used to describe a specific type of pyel/o/graphy. Retro/grade pyel/o/graphy (RP) consists of radi/o/graph/ic images taken after a contrast medium is injected through a urin/ary catheter directly into the urethra, bladder, and ureters. Identify two types of pyel/o/graphy. Pyel/o/graphy in which a contrast medium is injected within a vein is called _____ / _____ / _____ _____ / ___ / _____ (_____). Pyel/o/graphy in which a contrast medium is injected into the urethra is called _____ / _____ _____ / ___ / _____ (_____).
nephr/o/scope NĔF-rō-skōp **nephr/o/scopy** nĕ-FRŎ-skŏ-pē	**7–71** The nephr/o/scope, a fiber-optic instrument, is used to visualize the kidney and remove ren/al calculi. Use *nephr/o* to construct medical terms that mean *instrument for examining the kidney:* _____ / ___ / _____ *visual examination of the kidney:* _____ / ___ / _____
pyel/itis pī-ĕ-LĪ-tĭs **pyel/o/nephr/itis** pī-ĕ-lō-nĕ-FRĪ-tĭs	**7–72** Pyel/o/nephr/itis is a bacterial infection of the ren/al pelvis and kidney caused by bacterial invasion from the middle and lower urinary tract or bloodstream. Bacteria may gain access to the bladder via the urethra and ascend to the kidney. Form medical words that mean *inflammation of the renal pelvis:* _____ / _____ *inflammation of the renal pelvis and kidney:* _____ / ___ / _____ / _____

pyel/o/nephr/itis pǐ-ě-lō-ně-FRĪ-tǐs	**7-73** Pyel/o/nephr/itis is an extremely dangerous condition, especially in pregnant women, because it can cause premature labor. The medical term for bacterial infection of the renal pelvis and kidneys is _____ / _____ / _____ / _____.

Two combining forms that sound alike but have different meanings are **pyel/o** and **py/o**. Here is a useful clarification:

Combining Form	Meaning	Example
pyel/o	renal pelvis	pyel/o/pathy
py/o	pus	py/o/rrhea

pyel/o/plasty PĪ-ě-lō-plǎs-tē **pyel/o/gram** PĪ-ě-lō-grǎm	**7-74** Use *pyel/o (renal pelvis)* to form medical words that mean *surgical repair of the renal pelvis:* _____ / _____ / _____ *record (x-ray) of the renal pelvis:* _____ / _____ / _____

py/o/rrhea pī-ō-RĒ-ǎ **py/o/nephr/osis** pī-ō-něf-RŌ-sǐs	**7-75** Use *py/o (pus)* to build words that mean *discharge or flow of pus:* _____ / _____ / _____ *abnormal condition of pus from the kidney:* _____ / _____ / _____ / _____

Remember not to use *-iasis* because the pus is not produced by something specified; the term just denotes that there is pus in the kidneys.

py/uria pī-Ū-rē-ǎ	**7-76** An important diagnostic test that provides early detection of ren/al disease is urinalysis. Urine samples are analyzed for abnormalities, such as blood or pus in urine and other physical and chemical properties. Hemat/uria is a condition of blood in the urine. Form a word that means *pus in the urine:* _____ / _____

an/uria ǎn-Ū-rē-ǎ	**7-77** The prefixes *a-* and *an-* are used in words to mean *without* or *not.* The *a-* is usually used before a consonant; the *an-* is usually used before a vowel. Construct a word that literally means *without urine:* _____ / _____

Boldface indicates a word root or combining form. Blue indicates a suffix. Pink indicates a prefix.

proxim/al

dist/al

7–78   Hydr/o/nephr/osis is an enlargement of the kidney due to constant pressure from backed-up urine in the ureter. It may be caused by a stricture, tumor, or a stone in the proxim/al part of a ureter that obstructs urine flow. When obstruction occurs in the dist/al part of the ureter, the condition is called hydr/o/ureter *with* hydr/o/nephr/osis. (See Fig. 7–8.)

Identify the terms in this frame that mean

nearest the point of attachment: _____ / _____

farthest from the point of attachment: _____ / _____

hydr/o/nephr/osis
hī-drō-něf-RŌ-sĭs

7–79   Although partial obstruction in hydr/o/nephr/osis may not produce symptoms initially, the built-up pressure behind the area of obstruction eventually results in symptoms of ren/al dysfunction.

When calculi obstruction causes cessation of urine flow, it may result in a condition

called _____ / _____ / _____ / _____.

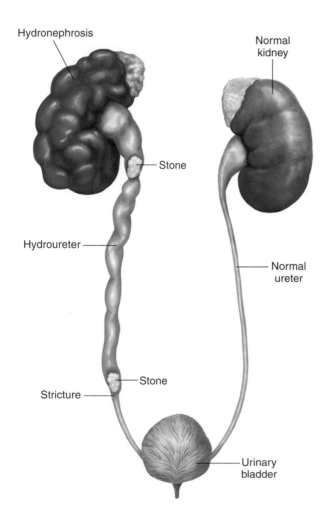

Hydronephrosis

Normal kidney

Stone

Hydroureter

Normal ureter

Stone

Stricture

Urinary bladder

Figure 7-8 Hydronephrosis and hydroureter.

hydr/o/nephr/osis hī-drō-nĕf-RŌ-sĭs	**7–80** Presence of ren/al calculi increases the risk of urinary tract infections (UTIs) because they obstruct the free flow of urine. Untreated obstruction of a stone in any of the urin/ary structures can also result in retention of urine and damage to the kidney. (See Fig. 7–8.) Build a word that means *abnormal condition of water (urine) in the kidney:* _____ / _____ / _____ / _____
hemat/uria hĕm-ă-TŪ-rē-ă **protein/uria** prō-tēn-Ū-rē-ă	**7–81** A person who suffers from hydr/o/nephr/osis may experience pain, hemat/uria, and py/uria. Blood or pus may be present in the urine. Build medical words that mean *blood in the urine:* _____ / _____ *protein in the urine:* _____ / _____
olig/uria ŏl-ĭg-Ū-rē-ă	**7–82** Kidney disease diminishes the kidney's capacity to form urine. Build a word that means *diminished or scanty amount of urine formation:* _____ / _____
py/uria pī-Ū-rē-ă	**7–83** Py/uria refers to the presence of an excessive number of white blood cells in urine. It is generally a sign of a urinary tract infection. A bacterial infection of the bladder and urethra may result in the condition called _____ / _____.
poly/uria pŏl-ē-Ū-rē-ă	**7–84** The prefix *poly-* means *many, much.* Combine *poly-* and *-uria* to build a word that means *excessive urination:* _____ / _____
poly/cyst/ic pŏl-ē-SĬS-tĭk **ren/al** RĒ-năl	**7–85** Poly/cyst/ic kidney disease (PKD) is a hereditary condition in which the kidneys are enlarged and contain many cysts. Renal failure commonly develops over time, requiring dialysis or kidney transplantation. Identify terms in this frame that mean *pertaining to many cysts:* _____ / _____ / _____ *pertaining to the kidney:* _____ / _____
noct/uria nŏk-TŪ-rē-ă	**7–86** Noct/uria refers to urination at night. If a child has a tendency to urinate at night, the condition is known as _____ / _____.
urination *or* urine ū-rĭ-NĀ-shŭn	**7–87** Continence is the ability to control urination and defecation. A person who has urinary continence is able to control urination. A person with urinary in/continence is not able to control _____.

Boldface indicates a word root or combining form. Blue indicates a suffix. Pink indicates a prefix.

in/continence ĭn-KŎN-tĭ-nĕns	**7–88** Elderly patients in nursing homes may experience uncontrolled loss of urine from the bladder. They may suffer from the condition known as urinary _____ / _____.
ur/o/logist ū-RŎL-ō-jĭst **nephr/o/logist** nĕ-FRŎL-ō-jĭst	**7–89** Ur/o/logists specialize in treating urin/ary tract disorders; nephr/o/logists specialize in management of kidney disease, kidney transplantation, and dia/lysis therapies. Persons with urin/ary disorders see the medical specialist called a _____ / _____ / _____. Persons with kidney disorders, including transplantations and dia/lysis, see the medical specialist called a _____/_____/_____.
hemat/uria hĕm-ă-TŪ-rē-ă	**7–90** Cyst/itis, an inflammatory condition of the urin/ary bladder, is commonly caused by bacterial infection and is characterized by pain, frequency of urination, urgency, and, sometimes, hemat/uria. If cyst/itis results in traces of blood in urine, the medical term for this condition is _____ / _____.
acute renal failure RĒ-năl	**7–91** Any condition that impairs flow of blood to the kidneys, such as shock, injury, and exposure to toxins, may result in acute renal failure (ARF). The abbreviation ARF refers to _____ _____ _____.

SECTION REVIEW 7-4

Using the following table, write the CF, suffix, or prefix that matches its definition in the space provided to the left of the definition. There may be more than one word element that matches a definition.

Combining Forms		Suffixes	Prefixes
azot/o	ren/o	-cele	a-
cyst/o	scler/o	-ist	an-
glomerul/o	ureter/o	-logist	intra-
hemat/o	urethr/o	-ptosis	poly-
nephr/o	ur/o		
noct/o	vesic/o		
olig/o			
pyel/o			
py/o			

1. _____ bladder

2. _____ blood

3. _____ specialist in the study of

4. _____ glomerulus

5. _____ hardening; sclera (white of the eye)

6. _____ specialist

7. _____ kidney

8. _____ pus

9. _____ nitrogenous compounds

10. _____ renal pelvis

11. _____ scanty

12. _____ ureter

13. _____ urethra

14. _____ urine; urinary tract

15. _____ night

16. _____ hernia, swelling

17. _____ many, much

18. _____ prolapse, downward displacement

19. _____ in, within

20. _____ without, not

Competency Verification: Check your answers in Appendix B: Answer Key, page 583. If you are not satisfied with your level of comprehension, go back to Frame 7–61 and rework the frames.

Correct Answers _____ × 5 = _____ % Score

ABBREVIATIONS

This section introduces urinary system–related abbreviations and their meanings. Included are abbreviations contained in the medical record activities that follow.

Abbreviation	Meaning	Abbreviation	Meaning
ARF	acute renal failure	IVP	intravenous pyelogram; intravenous pyelography
BNO	bladder neck obstruction	IVU	intravenous urogram; intravenous urography
BPH	benign prostatic hyperplasia; benign prostatic hypertrophy	KUB	kidney, ureter, bladder
BUN	blood urea nitrogen	PD	peritoneal dialysis
C&S	culture and sensitivity	PKD	polycystic kidney disease
Cath	catheter, catheterization	PSA	prostate-specific antigen
CRF	chronic renal failure	RP	retrograde pyelography
CT	computed tomography	TURP	transurethral resection of the prostate
cysto	cystoscopy	UA	urinalysis
ESRD	end-stage renal disease	US	ultrasonography, ultrasound
ESWL	extracorporeal shock-wave lithotripsy	UTI	urinary tract infection
EU	excretory urography	VCUG	voiding cystourethrogram; voiding cystourethrography
HD	hemodialysis	WBC	white blood cell

ADDITIONAL MEDICAL TERMS

The following are additional terms related to the urinary system. Recognizing and learning these terms will help you understand the connection between a pathological condition, its diagnosis, and the rationale behind the method of treatment selected for a particular disorder.

Diseases and Conditions

azoturia
ăz-ō-TŪ-rē-ă
  azot: nitrogenous
      compounds
  -uria: urine

Increase of nitrogenous substances, especially urea, in urine

diuresis dī-ū-RĒ-sĭs	Increased formation and secretion of urine
di-: double	
ur: urine	
-esis: condition	

end-stage renal disease (ESRD) RĒ-năl	Kidney disease that has advanced to the point that the kidneys can no longer adequately filter the blood and, ultimately, requires dialysis or renal transplantation for survival; also called *chronic renal failure* (CRF) (See Fig. 7–9.)
	Common diseases leading to ESRD include malignant hypertension, infections, diabetes mellitus, and glomerulonephritis. Diabetes is the most common cause of kidney transplantation.

enuresis ĕn-ū-RĒ-sĭs	Involuntary discharge of urine after the age at which bladder control should be established; also called *bed-wetting at night* or *nocturnal enuresis*
en-: in, within	*In children, voluntary control of urination is usually present by age 5.*
ur: urine	
-esis: condition	

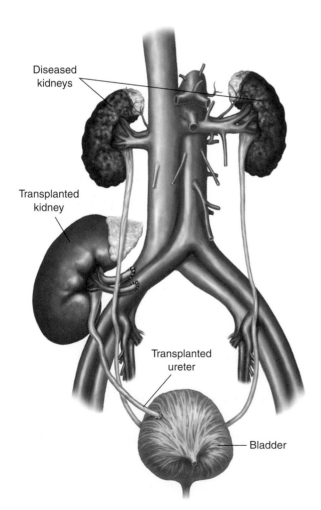

Figure 7-9 Renal transplantation.

hypospadias hī-pō-SPĀ-dē-ăs *hypo-:* under, below, deficient *-spadias:* slit, fissure	Abnormal congenital opening of the male urethra on the undersurface of the penis
interstitial nephritis ĭn-tĕr-STĬSH-ăl nĕf-RĪ-tĭs *nephr:* kidney *-itis:* inflammation	Condition associated with pathological changes in the renal interstitial tissue that may be primary or due to a toxic agent, such as a drug or chemical, which results in destruction of nephrons and severe impairment in renal function
renal hypertension RĒ-năl hī-pĕr-TĔN-shŭn *ren:* kidney *-al:* pertaining to *hyper-:* excessive, above normal *-tension:* to stretch	High blood pressure that results from kidney disease
uremia ū-RĒ-mē-ă *ur:* urine *-emia:* blood	Elevated levels of urea and other nitrogenous waste products in the blood as a result of the kidneys' failure to expel these waste products in the urine; also called *azotemia* *The term uremia usually describes the illness that accompanies renal or kidney failure.*
Wilms tumor VĬLMZ TOO-mŏr	Malignant neoplasm of the kidney that occurs in young children, usually before age 5 *The most common early signs of Wilms tumor are hypertension, a palpable mass, pain, and hematuria.*

Diagnostic Procedures

blood urea nitrogen (BUN) ū-RĒ-ă NĪ-trō-jĕn	Laboratory test that measures the amount of urea (nitrogenous waste product) in the blood and demonstrates the kidneys' ability to filter urea from the blood for excretion in urine *An increase in BUN level may indicate impaired kidney function.*
creatinine clearance krē–ĂT-ĭn-ĭn	Laboratory test that measures the rate at which creatinine is cleared from the blood by the kidney *Creatinine clearance is the most common, most precise test that uses a blood and urine sample to assess kidney function.*

computed tomography (CT) kŏm-PŪ-tĕd tō-MŎG-ră-fē *tom/o:* to cut, slice *-graphy:* process of recording	Radiographic study using a narrow beam of x-rays that rotates in a full arc around the patient to acquire multiple views of the body, which a computer interprets to produce cross-sectional images of an internal organ or tissue; also called *computerized axial tomography (CAT) scanning* *CT scanning of the urinary system, called CT KUB or abdominal and pelvic CT, produces images of the kidneys, ureters, and bladder (KUB) with or without a contrast medium. It helps detect kidney stones, obstructions, renal masses, and other urinary disorders.*
pyelography pī-ĕ-LŎG-ră-fē *pyel/o:* renal pelvis *-graphy:* process of recording	Radiographic study of the kidney, ureters, and, usually, the bladder after injection of a contrast agent *A contrast medium is injected into a vein (intravenous pyelography) or through a catheter placed through the urethra, bladder, or ureter and into the renal pelvis (retrograde pyelography).*
intravenous pyelography (IVP) ĭn-tră-VĒ-nŭs pī-ĕ-LŎG-ră-fē *intra:* in, within *ven:* vein *-ous:* pertaining to *pyel/o:* renal pelvis *-graphy:* process of recording	Radiographic imaging in which a contrast medium is injected intravenously and serial x-ray films are taken to provide visualization of the entire urinary tract; also called *intravenous urography* (IVU) or *excretory urography* (EU) *In IVP, the x-ray image produced is known as a pyelogram or urogram.*
retrograde pyelography (RP) RĔT-rō-grād pī-ĕ-LŎG-ră-fē *retro-:* backward, behind *-grade:* to go *pyel/o:* renal pelvis *-graphy:* process of recording	Radiographic imaging in which a contrast medium is introduced through a cystoscope directly into the bladder and ureters using small-caliber catheters *RP provides detailed visualization of the urinary collecting system (pelvis and calyces of the kidney as well as the ureters). It helps locate urinary tract obstruction. It may also serve as a substitute for IVP when a patient is allergic to the contrast medium.*
nuclear scan	Radiographic technique that produces images of an organ or area of the body by introducing a radionuclide substance (tracer or radiopharmaceutical) that releases a low level of radiation; also called nuclear scanning, radionuclide imaging, and nuclear medicine scan *The amount of radioactivity used in a nuclear scan is very small and is not known to cause harm.*
renal RĒ-năl *ren:* kidney *-al:* pertaining to	Nuclear scan that determines renal function and shape

ultrasonography (US)
ŭl-tră-sŏn-ŎG-ră-fē
   -ultra: excess, beyond
   son/o: sound
   -graphy: process of
       recording
	Radiographic technique using high-frequency sound waves (ultrasound) that bounce off body tissues and are recorded to produce an image of an internal organ or tissue; also called *ultrasound* and *echo*
	
	US provides images of urinary tract structures and detects such abnormalities as tumors, obstructions, and polycystic kidney disease. It also helps measure postvoid residual urine (urine that remains in the bladder after urinating).

urinalysis ū-rĭ-NĂL-ĭ-sĭs	Physical, chemical, and microscopic evaluation of urine

voiding cystourethrography (VCUG)
sĭs-tō-ū-rē-THRŎG-ră-fē
   cyst/o: bladder
   urethr/o: urethra
   -graphy: process of
       recording
	Radiography of the bladder and urethra while the bladder fills and empties
	
	VCUG involves placement of a radiopaque liquid (that can be seen on x-ray) in the bladder through a catheter. Radiographs taken before, during, and after voiding reveal interior abnormalities of the urethra and bladder and help determine whether urine flow is normal when the bladder empties.

Medical and Surgical Procedures

catheterization (Cath) kăth-ĕ-tĕr-ĭ-ZĀ-shŭn	Insertion of a catheter (hollow flexible tube) into a body cavity or organ to instill a substance or remove fluid, most commonly through the urethra into the bladder to withdraw urine (See Fig. 7–10.) *Catheters are available in two basic types: a straight catheter, which is used only for short-term drainage, and a Foley catheter, which is used for short-term and long-term (indwelling) drainage.*

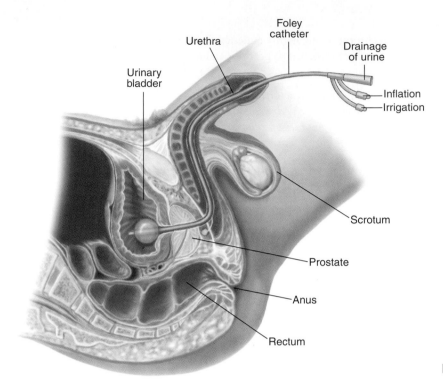

Figure 7-10 Catheterization.

dialysis dī-ĂL-ĭ-sĭs *dia-:* through, across *-lysis:* separation; destruction; loosening	Mechanical filtering process used to clean blood of high concentrations of metabolic waste products, draw off excess fluids, and regulate body chemistry when kidneys fail to function properly *Two primary methods of dialysis are used to dialyze the blood: hemodialysis and peritoneal dialysis.*
hemodialysis (HD) hē-mō-dī-ĂL-ĭ-sĭs	Process of removing excess fluids and toxins from the blood by continually shunting (diverting) the patient's blood from the body into a dialysis machine for filtering, and then returning the clean blood to the patient's body via tubes connected to the circulatory system (See Fig. 7–11.)
peritoneal dialysis (PD) pĕr-ĭ-tō-NĒ-ăl dī-ĂL -ĭ-sĭs	Dialysis in which the patient's own peritoneum is used as the dialyzing membrane (See Fig. 7–12.) *In peritoneal dialysis, dialyzing fluid passes through a tube into the peritoneal cavity and remains there for a prescribed period. During this time, wastes diffuse across the peritoneal membrane into the fluid. Contaminated fluid then drains out and is replaced with fresh solution. This process is repeated as often as required and may be continuous or intermittent.*

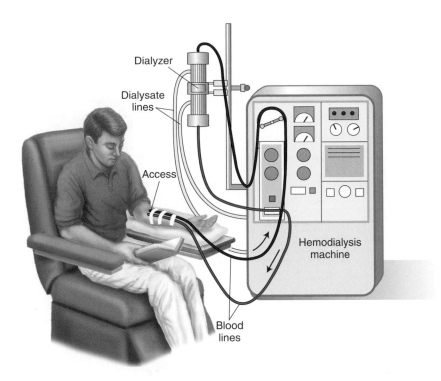

Figure 7-11 Hemodialysis.

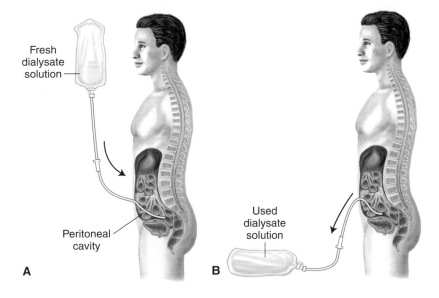

Figure 7-12 Peritoneal dialysis.
(**A**) Introducing dialysis fluid into the peritoneal cavity. (**B**) Draining dialysate with waste products from the peritoneal cavity.

renal transplantation RĒ-năl trăns-plăn-TĀ-shŭn *ren:* kidney *-al:* pertaining to	Organ transplant of a kidney in a patient with end-stage renal disease; also called *kidney transplantation*

ureteral stent
ū-RĒ-tĕr-ăl

   ureter: ureter
     -al: pertaining to

Placement of a thin tube into the ureter to prevent or treat obstruction of urine flow from the kidney

Indwelling stents require constant monitoring because they may lead to infections, blockages, or stone formations. To avoid complications, they must be removed or changed periodically. (See Fig. 7–13.)

urethrotomy
ū-rē-THRŎT-ō-mē

   urethr/o: urethra
     -tomy: incision

Incision of a urethral stricture

Urethrotomy corrects constrictions of the urethra that make voiding difficult.

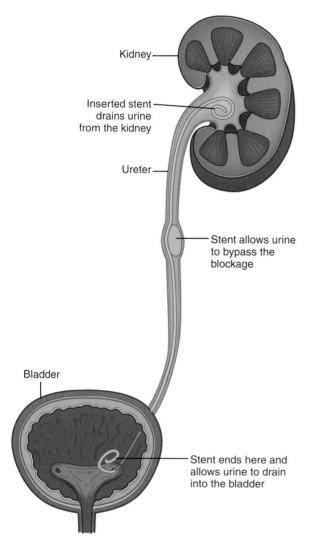

Kidney

Inserted stent drains urine from the kidney

Ureter

Stent allows urine to bypass the blockage

Bladder

Stent ends here and allows urine to drain into the bladder

Figure 7-13 Ureteral stent placement.

PHARMACOLOGY

The following table lists common drug categories used to treat urinary disorders, as well as their therapeutic actions.

Drug Category	Action
antibiotics ăn-tĭ-bī-ŎT-ĭks	Kill bacteria that commonly cause urinary tract infections (UTIs) *Most antibiotics come in pill or liquid form. Some may be administered as an injection or intravenously if the patient has a severe kidney infection.*
antispasmodics ăn-tĭ-spăz-MŌT-ĭks	Suppress spasms of the ureter, bladder, and urethra by relaxing the smooth muscles lining their walls, thus allowing normal emptying of the bladder
diuretics dī-ū-RĔT-ĭks	Block reabsorption of sodium by the kidneys, thereby increasing the amount of salt and water excreted in the urine *Diuretics promote a reduction of fluid retained in body tissues and also prevent edema.*
potassium supplements pō-TĂS-ē-ŭm	Replace potassium loss due to diuretic drugs *Diuretics increase sodium excretion and also potassium excretion.*

Pronunciation Help	Long sound	ā in rāte	ē in rēbirth	ī in īsle	ō in ōver	ū in ūnite
	Short sound	ă in ălone	ĕ in ĕver	ĭ in ĭt	ŏ in nŏt	ŭ in cŭt

ADDITIONAL MEDICAL TERMS REVIEW

Match the medical term(s) below with the definitions in the numbered list.

azoturia	diuresis	renal hypertension	US
BUN	enuresis	retrograde pyelography	VCUG
catheterization	hypospadias	uremia	Wilms tumor
dialysis	interstitial nephritis	urinalysis	

1. _____ refers to microscopic examination of urine.

2. _____ is a malignant neoplasm in the kidney that occurs in young children.

3. _____ is an increase in nitrogenous compounds in urine.

4. _____ is a radiographic technique that detects abnormalities of the kidneys and bladder using high-frequency sound waves.

5. _____ means increased formation and secretion of urine.

6. _____ is a radiologic technique in which a contrast medium is introduced through a cystoscope to provide detailed visualization of the urinary collecting system.

7. _____ is an abnormal congenital opening of the male urethra on the undersurface of the penis.

8. _____ is associated with pathological changes in the renal tissue, which may be primary or due to a toxic agent.

9. _____ is a test that measures the amount of urea excreted by kidneys into the blood.

10. _____ means urinary incontinence, including bed-wetting.

11. _____ refers to insertion of a hollow, flexible tube into a body cavity or organ to instill a substance or remove fluid.

12. _____ is radiography of the bladder and urethra after introduction of a contrast medium and during the process of urination.

13. _____ refers to an elevated level of urea and other nitrogenous waste products in the blood.

14. _____ refers to high blood pressure that results from kidney disease.

15. _____ is the mechanical filtering process used to clean blood of high concentrations of metabolic waste products.

Competency Verification: Check your answers in Appendix B: Answer Key, page 583. If you are not satisfied with your level of comprehension, review the pathological, diagnostic, and therapeutic terms and retake the review.

Correct Answers _____ × 6.67 = _____ % Score

MEDICAL RECORD ACTIVITIES

Medical reports included in the following activities reflect common, real-life clinical scenarios using medical terminology to document patient care.

MEDICAL RECORD ACTIVITY 7-1

CYSTITIS

Terminology

Terms listed in the table below come from the medical report Cystitis that follows. Use a medical dictionary such as Taber's Cyclopedic Medical Dictionary, the appendices of this book, or other resources to define each term. Then practice reading the pronunciations aloud for each term.

Term	Definition
cholecystectomy kō-lē-sĭs-TĔK-tō-mē	
choledocholithiasis kō-lĕd-ō-kō-lĭ-THĪ-ă-sĭs	
choledocholithotomy kō-lĕd-ō-kō-lĭth-ŎT-ō-mē	
cholelithiasis kō-lē-lĭ-THĪ-ă-sĭs	
cystoscopy sĭs-TŎS-kō-pē	
hematuria hĕm-ă-TŪ-rē-ă	
nocturia nŏk-TŪ-rē-ă	
polyuria pŏl-ē-Ū-rē-ă	
urinary incontinence Ū-rĭ-nār-ē ĭn-KŎNT-ĭn-ĕns	

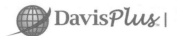 **DavisPlus.** | Visit the *Medical Terminology Simplified* online resource center at Davis*Plus* to hear pronunciation and meanings of selected terms in this medical report.

Reading

Practice pronunciation of medical terms by reading the following medical report aloud.

Cystitis

This 50-year-old white woman has been complaining of diffuse pelvic pain with urinary bladder spasm since cystoscopy 10 days ago, at which time marked cystitis was noted. She reports nocturia 3–4 times, urinary frequency, urgency, and epigastric discomfort. The patient has a history of polyuria, hematuria, and urinary incontinence. There is a history of numerous stones, large and small, in the gallbladder. In 20xx she was admitted to the hospital with cholecystitis, chronic and acute; cholelithiasis; and choledocholithiasis. Subsequently, cholecystectomy, choledocholithotomy, and incidental appendectomy were performed. My impression is that the urinary incontinence is due to cystitis and is temporary in nature.

Evaluation

Review the medical report above to answer the following questions. Use a medical dictionary such as Taber's Cyclopedic Medical Dictionary *and other resources if needed.*

1. What was found when the patient had a cystoscopy?

_____

_____

2. What are the symptoms of cystitis?

_____

_____

3. What is the patient's past surgical history?

_____

_____

4. What is the treatment for cystitis?

_____

_____

5. What are the dangers of untreated cystitis?

_____

_____

6. What instrument is used to perform a cystoscopy?

_____

_____

MEDICAL RECORD ACTIVITY 7-2

DYSURIA WITH BENIGN PROSTATIC HYPERTROPHY

Terminology

Terms listed in the table below come from the medical report Dysuria with Benign Prostatic Hypertrophy that follows. Use a medical dictionary such as Taber's Cyclopedic Medical Dictionary, *the appendices of this book, or other resources to define each term. Then practice reading the pronunciations aloud for each term.*

Term	Definition
asymptomatic ā-sĭmp-tō-MĂT-ĭk	
auscultation aws-kŭl-TĀ-shŭn	
basal cell carcinoma BĀ-săl SĔL kăr-sĭ-NŌ-mă	
benign prostatic hypertrophy bē-NĬN prŏs-TĂT-ĭk hī-PĔR-trŏ-fē	
bruits BRWĒZ	
catheterization kăth-ĕ-tĕr-ĭ-ZĀ-shŭn	
hemorrhoid HĔM-ō-royd	
hydrocele HĪ-drō-sēl	
impotence ĬM-pō-tĕns	

Continued

Term	Definition
inguinal hernia ĬNG-gwĭ-năl HĔR-nē-ă	
normocephalic nor-mō-sĕ-FĂL-ĭk	
palpable PĂL-pă-bl	
percussion pĕr-KŬSH-ŭn	
pneumothorax nū-mō-THŌ-răks	

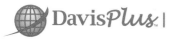 Visit the *Medical Terminology Simplified* online resource center at Davis*Plus* to hear pronunciation and meanings of selected terms in this medical report.

Reading

Practice pronunciation of medical terms by reading the following medical report aloud.

Dysuria with Benign Prostatic Hypertrophy

HISTORY OF PRESENT ILLNESS: Patient is a 72-year-old white man with symptoms of dysuria and frequency before this admission. He recently was found to have colon cancer and is being admitted for colectomy. Preoperative catheterization was not possible, and consultation with Dr. Moriarty was obtained.

PAST HISTORY: Negative for transurethral resection of the prostate or any urological trauma or venereal disease. Past medical history includes hemorrhoid symptoms, bilateral inguinal hernia repair, high cholesterol, retinal surgery, spontaneous pneumothorax ×2 requiring chest tube insertion. He also had a basal cell carcinoma.

PHYSICAL EXAMINATION: Head: Normocephalic. **Eyes, Ears, Nose, and Throat:** Within normal limits. **Neck:** No nodes. No bruits over carotids. **Chest:** Clear to auscultation and percussion. **Heart:** Normal heart sounds. No murmur. **Abdomen:** Soft and nontender. No masses are palpable. It is very distended. **Penis:** Normal. There is a right hydrocele. **Rectal:** Examination reveals benign prostatic hypertrophy.

ASSESSMENT: 1. Mild to moderate benign prostatic hypertrophy.
2. Status post colon resection for carcinoma of the colon.
3. Right hydrocele, asymptomatic.

Evaluation

Review the medical report to answer the following questions. Use a medical dictionary such as Taber's Cyclopedic Medical Dictionary *and other resources if needed.*

1. What prompted the consultation with the urologist, Dr. Moriarty?

   _____

   _____

2. What abnormality did the urologist discover?

   _____

   _____

3. Did the patient have any previous surgery on his prostate?

   _____

   _____

4. Where was the patient's hernia?

   _____

   _____

5. What in the patient's past medical history contributed to his present urological problem?

   _____

   _____

URINARY SYSTEM CHAPTER REVIEW

WORD ELEMENTS SUMMARY

The following table summarizes CFs, suffixes, and prefixes related to the urinary system. Study the word elements and their meanings before completing the Word Elements Chapter Review that follows.

Word Element	Meaning	Word Element	Meaning
Combining Forms			
aden/o	gland	nephr/o, ren/o	kidney
azot/o	nitrogenous compounds	noct/o	night
carcin/o	cancer	olig/o	scanty
cyst/o, vesic/o	bladder	py/o	pus
erythr/o	red	pyel/o	renal pelvis
glomerul/o	glomerulus	scler/o	hardening; sclera (white of the eye)
hemat/o	blood	ureter/o	ureter
lith/o	stone, calculus	urethr/o	urethra
meat/o	opening, meatus	ur/o, urin/o	urine
Suffixes			
-al, -ic, -ous	pertaining to	-megaly	enlargement
-algia, -dynia	pain	-oma	tumor
-cele	hernia, swelling	-osis	abnormal condition; increase (used primarily with blood cells)
-ectasis	dilation, expansion	-pathy	disease
-ectomy	excision, removal	-pepsia	digestion
-edema	swelling	-pexy	fixation (of an organ)
-emesis	vomiting	-phagia	swallowing, eating
-grade	to go	-phobia	fear
-gram	record, writing	-plasty	surgical repair
-graphy	process of recording	-ptosis	prolapse, downward displacement
-ia	condition	-rrhaphy	suture
-iasis	abnormal condition (produced by something specified)	-rrhea	discharge, flow
-ist	specialist	-stomy	forming an opening (mouth)
-lith	stone, calculus	-tome	instrument to cut
-logist	specialist in the study of	-tomy	incision
-logy	study of	-tripsy	crushing
-lysis	separation, destruction, loosening	-uria	urine

Prefixes

a-, an-	without, not	intra-	in, within
dia-	through, across	poly-	many, much
dys-	bad; painful; difficult	retro-	backward, behind
in-	in, not	supra-	above; excessive; superior

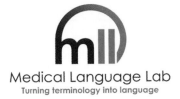

Medical Language Lab
Turning terminology into language

Visit the *Medical Language Lab* at the website *medicallanguagelab.com*. Use the flash-card exercise for this chapter to reinforce your study of word elements. We recommend you complete the flash-card exercise before starting the Word Elements Chapter Review that follows.

WORD ELEMENTS CHAPTER REVIEW

This review provides a verification of your knowledge of the word elements covered in this chapter. Write the meaning of the word element in the space provided. To reinforce your understanding of the word parts that make up a medical term, identify each word element as a prefix (P), word root (WR), combining form (CF), or suffix (S). The first word is completed for you.

Medical Term	Word Elements	Meaning
1. anuria	*an- (P)*	*without, not*
	-uria (S)	*urine*
2. azotemia		
3. dialysis		
4. dysuria		
5. glomeropathy		

Medical Term	Word Elements	Meaning
6. hypertension		
7. hypospadias		
8. lithotripsy		
9. meatus		
10. nephralgia		
11. nephrolithotomy		

Continued

Medical Term	Word Elements	Meaning
12. nephromegaly		
13. nephropexy		
14. nephroptosis		
15. nocturia		
16. polyuria		
17. pyeloplasty		

Medical Term	Word Elements	Meaning
18. pyelostomy		
19. suprarenal		
20. ureterolithiasis		
21. ureterocystoscopy		

Continued

Medical Term	Word Elements	Meaning
22. urography		
23. urethrocele		
24. urologist		
25. vesicocele		

Competency Verification: Check your answers in Appendix B: Answer Key, page 585. If you are not satisfied with your level of comprehension, review the chapter's flash-card exercise at *medicallanguagelab.com* and retake the review.

Correct Answers _____ × 4 = _____ % Score

VOCABULARY REVIEW

Match the medical term(s) with the definitions in the numbered list.

acute renal failure	cystocele	malignant	oliguria
anuria	diuretics	nephrolithotomy	polyuria
benign	edema	nephrons	renal pelvis
bilateral	hematuria	nephroptosis	ureteropyeloplasty
cholelithiasis	IVP	nocturia	urinary incontinence

1. _____ refers to cancerous growths.

2. _____ are microscopic filtering units in the kidney that are responsible for keeping body fluids in balance.

3. _____ refers to formation of gallstones.

4. _____ is a funnel-shaped reservoir that is the basin of the kidney.

5. _____ is an x-ray film of the kidneys after injection of dye.

6. _____ are drugs that stimulate urine flow.

7. _____ means swelling (of body tissues).

8. _____ refers to noncancerous growths.

9. _____ is an incision into a kidney to remove a stone.

10. _____ is a condition that results from lack of blood flow to the kidneys.

11. _____ is downward displacement of a kidney.

12. _____ is surgical repair of a ureter and renal pelvis.

13. _____ means pertaining to two sides.

14. _____ means excessive urination at night.

15. _____ refers to the inability to hold urine.

16. _____ refers to the presence of red blood cells in urine.

17. _____ means excessive discharge of urine.

18. _____ is a diminished amount of urine formation.

19. _____ is an absence of urine formation.

20. _____ is a herniation of the urinary bladder.

Competency Verification: Check your answers in Appendix B: Answer Key, page 586. If you are not satisfied with your level of comprehension, review the chapter vocabulary and retake the review.

Correct Answers _____ × 5 = _____ % Score

Reproductive Systems

OBJECTIVES

Upon completion of this chapter, you will be able to:

- Describe the type of medical treatment gynecologists and obstetricians provide.
- Identify female and male reproductive structures by labeling them on the anatomical illustrations.
- Describe primary functions of the female and male reproductive systems.
- Describe diseases, conditions, and procedures related to the female and male reproductive systems.
- Apply your word-building skills by constructing medical terms related to the female and male reproductive systems.
- Describe common abbreviations and symbols related to the female and male reproductive systems.
- Recognize, define, pronounce, and spell terms correctly.
- Demonstrate your knowledge of this chapter by successfully completing the frames, reviews, and medical report evaluations.

MEDICAL SPECIALTIES

Gynecology

Gynecology is the medical specialty concerned with diagnosis and treatment of female reproductive disorders, including the breasts. Unlike most medical specialties, gynecology encompasses surgical and nonsurgical expertise of the physician. The **gynecologist** is a physician who specializes in gynecology.

Obstetrics

Obstetrics is the branch of medicine concerned with pregnancy and childbirth, including the study of the physiological and pathological functions of the female reproductive tract. It also involves the care of the mother and fetus throughout pregnancy, childbirth, and the immediate **postpartum** (after birth) period. An **obstetrician** is a physician who specializes in obstetrics. The branch of medicine that concentrates on the care of the neonate (newborn) and in the diagnosis and treatment of disorders of the neonate is known as **neonatology**. Once the infant is born, physicians called **neonatologists** specialize in providing their medical care.

Obstetrics and Gynecology

Because obstetrics is studied in conjunction with gynecology, the physician's medical practice commonly includes both areas of expertise. This branch of medicine is called **obstetrics and gynecology (OB-GYN)**. The OB-GYN physician possesses knowledge of endocrinology, because hormones play an important role in the function of the female reproductive system, especially the process of secondary sex characteristics, menstruation, pregnancy, and menopause. Therefore, infertility, birth control, and hormone imbalance are all part of the treatment provided by an OB-GYN physician.

Urology

Urology is the branch of medicine concerned with disorders and care of the urinary tract in men and women and of the male reproductive system. **Urologists** diagnose and treat disorders of the male reproductive system, such as sexual dysfunction and infertility. Their scope of practice includes various surgeries, such as transurethral resection of the prostate and cystoscopy. In addition, urologists treat genitourinary tract diseases that affect the urinary systems of men and women.

ANATOMY AND PHYSIOLOGY OVERVIEW

Although structures of the female and male reproductive systems differ, both have a common purpose. They are specialized to produce and unite gametes (reproductive cells) and transport them to sites of fertilization. Reproductive systems of both sexes are designed specifically to perpetuate the species and pass genetic material from generation to generation. In addition, both sexes produce hormones, which are vital in the development and maintenance of sexual characteristics and regulation of reproductive physiology.

FEMALE REPRODUCTIVE SYSTEM

The female reproductive system is composed of internal organs of reproduction and external genitalia. The internal organs are the ovaries, fallopian tubes (oviducts, uterine tubes), uterus, and vagina. External organs, also called the **genitalia,** are known collectively as the **vulva.** Included in the vulva are the mons pubis, labia majora, labia minora, clitoris, and Bartholin glands. (See Fig. 8–1.) The combined organs of the female reproductive system are designed to produce and transport ova (female sex cells), discharge ova from the body if fertilization does not occur, and nourish and provide a place for the developing fetus throughout pregnancy if fertilization occurs. The female reproductive system also produces the female sex hormones estrogen and progesterone, which are responsible for development of secondary sex characteristics, such as breast development and regulation of the menstrual cycle.

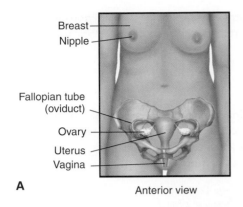

Breast
Nipple

Fallopian tube
(oviduct)

Ovary
Uterus
Vagina

A

Anterior view

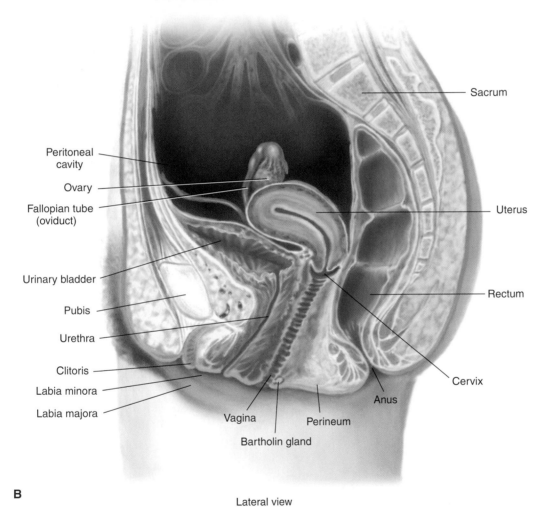

Peritoneal
cavity

Ovary

Fallopian tube
(oviduct)

Urinary bladder

Pubis

Urethra

Clitoris

Labia minora

Labia majora

Vagina

Bartholin gland

Perineum

Anus

Cervix

Rectum

Uterus

Sacrum

B

Lateral view

Figure 8-1 Female reproductive system. (**A**) Anterior view. (**B**) Lateral view.

WORD ELEMENTS

This section introduces combining forms (CFs) related to the female reproductive system. Included are key suffixes; prefixes are defined in the right-hand column as needed. Review the following table and pronounce each word in the word analysis column aloud before you begin to work the frames.

Word Element	Meaning	Word Analysis
Combining Forms		
amni/o	amnion (amniotic sac)	**amni/o**/centesis (ăm-nē-ō-sĕn-TĒ-sĭs): surgical puncture of the amniotic sac *-centesis:* surgical puncture *The sample of amniotic fluid obtained in amniocentesis is studied chemically and cytologically to detect genetic abnormalities, biochemical disorders, and maternal–fetal blood incompatibility.*
cervic/o	neck; cervix uteri (neck of the uterus)	**cervic**/itis (sĕr-vĭ-SĪ-tĭs): inflammation of the cervix uteri *-itis:* inflammation *Cervicitis is usually the result of infection or a sexually transmitted infection. It may also become chronic because, unlike the uterine lining, the cervical lining is not renewed each month during menstruation.*
colp/o	vagina	**colp/o**/scopy (kŏl-PŎS-kō-pē): examination of the vagina and cervix with an optical magnifying instrument (colposcope) *-scopy:* visual examination *Colposcopy is commonly performed after a Papanicolaou (Pap) test for treatment of cervical dysplasia and to obtain biopsy specimens of the cervix.*
vagin/o		**vagin/o**/cele (VĂJ-ĭn-ō-sēl): herniation into the vagina; also called a *colpocele* *-cele:* hernia; swelling
galact/o	milk	**galact/o**/rrhea (gă-lăk-tō-RĒ-ă): discharge or flow of milk *-rrhea:* discharge, flow
lact/o		**lact/o**/gen (LĂK-tō-jĕn): production and secretion of milk *-gen:* forming, producing, origin
gynec/o	woman, female	**gynec/o**/logist (gī-nĕ-KŎL-ō-jĭst): physician specializing in treating disorders of the female reproductive system *-logist:* specialist in the study of
hyster/o	uterus (womb)	**hyster**/ectomy (hĭs-tĕr-ĔK-tō-mē): excision of the uterus *-ectomy:* excision, removal

uter/o		**uter/o**/vagin/al (ū-tĕr-ō-VĂJ-ĭ-năl): pertaining to the uterus and vagina
		    vagin: vagina
		        -al: pertaining to

mamm/o	breast	**mamm/o**/gram (MĂM-ō-grăm): radiograph of the breast *-gram:* record, writing
mast/o		**mast/o**/pexy (MĂS-tō-pĕks-ē): surgical fixation of the breast(s) *-pexy:* fixation (of an organ) *Mastopexy is a cosmetic surgery to affix sagging breasts in a more elevated position, commonly improving their shape.*
men/o	menses, menstruation	**men/o**/rrhagia (mĕn-ō-RĂ-jē-ă): excessive amount of menstrual flow over a longer duration than normal *-rrhagia:* bursting forth (of)

metr/o	uterus (womb); measure	endo/**metr**/itis (ĕn-dō-mē-TRĪ-tĭs): inflammation of the endometrium
		    endo-: in, within
		        -itis: inflammation

Word Element	Meaning	Word Analysis
nat/o	birth	pre/**nat**/al (prē-NĀ-tl): pertaining to (the period) before birth 　*pre-:* before, in front of 　　*-al:* pertaining to
oophor/o	ovary	**oophor**/oma (ō-ŏf-ōr-Ō-mă): ovarian tumor 　*-oma:* tumor
ovari/o		**ovari**/o/rrhexis (ō-văr-rē-ō-RĔK-sĭs): rupture of an ovary 　*-rrhexis:* rupture
perine/o	perineum	**perine**/o/rrhaphy (pĕr-ĭ-nē-OR-ă-fē): suture of the perineum 　*-rrhaphy:* suture *Perineorrhaphy is performed to repair a laceration that occurs spontaneously or is made surgically during the delivery of the fetus.*
salping/o	tube (usually fallopian or eustachian [auditory] tubes)	**salping**/ectomy (săl-pĭn-JĔK-tō-mē): excision of a fallopian tube 　*-ectomy:* excision, removal
vulv/o	vulva	**vulv**/o/pathy (vŭl-VŎP-ă-thē): disease of the vulva 　*-pathy:* disease
episi/o		**episi**/o/tomy (ĕ-pēs-ē-ŎT-ō-mē): incision of the perineum 　*-tomy:* incision *Episiotomy is performed to enlarge the vaginal opening for delivery of the fetus. The perineum is the region between the vaginal orifice and the anus.*

Suffixes

Word Element	Meaning	Word Analysis
-arche	beginning	men/**arche** (mĕn-ĂR-kē): initial menstrual period 　*men:* menses, menstruation *Menarche usually occurs between ages 9 and 17.*
-gravida	pregnant woman	primi/**gravida** (prī-mĭ-GRĂV-ĭ-dă): woman during her first pregnancy 　*primi-:* first
-para	to bear (offspring)	multi/**para** (mŭl-TĬP-ă-ră): woman who has delivered more than one viable infant 　*multi-:* many, much
-salpinx	tube (usually fallopian or eustachian [auditory] tubes)	hemat/o/**salpinx** (hĕm-ă-tō-SĂL-pinks): collection of blood in a fallopian tube; also called *hemosalpinx* 　*hemat/o:* blood *Hematosalpinx is commonly associated with a tubal pregnancy.*
-tocia	childbirth, labor	dys/**tocia** (dĭs-TŌ-sē-ă): childbirth that is painful and difficult 　*dys-:* bad; painful; difficult *Dystocia may be caused by an obstruction or constriction of the birth passage or abnormal size, shape, position, or condition of the fetus.*
-version	turning	retro/**version** (rĕt-rō-VĔR-shŭn): tipping back of an organ 　*retro-:* backward, behind *Uterine retroversion is measured as first-, second-, or third-degree, depending on the angle of tilt in relationship to the vagina.*

Pronunciation Help	Long sound	ā in rāte	ē in rēbirth	ī in īsle	ō in ōver	ū in ūnite
	Short sound	ă in ălone	ĕ in ĕver	ĭ in ĭt	ŏ in nŏt	ŭ in cŭt

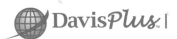

Visit the *Medical Terminology Simplified* online resource center at Davis*Plus* for an audio exercise of the terms in this table. It will help you master pronunciations and meanings of medical terms.

SECTION REVIEW 8-1

For the following medical terms, first write the suffix and its meaning. Then translate the meaning of the remaining elements starting with the first part of the word. The first word is completed for you.

Term	Definition
1. primi/gravida	-gravida: pregnant woman; first
2. colp/o/scopy	
3. gynec/o/logist	
4. perine/o/rrhaphy	
5. hyster/ectomy	
6. oophor/oma	
7. dys/tocia	
8. endo/metr/itis	
9. mamm/o/gram	
10. amni/o/centesis	

Competency Verification: Check your answers in Appendix B: Answer Key, page 587. If you are not satisfied with your level of comprehension, review the vocabulary and retake the review.

Correct Answers _____ × 10 = _____ % Score

Internal Structures

8-1   The female reproductive system is composed of internal and external organs of reproduction. The internal reproductive organs are the (1) **ovaries**, (2) **fallopian tubes**, (3) **uterus**, and (4) **vagina**. Label these organs in Figures 8–2 and 8–3 as you learn the names of the internal reproductive organs.

tumor TOO-mŏr	**8-2** An oophor/oma is an ovarian _____. Pronounce the initial *o* and the second *o* in words with *oophor/o*.
oophor/o	**8-3** The main purpose of the ovaries is to produce an ovum, the female reproductive cell. This process is called **ovulation**. Another important function of the ovaries is to produce the hormones estrogen and progesterone. From oophor/oma, construct the CF for ovary. _____ / _____

Boldface indicates a word root or combining form. Blue indicates a suffix. Pink indicates a prefix.

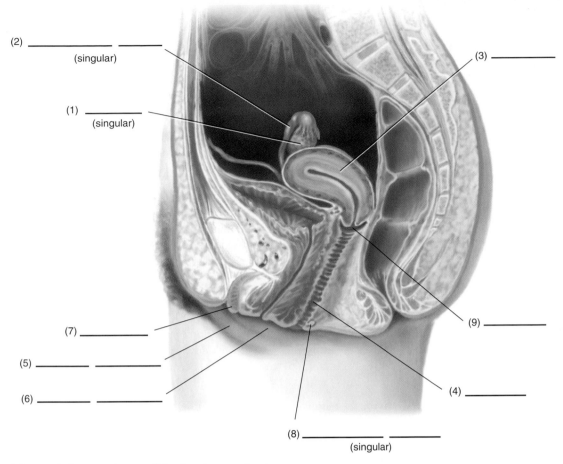

(2) _____ _____ _____
(singular)

(1) _____ _____
(singular)

(3) _____ _____

(7) _____ _____

(5) _____ _____ _____

(6) _____ _____ _____

(9) _____ _____

(4) _____ _____

(8) _____ _____ _____
(singular)

Figure 8-2 Lateral view of the female reproductive system.

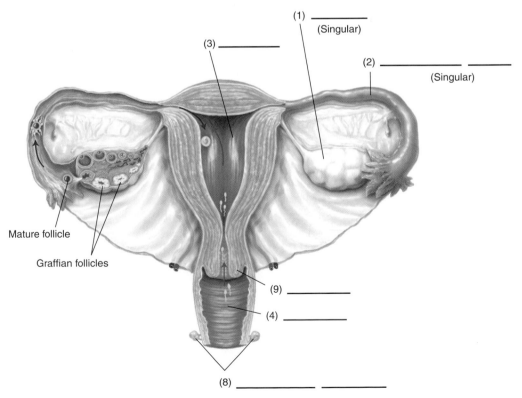

(1) _____ _____
(Singular)

(3) _____ _____

(2) _____ _____ _____
(Singular)

Mature follicle

Graffian follicles

(9) _____ _____

(4) _____ _____

(8) _____ _____ _____

Figure 8-3 Anterior view of the female reproductive system, showing developing follicles in the cross section of the right ovary with red arrows indicating movement of the ovum toward the uterus and blue arrows indicating movement of the sperm toward the fallopian tube.

oophor/o/pathy ō-ŏf-ŏr-ŎP-ă-thē **oophor/o/plasty** ō-ŎF-ŏr-ō-plăs-tē **oophor/o/pexy** ō-ŏf-ō-rō-PĔK-sē	**8–4** Use *oophor/o* to build medical words that mean *disease of the ovaries:* _____ / _____ / _____ *surgical repair of an ovary:* _____ / _____ / _____ *fixation of a displaced ovary:* _____ / _____ / _____
salping/o/plasty săl-PĬNG-gō-plăs-tē	**8–5** The CF *salping/o* means *tube (usually fallopian or eustachian [auditory] tube)* and is related to the female reproductive system. Eustachian (auditory) tubes are related to the sense of hearing and are discussed in Chapter 11. Surgical repair of a fallopian tube (also known as an oviduct) is called _____ / _____ / _____.
salping/o	**8–6** Approximately once per month, maturation of the ovum, or ovulation, occurs when the egg leaves the ovary and slowly travels down the fallopian tube to the uterus. (See Fig. 8–3.) If union of the ovum with sperm takes place during this time, fertilization (pregnancy) results. To form words for the fallopian tube(s), uterine tube(s), or oviduct(s), use the CF _____ / _____.
salping/ectomy săl-pĭn-JĔK-tō-mē	**8–7** If the fertilized egg attaches to the wall of the fallopian tube (instead of the uterus), the tube must be removed to prevent serious bleeding or possible death of the mother. When a fallopian tube is removed, the surgical procedure is called _____ / _____.
instrument	**8–8** A salping/o/scope is an _____ for viewing the fallopian tube(s).
salping/o/scopy săl-pĭng-GŎS-kō-pē	**8–9** Visual examination of the fallopian tube(s) is called _____ / _____ / _____.
salping/o/cele săl-PĬNG-ō-sēl	**8–10** Herniation of a fallopian tube(s) is known as _____ / _____ / _____.
oviducts Ŏ-vĭ-dŭkts	**8–11** Locate the two small tubes in Figure 8–3 that lead to each ovary. They are called fallopian tubes, uterine tubes, or _____.

Boldface indicates a word root or combining form. Blue indicates a suffix. Pink indicates a prefix.

hernia *or* **herniation, uterus** HĔR-nē-ă, hĕr-nē-Ā-shŭn, Ū-tĕr-ŭs	**8-12** The uterus, also called the womb, is the organ that contains and nourishes the embryo and fetus from the time the fertilized egg is implanted to the time of birth. The CF *hyster/o* is used to form words about the uterus as an organ. A hyster/o/cele is a _____ of the _____.
hyster/o/pathy hĭs-tĕr-ŎP-ă-thē **hyster/algia, hyster/o/dynia** hĭs-tĕr-ĂL-jē-ă, hĭs-tĕr-ō-DĬN-ē-ă **hyster/o/spasm** HĬS-tĕr-ō-spăzm	**8-13** Use *hyster/o* to build medical words that mean *disease of the uterus:* _____ / _____ / _____ *pain in the uterus:* _____ / _____ *or* _____ / _____ / _____ *involuntary contraction, twitching of the uterus:* _____ / _____ / _____
hyster/ectomy hĭs-tĕr-ĔK-tō-mē **hyster/o/tomy** hĭs-tĕr-ŎT-ō-mē	**8-14** Presence of one or more tumors (either benign or malignant) in the uterus may necessitate its removal. (See Fig. 8–4.) Use *hyster/o* to form surgical terms that mean *excision of the uterus:* _____ / _____ *incision of the uterus:* _____ / _____ / _____
dictionary	**8-15** Besides *hyster/o,* the CFs *metr/o* and *uter/o* are also used to denote the uterus. When in doubt about forming medical words with **hyster/o, uter/o,** or **metr/o,** refer to your medical _____.

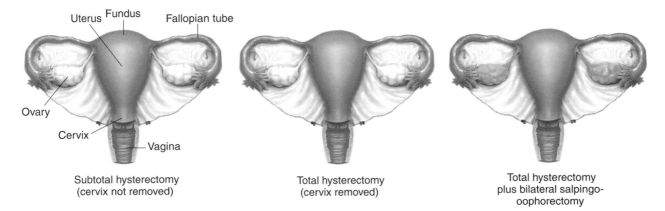

Figure 8-4 Hysterectomy, showing the excised structure in purple.

hyster/o/scopy hĭs-tĕr-ŎS-kō-pē **uter/o/scopy** Ū-tĕr-ŏs-kō-pē	**8-16** The uterus is a muscular, hollow, pear-shaped structure located in the pelvic area between the bladder and rectum. (See Fig. 8–1.) Use *hyster/o* to form a word that means *visual examination of the uterus.* _____ / _____ / _____ Use *uter/o* to form another word that means *visual examination of the uterus.* _____ / _____ / _____
hyster/o/ptosis hĭs-tĕr-ŏp-TŌ-sĭs	**8-17** The uterus is supported and held in place by ligaments. Weakening of these ligaments may cause a downward displacement, or prolapse, of the uterus. Combine *hyster/o* and *-ptosis* to form a word that means *prolapse or downward displacement of the uterus.* _____ / _____ / _____
hyster/o, uter/o **-pexy**	**8-18** A prolapsed uterus may be caused by heavy physical exertion, pregnancy, or an inherent weakness. The surgical procedure to correct a prolapsed uterus is known as hyster/o/pexy or uter/o/pexy. Write the elements in this frame that mean *uterus:* _____ / _____, _____ / _____ *fixation (of an organ):* _____
surgical repair, uterus Ū-tĕr-ŭs	**8-19** Surgical repair is denoted by the suffix *-plasty*. Hyster/o/plasty, uter/o/plasty, and metr/o/plasty all refer to _____ _____ of the _____.
hyster/o/cele HĬS-tĕr-ō-sēl	**8-20** Hyster/o/cele, a protrusion of uter/ine contents into a weakened area of the uterine wall, may occur as a result of pregnancy. A diagnosis (Dx) of herniation of the uterus would be documented in the medical chart as _____ / _____ / _____.
estrogen, progesterone ĔS-trō-jĕn, prō-JĔS-tĕr-ōn	**8-21** The ovaries secrete two important hormones: estrogen and progesterone. These hormones play an important role in the processes of menstruation and pregnancy, as well as the development of secondary sex characteristics. When ovaries are diseased and necessitate removal, the body becomes deficient in the hormones known as _____ and _____.

Boldface indicates a word root or combining form. Blue indicates a suffix. Pink indicates a prefix.

men/o/pause MĔN-ō-pawz **trans/derm/al** trănz-DĔR-măl	**8–22**　Men/o/pause, a natural process, is the gradual ending of the menstrual cycle, which also results in an estrogen hormone deficiency. Hormone replacement therapy (HRT) given orally or as a trans/derm/al patch may be used to relieve uncomfortable symptoms of men/o/pause. Identify terms in this frame that mean *cessation of the menses:* _____ / _____ / _____ *through, across the skin:* _____ / _____ / _____
post/men/o/pause PŌST-mĕn-ō-pawz	**8–23**　The term pre/men/o/pause refers to a time period before men/o/pause. Can you build a word that refers to a time period *after* men/o/pause? _____ / _____ / _____ / _____
bursting forth	**8–24**　The suffixes *-rrhage* and *-rrhagia* mean *bursting forth (of).* Hem/o/rrhage denotes a _____ _____ (of) blood.
hem/o	**8–25**　The CF in hem/o/rrhage that denotes blood is _____ / _____.
blood	**8–26**　The elements **hemat/o, hem/o**, and *-emia* mean _____.
blood	**8–27**　Hemat/o/logy is the study of _____.
blood **tumor** TOO-mŏr	**8–28**　A hemat/oma is a localized collection or swelling of blood, usually clotted, in an organ, space, or tissue, caused by a break in the wall of a blood vessel. Analyze hemat/oma by defining the elements. *hemat:* _____ *-oma:* _____
hemat/o/logist hē-mă-TŎL-ō-jĭst **hemat/o/pathy** hē-mă-TŎP-ă-thē **hemat/emesis** hĕm-ăt-ĔM-ĕ-sĭs	**8–29**　Use **hemat/o** to build medical words that mean *specialist in the study of blood:* _____ / _____ / _____ *disease of the blood:* _____ / _____ / _____ *vomiting blood:* _____ / _____

curet kū-RĔT	**8–30** Dilation and curettage (D&C) is a surgical procedure to widen (dilate) the cervic/al canal of the uterus and scrape (curet) the endo/metri/um of the uterus. The uterine cavity is examined with a uterine sound to prevent perforation during dilation and to measure depth of the uterus. The instrument used to scrape the endo/metri/um is known as a _____. (See Fig. 8–5.)
uterine sound **serrated**	**8–31** Review Figure 8–5 to learn about the surgical procedure and instruments used to perform D&C. The instrument that is used to measure the uterus and prevent perforation during dilation is called a _____ _____. Scraping the uterine lining requires the use of a _____ curet.
inflammation, vagina vă-JĪ-nă	**8–32** The vagina is a muscular tube that extends from the cervix (neck of the uterus) to the exterior of the body. (See Fig. 8–3.) In addition to serving as the organ of sexual intercourse and the receptor of semen, the vagina discharges menstrual flow and acts as a passageway for the delivery of the fetus. The CFs *colp/o* and *vagin/o* refer to the vagina. Colp/itis is an _____ of the _____.

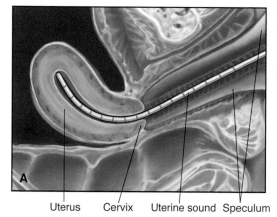

A

Uterus   Cervix   Uterine sound   Speculum

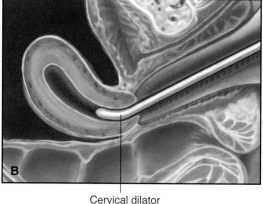

B

Cervical dilator

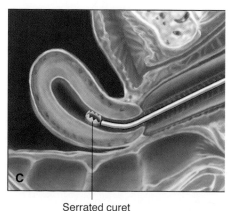

C

Serrated curet

Figure 8-5 Dilation and curettage of the uterus. (**A**) Examination of the uterine cavity with a uterine sound. (**B**) Dilation of the cervix using dilators of increasing size to enable insertion of a curet. (**C**) Curettage of the uterine lining with a serrated uterine curet.

Boldface indicates a word root or combining form. Blue indicates a suffix. Pink indicates a prefix.

vagin/itis văj-ĭn-Ī-tĭs	**8-33** Form another word in addition to colp/itis that means *inflammation of the vagina*. _____ / _____
colp/algia kŏl-PĂL-jē-ā	**8-34** Colp/o/dynia denotes a *pain in the vagina*. Use *colp/o* to build another term for *pain in the vagina*. _____ / _____
colp/o/spasm KŎL-pō-spăzm **colp/o/ptosis** kŏl-pŏp-TŌ-sĭs **colp/o/pexy** KŎL-pō-pĕk-sē	**8-35** Use *colp/o* to construct medical words that mean *spasm or twitching of the vagina:* _____ / _____ / _____ *prolapse or downward displacement of the vagina:* _____ / _____ / _____ *fixation of the vagina:* _____ / _____ / _____
vagin/o/plasty VĂJ-ĭ-nō-plăs-tē **vagin/o/scope** VĂJ-ĭn-ō-skōp **vagin/o/tomy** văj-ĭ-NŎT-ō-mē	**8-36** Use *vagin/o* to form medical words that mean *surgical repair of the vagina:* _____ / _____ / _____ *instrument to view the vagina:* _____ / _____ / _____ *incision of the vagina:* _____ / _____ / _____
suture, vagina SŪ-chŭr, vă-JĪ-nă	**8-37** A prolapsed vagina is usually sutured to the abdominal wall. Colp/o/rrhaphy is a _____ of the _____.
vesic/o/vagin/al fistula vĕs-ĭ-kō-VĂJ-ĭ-năl, FĬS-tū-lă	**8-38** A vesic/o/vagin/al fistula is another type of path/o/logy that can develop in the female reproductive system. This is an abnormal passage between the urinary bladder and the vagina. (See Fig. 8–6.) An abnormal connection that develops between the bladder and vagina is known as a _____ / _____ / _____ / _____ _____.
vagina vă-JĪ-nă	**8-39** The term **fistula** refers to an abnormal passage from one epithelial surface to another epithelial surface. It can occur in any body system. Thus, a vesic/o/vagin/al fistula is only one type of fistula. A ureter/o/vagin/al fistula occurs between the lower ureter and the _____.

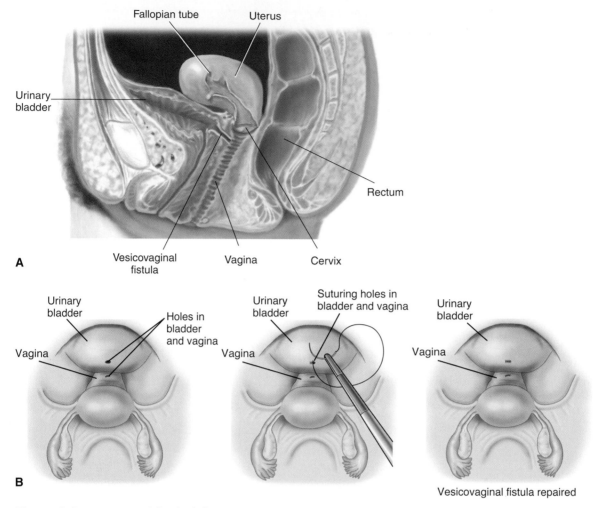

Figure 8-6 Vesicovaginal fistula. (**A**) Lateral view of the female reproductive system with a vesicovaginal fistula. (**B**) Frontal view of the urinary bladder and vagina with vesicovaginal fistula repair.

vagina vă-JĪ-nă	**8–40** A rect/o/vagin/al fistula is one that develops between the rectum and the _____.
-rrhagia, -rrhage	**8–41** Colp/o/rrhagia refers to a *vagin/al hem/o/rrhage*. The elements in these words that mean *bursting forth (of)* are _____ and _____.
hem/o/rrhage HĔM-ĕ-rĭj	**8–42** Form a word that means *bursting forth (of) blood*. _____ / ____ / _____

Boldface indicates a word root or combining form. Blue indicates a suffix. Pink indicates a prefix.

hernia, swelling HĔR-nē-ă	**8–43** Recall that *-cele* means _____ or _____ .
vagina vă-JĪ-nă	**8–44** A colp/o/cyst/o/cele is swelling or herniation of the bladder into the _____ .
vagina vă-JĪ-nă **bladder** **hernia, swelling** HĔR-nē-ă	**8–45** Women who have had several vagin/al childbirths may suffer from hernia- tion of the bladder, or colp/o/cyst/o/cele. Identify the elements in colp/o/cyst/o/cele. *colp/o:* _____ *cyst/o:* _____ *-cele:* _____ or _____
vagin/al VĂJ-ĭn-ăl **hyster/ectomy** hĭs-tĕr-ĔK-tō-mē	**8–46** When the uterus is removed through the vagina, the surgical procedure is known as a vagin/al hyster/ectomy or a colp/o/hyster/ectomy. Identify words in this frame that mean *pertaining to the vagina:* _____ / _____ *excision of the uterus:* _____ / _____
muc/ous MŪ-kŭs	**8–47** The vagina is lubricated by mucus. ***Muc/o*** is the CF for *mucus*. Use the ad- jective ending *-ous* to form a word that means *pertaining to mucus*. _____ / _____
-oid	**8–48** The term muc/oid means *resembling mucus*. The adjective element that means *resembling* is _____ .
resembling fat	**8–49** Lip/oid means _____ _____ .
adip/oid ĂD-ĭ-poyd	**8–50** Use adip/o to form another term that means *resembling fat*. _____ / _____

SECTION REVIEW 8-2

Using the following table, write the CF and suffix that matches its definition in the space provided to the left of the definition. There may be more than one word element that matches a definition.

Combining Forms

colp/o	oophor/o
cyst/o	ovari/o
hemat/o	salping/o
hem/o	uter/o
hyster/o	vagin/o
metr/o	
muc/o	

Suffixes

-arche	-ptosis
-cele	-rrhage
-logist	-rrhagia
-logy	-salpinx
-oid	-scope
-pexy	-tome
-plasty	-tomy

1. _____ bladder

2. _____ blood

3. _____ bursting forth (of)

4. _____ uterus (womb)

5. _____ hernia; swelling

6. _____ incision

7. _____ instrument to cut

8. _____ instrument for examining

9. _____ tube (usually fallopian or eustachian [auditory] tubes)

10. _____ fixation (of an organ)

11. _____ mucus

12. _____ ovary

13. _____ beginning

14. _____ uterus (womb); measure

15. _____ prolapse, downward displacement

16. _____ resembling

17. _____ specialist in the study of

18. _____ study of

19. _____ surgical repair

20. _____ vagina

Competency Verification: Check your answers in Appendix B: Answer Key, page 587. If you are not satisfied with your level of comprehension, go back to Frame 8–1 and rework the frames.

Correct Answers _____ × 5 = _____ % Score

External Structures

8-51   The external structures, or **genitalia**, include the (5) **labia majora** (the outer lips of the vagina), (6) **labia minora** (the smaller, inner lips of the vagina), (7) **clitoris**, and (8) **Bartholin glands.** Label Figures 8–2 and 8–3 to locate the structures of the genitalia.

---

vulva
VŬL-vă

8-52   The CF *vulv/o* refers to the vulva, the combined external structures of the female reproductive system. Vulv/o/uter/ine refers to the uterus and

_____ .

---

clitoris, Bartholin glands
KLĬT-ō-rĭs, BĂR-tō-lĭn

8-53   The external structures, or genitalia (also known as the vulva), include the

labia majora, labia minora, _____ , and _____

_____ .

---

muc/ous
MŪ-kŭs

8-54   Mucus secretions from Bartholin glands help keep the vagina moist and lubricated, facilitating intercourse.

Use *-ous* to build a word that means *pertaining to mucus.*

_____ / _____ (adjective ending)

---

vulv/itis
vŭl-VĪ-tĭs

vulv/o/pathy
vŭl-VŎP-ă-thē

8-55   Use *vulv/o* to construct words that mean

inflammation of the vulva: _____ / _____

disease of the vulva: _____ / _____ / _____

8-56   The (9) **cervix** is the neck of the uterus and extends into the upper portion of the vagina. Examine the position of the cervix in the lateral and anterior view as you label Figures 8–2 and 8–3.

---

cervic/itis
sĕr-vĭ-SĪ-tĭs

8-57   The CF *cervic/o* refers to the cervix uteri or the neck. Inflammation of the

cervix uteri is called _____ / _____ .

---

vagina, uteri
vă-JĪ-nă, Ū-tĕ-rī

8-58   When *cervic/o* is used in a word, you can determine whether it refers to the neck or the cervix uteri by reviewing the other parts of the word.

Colp/o/cervic/al refers to the _____ and cervix

_____ .

---

colp/o/scopy
kŏl-PŎS-kō-pē

8-59   A colp/o/scope is an instrument with a magnifying lens that is used to examine vagin/al and cervic/al tissue. Visual examination of vagin/al and cervic/al

tissue using a colposcope is called _____ / _____ / _____ .

---

colp/o/scope KŎL-pō-skōp **colp/o/scopy** kŏl-PŎS-kō-pē **vagin/al** VĂJ-ĭn-ăl **cervic/al** SĔR-vĭ-kăl	**8-60** Determine the words in Frame 8–59 that mean *instrument for examining the vagina and cervix uteri:* _____ / _____ / _____ *visual examination of the vagina and cervix uteri using a colp/o/scope:* _____ / _____ / _____ *pertaining to the vagina:* _____ / _____ *pertaining to the cervix uteri:* _____ / _____

uterus Ū-tĕr-ŭs	**8-61** Cervix uteri refers to the neck of the _____.

Competency Verification: Check your labeling of Figures 8–2 and 8–3 in Appendix B: Answer Key, page 587.

gynec/o/logist gī-nĕ-KŎL-ō-jĭst	**8-62** The term gynec/o/logy means *study of females or women* and is the medical specialty for treating female reproductive disorders. A specialist in the study of female reproductive disorders is called a _____ / _____ / _____.

gynec/o	**8-63** The CF in gynec/o/logy that means *woman* or *female* is _____ / _____.

gynec/o/pathy gī-nĕ-KŎP-ă-thē	**8-64** Use *-pathy* to form a word that means *disease of a female.* _____ / _____ / _____

gynec/o/logy gī-nĕ-KŎL-ō-jē	**8-65** GYN is the abbreviation for gynec/o/logy. OB-GYN refers to *obstetrics and* _____ / _____ / _____.

menses, menstruation MĔN-sēz, mĕn-stroo-Ā-shŭn	**8-66** The CF *men/o* means *menses* or *menstruation,* which is the monthly flow of blood and tissue from the uterus. Men/o/rrhea is a flow of _____ or _____.

dys/men/o/rrhea dĭs-mĕn-ō-RĒ-ă	**8-67** Use *dys-* and men/o/rrhea to develop a word that means *painful or difficult menstrual flow.* _____ / _____ / _____ / _____

Boldface indicates a word root or combining form. Blue indicates a suffix. Pink indicates a prefix.

dys/men/o/rrhea dĭs-mĕn-ō-RĒ-ă	**8-68** Dys/men/o/rrhea is pain associated with menstruation. Primary dys/men/o/rrhea is menstrual pain that results from factors intrinsic to the uterus and the process of menstruation. It is extremely common, occurring at least occasionally in almost all women. If the painful episode is mild and brief, it is considered functional and normal and requires no treatment. The symptomatic term that literally means *bad, painful, difficult menstruation* is _____ / _____ / _____ / _____ .
bursting forth, menses *or* **menstruation** MĔN-sēz, mĕn-stroo-Ā-shŭn	**8-69** Men/o/rrhagia is *excessive bleeding at the time of a menstrual period.* Literally, it means _____ _____ of _____ .
menstruation mĕn-stroo-Ā-shun	**8-70** Men/o/pause terminates the reproductive period of life and is a permanent cessation of menses or _____ .
menstruation mĕn-stroo-Ā-shun	**8-71** A/men/o/rrhea is the *absence or abnormal stoppage of menstruation.* Men/o/rrhea is a *flow of the menses, or* _____ .
-pause	**8-72** Identify the element in men/o/pause that means *cessation.* _____
after, before	**8-73** The terms post/men/o/paus/al and pre/men/o/paus/al refer to bleeding occurring at times other than during the normal menstrual flow. *Post-* means _____ , or *behind. Pre* means _____ , or *in front of.*

Breasts

mamm/o, mast/o	**8-74** The breasts, also called mamm/ary glands, are present in both sexes but they normally function only in females. The biological role of the mammary glands is to secrete milk for the nourishment of the infant, a process called lactation. The CFs that refer to the breast are _____ / _____ and _____ / _____ .
excision *or* **removal** ĕk-SĬ-zhŭn	**8-75** Mast/ectomy is the _____ of a breast.

mast/o/dynia, mast/algia măst-ō-DĬN-ē-ă, măst- ĂL-jē-ă	**8–76** Use *mast/o* to form a word that means *pain in the breast*. _____ / _____ / _____ *or* _____ / _____
mast/ectomy măs-TĔK-tō-mē	**8–77** To prevent the spread of cancer (CA), a malignant breast tumor may be treated with a partial or complete excision. When a breast has to be removed, the patient undergoes a _____ / _____ .
	8–78 During puberty, the female's breasts develop as a result of periodic stimulation of the ovarian hormones estrogen and progesterone. Estrogen is responsible for the development of (1) **adipose tissue,** which enlarges the size of the breasts until they reach full maturity around age 16. Breast size is primarily determined by the amount of fat around the (2) **glandular tissue,** but is not a factor in the ability to produce and secrete milk. Label the adipose and glandular tissues in Figure 8–7.
	8–79 During pregnancy, high levels of estrogen and progesterone prepare the mammary glands for milk production. Each breast has approximately 20 lobes. Each (3) **lobe** is drained by a (4) **lactiferous duct** that opens on the tip of the raised (5) **nipple.** Circling the nipple is a border of slightly darker skin called the (6) **areola.** Label the structures of the mammary glands in Figure 8–7.
lactation lăk-TĀ-shŭn	**8–80** During pregnancy, the breasts enlarge and remain so until lactation ceases. At menopause, breast tissue begins to atrophy. The ability of mammary glands to secrete milk for the nourishment of the infant is a process called _____ .
-graphy **mamm/o**	**8–81** Mamm/o/graphy, an x-ray examination of the breast, is used in the Dx of CA. Determine the elements in this frame that mean *process of recording:* _____ *breast:* _____ / _____
mamm/o/plasty MĂM-ō-plăs-tē	**8–82** Use mamm/o to construct a word that means *surgical reconstruction or repair of a breast*. _____ / _____ / _____
mast/o/plasty MĂS-tō-plăs-tē **mast/o/pexy** MĂS-to-pĕk-sē	**8–83** Correction of pendulous breasts can be performed by reconstructive cosmetic surgery to lift the breasts. Use mast/o to develop surgical terms that mean *surgical repair of the breast:* _____ / _____ / _____ *fixation of the breast:* _____ / _____ / _____

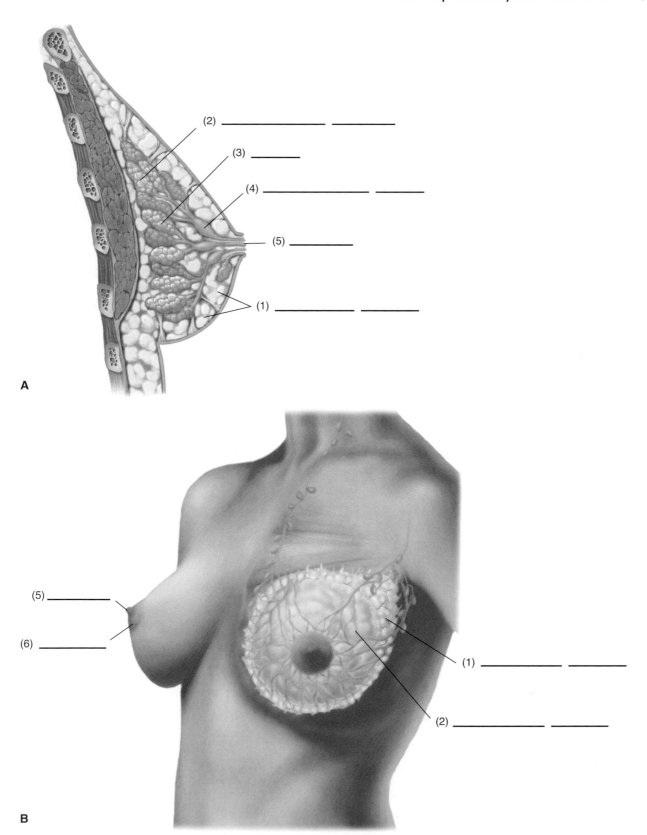

A

B

Figure 8-7 Structure of mammary glands. (**A**) Saggital section of the breast. (**B**) Anterior view showing lymph nodes and structures of the breast.

8–84   When a small primary tumor is localized, the surgeon performs a lumpectomy. In these instances, the tumor and some of the normal tissue surrounding it are excised. All tissue removed from the breast is biopsied to determine if CA cells are present in the normal tissue surrounding the tumor. (See Fig. 8–8.)

Competency Verification: Check your labeling of Figure 8–7 in Appendix B: Answer Key, page 587.

---

before, after	**8–85** The term nat/al means *pertaining to birth.* Pre/nat/al refers to the time period _____ birth; post/nat/al refers to the time period _____ birth.
neo- **nat/o** **-logy**	**8–86** Identify elements in neo/nat/o/logy that mean *new:* _____ *birth:* _____ / _____ *study of:* _____
neo/nat/o/logist nē-ō-nā-TŎL-ō-jĭst	**8–87** Neo/nat/o/logy is the *study and treatment of the neonate (newborn infant).* A physician who specializes in the care and treatment of the neonate is called a _____ / _____ / _____ / _____.
woman	**8–88** Gravida is used to describe a pregnant woman, as is the suffix *-gravida.* A primi/gravida is a woman pregnant for the first time; a multi/gravida is a woman who has been pregnant more than once. Whenever you see gravida in a word, you will know it denotes a pregnant _____.

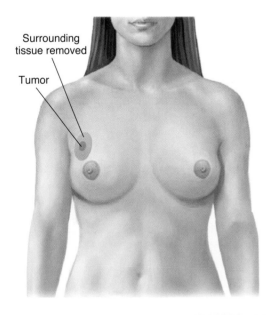

Surrounding
tissue removed

Tumor

Figure 8-8 Lumpectomy, with primary tumor in red and the surrounding tissue removed during lumpectomy highlighted in pink.

Boldface indicates a word root or combining form. Blue indicates a suffix. Pink indicates a prefix.

Female Reproductive System • CHAPTER 8

fourth **second**	**8-89** Gravida may also be followed by numbers to denote the number of pregnancies, as in gravida 1, gravida 2, gravida 3, and gravida 4 (or gravida I, II, III, and IV). Gravida 4 is a woman in her _____ pregnancy. Gravida 2 is a woman in her _____ pregnancy.
gravida 3 GRĂV-ĭ-dă **gravida 5** GRĂV-ĭ-dă	**8-90** A woman in her third pregnancy is a _____ _____. A woman in her fifth pregnancy is a _____ _____.
two, five	**8-91** The word para refers to a woman who has given birth to an infant, regardless of whether or not the offspring was alive at birth. It also may be followed by numbers to indicate the number of deliveries, as in para 1, 2, 3, or 4 (or I, II, III, or IV). Para 2 means _____ deliveries; para 5 means _____ deliveries.
para 6 PĂR-ă	**8-92** A woman who has delivered three infants would be described as para 3. A woman who has delivered six infants would be described as _____ _____.
PID	**8-93** Pelvic inflammatory disease (PID) is a collective term for inflammation of the uterus, fallopian tubes, ovaries, and adjacent pelvic structures. This disease is usually caused by bacterial infection. The abbreviation for pelvic inflammatory disease is _____.
path/o/gen PĂTH-ō-jĕn	**8-94** In the female reproductive system, an infection may be confined to a single organ or it may involve all of the internal female reproductive organs. Path/o/gens generally enter through the vagina during coitus, induced abortion, childbirth, or the postpartum period. As an ascending infection, pathogens spread from the vagina and cervix to the upper structures of the female reproductive tract. A term in this frame that means *forming, producing, or origin of disease* is _____ / _____ / _____.
sexually transmitted infection **pelvic inflammatory disease**	**8-95** The two most common causes of PID are gonorrhea and chlamydia, both of which are sexually transmitted infections (STIs). Unless treated promptly, PID may result in sterility, because the fallopian tubes and ovaries become scarred. Widespread infection of reproductive structures may also lead to fatal septicemia. The abbreviation STI refers to _____ _____ _____. The abbreviation PID refers to _____ _____ _____.

pelvic inflammatory disease	**8-96** Because regions of the fallopian tubes have an internal diameter as small as the width of a human hair, the scarring and closure of the tubes caused by PID is one of the major causes of female sterility (infertility). Chlamydia and gonorrhea are two main causes of PID. The abbreviation PID means _____ _____ _____ .
oophor/itis ō-ŏf-ō-RĪ-tĭs **oophor/oma** ō-ŏf-ō-RŌ-mă	**8-97** A pelvic infection that involves the ovaries is known as oophor/itis. Use *oophor/o* to build a term that means *inflammation of the ovaries:* _____ / _____ *tumor of the ovaries:* _____ / _____
salping/ectomy săl-pĭn-JĔK-tō-mē	**8-98** The CF *salping/o* means *tube (usually fallopian or eustachian [auditory] tubes)*. A tumor or cyst in a fallopian tube may necessitate the removal of a fallopian tube. Build a surgical term that means excision of a fallopian tube. _____ / _____
uterus Ū-tĕr-ŭs	**8-99** A hyster/o/tome is an instrument for incising the _____ .
incision, uterus	**8-100** Abdominal incision of the uterus (hyster/o/tomy) is performed to remove the fetus during a cesarean section (CS), also called C-section. Hyster/o/tomy is an _____ into the _____ .
CS, C-section	**8-101** Abbreviations for cesarean section are _____ and _____ .

Boldface indicates a word root or combining form. Blue indicates a suffix. Pink indicates a prefix.

SECTION REVIEW 8-3

Using the following table, write the CF, suffix, or prefix that matches its definition in the space provided to the left of the definition. There may be more than one word element that matches a definition.

Combining Forms		Suffixes		Prefixes
cervic/o	men/o	-algia	-ous	dys-
colp/o	salping/o	-ary	-pathy	post-
episi/o	vagin/o	-dynia	-rrhea	pre-
gynec/o	vulv/o	-ectomy	-scope	
mamm/o		-itis	-scopy	
mast/o		-logist	-tome	

1. _____ after, behind

2. _____ woman, female

3. _____ before, in front of

4. _____ breast

5. _____ disease

6. _____ excision, removal

7. _____ discharge, flow

8. _____ inflammation

9. _____ instrument to cut

10. _____ instrument for examining

11. _____ visual examination

12. _____ menses, menstruation

13. _____ neck; cervix uteri (neck of uterus)

14. _____ pain

15. _____ pertaining to

16. _____ specialist in study of

17. _____ tube (usually fallopian or eustachian [auditory] tubes)

18. _____ vagina

19. _____ vulva

20. _____ bad; painful; difficult

Competency Verification: Check your answers in Appendix B: Answer Key, page 587. If you are not satisfied with your level of comprehension, go back to Frame 8–51 and rework the frames.

Correct Answers _____ × 5 = _____ % Score

MALE REPRODUCTIVE SYSTEM

The primary sex organs of the male are called **gonads**, specifically the **testes** (singular, **testis**). Gonads produce gametes (sperm) and secrete sex hormones. The remaining accessory reproductive organs are the structures that are essential in caring for and transporting sperm. All of these organs and structures are designed to accomplish the male's reproductive role of producing and delivering sperm to the female reproductive tract, where fertilization can occur.

These structures can be divided into three categories:

- **Sperm-transporting ducts**, which include the epididymis, vas deferens (or ductus deferens), ejaculatory duct, and urethra
- **Accessory glands**, which include the seminal vesicles, prostate gland, and bulbourethral glands
- **Copulatory organ**, called the **penis**, which contains erectile tissue. (See Fig. 8–9.)

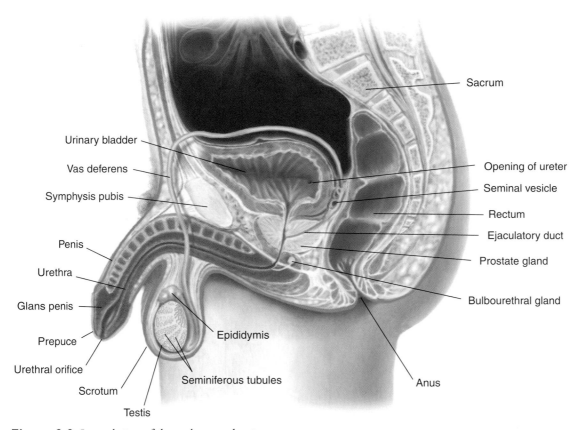

Figure 8-9 Lateral view of the male reproductive system.

WORD ELEMENTS

This section introduces combining forms related to the male reproductive system. Included are key suffixes; prefixes are defined in the right-hand column as needed. Review the following table and pronounce each word in the word analysis column aloud before you begin to work the frames.

Word Element	Meaning	Word Analysis
Combining Forms		
andr/o	male	**andr/o/gen** (ĂN-drō-jĕn): forming or producing male (hormones) *-gen:* forming, producing, origin *Such hormones as testosterone and androsterone produce or stimulate the development of male characteristics (masculinization).*

Word Element	Meaning	Word Analysis
balan/o	glans penis	**balan**/itis (băl-ă-NĪ-tĭs): inflammation of the glans penis *-itis:* inflammation
gonad/o	gonads, sex glands	**gonad**/o/tropin (gŏn-ă-dō-TRŌ-pĭn): hormone that stimulates the gonads *-tropin:* stimulate *Gonadotropin is a hormone that stimulates the function of the testes and ovaries (gonads).*

orch/o	testis (plural,
	testes)
		crypt/**orch**/ism (krĭpt-OR-kĭzm): condition of undescended testicles; also called *cryptorchidism*
		    crypt: hidden
		    -ism: condition
		
		In cryptorchism, the testicles are retained in the abdomen or inguinal canal. If spontaneous descent does not occur by age 1, hormone therapy or surgery may be performed.

orchi/o		**orchi**/o/pexy (OR-kē-ō-pĕk-sē): surgical fixation of a testis *-pexy:* fixation (of an organ) *An orchiopexy is performed to mobilize an undescended testis, bring it into the scrotum, and attach it so that it will not retract.*
orchid/o		**orchid**/ectomy (or-kĭ-DĔK-tō-mē): excision of one or both testes *-ectomy:* excision, removal
test/o		**test**/algia (tĕs-TĂL-jē-ă): pain in the testes *-algia:* pain
prostat/o	prostate gland	**prostat**/itis (prŏs-tă-TĪ-tĭs): inflammation of the prostate gland, usually as a result of infection *-itis:* inflammation
spermat/o	spermatozoa, sperm cells	**spermat**/o/cyte (spĕr-MĂT-ō-sīt): sperm cell *cyte:* cell
sperm/i*		**sperm**/i/cide (SPĔR-mĭ-sīd): agent that kills spermatozoa; also called *spermatocide* *-cide:* killing

sperm/o		a/**sperm**/ia (ă-SPĔR-mē-ă): without semen
		    a-: without, not
		    -ia: condition
		
		In aspermia, semen fail to form or ejaculate.

varic/o	dilated vein	**varic**/o/cele (VĂR-ĭ-kō-sēl): dilated or enlarged vein of the spermatic cord *-cele:* hernia; swelling
vas/o	vessel; vas deferens; duct	**vas**/ectomy (văs-ĔK-tō-mē): removal of all or part of the vas deferens *-ectomy:* excision, removal

*Using the combining vowel *i* instead of *o* is an exception to the rule.

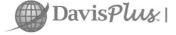

Visit the *Medical Terminology Simplified* online resource center at Davis*Plus* for an audio exercise of the terms in this table. It will help you master pronunciations and meanings of medical terms.

SECTION REVIEW 8-4

For the following medical terms, first write the suffix and its meaning. Then translate the meaning of the remaining elements starting with the first part of the word. The first word is completed for you.

Term	Meaning
1. vas/ectomy	-ectomy: excision, removal; vessel, vas deferens, duct
2. balan/itis	
3. spermat/i/cide	
4. gonad/o/tropin	
5. orchi/o/pexy	
6. a/sperm/ia	
7. vesicul/itis	
8. orchid/ectomy	
9. andr/o/gen	
10. crypt/orch/ism	

Competency Verification: Check your answers in Appendix B: Answer Key, page 588. If you are not satisfied with your level of comprehension, review the word elements tables and retake the review.

Correct Answers _____ × 10 = _____ % Score

8-102   The (1) **testes** (singular, testis), also called testicles (singular, testicle), are paired oval glands that descend into the (2) **scrotum**. At the onset of puberty, the testes produce the hormone testosterone. Label Figure 8–10 as you learn about the organs of reproduction.

---

disease, testes *or* testicles
TĔS-tēz, TĔS-tĭ-klz

8-103   The CF *test/o* refers to the testis. Test/o/pathy is a

_____ of the _____ (plural).

---

testis
TĔS-tĭs

testicle
TĔS-tĭ-kl

8-104   The male hormone testosterone stimulates and promotes the growth of secondary sex characteristics in the male. This hormone is produced by the testes (plural).

The singular form of testes is _____.

The singular form of testicles is _____.

Boldface indicates a word root or combining form. Blue indicates a suffix. Pink indicates a prefix.

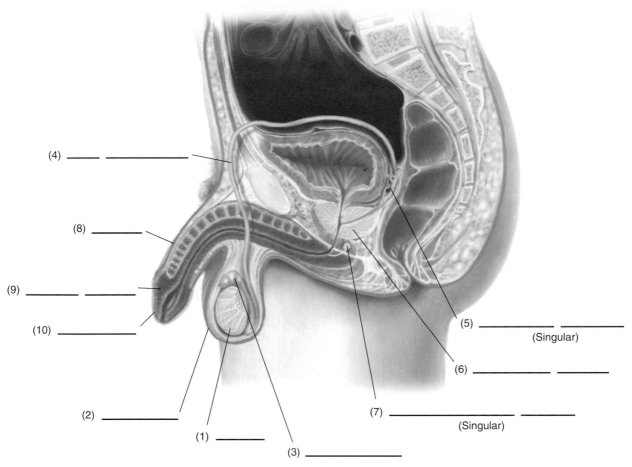

Figure 8-10 Lateral view of the male reproductive system.

---

test/itis
tĕs-TĪ-tĭs

test/ectomy
tĕs-TĔK-tō-mē

test/o/pathy
tĕs-TŎP-ă-thē

8–105   Use *test/o* to form medical words that mean

inflammation of the testis: _____ / _____

excision of the testis: _____ / _____

disease of the testis: _____ / _____ / _____

---

spermatozoa
spĕr-măt-ō-ZŌ-ă

8–106   The CF *spermat/o* means *spermatozoa, sperm cells,* which are the male sex cell produced by the testes.

Spermat/o/genesis is the *beginning or formation of sperm cells, or*

_____.

stone, calculus KĂL-kū-lŭs	**8-107** A spermat/o/lith is a _____, or _____, in the spermatic duct.
spermat/o/genesis spĕr-măt-ō-JĔN-ĕ-sĭs	**8-108** The suffix *-genesis* is used in words to mean *forming, producing, origin.* Construct a word that means *producing or forming sperm.* _____ / _____ / _____
spermat/o/cyte spĕr-MĂT-ō-sīt **spermat/oid** SPĔR-mă-toyd	**8-109** Use *spermat/o* to form a word that means *spermatozoa, or sperm cell:* _____ / _____ / _____ *resembling spermatozoa, or sperm:* _____ / _____
spermat/uria spĕr-mă-TŪ-rē-ă	**8-110** Spermat/uria is a condition in which there is sperm in the urine. A discharge of semen in urine is also called _____ / _____.
without	**8-111** A/spermat/ism is a condition in which a male lacks sperm. A/spermat/ism literally means _____ sperm.
olig/o/sperm/ia ŏl-ĭ-gō-SPĔR-mē-ă	**8-112** Olig/o/sperm/ia, also known as a low sperm count, is a condition in which there are fewer sperm cells in the ejaculate than normal. It is one of the main causes of male infertility. Use *olig/o* to build a word that means *condition of scanty sperm.* _____ / _____ / _____
olig/o/sperm/ia ŏl-ĭ-gō-SPĔR-mē-ă	**8-113** When the physician detects a low sperm count, the Dx is noted in the medical record as _____ / _____ / _____ / _____.
	8-114 A comma-shaped organ, the (3) **epididymis**, stores and propels sperm toward the urethra during ejaculation. The (4) **vas deferens**, also called ductus deferens, is a duct that transports sperm from the testes to the urethra. The sperm is excreted in the semen, or seminal fluid. Semen is a mixture of secretions from the (5) **seminal vesicles**, (6) **prostate gland**, and (7) **bulbourethral glands**, also known as Cowper glands. Label Figure 8–10 as you continue to learn about the male reproductive organs.
muc/o	**8-115** Ducts of bulbourethral (Cowper) glands open into the urethra and secrete thick mucus that acts as a lubricant during sexual stimulation. Write the CF that refers to mucus. _____ / _____

Boldface indicates a word root or combining form. Blue indicates a suffix. Pink indicates a prefix.

adjective	**8-116** Muc/us is a noun. Muc/ous is a(n) (noun, adjective) _____ .
muc/oid MŪ-koyd	**8-117** Use *-oid* to construct a medical term that means *resembling mucus*. _____ / _____
orchi/o/plasty OR-kē-ō-plăs-tē **orchi/o/rrhaphy** or-kē-OR-ă-fē **orchi/o/pexy** or-kē-ō-PĔK-sē	**8-118** In addition to *test/o,* two other CFs that refer to the testes are *orchi/o* and *orchid/o.* Use *orchi/o* to develop medical words that mean *surgical repair of the testicle:* _____ / _____ / _____ *suture of a testicle:* _____ / _____ / _____ *fixation of a testicle:* _____ / _____ / _____
enlargement	**8-119** The CF *prostat/o* means *prostate gland.* The prostate gland secretes a thick fluid that, as part of the semen, helps the sperm to move spontaneously. Prostat/o/megaly is a(n) _____ of the prostate gland.
prostat/o/megaly prŏs-tă-tō-MĔG-ă-lē	**8-120** Benign prostatic hyperplasia (BPH), also called benign prostatic hypertor-phy, is a gradual enlargement of the prostate gland that normally occurs as a man ages. It is a common disorder in men older than age 60. The enlarged prostate com-presses the urethra and causes the bladder to retain urine. Symptoms include an in-ability to empty the bladder completely and a weak urine stream. (See Fig. 8–11.) Construct a medical word that means *enlargement of the prostate gland.* _____ / _____ / _____
growth, nourishment	**8-121** The abbreviation BPH refers to benign prostat/ic hyper/plasia, or benign prostat/ic hyper/trophy. The suffix *-plasia* means *formation,* _____ . The suffix *-trophy* means *development,* _____ .
trans/urethr/al trăns-ū-RĒ-thrăl	**8-122** Common symptoms of BPH include hesitancy and dribbling on urination and a weak urine stream. Treatment includes drugs to decrease prostate size or a trans/urethr/al resection of the prostate (TURP), in which the obstructing tissue is removed. TURP makes it possible to perform surgery on certain organs that lie near the urethra without having an abdominal incision. (See Fig. 8–12.) Because this surgery is performed by passing a resect/o/scope through the urethra, it is called _____ / _____ / _____ *resection of the prostate.*

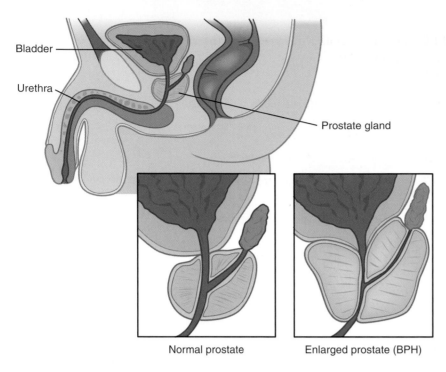

Figure 8-11 Benign prostatic hyperplasia.

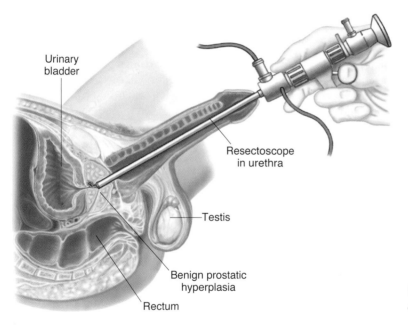

Figure 8-12 Transurethral resection of the prostate.

resect/o/scope
rē-SĔK-tō-skōp

8-123 The resect/o/scope (special type of endoscope) contains a light, valves for controlling irrigating fluid, and an electrical loop that cuts tissue and seals blood vessels. The wire loop is used to remove obstructing tissue piece-by-piece through the resectoscope. The chips of tissue are irrigated into the bladder and then flushed out at the end of the surgical procedure.

The endo/scop/ic instrument used by the urologist to perform TURP is called a

_____ / _____ / _____.

PSA	**8-124** The prostate-specific antigen (PSA) test is a blood test that screens for prostate abnormalities. Elevated levels of PSA are associated with prostate enlargement and cancer. The abbreviation for *prostate-specific antigen* is _____ .
prostat/itis prŏs-tă-TĪ-tĭs **prostat/o/cyst/itis** prŏs-tă-tō-sĭs-TĪ-tĭs	**8-125** Build medical words that mean *inflammation of the prostate gland:* _____ / _____ *inflammation of the prostate gland and bladder:* _____ / _____ / _____ / _____
prostate, bladder PRŎS-tāt	**8-126** Prostat/o/cyst/o/tomy is an incision of the _____ and _____ .
	8-127 The (8) **penis** is the male sex organ that transports the sperm into the female vagina. A slightly enlarged region at the tip of the penis is the (9) **glans penis.** The tip of the penis is covered by a fold of skin called the (10) **foreskin**, or prepuce. Label Figure 8–10 as you learn the names of organs of reproduction.
water **hernia, swelling** HĔR-nē-ă	**8-128** Hydr/o/cele is a collection of fluid in a saclike cavity, specifically the testis. Analyze hydr/o/cele by defining the elements. *hydr/o:* _____ *-cele:* _____ , _____

Competency Verification: Check your labeling of Figure 8–10 in Appendix B: Answer Key, page 588.

prostat/ectomy prŏs-tă-TĔK-tō-mē	**8-129** Prostate CA is the third leading cause of cancer deaths in men (after lung and colon CA). Surgery may be performed to remove the prostate and adjacent affected tissues. Develop a surgical term that means *excision of the prostate gland.* _____ / _____
cancer	**8-130** Currently, PSA is considered the most sensitive tumor marker for prostate _____ .
threatening	**8-131** Tumors may be benign or malignant. Benign tumors are not malignant (cancerous) and not life-threatening. A malignant tumor, however, is cancerous and life- _____ .

benign bē-NĬN	**8–132** Tumors are also called neo/plasms (new growths or formations). Similar to tumors, neo/plasms can be malignant or _____.
cancer/ous KĂN-sĕr-ŭs	**8–133** A benign tumor is non/cancer/ous. A malignant tumor is _____ / _____.
neo/plasm NĒ-ō-plăzm	**8–134** A new growth in any body system or organ is called a _____ / _____.
prostat/itis prŏs-tă-TĬ-tĭs	**8–135** Prostat/itis, an acute or chronic inflammation of the prostate gland, is usually the result of infection. The patient usually complains of burning, urinary frequency, and urgency. Build a symptomatic term that means _inflammation of the prostate gland._ _____ / _____
growth	**8–136** The suffixes _-plasm_ and _-plasia_ refer to _formation or_ _____.
dys- **-plasia**	**8–137** Dys/plasia is an abnormal development of tissue. Identify the element in dys/plasia that means _bad, painful, or difficult:_ _____ _formation, growth:_ _____
without, not **formation, growth**	**8–138** A/plasia means _without formation,_ and is a condition that is due to failure of an organ to develop or form normally. Analyze a/plasia by defining the elements. _a-:_ _____, _____ _-plasia:_ _____, _____
hyper- **-plasia**	**8–139** Hyper/plasia is an excessive increase in the number of cells in a tissue or organ, as shown in Figure 8–11. Determine the element in hyper/plasia that means _excessive:_ _____ _formation or growth:_ _____

Boldface indicates a word root or combining form. Blue indicates a suffix. Pink indicates a prefix.

vas/o	**8–140** Vas/ectomy, a sterilization procedure, involves bi/later/al cutting and tying of the vas deferens to prevent the passage of sperm. This sterilization procedure is most commonly performed at an outpatient surgery center using local an/esthesia. (See Fig. 8–13.) From the term vas/ectomy, construct the combining form that means vessel, vas deferens, or duct. _____ / _____
an/esthesia ăn-ĕs-THĒ-zē-ă **bi/later/al** bī-LĂT-ĕr-ăl **vas/ectomy** văs-ĔK-tō-mē	**8–141** Identify the terms in Frame 8–140 that mean *without feeling:* _____ / _____ *pertaining to two sides:* _____ / _____ / _____ *excision of the vas deferens:* _____ / _____
prostat/itis prŏs-tă-TĪ-tĭs	**8–142** Vas/ectomy is also performed routinely before removal of the prostate gland to prevent inflammation of the testes and epididymides. Potency is not affected. (See Fig. 8–13.) Inflammation of the prostate gland is called _____ / _____.

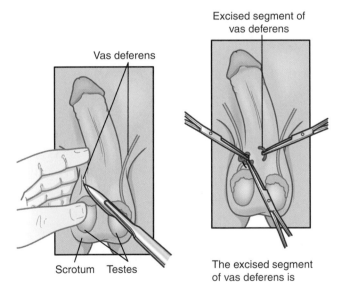
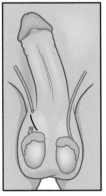

Excised segment of vas deferens

Vas deferens

Scrotum   Testes

An incision of vas deferens on each side.

The excised segment of vas deferens is withdrawn and ends are tied (ligation).

Vas deferens is returned and scrotum incision is closed with sutures. This procedure is performed for both the right and left vas deferens.

Figure 8-13 Vasectomy.

vas/ectomy reversal
văs-ĔK-tō-mē

8-143   Vas/o/vas/o/stomy, also called vas/ectomy reversal, is a surgical procedure in which the function of the vas deferens on each side of the testes is restored, having been cut and ligated in a preceding vasectomy.

Another term for vas/o/vas/o/stomy is

_____ / _____ _____.

patency
PĀ-tĕn-sē

vas/o/vas/o/stomy
văs-ō-vă-SŎS-tō-mē

8-144   Vas/o/vas/o/stomy may be performed if a man wants to regain his fertility. In most cases, patency (opening up) of the canals is achieved, but fertility is not always regained.

The term in this frame that refers to *the state of being open* is

_____.

The surgical term in this frame that is synonymous with vas/ectomy reversal is

_____ / _____ / _____ / _____ / _____.

SECTION REVIEW 8 - 5

Using the following table, write the CF, suffix, or prefix that matches its definition in the space provided to the left of the definition. There may be more than one word element that matches a definition.

Combining Forms		Suffixes		Prefixes
carcin/o	prostat/o	-cele	-pexy	dys-
cyst/o	spermat/o	-cyte	-rrhaphy	hyper-
muc/o	sperm/o	-genesis	-tome	neo-
olig/o	test/o	-itis		
orchid/o	vas/o	-megaly		
orchi/o		-pathy		

1. _____ suture

2. _____ bad; painful; difficult

3. _____ bladder

4. _____ cancer

5. _____ cell

6. _____ disease

7. _____ enlargement

8. _____ hernia; swelling

9. _____ inflammation

10. _____ instrument to cut

11. _____ vessel; vas deferens; duct

12. _____ mucus

13. _____ new

14. _____ forming, producing, origin

15. _____ prostate gland

16. _____ testes

17. _____ scanty

18. _____ spermatozoa, sperm cells

19. _____ fixation (of an organ)

20. _____ excessive, above normal

Competency Verification: Check your answers in Appendix B: Answer Key, page 588. If you are not satisfied with your level of comprehension, go back to Frame 8–102 and rework the frames.

Correct Answers _____ × 5 = _____ % Score

ABBREVIATIONS

This section introduces reproductive system–related abbreviations and their meanings. Included are abbreviations contained in the medical record activities that follow.

Abbreviation	Meaning	Abbreviation	Meaning
Female Reproductive System			
CS, C-section	cesarean section	OCP	oral contraceptive pill
D&C	dilation and curettage	Pap	Papanicolaou (test)
Dx	diagnosis	para 1, 2, 3	unipara, bipara, tripara (number of viable births)
G	gravida (pregnant)	PID	pelvic inflammatory disease
GYN	gynecology	PSA	prostate-specific antigen
HRT	hormone replacement therapy	TAH	total abdominal hysterectomy
IVF	in vitro fertilization	TRAM	transverse rectus abdominis muscle
LMP	last menstrual period	TSS	toxic shock syndrome
OB	obstetrics	TVH	total vaginal hysterectomy
OB-GYN	obstetrics and gynecology		
Male Reproductive System			
BPH	benign prostatic hyperplasia, benign prostatic hypertrophy	TURP	transurethral resection of the prostate
DRE	digital rectal examination	TRUS	transrectal ultrasonography
Sexually Transmitted Infections			
GC	gonorrhea	STI	sexually transmitted infection
HPV	human papillomavirus	VD	venereal disease

ADDITIONAL MEDICAL TERMS

The following are additional terms related to the female and male reproductive systems. Recognizing and learning these terms will help you understand the connection between a pathological condition, its diagnosis, and the rationale behind the method of treatment selected for a particular disorder.

Diseases and Conditions

Female Reproductive System

candidiasis kăn-dĭ-DĪ-ă-sĭs	Vaginal fungal infection caused by *Candida albicans* and characterized by a curdy, or cheeselike, discharge and extreme itching

ectopic pregnancy ĕk-TŎP-ik	Implantation of the fertilized ovum outside of the uterine cavity, such as a fallopian tube, an ovary, the abdomen, or the cervix uteri (See Fig. 8–14.) *Ectopic pregnancy occurs in approximately 1% of pregnancies, most commonly in the oviducts (tubal pregnancy). Some types of ectopic pregnancies include ovarian, interstitial, and isthmic.*

endometriosis
ĕn-dō-mē-trē-Ō-sĭs
  endo: in, within
  metri: uterus (womb)
  -osis: abnormal condi-
       tion; increase
       (used primarily
       with blood cells)
	Presence of endometrial tissue outside the uterine cavity, such as the pelvis or abdomen (See Fig. 8–15.)

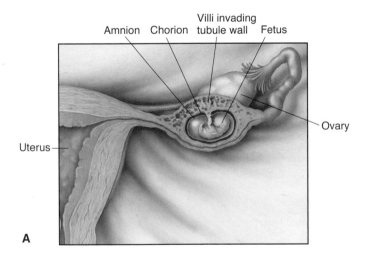

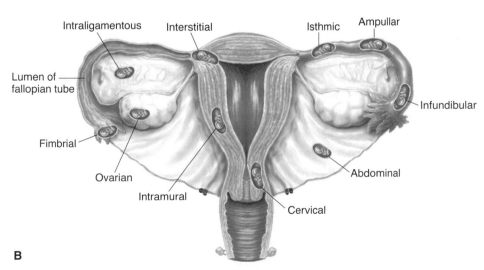

Figure 8-14 (A) Tubal pregnancy. (B) Other sites of ectopic pregnancy.

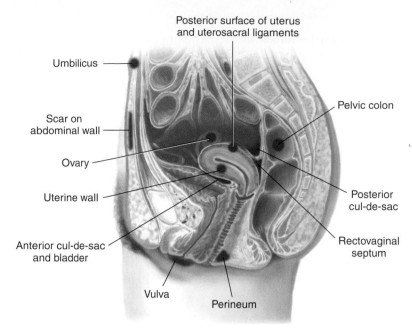

Posterior surface of uterus
and uterosacral ligaments

Umbilicus

Pelvic colon

Scar on
abdominal wall

Ovary

Uterine wall

Posterior
cul-de-sac

Anterior cul-de-sac
and bladder

Rectovaginal
septum

Vulva

Perineum

Figure 8-15 Endometriosis.

fibroid
FĪ-broyd
   fibr: fiber, fibrous
       tissue
   -oids: resembling
	Benign neoplasm in the uterus that is composed largely of fibrous tissue; also called *leiomyoma*
	
	Uterine fibroids are the most common tumors in women. If fibroids grow too large and cause such symptoms as pelvic pain or menorrhagia, hysterectomy may be indicated.

gestational hypertension
jĕs-TĀ-shŭn-ăl hī-pĕr-
TĔN-shŭn
 	
   preeclampsia
   prē-ē-KLĂMP-sē-ă
 	
   eclampsia
   ē-KLĂMP-sē-ă
	Potentially life-threatening disorder that usually develops after the 20th week of pregnancy and is characterized by edema and proteinuria
	
	Gestational hypertension may occur in nonconvulsive or convulsive forms.
	
	Nonconvulsive form of gestational hypertension that, if left untreated, may progress to eclampsia
	
	Treatment includes bedrest and blood pressure monitoring.
	
	Convulsive form of gestational hypertension that is a medical emergency and life-threatening to the mother and/or baby
	
	Treatment includes bedrest, blood pressure monitoring, and antiseizure drugs.

leukorrhea
loo-kō-RĒ-ă
   leuk/o: white
   -rrhea: discharge, flow
	White discharge from the vagina
	
	A greater than usual amount of leukorrhea is normal in pregnancy, and a decrease is to be expected after delivery, during lactation, and after menopause. Leukorrhea is the most common reason women seek gynecological care.

oligomenorrhea
ŏl-ĭ-gō-měn-ō-RĒ-ă
  olig/o: scanty
  men/o: menses,
        menstruation
  -rrhea: discharge, flow
	Scanty or infrequent menstrual flow

sterility stěr-ĬL-ĭ-tē	Inability of a woman to become pregnant or for a man to impregnate a woman

toxic shock syndrome (TSS)
TŎK-sĭk shŏk SĬN-drōm
  tox: poison
  -ic: pertaining to
	Rare and sometimes fatal *Staphylococcus* infection that generally occurs in menstruating women, most of whom use vaginal tampons for menstrual protection
	
	In TSS, the normally harmless vaginal bacterium Staphylococcus aureus multiplies in the old blood in the tampon and releases toxins. The tampon itself creates small tears in the vaginal wall that allow the toxins to enter the bloodstream.

Male Reproductive System

anorchism
ăn-ŎR-kĭzm
  an: without, not
  orch: testis (plural,
        testes)
  -ism: condition
	Congenital absence of one or both testes; also called *anorchidism* or *anorchia*

balanitis
băl-ă-NĪ-tĭs
  balan: glans penis
  -itis: inflammation
	Inflammation of the skin covering the glans penis
	
	Balanitis is caused by irritation and invasion of microorganisms. It is commonly associated with inadequate hygiene of the prepuce and phimosis.

cryptorchism
krĭpt-OR-kĭ-zm
  crypt: hidden
  orch: testis (plural,
        testes)
  -ism: condition
	Failure of one or both testicles to descend into the scrotum; also called *cryptorchidism*
	
	Cryptorchism is associated with a high risk of sterility, causing a low sperm count and male infertility. If testes do not descend on their own at an early age, orchiopexy is performed to bring the testicles into the scrotum.

epispadias
ĕp-ĭ-SPĀ-dē-ăs
    epi-: above, upon
  -spadias: slit, fissure
	Congenital defect in which the urethra opens on the upper side of the penis near the glans penis instead of the tip

hypospadias
hī-pō-SPĀ-dē-ăs
    hypo: under, below,
        deficient
  -spadias: slit, fissure
	Congenital defect in which the male urethra opens on the undersurface of the penis instead of the tip

impotence ĬM-pŏ-tĕns	Inability of a man to achieve or maintain a penile erection; commonly called *erectile dysfunction*

phimosis
fĭ-MŌ-sĭs
  phim: muzzle
    -osis: abnormal condi-
       tion; increase
       (used primarily
       with blood cells)
	Stenosis or narrowness of the preputial orifice so that the foreskin cannot be pushed back over the glans penis

sexually transmitted infections (STIs)	Any disease that may be acquired as a result of sexual intercourse or other intimate contact with an infected individual and affects the male and female reproductive systems.
chlamydia klă-MĬD-ē-ă	Sexually transmitted bacterial infection that causes cervicitis in women and urethritis and epididymitis in men *Chlamydial infection is now highly prevalent and is among the most potentially damaging of all STIs. Antibiotics are prescribed to cure the infection. If left untreated, chlamydia can cause pelvic inflammatory disease (PID) and infertility in women.*

gonorrhea
gŏn-ō-RĒ-ă
  gon/o: seed (ovum or
      spermatozoon)
  -rrhea: discharge,
      flow
	Sexually transmitted bacterial infection of the mucous membrane of the genital tract in men and women
	
	Gonorrheal infection results from anal, vaginal, or oral sex with an infected partner. It can also be passed on from an infected mother to her infant during the birth process (as the baby passes through the vaginal canal). Gonorrhea and chlamydia infections commonly occur together. Both partners are treated for these infections with antibiotics.

herpes genitalis HĔR-pēz jĕn-ĭ-TĂL-ĭs	Highly contagious viral infection of the male and female genitalia that is transmitted by direct contact with infected body secretions (usually through sexual intercourse) and differs from other STIs in that it can recur spontaneously once the virus has been acquired; also called *venereal herpes* *Herpes genitalis is most commonly caused by herpes simplex virus (HSV) type 2. Treatment is symptomatic, which means that medications are given to reduce the symptoms of swelling and pain. There is no cure for genital herpes. A particularly life-threatening form of the disease can occur in infants infected by the virus during vaginal birth.*
human papillomavirus (HPV)	Infection of the genital areas of men and women, including the penis, vulva, anus, and the rectal, cervical, and vaginal linings *There are over 40 types of HPV. One type, genital warts, causes cancer of the cervix, as well as cancer in men. A vaccine is available for young girls and women that protects against four types of HPV.*
syphilis SĬF-ĭ-lĭs	Infectious, chronic STI characterized initially by a skin lesions (chancres), typically on the genitals, rectum, or mouth *Syphilis may exist without symptoms for years and cause long-term complications, including death, if not treated. It can also be transmitted from mother to fetus, causing multiple, severe health problems for the baby. Penicillin, intramuscularly or IV, is the antibiotic of choice for the treatment of all stages of syphilis.*
trichomoniasis trĭk-ō-mō-NĪ-ă-sĭs	Infection of the vagina or male genital tract that commonly causes vaginitis, urethritis, and cystitis *Trichomoniasis is the most common sexually transmitted infection that is asymptomatic. Treatment consists of a single oral dose of a combined antibacterial and antiprotozoal medication.*

Diagnostic Procedures

Female Reproductive System

amniocentesis ăm-nē-ō-sĕn-TĒ-sĭs *amni/o:* amnion (amniotic sac) *-centesis:* surgical puncture	Obstetric procedure that involves surgical puncture of the amniotic sac under ultrasound guidance to remove amniotic fluid *In amniocentesis, cells of the fetus found in the fluid are cultured and studied to detect genetic abnormalities and maternal–fetal blood incompatibility. (See Fig. 8–16.)*
colposcopy kŏl-PŎS-kō-pē *colp/o:* vagina *-scopy:* visual examination	Examination of the vagina and cervix with an optical magnifying instrument (colposcope) *Colposcopy is commonly performed after a Papanicolaou test to obtain biopsy specimens of the cervix and identify abnormal cervical tissue. (See Fig. 8–17.)*
laparoscopy lăp-ăr-ŎS-kō-pē *lapar/o:* abdomen *-scopy:* visual examination	Visual examination of the abdominal cavity with a laparoscope through one or more small incisions in the abdominal wall, usually at the umbilicus (See Fig. 8–18.) *Laparoscopy is used for inspection of the ovaries and fallopian tubes, diagnosis of endometriosis, destruction of uterine leiomyomas, myomectomy, and gynecological sterilization.*

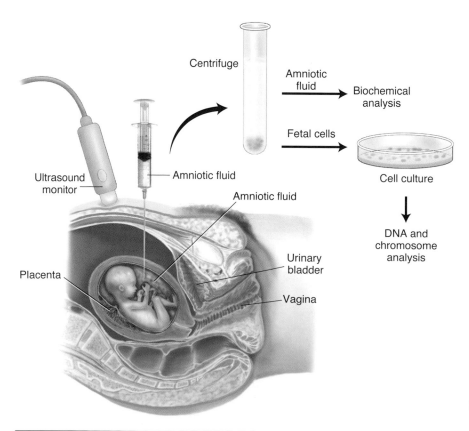

Figure 8-16 Amniocentesis.

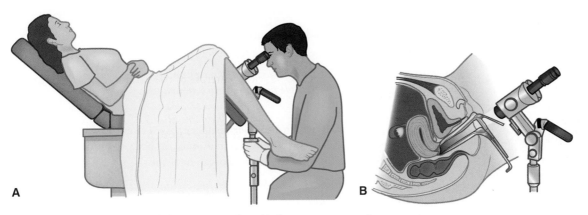

Figure 8-17 Colposcopy. (**A**) Woman in dorsal lithotomy position for examination.
(**B**) Colposcope illuminating the cervix for biopsy.

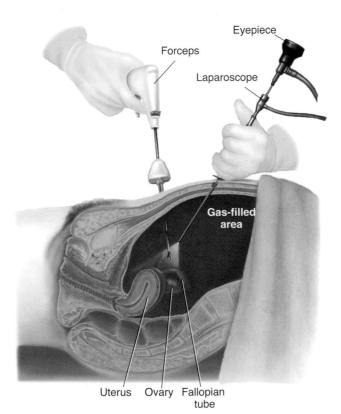

Figure 8-18 Laparoscopy.

mammography măm-ŎG-ră-fē *mamm/o:* breast *-graphy:* process of recording	Radiography of the breast used to diagnose benign and malignant tumors

Papanicolaou (Pap) test pă-pă-NĬ-kō-lŏw	Microscopic analysis of cells taken from the cervix and vagina to detect the presence of carcinoma *Cells are obtained for a Pap test via insertion of a vaginal speculum and the use of a swab to scrape a small tissue sample from the cervix and vagina.*
ultrasonography (US) ŭl-tră-sŏn-ŎG-ră-fē *ultra-:* excess, beyond *son/o:* sound *-graphy:* process of recording	Radiographic procedure in which a small transducer passed over the skin transmits high-frequency sound waves (ultrasound) that bounce off body tissues and are then recorded to produce an image of an internal organ or tissue *Pelvic US is used to evaluate the female reproductive organs and the fetus during pregnancy. Transvaginal US places the sound probe in the vagina instead of across the pelvis or abdomen, producing a sharper examination of normal and pathological structures within the pelvis.*

Male Reproductive System

digital rectal examination (DRE) DĬJ-ĭ-tăl RĔK-tăl *rect:* rectum *-al:* pertaining to	Examination of the prostate gland by finger palpation through the anal canal and the rectum (See Fig. 8–19.) *DRE is usually performed during physical examination to detect prostate enlargement. It is also used to check for problems with organs or other structures in the pelvis and lower abdomen.*

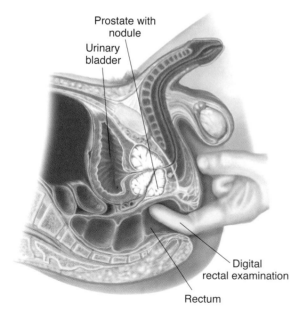

Prostate with nodule

Urinary bladder

Digital rectal examination

Rectum

Figure 8-19 Digital rectal examination.

transrectal ultrasound (TRUS) and biopsy of the prostate *trans:* across, through *rect:* rectum *al:* pertaining to *bi-:* two *-opsy:* view of	An ultrasound probe is inserted into the rectum to obtain an image of the prostate gland and collect multiple needle biopsy specimens of the prostate gland tissues where abnormalities are detected (See Fig. 8–20.) *High-frequency sound waves are recorded and transformed into video or photographic images of the prostate gland. If cancer is identified, the physician will be able to grade the cancer and determine its aggressiveness or likelihood of spreading.*

Medical and Surgical Procedures

Female Reproductive System

cerclage sāir-KLŎZH	Obstetric procedure in which a nonabsorbable suture is used for holding the cervix closed to prevent spontaneous abortion in a woman who has an incompetent cervix

dilation and curettage (D&C) DĬ-lă-tā-shŭn, kū-rĕ-TĂZH	Surgical procedure that widens the cervical canal of the uterus (dilatation) so that the endometrium of the uterus can be scraped (curettage) (See Fig. 8–5) *D&C is performed to stop prolonged or heavy uterine bleeding, diagnose uterine abnormalities, and obtain tissue for microscopic examination. It is also performed to remove tumors, rule out carcinoma of the uterus, remove retained placental fragments after delivery or after an incomplete abortion, and determine the cause of infertility.*

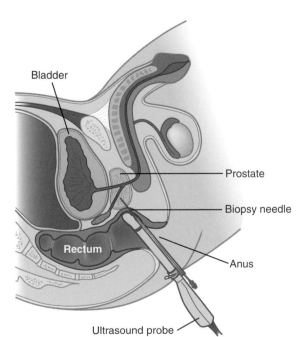

Figure 8-20 Transrectal ultrasound and biopsy of the prostate.

hysterosalpingo-oophorectomy hĭs-tĕr-ō-săl-pĭng-gō-ō-ŏ-for-ĔK-tō-mē *hyster/o:* uterus (womb) *salping/o:* tube (usually fallopian or eustachian [auditory] tube) *oophor:* ovary *-ectomy:* excision	Surgical removal of a uterus, a fallopian tube, and an ovary (See Fig. 8–4)
lumpectomy lŭm-PĔK-tō-mē	Excision of a small, primary breast tumor ("lump") and some of the normal tissue that surrounds it (See Fig. 8–8) *In lumpectomy, lymph nodes may also be removed because they are located within the breast tissue taken during surgery. All tissue removed from the breast is biopsied to determine whether cancer cells are present in the normal tissue surrounding the tumor. Lumpectomy is the most common form of breast cancer surgery today.*
mastectomy măs-TĔK-tō-mē *mast:* breast *-ectomy:* excision, removal	Complete or partial excision of one or both breasts, most commonly performed to remove a malignant tumor *Mastectomy may be simple, radical, or modified depending on the extent of the malignancy and amount of breast tissue excised.*
total	Excision of an entire breast, nipple, areola, and the involved overlying skin; also called *simple mastectomy* *In total mastectomy, lymph nodes are removed only if they are included in the breast tissue being removed.*
modified radical	Excision of an entire breast, including lymph nodes in the underarm (axillary dissection) (See Fig. 8–21.) *Most women who have mastectomies today have modified radical mastectomies.*
radical	Excision of an entire breast, all underarm lymph nodes, and chest wall muscles under the breast

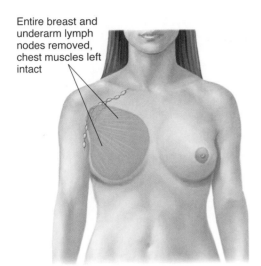

Entire breast and underarm lymph nodes removed, chest muscles left intact

Figure 8-21 Modified radical mastectomy.

reconstructive breast surgery	Reconstruction of a breast that has been removed due to cancer or other disease *Reconstruction is commonly possible immediately following mastectomy so the patient awakens from anesthesia with a breast mound already in place.*
tissue (skin) expansion	Common breast reconstruction technique in which a balloon expander is inserted beneath the skin and chest muscle, saline solution is gradually injected to increase size, and the expander is then replaced with a more permanent implant (See Fig. 8–22.)
transverse rectus abdominis muscle (TRAM) flap	Surgical creation of a skin flap (using skin and fat from the lower half of the abdomen), which is passed under the skin to the breast area, shaped into a natural-looking breast, and sutured into place (See Fig. 8–23.) *The TRAM flap procedure is one of the most popular reconstruction options.*
tubal ligation TŪ-băl lī-GĀ-shŭn	Sterilization procedure that involves blocking both fallopian tubes by cutting or burning them and tying them off

Male Reproductive System

circumcision sĕr-kŭm-SĬ-zhŭn	Surgical removal of the foreskin or prepuce of the penis, usually performed on the male as an infant
transurethral resection of the prostate (TURP)	Surgical procedure to relieve obstruction caused by benign prostatic hyperplasia (excessive overgrowth of normal tissue) by insertion of a resectoscope into the penis and through the urethra to "chip away" at prostatic tissue and flush out chips (using an irrigating solution) (See Fig. 8–12) *The pieces of prostatic tissue obtained through TURP are sent to the laboratory to be analyzed for possible evidence of CA. Although TURP relieves the obstruction, overgrowth of tissue may recur over several years. Lasers may also be used to destroy prostatic tissue and relieve obstruction.*

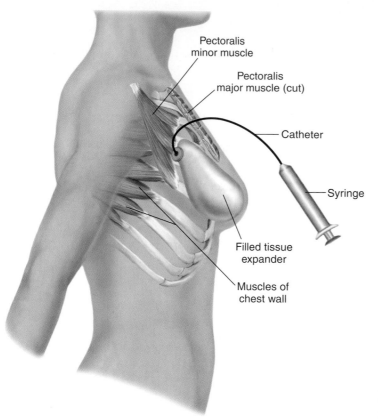

Pectoralis
minor muscle

Pectoralis
major muscle (cut)

Catheter

Syringe

Filled tissue
expander

Muscles of
chest wall

Figure 8-22 Tissue expander for breast reconstruction.

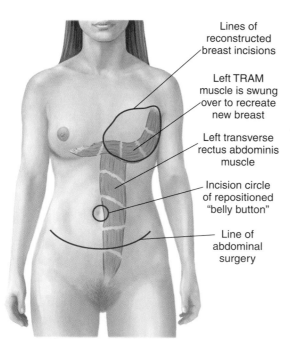

Lines of
reconstructed
breast incisions

Left TRAM
muscle is swung
over to recreate
new breast

Left transverse
rectus abdominis
muscle

Incision circle
of repositioned
"belly button"

Line of
abdominal
surgery

Figure 8-23 TRAM flap.

PHARMACOLOGY

The following table lists common drug categories used to treat reproductive disorders, as well as their therapeutic actions.

Drug Category	Action
Female Reproductive System	
antifungals ăn-tĭ-FŬN-gălz	Treat vaginal fungal infection, such as candidiasis
estrogens ĔS-trō-jĕnz	Treat symptoms of menopause (hot flashes, vaginal dryness) through hormone replacement therapy (HRT)
contraceptives kŏn-tră-SĔP-tĭvz	Prevent ovulation in order to avoid pregnancy *The most common female contraceptives are oral contraceptive pills (OCPs), also known as birth control pills.*
oxytocics ŏk-sē-TŌ-sĭks	Induce labor at term by increasing the strength and frequency of uterine contractions.
spermicides SPĔR-mĭ-sīdz	Destroy sperm by creating a highly acidic environment in the uterus *Spermicides are used as a method of birth control.*
Male Reproductive System	
erectile agents ĕ-RĔK-tīl	Treat erectile dysfunction (impotence) by increasing blood flow to the penis, resulting in an erection
gonadotropins gŏn-ă-dō-TRŌ-pĭnz	Increase sperm count in infertility cases

Pronunciation Help	Long sound	ā in rāte	ē in rēbirth	ī in īsle	ō in ōver	ū in ūnite
	Short sound	ă in ălone	ĕ in ĕver	ĭ in ĭt	ŏ in nŏt	ŭ in cŭt

ADDITIONAL MEDICAL TERMS REVIEW

Match the medical term(s) below with the definitions in the numbered list.

anorchism	cryptorchidism	impotence	fibroid
candidiasis	D&C	leukorrhea	sterility
cerclage	endometriosis	mammography	syphilis
chlamydia	gonadotropins	oligomenorrhea	toxic shock
circumcision	gonorrhea	phimosis	trichomoniasis

1. _____ refers to the failure of the testicles to descend into the scrotum.

2. _____ is a benign neoplasm in the uterus composed largely of leiomyomas.

3. _____ refers to the inability of a woman to become pregnant or for a man to impregnate a woman.

4. _____ refers to the congenital absence of one or both testes.

5. _____ is a vaginal fungal infection caused by *Candida albicans* and is characterized by a curdy discharge and extreme itching.

6. _____ is a sexually transmitted bacterial infection that causes cervicitis in women and urethritis and epididymitis in men.

7. _____ is the surgical removal of the foreskin, or prepuce, of the penis.

8. _____ is an obstetric procedure to prevent spontaneous abortion in a woman who has an incompetent cervix.

9. _____ is a discharge from the vagina and a common reason for women to seek gynecological care.

10. _____ is a condition in which endometrial tissue is found in various abnormal sites throughout the pelvis or in the abdominal wall.

11. _____ refers to radiography of the breast and is used to diagnose benign and malignant tumors.

12. _____ is a sexually transmitted bacterial infection that most commonly affects the genitourinary tract and, occasionally, the pharynx or rectum.

13. _____ is a sexually transmitted infection that is characterized by lesions that change to a chancre and, eventually, serious organ damage.

14. _____ is a rare and sometimes fatal staphylococcal infection that occurs in menstruating women who use vaginal tampons.

15. _____ is an infection of the vagina or male genital tract that commonly causes vaginitis, urethritis, and cystitis.

16. _____ refers to a widening of the uterine cervix so that the surface lining of the uterus can be scraped.

17. _____ means stenosis of the preputial orifice so that the foreskin does not retract over the glans penis.

18. _____ refers to the inability of a man to achieve a penile erection.

19. _____ refers to scanty or infrequent menstrual flow.

20. _____ are hormonal preparations used to increase the sperm count in cases of infertility.

Competency Verification: Check your answers in Appendix B: Answer Key, page 588. If you are not satisfied with your level of comprehension, review the pathological, diagnostic, and therapeutic terms and retake the review.

Correct Answers _____ × 5 = _____ % Score

MEDICAL RECORD ACTIVITIES

The following medical reports reflect common, real-life clinical scenarios using medical terminology to document patient care.

MEDICAL RECORD ACTIVITY 8-1

POSTMENOPAUSAL BLEEDING

Terminology

Terms listed in the table below come from the medical report Postmenopausal Bleeding that follows. Use a medical dictionary such as Taber's Cyclopedic Medical Dictionary, *the appendices of this book, or other resources to define each term. Then practice reading the pronunciations aloud for each term.*

Term	Definition
axilla ăk-SĬL-ă	
gravida 4 GRĂV-ĭ-dă	
laparoscopy lăp-ăr-ŎS-kō-pē	
lesion LĒ-zhŭn	
metastases mě-TĂS-tă-sēz	
neoplastic nē-ō-PLĂS-tĭk	
para 4 PĂR-ă	
postmenopausal pōst-měn-ō-PAW-zăl	
Premarin PRĔM-ă-rĭn	

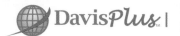 **DavisPlus** | Visit the *Medical Terminology Simplified* online resource center at Davis*Plus* to hear pronunciation and meanings of selected terms in this medical report.

Reading

Practice pronunciation of medical terms by reading the following medical report aloud.

Postmenopausal Bleeding

A 52-year-old gravida 4, para 4 woman had her last menstrual period at age 48. She was in our office last month for an evaluation because of postmenopausal bleeding. She has been taking Premarin and has had vaginal bleeding. The patient is currently admitted for gynecological laparoscopy and diagnostic D&C to rule out the possibility of a neoplastic process.

Last year this patient was admitted to the hospital for a simple mastectomy. The patient had a large preulcerating lesion of the left breast with metastases to the axilla, liver, and bone. Further medical evaluation will be performed next week.

Evaluation

Review the medical record to answer the following questions. Use a medical dictionary such as Taber's Cyclopedic Medical Dictionary *and other resources if needed.*

1. How many times has the patient been pregnant? How many children has the patient given birth to?

_____

_____

2. Why is the patient being admitted to the hospital?

_____

_____

3. What is a D&C?

_____

_____

4. What is the patient's past surgical history?

_____

_____

5. At what sites did the patient have malignant growth?

_____

_____

MEDICAL RECORD ACTIVITY 8-2

BILATERAL VASECTOMY

Terminology

Terms listed in the table below come from the medical report Bilateral Vasectomy that follows. Use a medical dictionary such as Taber's Cyclopedic Medical Dictionary, *the appendices of this book, or other resources to define each term. Then practice reading the pronunciations aloud for each term.*

Term	Definition
bilateral bī-LĂT-ĕr-ăl	
cauterized KAW-tĕr-īzd	
Darvocet-N DĂHR-vō-sĕt	
hemostat HĒ-mō-stăt	
semen SĒ-mĕn	
supine sū-PĬN	
vasectomy văs-ĔK-tō-mē	
Xylocaine ZĪ-lō-kān	

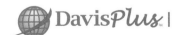 | Visit the *Medical Terminology Simplified* online resource center at Davis*Plus* to hear pronunciation and meanings of selected terms in this medical report.

Reading

Practice pronunciation of medical terms by reading the following medical report aloud.

Bilateral Vasectomy

Patient was placed on the table in supine position and prepped, scrotum shaved, and draped in the usual fashion. The right testicle was grasped and brought to skin level. This area was injected with 1% Xylocaine anesthesia. After a few minutes, a small incision was made, and the right vas was located. A hemostat was used and clamped on the right and left vas. A segment of the right vas was removed, and both ends were cauterized and tied independently with 3-0 silk suture. The skin was closed with 2-0 chromic suture. The same procedure was performed on the left side. The hemostats were removed. There were no complications or bleeding. Patient was discharged to home in care of his wife. Postoperative care instruction sheet was given along with prescription of Darvocet-N 100 mg, 1 q4h as required for pain. Patient will be seen for follow-up semen analysis in 6 weeks.

Evaluation

Review the medical record to answer the following questions. Use a medical dictionary such as Taber's Cyclopedic Medical Dictionary *and other resources if needed.*

1. What is the end result of a bilateral vasectomy?

   _____

   _____

2. Was the patient awake during the surgery? What type of anesthesia was used?

   _____

   _____

3. What was used to prevent bleeding?

   _____

   _____

4. What type of suture material was used to close the incision?

   _____

   _____

5. What was the patient given for pain relief at home?

   _____

   _____

6. Why is it important for the patient to go for a follow-up visit?

   _____

   _____

REPRODUCTIVE SYSTEMS CHAPTER REVIEW

WORD ELEMENTS SUMMARY

The following table summarizes CFs, suffixes, and prefixes related to the reproductive system. Study the word elements and their meanings before completing the Word Elements Chapter Review that follows.

Word Element	Meaning	Word Element	Meaning
Combining Forms			
Female Reproductive System			
amni/o	amnion (amniotic sac)	metr/o	uterus (womb); measure
cervic/o	neck; cervix uteri (neck of the uterus)	mamm/o, mast/o	breast
colp/o, vagin/o	vagina	men/o	menses, menstruation
episi/o, vulv/o	vulva	nat/o	birth
galact/o, lact/o	milk	oophor/o, ovari/o	ovary
gynec/o	woman, female	path/o	disease
hyster/o, uter/o	uterus (womb)	perine/o	perineum
lapar/o	abdomen	salping/o	tube (usually fallopian or eustachian [auditory] tubes)
Male Reproductive System			
andr/o	male	orchid/o, orchi/o, orch/o, test/o	testis (plural, testes)
balan/o	glans penis	prostat/o	prostate gland
gonad/o	gonads, sex glands	spermat/o, sperm/i, sperm/o	spermatozoa, sperm cells
muc/o	mucus	varic/o	dilated vein
olig/o	scanty	vas/o	vessel; vas deferens; duct
Suffixes			
-al, -ic, -ous	pertaining to, relating to	-para	to bear (offspring)
-algia, -dynia	pain	-pathy	disease
-arche	beginning	-pexy	fixation (of an organ)
-cele	hernia; swelling	-plasia, -plasm	formation, growth
-cyesis	pregnancy	-plasty	surgical repair
-ectomy	excision, removal	-ptosis	prolapse, downward displacement
-genesis	forming, producing, origin	-rrhage, -rrhagia	bursting forth (of)
-gravida	pregnant woman	-rrhaphy	suture
-ia	condition	-rrhea	discharge, flow
-ist	specialist	-salpinx	tube (usually fallopian or eustachian [auditory] tubes)

Continued

Word Element	Meaning	Word Element	Meaning
-itis	inflammation	-scope	instrument for examining
-lith	stone, calculus	-spasm	involuntary contraction, twitching
-logist	specialist in the study of	-tocia	childbirth, labor
-logy	study of	-tome	instrument to cut
-megaly	enlargement	-tomy	incision
-oid	resembling	-uria	urine
-oma	tumor	-version	turning
Prefixes			
a-, an-	without, not	neo-	new
dys-	bad; painful; difficult	post-	after, behind
hyper-	excessive, above normal	pre-	before, in front of

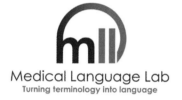

Medical Language Lab
Turning terminology into language

Visit the *Medical Language Lab* at the website *medicallanguagelab.com*. Use the flash-card exercise for this chapter to reinforce your study of word elements. We recommend you complete the flash-card exercise before starting the Word Elements Chapter Review that follows.

WORD ELEMENTS CHAPTER REVIEW

This review provides a verification of your knowledge of the word elements covered in this chapter. Write the meaning of the word element in the space provided. To reinforce your understanding of the word parts that comprise a medical term, identify each word element as a prefix (P), word root (WR), combining form (CF), or suffix (S). The first word is completed for you.

Medical Term	Word Elements	Meaning
1. hyster/ectomy	*hyster (WR)*	*uterus (womb)*
	-ectomy (S)	*excision, removal*
2. amni/o/centesis		
3. andr/o/gen		
4. balan/itis		
5. dys/tocia		

Continued

Medical Term	Word Elements	Meaning
6. episi/o/tomy		
7. galact/o/rrhea		
8. gynec/o/logist		
9. mamm/o/gram		
10. men/o/rrhagia		
11. multi/para		

Medical Term	Word Elements	Meaning
12. oophor/oma		
13. orchi/o/rrhaphy		
14. primi/gravida		
15. prostat/o/megaly		
16. rect/o/scope		
17. salping/ectomy		

Continued

Medical Term	Word Elements	Meaning
18. vagin/o/cele		
19. vas/ectomy		
20. vas/o/vas/o/stomy		

Competency Verification: Check your answers in Appendix B: Answer Key, page 589. If you are not satisfied with your level of comprehension, review the chapter's flash-card exercise at *medicallanguagelab.com* and retake the review.

Correct Answers _____ × 5 = _____ % Score

VOCABULARY REVIEW

Match the medical terms below with the definitions in the numbered list.

amenorrhea	estrogen	PID	testopathy
aplasia	gravida 4	postmenopausal	testosterone
aspermatism	hydrocele	progesterone	uterus
cervix uteri	oophoritis	prostatic cancer	vas deferens
dysmenorrhea	para 4	prostatomegaly	vasectomy
epididymis			

1. _____ means *enlargement of the prostate gland.*

2. _____ refers to a disease of the testes.

3. _____ is a male hormone produced by the testes.

4. _____ is an absence or abnormal stoppage of the menses.

5. _____ is a female hormone produced by the ovaries.

6. _____ is an inflamed condition of the ovaries.

7. _____ is a condition in which there is a lack of male sperm.

8. _____ refers to a woman in her fourth pregnancy.

9. _____ is an organ that nourishes the embryo.

10. _____ is a malignant neoplasm of the prostate.

11. _____ is a tube that temporarily stores sperm.

12. _____ is a collection of fluid in a saclike cavity.

13. _____ is a duct that transports sperm from the testes to the urethra.

14. _____ refers to a woman who has delivered four infants.

15. _____ means *neck of the uterus.*

16. _____ refers to painful menstruation.

17. _____ means *occurring after menopause.*

18. _____ is failure or lack of formation or growth.

19. _____ is a procedure to sterilize a man by cutting the vas deferens, preventing the release of sperm.

20. _____ is a collective term for any extensive bacterial infection of the pelvic organs, especially the uterus, uterine tubes, or ovaries.

Competency Verification: Check your answers in Appendix B: Answer Key, page 590. If you are not satisfied with your level of comprehension, review the chapter vocabulary and retake the review.

Correct Answers _____ × 5 = _____ % Score

Endocrine and Nervous Systems

OBJECTIVES

Upon completion of this chapter, you will be able to:

- Describe the type of medical treatment endocrinologists and neurologists provide.

- Identify the structures of the endocrine and nervous systems by labeling them on the anatomical illustrations.

- Describe the primary functions of the endocrine and nervous systems.

- Describe diseases, conditions, and procedures related to the endocrine and nervous systems.

- Apply your word-building skills by constructing medical terms related to the endocrine and nervous systems.

- Describe common abbreviations and symbols related to the endocrine and nervous systems.

- Recognize, define, pronounce, and spell terms correctly.

- Demonstrate your knowledge of this chapter by successfully completing the frames, reviews, and medical report evaluations.

MEDICAL SPECIALTIES

Endocrinology

Endocrinology is the medical specialty concerned with diagnosis and treatment of endocrine gland disorders. **Endocrinologists** evaluate the body's overall metabolic function and diagnose and treat hormone imbalances due to underproduction or overproduction of hormones. Endocrinologists treat such disorders as diabetes, osteoporosis, and other disorders of the endocrine glands. When surgery is required, the endocrinologist works closely with the surgeon to provide the most beneficial patient care. Endocrinologists also play important roles related to their field of expertise in university academic research and in the pharmaceutical industry.

Neurology

Neurology is the medical specialty concerned with the diagnosis and treatment of diseases of the nervous system, which includes the brain, spinal cord, and peripheral nerves. **Neurologists** use specialized examination procedures and employ diagnostic tests, medical and surgical procedures, and drugs to treat nervous system diseases. The branch of surgery involving the nervous system, including the brain and spinal cord, is called **neurosurgery.** The physician who specializes in neurosurgery is a **neurosurgeon.**

ANATOMY AND PHYSIOLOGY OVERVIEW

The endocrine and nervous systems work together like interlocking supersystems to control many intricate activities of the body. Together they monitor changes in the body and in the external environment, interpret these changes, and coordinate appropriate responses to reestablish and maintain a relative equilibrium in the internal environment of the body (**homeostasis**).

The endocrine system consists of a network of glandular structures that slowly discharge hormones into the bloodstream. In contrast, the nervous system is designed to act instantaneously by transmitting electrical impulses to specific body locations, which helps control all critical body activities and reactions.

ENDOCRINE SYSTEM

The endocrine system is a network of ductless glands that have a rich blood supply, which enables the hormones they produce to enter the bloodstream. Although hormone production occurs at one site, the effects of these hormones take place at various other sites in the body. Processes under direct endocrine control include growth, reproduction, cellular metabolism, and the regulation of blood levels of many important nutrients. The tissues or organs that respond to the effects of a hormone are called **target tissues,** or **target organs**. (See Fig. 9–1.)

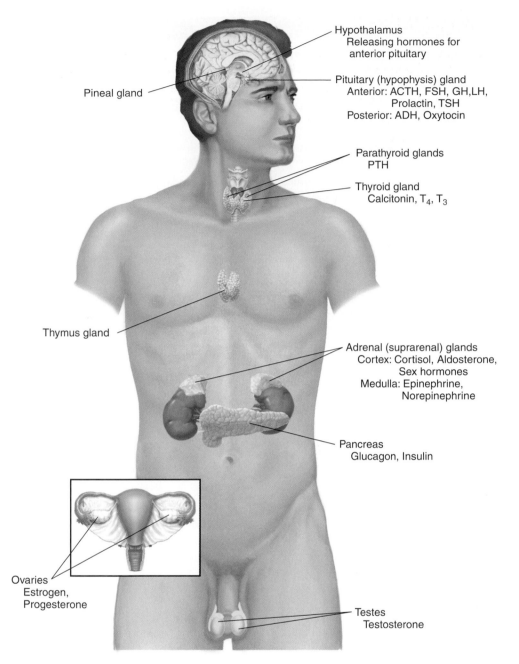

Hypothalamus
  Releasing hormones for
  anterior pituitary

Pituitary (hypophysis) gland
  Anterior: ACTH, FSH, GH,LH,
    Prolactin, TSH
  Posterior: ADH, Oxytocin

Pineal gland

Parathyroid glands
  PTH

Thyroid gland
  Calcitonin, T$_4$, T$_3$

Thymus gland

Adrenal (suprarenal) glands
  Cortex: Cortisol, Aldosterone,
    Sex hormones
  Medulla: Epinephrine,
    Norepinephrine

Pancreas
  Glucagon, Insulin

Ovaries
  Estrogen,
  Progesterone

Testes
  Testosterone

Figure 9-1 Locations of major endocrine glands.

WORD ELEMENTS

This section introduces CFs related to the endocrine system. Included are key suffixes; prefixes are defined in the right-hand column as needed. Review the following table, and pronounce each word in the word analysis column aloud before you begin to work the frames.

Word Element	Meaning	Word Analysis
Combining Forms		
aden/o	gland	**aden**/oma (ăd-ĕ-NŌ-mă): tumor composed of glandular tissue *-oma:* tumor
adren/o		**adren**/al (ăd-RĒ-năl): pertaining to the adrenal glands *-al:* pertaining to
adrenal/o	adrenal glands	**adrenal**/ectomy (ăd-rē-năl-ĚK-tō-mē): excision of adrenal gland(s) *-ectomy:* excision, removal *Adrenalectomy involves surgical removal of one or both adrenal glands to remove a tumor, aid in correcting a hormone imbalance, or prevent metastasis.*

calc/o	calcium	hypo/**calc**/emia (hī-pō-kăl-SĒ-mē-ă): deficiency of calcium in the blood
		    hypo-: under, below, deficient
		    -emia: blood condition

gluc/o	sugar, sweetness	**gluc**/o/genesis (gloo-kō-JĔN-ĕ-sĭs): formation of glucose *-genesis:* forming, producing, origin

glyc/o		hyper/**glyc**/emia (hī-pĕr-glī-SĒ-mē-ă): excessive glucose in the blood
		    hyper-: excessive, above normal
		     -emia: blood condition
		
		 Hyperglycemia is most commonly associated with diabetes mellitus.

pancreat/o	pancreas	**pancreat**/itis (păn-krē-ă-TĪ-tĭs): inflammation of the pancreas *itis:* inflammation *Pancreatitis occurs when pancreatic enzymes that digest food are activated in the pancreas instead of the duodenum and attack pancreatic tissue, causing damage to the gland.*
parathyroid/o	parathyroid glands	**parathyroid**/ectomy (păr-ă-thī-royd-ĚK-tō-mē): excision of the parathyroid gland(s) *-ectomy:* excision, removal
pituitar/o	pituitary gland	hypo/**pituitar**/ism (hī-pō-pĭ-TŪ-ĭ-tă-rĭzm): condition of inadequate levels of pituitary hormone in the body *-ism:* condition
thym/o	thymus gland	**thym**/oma (thī-MŌ-mă): tumor of the thymus gland *-oma:* tumor
thyr/o	thyroid gland	**thyr**/o/megaly (thī-rō-MĔG-ă-lē): enlargement of the thyroid gland *-megaly:* enlargement
thyroid/o		**thyroid**/ectomy (thī-royd-ĚK-tō-mē): excision of the thyroid gland *-ectomy:* excision, removal *Thyroidectomy is the complete removal of the thyroid gland (total thyroidectomy) or removal of half of the thyroid gland (subtotal, or partial, thyroidectomy).*
toxic/o	poison	**toxic**/o/logist (tŏks-ĭ-KŎL-ō-jĭst): specialist in the study of poisons (toxins) *-logist:* specialist in study of *The toxicologist studies the effects that poisons or chemicals have on humans, animals, plants, and other living organisms, as well as subsequent treatments.*

Word Element	Meaning	Word Analysis
Suffixes		
-dipsia	thirst	poly/**dipsia** (pŏl-ē-DĬP-sē-ă): excessive thirst *poly-:* many, much *Polydipsia is a characteristic symptom of diabetes mellitus.*
-trophy	development, nourishment	hyper/**trophy** (hī-PĔR-trŏ-fē): increase in the size of an organ *hyper-:* excessive, above normal *Hypertrophy is due to an increase in the size of the cells of an organ, rather than an increase in the number of cells, as in carcinoma.*

Pronunciation Help	Long sound	ā in rāte	ē in rēbirth	ī in īsle	ō in ōver	ū in ūnite
	Short sound	ă in ălone	ĕ in ĕver	ĭ in ĭt	ŏ in nŏt	ŭ in cŭt

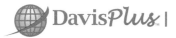 Visit the *Medical Terminology Simplified* online resource center at Davis*Plus* for an audio exercise of the terms in this table. It will help you master pronunciations and meanings of medical terms.

acr/o/megaly
ăk-rō-MĔG-ă-lē

9-26 The CF *acr/o* means *extremity*. Acr/o/megaly, a chronic metabolic condition, is characterized by a gradual, marked enlargement and thickening of the bones of the face and jaw. This condition, which afflicts middle-aged and older persons, is caused by overproduction of growth hormone and is treated by radiation, pharmacological agents, or surgery, commonly involving partial resection of the pituitary gland.

A term that literally means *enlargement of the extremities* is

_____ / _____ / _____.

TABLE 9-1 PITUITARY HORMONES

This table identifies pituitary hormones, their target organs and functions, and associated disorders.

Hormone	Target Organ and Functions	Disorders
Anterior Pituitary Hormones (Adenohypophysis)		
Adrenocorticotropic hormone (ACTH)	• Adrenal cortex—promotes secretions of some hormones by adrenal cortex, especially cortisol	• Hyposecretion is rare. • Hypersecretion causes Cushing disease.
Follicle-stimulating hormone (FSH)	• Ovaries in females—stimulates egg production; increases secretion of estrogen • Testes in males—stimulates sperm production	• Hyposecretion causes failure of sexual maturation. • Hypersecretion has no known significant effects.
Growth hormone (GH), or somatotropin	• Bone, cartilage, liver, muscle, and other tissues—stimulates somatic growth; increases use of fats for energy	• Hyposecretion in children causes pituitary dwarfism. • Hypersecretion in children causes gigantism; hypersecretion in adults causes acromegaly.
Luteinizing hormone (LH)	• Ovaries in females—promotes ovulation; stimulates production of estrogen and progesterone • Testes in males—promotes secretion of testosterone	• Hyposecretion causes failure of sexual maturation. • Hypersecretion has no known significant effects.
Prolactin	• Breast—promotes lactation in conjunction with other hormones	• Hyposecretion in nursing mothers causes poor lactation. • Hypersecretion in nursing mothers causes galactorrhea.
Thyroid-stimulating hormone (TSH)	• Thyroid gland—stimulates secretion of thyroid hormone	• Hyposecretion in infants causes cretinism; hyposecretion in adults causes myxedema. • Hypersecretion causes Graves disease, indicated by exophthalmos. (See Fig. 9–4.)
Posterior Pituitary Hormones (Neurohypophysis)		
Antidiuretic hormone (ADH)	• Kidney—increases water reabsorption (water returns to the blood)	• Hyposecretion causes diabetes insipidus. • Hypersecretion causes syndrome of inappropriate antidiuretic hormone (SIADH).
Oxytocin	• Uterus—stimulates uterine contractions; initiates labor • Breast—promotes milk secretion from the mammary glands	• Unknown

Boldface indicates a word root or combining form. Blue indicates a suffix. Pink indicates a prefix.

Thyroid Gland

9–27   The (2) **thyroid gland** contains two lobes connected by a thin bridge of tissue called the isthmus. Locate and label the thyroid gland in Figure 9–3.

---

thyroid/ectomy
thī-royd-ĔK-tō-mē

9–28   The CFs for thyroid gland are *thyr/o* and *thyroid/o.* Use *thyroid/o* to form a word that means *excision of the thyroid gland.*

_____ / _____

---

thyr/o/megaly
thī-rō-MĔG-ă-lē

thyr/o/pathy
thī-RŎP-ă-thē

thyr/o/tomy
thī-RŎT-ō-mē

9–29   Use *thyr/o* to construct words that mean

enlargement of the thyroid gland: _____ / _____ / _____

disease of the thyroid gland: _____ / _____ / _____

incision of the thyroid gland: _____ / _____ / _____

9–30   Table 9–2 on page 407 outlines thyroid hormones along with their functions and selected associated disorders. Refer to the table to complete Frames 9–30 through 9–32.

The thyroid gland secretes three hormones, two of which regulate the body's metabolism (rate at which food is converted into heat and energy). These hormones are called _____ and _____.

9–31   In conjunction with parathyroid hormone (PTH), calcium levels in the blood are regulated by secretion of the thyroid hormone called _____.

To check answers for Frames 9–30 through 9–32, refer to Table 9–2 on page 407.

9–32   When does calcitonin exert its most important effects in the body?

_____

_____

_____

---

excessive, above normal

thyroid gland
THĪ-royd

condition

9–33   Hyper/thyroid/ism is caused by excessive secretion of the thyroid gland. The gland increases the body's metabolism and intensifies the demand for food. Analyze hyper/thyroid/ism by defining the elements.

hyper-: _____, _____ _____

thyroid: _____ _____

-ism: _____

ex/ophthalm/os *or*
ex/ophthalm/ic
ĕks-ŏf-THĂL-mŏs,
ĕks-ŏf-THĂL-mĭc

thyr/o/toxic/osis
thī-rō-tŏks-ĭ-KŌ-sĭs

9–34   Hyper/thyroid/ism involves enlargement of the thyroid gland associated with hypersecretion of thyroxine. It is characterized by exophthalmos (bulging of the eyes), which develops because of edema in the tissues of the eye sockets and swelling of the extrinsic eye muscles. (See Fig. 9–4.) Hyper/thyroid/ism is also called Graves disease, ex/ophthalm/ic goiter, thyr/o/toxic/ osis, and tox/ic goiter. (See Fig. 9–5.)

Identify the terms in this frame that mean

bulging of the eyes: _____ / _____ / _____

abnormal condition of thyroid gland poisoning:

_____ / _____ / _____ / _____

toxic/o/logist
tŏks-ĭ-KŎL-ō-jĭst

9–35   Toxic/o/logy is the scientific study of poisons and treatment of conditions produced by them.

A specialist in the study of poisons is called a

_____ / _____ / _____.

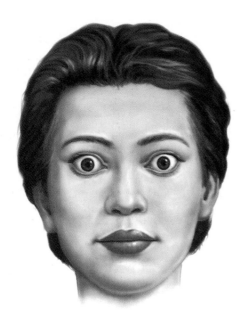

Figure 9-4 Exophthalmos caused by Graves disease.

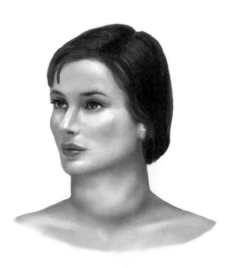

Figure 9-5 Enlargement of the thyroid gland in goiter.

Boldface indicates a word root or combining form. Blue indicates a suffix. Pink indicates a prefix.

poison	**9–36** Toxic/o/pathy is any disease caused by _____.
thyroid/o/tomy thī-royd-ŎT-ō-mē **thyroid/o/tome** thī-ROYD-ō-tōm	**9–37** Use *thyroid/o* to form words that mean *incision of the thyroid gland:* _____ / _____ / _____ *instrument to incise the thyroid:* _____ / _____ / _____
blood	**9–38** The CF *calc/o* means *calcium. Calc/emia* indicates an abnormal presence of calcium in the _____.
hyper/calc/emia hī-pĕr-kăl-SĒ-mē-ă	**9–39** Hypo/calc/emia is a condition of abnormally low blood calcium. A person with excessively high blood calcium has a condition called _____ / _____ / _____.

TABLE 9-2   THYROID HORMONES

This table identifies thyroid hormones, their functions, and associated disorders.

Hormone	Functions	Disorders
Calcitonin	• Regulates calcium levels in the blood in conjunction with parathyroid hormone • Secreted when calcium levels in the blood are high in order to maintain homeostasis	• The most significant effects are exerted in childhood when bones are growing and changing dramatically in mass, size, and shape. • At best, calcitonin is a weak hypocalcemic agent in adults.
Thyroxine (T_4) and triiodothyronine (T_3)	• Increases energy production from all food types • Increases rate of protein synthesis	• Hyposecretion in infants causes cretinism; hyposecretion in adults causes myxedema. • Hypersecretion causes Graves disease, indicated by exophthalmos. (See Fig. 9-4.)

SECTION REVIEW 9-2

Using the following table, write the CF, suffix, or prefix that matches its definition in the space provided to the left of the definition. There may be more than one word element that matches a definition.

Combining Forms		Suffixes		Prefixes
acr/o	poster/o	-emia	-tome	dys-
aden/o	radi/o	-logist	-tomy	hyper-
anter/o	thyr/o	-megaly		hypo-
calc/o	thyroid/o	-osis		poly-
neur/o	toxic/o	-pathy		

1. _____ abnormal condition; increase (used primarily with blood cells)

2. _____ excessive, above normal

3. _____ back (of body), behind, posterior

4. _____ bad; painful; difficult

5. _____ blood condition

6. _____ calcium

7. _____ disease

8. _____ enlargement

9. _____ extremity

10. _____ anterior, front

11. _____ gland

12. _____ incision

13. _____ instrument to cut

14. _____ nerve

15. _____ poison

16. _____ radiation, x-ray; radius (lower arm bone on thumb side)

17. _____ specialist in the study of

18. _____ many, much

19. _____ thyroid gland

20. _____ under, below, deficient

Competency Verification: Check your answers in Appendix B: Answer Key, page 591. If you are not satisfied with your level of comprehension, go back to Frame 9–1 and rework the frames.

Correct Answers _____ × 5 = _____ % Score

Parathyroid Glands

9–40   The (3) **parathyroid glands** are located on the posterior surface of the thyroid gland. The parathyroid glands are so called because they are located around the thyroid gland. Label the parathyroid glands in Figure 9–3.

Boldface indicates a word root or combining form. Blue indicates a suffix. Pink indicates a prefix.

para/thyr/oid glands păr-ă-THĪ-royd	**9–41** The parathyroid glands secrete parathyroid hormone (PTH), which helps regulate the amount of calcium in the blood. When we discuss the two pairs of glands located in the posterior aspect of the thyroid glands, we are talking about the _____ / _____ / _____ _____.
para-	**9–42** Identify the element in the previous frame that means *located near, beside; beyond.* _____
PTH	**9–43** The hormone produced by the parathyroid glands is called para/thormone or para/thyroid hormone (PTH). The abbreviation for para/thormone or para/thyr/oid hormone is _____.
To check answers for this frame, refer to Table 9–3 on page 409.	**9–44** Table 9–3 on page 409 outlines parathyroid hormone along with its target organs and functions and associated disorders. Refer to the table to complete this frame. The major function of PTH is to regulate levels of _____ and _____.
hyper/para/thyroid/ism hī-pěr-păr-ă-THĪ-roy-dĭzm	**9–45** Oste/itis fibrosa cystica is an inflammatory degenerative condition in which normal bone is replaced by cysts and fibrous tissue. It is usually associated with hyper/para/thyroid/ism. The term in this frame that means *abnormal condition characterized by hypersecretion of PTH* is _____ / _____ / _____ / _____.
hyper/calc/emia hī-pěr-kăl-SĒ-mē-ă **hypo/calc/emia** hī-pō-kăl-SĒ-mē-ă	**9–46** Calc/emia refers to *calcium in the blood.* Use *hypo-* and *hyper-* to form words that mean *excessive calcium in the blood:* _____ / _____ / _____ *deficiency of calcium in the blood:* _____ / _____ / _____

TABLE 9-3 PARATHYROID HORMONE

This table identifies parathyroid hormone along with its target organs and functions and associated disorders.

Hormone	Target Organ and Functions	Disorder
Parathyroid hormone (PTH)	• Bones—increases reabsorption of calcium and phosphate from bone to blood • Kidneys—increases calcium absorption and phosphate excretion • Small intestine—increases absorption of calcium and phosphate	• Hyposecretion causes tetany. • Hypersecretion causes osteitis fibrosa cystica.

Adrenal Glands

9-47   The (4) **adrenal glands,** also known as the supra/ren/al glands, are paired structures located super/ior to the kidneys. Label Figure 9–3 as you continue to learn about the endocrine system.

---

supra/ren/al
soo-prǎ-RĒ-nǎl

super/ior

9-48   Indicate the words in Frame 9–47 that mean

above or superior to a kidney: _____ / _____ / _____

pertaining to upper or above: _____ / _____

---

enlargement, adrenal

adrenal/ectomy
ăd-rē-nǎl-ĔK-tō-mē

9-49   *Adren/o* and *adrenal/o* are CFs for the adrenal glands. Adren/o/megaly is

an _____ of the _____ glands.

Use *adrenal/o* to form a word that means *excision of an adrenal gland.*

_____ / _____

---

kidneys

9-50   Each adrenal gland is structurally and functionally differentiated into two sections: the outer adrenal cortex, which comprises the bulk of the gland, and the inner portion, the adrenal medulla. The hormones produced by each part have different functions.

The adrenal glands are perched atop the _____.

9-51   Table 9–4 outlines adrenal hormones, along with their target organs and functions and selected associated disorders. Review the table to learn about hormones and their effects on target organs.

To check answers for Frames 9–52 through 9–57, refer to Table 9–4 on page 411.

9-52

To complete Frames 9–52 through 9–57, refer to Table 9–4 on page 411.

Three hormones produced by the adrenal cortex are

_____, _____, and _____.

9-53   Identify two hormones produced by the adrenal cortex that maintain secondary sex characteristics.

_____ and _____

9-54   Epinephrine helps the body cope with dangerous situations. Nerves transmit the message of fear to the glands, which react by rushing adrenaline to all parts of the system. Epinephrine is also called _____.

9-55   When a person is experiencing a stressful situation, the adrenal medulla produces adrenaline, which is also called _____.

Boldface indicates a word root or combining form. Blue indicates a suffix. Pink indicates a prefix.

TABLE 9-4 ADRENAL HORMONES

This table identifies adrenal hormones, their target organs and functions, and associated disorders.

Hormone	Target Organ and Functions	Disorders
Adrenal Cortex Hormones		
Glucocorticoids (mainly cortisol)	• Body cells—promote gluconeogenesis; regulate metabolism of carbohydrates, proteins, and fats; help depress inflammatory and immune responses	• Hyposecretion causes Addison disease. • Hypersecretion causes Cushing syndrome. (See Fig. 9–6.)
Mineralocorticoids (mainly aldosterone)	• Kidneys—increase blood levels of sodium and decrease blood levels of potassium in the kidneys	• Hyposecretion causes Addison disease. • Hypersecretion causes aldosteronism.
Sex hormones (any of the androgens, estrogens, or related steroid hormones) produced by the ovaries, testes, and adrenal cortices	• In females, possibly responsible for female libido and source of estrogen after menopause (otherwise, effects in adults are insignificant)	• Hypersecretion of adrenal androgen in females leads to virilism (development of male characteristics). • Hypersecretion of adrenal estrogen and progestin secretion in males leads to feminization (development of feminine characteristics). • Hyposecretion has no known significant effects.
Adrenal Medullary Hormones		
Epinephrine (adrenaline) and norepinephrine	• Sympathetic nervous system target organs—hormone effects mimic sympathetic nervous system activation (sympathomimetic), increase metabolic rate and heart rate, and raise blood pressure by promoting vasoconstriction	• Hyposecretion has no known significant effects. • Hypersecretion causes prolonged "fight-or-flight" reaction and hypertension.

9–56 Hormones produced by the adrenal medulla that increase blood pressure are _____ and _____.

9–57 The main glucocorticoid hormone secreted by the adrenal cortex is _____.

Pancreas (Islets of Langerhans)

9–58 The (5) **pancreas** is located posterior to the stomach. Hormone-producing cells of the pancreas are called islets of Langerhans. The islets produce two distinct hormones: alpha cells, which produce glucagons, and beta cells, which produce insulin. Both hormones play an important role in the proper metabolism of sugars and starches in the body. Label the pancreas in Figure 9–3.

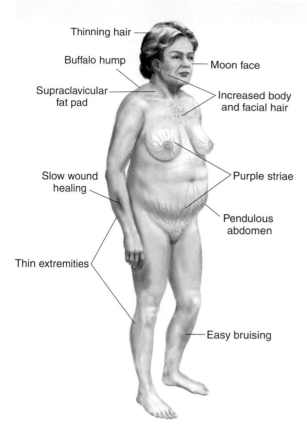

Thinning hair

Buffalo hump

Moon face

Supraclavicular fat pad

Increased body and facial hair

Slow wound healing

Purple striae

Pendulous abdomen

Thin extremities

Easy bruising

Figure 9-6 Physical manifestations seen in Cushing syndrome.

pancreat/oma păn-krē-ă-TŌ-mă	**9–59** Use *pancreat/o* (pancreas) to build medical words that mean *tumor of the pancreas:* _____ / _____ *calculus or stone in the pancreas:* _____ / _____ / _____ *abnormal condition of a pancreatic stone:* _____ / _____ / _____ / _____ *disease of the pancreas:* _____ / _____ / _____
pancreat/o/lith păn-krē-ĂT-ō-lĭth	
pancreat/o/lith/iasis păn-krē-ă-tō-lĭ-THĪ-ă-sĭs	
pancreat/o/pathy păn-krē-ă-TŎP-ă-thē	

pancreas PĂN-krē-ăs	**9–60** The suffix *-lysis* is used in words to mean *separation, destruction, loosening.* Pancreat/o/lysis is a destruction of the _____.

To check answers to Frames 9–61 through 9–63, refer to Table 9–5 on page 413.	**9–61** Refer to Table 9–5 on page 413 to complete Frames 9–61 through 9–63. Two hormones produced by the pancreas are _____ and _____.

Boldface indicates a word root or combining form. Blue indicates a suffix. Pink indicates a prefix.

TABLE 9-5 PANCREATIC HORMONES

This table identifies pancreatic hormones, their target organs and functions, and associated disorders.

Hormone	Target Organ and Functions	Disorders
Glucagon	• Liver and blood—increases blood glucose level by accelerating conversion of glycogen into glucose in the liver (glycogenolysis) and conversion of other nutrients into glucose in the liver (gluconeogenesis) and releasing glucose into the blood; converts glycogen to glucose	• Persistently low blood sugar levels (hypoglycemia) may be caused by a deficiency in glucagon.
Insulin	• Tissue cells—lowers blood glucose level by accelerating glucose transport into cells; converts glucose to glycogen	• Hyposecretion of insulin causes diabetes mellitus. • Hypersecretion of insulin causes hyperinsulinism.

9-62 Determine the pancreat/ic hormone that

lowers blood glucose: _____

increases blood glucose: _____

9-63 How does insulin lower blood glucose?

_____

_____

_____

glyc/o/gen
GLĪ-kō-jĕn

9-64 Gluc/ose is the chief source of energy for living organisms. *Gluc/o* and *glyc/o* are CFs that mean *sugar, sweetness.* The suffixes *-gen* and *-genesis* mean *forming, producing, origin.*

Combine *glyc/o* and *-gen* to form a word that means *forming or producing sugar.*

_____ / ____ / _____

gluc/o/genesis
gloo-kō-JĔN-ĕ-sĭs

glyc/o/genesis
glī-kō-JĔN-ĕ-sĭs

9-65 Use *-genesis* to build words that mean *forming, producing, or origin of sugar.*

_____ / ____ / _____

_____ / ____ / _____

gluc/o/meter
gloo-KŎM-tĕr

9-66 A gluc/o/meter is used to calculate blood glucose from one drop of blood. An instrument used by patients with diabetes to monitor their blood glucose levels is

known as a _____ / ____ / _____.

-emia **hyper-** **hypo-** **glyc**	**9–67** Hyper/glyc/emia is a condition of excessive amounts of glucose in the blood. Deficiency of glucose in the blood is known as hypo/glyc/emia. Identify the elements in this frame that mean *blood condition:* _____ *excessive, above normal:* _____ *under, below, deficient:* _____ *sugar, sweetness:* _____
hypo/glyc/emia hī-pō-glī-SĒ-mē-ă **intravenous**	**9–68** Insufficient amounts of gluc/ose in the blood, usually caused by excessive secretion of insulin by the pancreas, administration of too much insulin, or dietary deficiency, is called hypo/glyc/emia. Treatment for hypo/glyc/emia is administration of gluc/ose by mouth if the person is conscious or an IV solution if the person is unconscious. Deficiency of blood glucose is called _____ / _____ / _____. The abbreviation IV means _____.
-gen, -genesis	**9–69** Write the elements that mean *forming, producing, origin* in the terms glyc/o/gen and glyc/o/genesis. _____ , _____
insulin ĬN-sū-lĭn	**9–70** Diabetes causes hyper/glyc/emia and occurs if the pancreas does not produce sufficient amounts of insulin. It also occurs if the cells of the body become resistant to insulin and do not utilize insulin properly. Insulin is an essential hormone for the conversion of sugar, starches, and other food into energy. If hyper/glyc/emia occurs, diabetic patients can reduce the amount of gluc/ose in the blood by injecting themselves with the hormone called _____.
hyper/glyc/emia hī-pĕr-glī-SĒ-mē-ă **hypo/glyc/emia** hī-pō-glī-SĒ-mē-ă	**9–71** Diabetes is a general term that, when used alone, refers to diabetes mellitus (DM), a disease that occurs in two primary forms: type 1 diabetes and type 2 diabetes. When insulin is lacking, glucose does not enter cells but returns to the bloodstream with a subsequent rise in its concentration in the blood, a condition known as hyper/glyc/emia. Low blood glucose levels cause the opposite condition, called hypo/glyc/emia. Identify the terms in this frame that mean *excessive gluc/ose in the blood:* _____ / _____ / _____ *low or insufficient gluc/ose in the blood:* _____ / _____ / _____
hypo/glyc/emia hī-pō-glī-SĒ-mē-ă	**9–72** Hyper/glyc/emia can cause numerous complications, such as impairing wound healing, decreasing the body's ability to fight infection, and causing damage to the kidneys. The opposite of hyper/glyc/emia is _____ / _____ / _____.

poly/dipsia pŏl-ē-DĬP-sē-ă **poly/uria** pŏl-ē-Ū-rē-ă **poly/phagia** pŏl-ē-FĀ-jē-ă	**9–73** The suffix *-dipsia* denotes *a condition of thirst*. Poly/dipsia, poly/uria, and poly/phagia are three cardinal signs of diabetes mellitus. Write the words in this frame that mean *excessive thirst:* _____ / _____ *excessive urination:* _____ / _____ *excessive eating:* _____ / _____
poly/uria pŏl-ē-Ū-rē-ă	**9–74** When a person drinks too much water, he or she may experience a condition of excessive urine production (urination). The medical term for this condition is _____ / _____.

Pineal and Thymus Glands

9–75   The (6) **pineal gland** and (7) **thymus gland** are classified as endocrine glands, but little is known about their endocrine function. Label these structures in Figure 9–3.

thym/ectomy thī-MĔK-tō-mē **thym/oma** thī-MŌ-mă **thym/o/pathy** thī-MŎP-ă-thē **thym/o/lysis** thī-MŎL-ĭ-sĭs	**9–76** The CF *thym/o* means *thymus gland*. Build medical words that mean *excision of the thymus gland:* _____ / _____ *tumor of the thymus gland:* _____ / _____ *disease of the thymus gland:* _____ / _____ / _____ *destruction of the thymus gland:* _____ / _____ / _____

Ovaries and Testes

9–77   The (8) **ovaries** are a pair of small, almond-shaped glands positioned in the upper pelvic cavity, one on each side of the uterus. The (9) **testes** are paired oval glands surrounded by the scrotal sac. The functions of the ovaries and testes are covered in Chapter 8. Label the ovaries and testes in Figure 9–3.

oophor/o, ovari/o **orchid/o, orchi/o,** **orch/o, test/o**	**9–78** Recall the CFs for *ovaries:* _____ / _____ or _____ / _____ *testes:* _____ / _____, _____ / _____, _____ / _____, or _____ / _____

oophor/o/pathy ō-ŏf-or-ŎP-ă-thē **oophor/o/tomy** ō-ŏf-or-ŎT-ō-mē	**9–79** Use *oophor/o* to construct medical words that mean *disease of an ovary:* _____ / _____ / _____ *incision of an ovary:* _____ / _____ / _____

orchid/o/pexy OR-kĭd-ō-pĕk-sē	**9–80** Use *orchid/o* to form a word that means *surgical fixation of a testis.* _____ / _____ / _____

Competency Verification: Check your labeling of Figure 9–3 in Appendix B: Answer Key, page 591.

Boldface indicates a word root or combining form. Blue indicates a suffix. Pink indicates a prefix.

SECTION REVIEW 9-3

Using the following table, write the CF, suffix, or prefix that matches its definition in the space provided to the left of the definition. There may be more than one word element that matches a definition.

Combining Forms		Suffixes		Prefixes
adrenal/o	orch/o	-dipsia	-pathy	hypo-
adren/o	pancreat/o	-gen	-pexy	para-
gluc/o	thym/o	-genesis	-phagia	poly-
glyc/o	toxic/o	-iasis	-rrhea	supra-
orchid/o		-lith	-uria	
orchi/o		-lysis		

1. _____ abnormal condition (produced by something specified)

2. _____ above; excessive; superior

3. _____ adrenal glands

4. _____ disease

5. _____ fixation (of an organ)

6. _____ discharge, flow

7. _____ many, much

8. _____ near, beside; beyond

9. _____ pancreas

10. _____ forming, producing, origin

11. _____ separation; destruction; loosening

12. _____ stone, calculus

13. _____ sugar, sweetness

14. _____ swallowing, eating

15. _____ testis (plural, testes)

16. _____ thirst

17. _____ thymus gland

18. _____ under, below, deficient

19. _____ urine

20. _____ poison

Competency Verification: Check your answers in Appendix B: Answer Key, page 591. If you are not satisfied with your level of comprehension, go back to Frame 9–40 and rework the frames.

Correct Answers _____ × 5 = _____ % Score

NERVOUS SYSTEM

The nervous system is an extensive, intricate network of structures that activates, coordinates, and controls the functions of all other body systems. It can be grouped into two main divisions: the **central nervous system (CNS)** and the **peripheral nervous system (PNS).** The CNS consists of the brain and spinal cord and is the control center of the body. The PNS consists of the peripheral nerves, which include the cranial nerves (emerging from the base of the skull) and the spinal nerves (emerging from the spinal cord). The PNS connects the CNS to remote body parts to relay and receive messages, and its autonomic nerves regulate involuntary functions of the internal organs.

Despite the complex organization of the nervous system, it consists of only two principal types of cells, **neurons** and **neuroglia.** Neurons are the basic structural and functional units of the nervous system. (See Fig. 9–7.) They are specialized to respond to physical and chemical stimuli, conduct electrochemical impulses, and release specific chemical regulators. Through these activities, neurons perform such functions as perceiving sensory stimuli, learning, remembering, and controlling muscles and glands. Neuroglia do not carry impulses, but perform the functions of support and protection. Many neuroglial (glial) cells form a supporting network by twining around nerve cells or lining certain structures in the brain and spinal cord. Others bind nervous tissue to supporting structures and attach the neurons to their blood vessels. Specialized glial cells are phagocytic. In other words, they protect the CNS from disease by engulfing invading microbes and clearing away debris. Neuroglia are of clinical interest because they are a common source of tumors (gliomas) of the nervous system.

As illustrated in Figure 9–7, the (1) **dendrites** are branching processes (extensions) that transmit impulses toward the (2) **cell body,** which contains the (3) **nucleus.** The integrated signals in the cell body are then transmitted to the (4) **axon,** a single projection which extends to the neuron's target cell or tissue. Surrounding the axon is a fatty coating called the (5) **myelin sheath.** The sheath insulates the axon and speeds the transmission of electrical impulses. Due to their fatty coating, myelinated axons take on a whitish appearance. Because of this, groups of myelinated axons constitute the "white matter" of the brain and spinal cord, while cell bodies of neurons that are not covered by a myelin sheath appear gray and are referred to as the "gray matter."

The axon of one neuron does not actually touch the dendrite of the next neuron. Instead, there is a space or (6) **synapse** between the two neurons. The transmission of the impulse across the synapse depends on the release of a chemical substance called a (7) **neurotransmitter.** The neurotransmitter crosses the synapse and binds to (8) **receptor sites** on the dendrites of the next neuron. Ultimately this creates another electrical impulse that continues through the next neuron until the target cell is reached. All of this occurs within a fraction of a second.

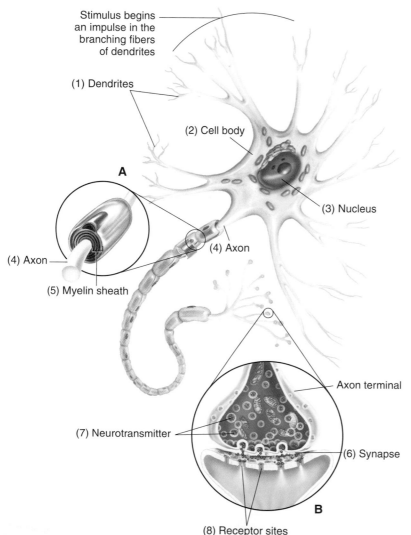

Stimulus begins an impulse in the branching fibers of dendrites

(1) Dendrites

(2) Cell body

(3) Nucleus

A

(4) Axon

(4) Axon

(5) Myelin sheath

Axon terminal

(7) Neurotransmitter

(6) Synapse

B

(8) Receptor sites

Figure 9-7 Neuron. (**A**) Myelin sheath. (**B**) Axon terminal synapse.

WORD ELEMENTS

This section introduces CFs related to the nervous system. Included are key suffixes; prefixes are defined in the right-hand column as needed. Review the following table and pronounce each word in the word analysis column aloud before you begin to work the frames.

Word Element	Meaning	Word Analysis
Combining Forms		
cephal/o	head	**hydro/cephal/us** (hī-drō-SĔF-ă-lŭs): condition of an enlarged cranium (portion of the skull that encloses the brain) *hydro:* water *-us:* condition; structure *Hydrocephalus is caused by an accumulation of fluid within the ventricles of the brain.*
cerebr/o	cerebrum	**cerebr/o/spin/al** (sĕr-ĕ-brō-SPĪ-năl): pertaining to the brain and spinal cord *spin:* spine *-al:* pertaining to
encephal/o	brain	**encephal/itis** (ĕn-sĕf-ă-LĪ-tĭs): inflammation of the brain (tissue) *-itis:* inflammation
gli/o	glue; neuroglial tissue	**gli/oma** (glī-Ō-mă): tumor composed of neuroglial tissue (supportive tissue of the nervous system) *-oma:* tumor
mening/o	meninges (membranes covering the brain and spinal cord)	**mening/o/cele** (mĕn-ĬN-gō-sēl): saclike protrusion of the meninges through the skull or vertebral column *-cele:* hernia, swelling *Meningocele is a congenital defect (occurs at birth) and can be repaired by surgery.*
meningi/o		**meningi/oma** (mĕn-ĭn-jē-Ō-mă): tumor composed of meninges *-oma:* tumor
myel/o	bone marrow; spinal cord	**myel/algia** (mī-ĕl-ĂL-jē-ă): pain of the spinal cord or its membranes *-algia:* pain
neur/o	nerve	**neur/o/lysis** (nū-RŎL-ĭs-ĭs): destruction of a nerve *-lysis:* separation; destruction; loosening
Suffixes		
-paresis	partial paralysis	**hemi/paresis** (hĕm-ē-pă-RĒ-sĭs): paralysis of one half of the body (right half or left half) *hemi-:* one half
-phasia	speech	**a/phasia** (ă-FĀ-zē-ă): absence of speech *a-:* without, not *Aphasia is an abnormal neurological condition in which language function is defective or absent because of an injury to certain areas of the cerebral cortex.*
-plegia	paralysis	**quadri/plegia** (kwŏd-rĭ-PLĒ-jē-ă): paralysis of all four extremities *quadri-:* four

Pronunciation Help	Long sound	ā in rāte	ē in rēbirth	ī in īsle	ō in ōver	ū in ūnite
	Short sound	ă in ălone	ĕ in ĕver	ĭ in ĭt	ŏ in nŏt	ŭ in cŭt

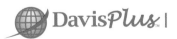 | Visit the *Medical Terminology Simplified* online resource center at Davis*Plus* for an audio exercise of the terms in this table. It will help you master pronunciations and meanings of medical terms.

SECTION REVIEW 9-4

For the following medical terms, first write the suffix and its meaning. Then translate the meaning of the remaining elements starting with the first part of the word. The first word is completed for you.

Term	Meaning
1. meningi/oma	-oma: tumor; meninges
2. neur/o/lysis	
3. hemi/paresis	
4. myel/algia	
5. cerebr/o/spin/al	
6. a/phasia	
7. mening/o/cele	
8. encephal/itis	
9. gli/oma	
10. quadri/plegia	

Competency Verification: Check your answers in Appendix B: Answer Key, page 591. If you are not satisfied with your level of comprehension, review the terms in the word elements table and retake the review.

Correct Answers _____ × 10 = _____ % Score

Brain

The brain is one of the most complicated organs in the human body, as it coordinates almost every physical and mental activity of the body. Although little is known about the mechanisms by which the brain regulates and coordinates all of the body's voluntary and involuntary activities, it is clear that the primary control over various functional activities is localized to different areas of the brain.

encephala/itis ĕn-sĕf-ă-LĪ-tĭs **encephala/oma** ĕn-sĕf-ă-lō-mă	**9-81** The CF *encephal/o* refers to the brain. Build a word that means *inflammation of brain (tissue):* _____ / _____ *tumor of the brain:* _____ / _____

9-82   The brain is divided into three major divisions for discussion. The first is the (1) **cerebrum,** which is the largest and uppermost portion of the brain. A thin layer known as the **cerebral cortex** covers the entire cerebrum and is composed of gray matter. Different areas of the cerebral cortex are responsible for most higher mental functions, including vision, speech, voluntary movements, memory, and reasoning. Label the cerebrum in Figure 9–8.

Boldface indicates a word root or combining form. Blue indicates a suffix. Pink indicates a prefix.

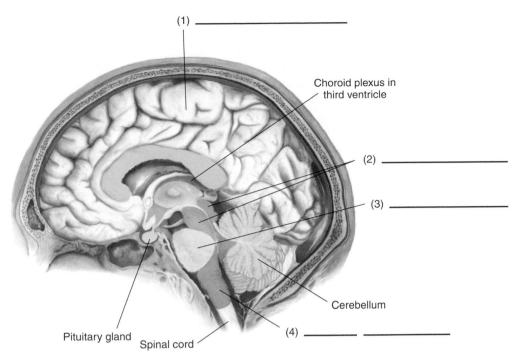

(1) _____

Choroid plexus in
third ventricle

(2) _____

(3) _____

Cerebellum

Pituitary gland

Spinal cord

(4) _____ _____

Figure 9-8 Structures of the brain.

---

cerebr/al sĕ-RĒ-brăl	**9–83** The CF *cerebr/o* refers to the cerebrum. Build a word that means *pertaining to the cerebrum.* _____ / _____
cerebr/o/tomy sĕr-ĕ-BRŎT-ō-mē	**9–84** Combine *cerebr/o* and *-tomy* to form a surgical procedure that means *incision of the cerebrum.* _____ / _____ / _____
	9–85 The more rudimentary processes are regulated by the **brainstem**, which consists of the (2) **midbrain**, the (3) **pons**, and the (4) **medulla.** Attached to the brainstem is the cerebellum, which plays a role in equilibrium, posture, and muscular coordination. Locate and label these structures in Figure 9–8.
inferior	**9–86** The **brainstem** is the site where motor neurons cross from one side of the body to the other, so that the right half of the brain controls movement involving the left side of the body and vice versa. Locate the brainstem in Figure 9-8. The brainstem lies (inferior or superior) _____ to the cerebrum.
superior	**9–87** The **pons** is part of the brainstem that literally means *bridge*. It contains nerve tracts that connect the cerebellum and cerebrum with the rest of the brain. Nerves to the eyes and face lie in the pons. Locate the pons in Figure 9–8. The pons lies (inferior or superior) _____ to the spinal cord.

vasomotor VĂ-sō-mō-tor **cardiac** KĂR-dē-ăk **respiratory** RĔS-pĭ-ră-tor-ē	**9–88** The **medulla** contains three vital centers that regulate internal activities of the body. The **cardiac center** slows the heart rate when the heart is beating too rapidly; the **respiratory center** controls muscles of respiration in response to chemicals or other stimuli; and the **vasomotor center** affects (constricts or dilates) the muscles in the walls of blood vessels, thus influencing blood pressure. The vital center that influences blood pressure by dilating or constricting blood vessel walls is the _____ center. The _____ center slows heart rate when it is beating too rapidly. The _____ center controls respiratory muscles in response to chemicals or other stimuli.

Competency Verification: Check your labeling of Figure 9–8 in Appendix B: Answer Key, page 592.

Spinal Cord

The spinal cord is a long, narrow cable of nervous tissue within the spinal canal and is part of the CNS. It descends from the brainstem to the lumbar part of the back and contains about 100 million neurons. Thirty-one pairs of spinal nerves originate from the spinal cord. (See Fig. 9–9.) Each pair of nerves serves a specific region on the right or left side of the body. Spinal nerves are mixed nerves that provide a two-way communication between the spinal cord and parts of the upper and lower limbs, neck, and trunk.

	9–89 Spin/al nerves are named according to locations of their respective vertebrae. As shown in Figure 9–9, there are 8 pairs of cervic/al nerves, identified as C1–C8; 12 pairs of thorac/ic nerves, identified as T1–T12; 5 pairs of lumb/ar nerves, identified as L1–L5; 5 pairs of sacr/al nerves, identified as S1–S5; and 1 pair of coccyg/eal nerves, identified as Co1. In Figure 9–9, label the (1) **cervical nerves**, (2) **thoracic nerves**, (3) **lumbar nerves**, (4) **sacral nerves**, and (5) **coccygeal nerve**.
cervic/al nerves SĔR-vĭ-kăl **thorac/ic nerves** thō-RĂS-ĭk **sacr/al nerves** SĀ-krăl	**9–90** Build medical words that mean *pertaining to nerves* *of the neck:* _____ / _____ _____ *in back of the chest:* _____ / _____ _____ *of the sacrum:* _____ / _____ _____
spin/al SPĪ-năl **cerebr/o/spin/al** sĕr-ē-brō-SPĪ-năl	**9–91** The spin/al cord, like the brain, is protected and nourished by the meninges, which consist of three layers: **dura mater,** the outermost membrane; **arachnoid membrane,** the second layer, which surrounds the brain and spin/al cord; and **pia mater,** the third layer, which is closest to the brain and spinal cord. Additional protection is provided by cerebr/o/spin/al fluid circulating in the subarachnoid space. (See Fig. 9–9.) Identify terms in this frame that mean *pertaining to* *the spine:* _____ / _____ *the cerebrum and the spine:* _____ / _____ / _____

Boldface indicates a word root or combining form. Blue indicates a suffix. Pink indicates a prefix.

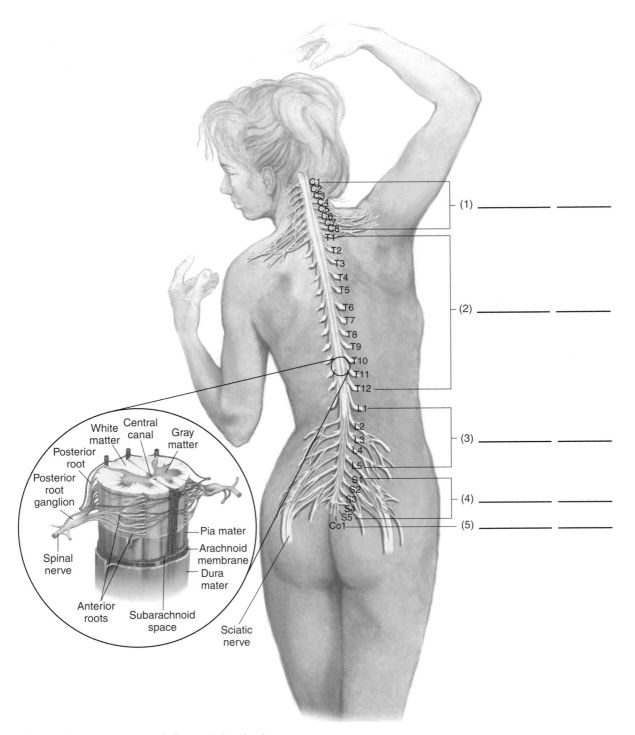

Figure 9-9 Spinal nerves. (A) Spinal chord enlargement.

mening/itis měn-ĭn-JĪ-tĭs **mening/o/cele** měn-ĬN-gō-sēl **meningi/oma** měn-ĭn-jē-Ō-mă	**9–92** *Mening/o* and *meningi/o* refer to the meninges (membranes covering the brain and spinal cord). Use *mening/o* to build a word that means *inflammation of the meninges:* _____ / _____ *hernia or swelling of the meninges:* _____ / _____ / _____ Use *meningi/o* to build a word that means *tumor of the meninges.* _____ / _____
cerebr/o/spin/al sĕr-ē-brō-SPĪ-năl	**9–93** The outer layer of the spinal cord, the **dura mater,** is a tough, fibrous membrane that covers the entire length of the spinal cord and contains channels for blood to enter brain tissue. The middle layer, the **arachnoid,** runs across the space known as the **sub/dur/al space,** which contains cerebr/o/spin/al fluid (CSF). The innermost layer, the **pia mater,** is a thin membrane containing many blood vessels that nourish the spinal cord. The fluid that circulates in the subarachnoid space and protects the brain and spinal cord is known as _____ / _____ / _____ / _____ fluid.
epi- **dur** **-al**	**9–94** The space between the pia mater and the bones of the spinal cord is called the epi/dur/al space. It contains blood vessels and some fat. It is the space into which anesthetics may be injected to dull pain or contrast material may be injected for certain diagnostic procedures. Identify the elements in this frame that mean *above, upon:* _____ *dura mater; hard:* _____ *pertaining to:* _____
mening/o/cele měn-ĬN-gō-sēl	**9–95** Herniation of the meninges may occur through a defect in the skull or spinal cord. When herniation of the meninges occurs, the condition is called _____ / _____ / _____ .
myel/itis mī-ě-LĪ-tĭs **myel/o/pathy** mī-ě-LŎP-ă-thē **myel/o/tome** mī-ĚL-ō-tōm	**9–96** The CF *myel/o* means *bone marrow; spinal cord.* Build medical words that mean *inflammation of the spinal cord:* _____ / _____ *any disease of the spinal cord:* _____ / _____ / _____ *instrument to cut or dissect the spinal cord:* _____ / _____ / _____

Competency Verification: Check your labeling of Figure 9–9 in Appendix B: Answer Key, page 592.

Boldface indicates a word root or combining form. Blue indicates a suffix. Pink indicates a prefix.

back (of body)

nerve

belly, belly side

9-97 Each spin/al nerve has two roots, which are neurons entering or leaving the spinal cord. The dors/al root is made of sensory neurons that carry impulses into the spinal cord. The ventr/al root is the motor root. It is made of motor neurons carrying impulses from the spin/al cord to muscles or glands. The cell bodies of these motor neurons are in the gray matter of the spin/al cord. When the two nerve roots merge, the spin/al nerve formed is a mixed nerve.

Provide the meaning for the following CFs:

dors/o: _____ (_____ _____)

neur/o: _____

ventr/o: _____, _____ _____

---

neur/algia
nū-RĂL-jē-ă

neur/itis
nū-RĪ-tĭs

neur/oma
nū-RŌ-mă

neur/o/pathy
nū-RŎP-ă-thē

9-98 Use *neur/o* to form medical terms that mean

pain in a nerve: _____ / _____

inflammation of a nerve: _____ / _____

tumor of nerve (tissue): _____ / _____

any disease of nerves: _____ / _____ / _____

---

myel/itis
mī-ĕ-LĪ-tĭs

myel/o/malacia
mī-ĕ-lō-mă-LĀ-shē-ă

myel/oma
mī-ĕ-LŌ-mă

9-99 Use *myel/o* to form medical words that mean

inflammation of the spinal cord: _____ / _____

softening of the spinal cord: _____ / _____ / _____

tumor of bone marrow: _____ / _____

---

cell

thromb/o/cyte
THRŎM-bō-sīt

9-100 The CF *thromb/o* refers to a blood clot. A thromb/o/cyte is a blood-clotting _____.

A thromb/o/cyte (platelet) promotes the formation of clots and prevents bleeding. Another name for platelet is _____ / _____ / _____.

---

clot

9-101 Although the terms embolus and thrombus denote a disorder related to a clot, they both have different meanings. An **embolus** is a clot present in blood or lymphatic vessels and brought there by blood or lymph. A **thrombus** is a clot that adheres to the wall of a blood vessel or organ and may obstruct the vessel or organ in which it resides, preventing the flow of blood.

The term thromb/o/lysis refers to the destruction or loosening of a blood _____.

---

thromb/o/genesis
thrŏm-bō-JĔN-ĕ-sĭs

9-102 Use *-genesis* to form a word that means *producing, forming, or origin of a blood clot.*

_____ / _____ / _____

hem/o/rrhage
HĔM-ĕ-rĭj

cerebr/o/vascul/ar
sĕr-ĕ-brō-VĂS-kū-lăr

thrombus
THRŎM-bŭs

9–103   A **stroke**, also called **cerebr/o/vascul/ar accident (CVA)**, is the rapid loss of brain function due to disturbance of the normal blood supply (**ischemia**) to the brain. This can be due to occlusion from an embolus or thrombus (**ischemic stroke**) or a ruptured blood vessel (**hemorrhagic stroke**). The resulting neur/o/logic/al symptoms vary according to the location of the obstruction and extent of brain tissue affected.

Write the terms in this frame that mean

bursting forth (of) blood: _____ / _____ / _____

pertaining to the cerebrum and blood vessels:

_____ / _____ / _____ / _____

stationary blood clot: _____

---

aneurysm/ectomy
ăn-ū-rĭz-MĔK-tō-mē

9–104   Stroke caused by hem/o/rrhage from a cerebral artery is commonly fatal. It usually results from high blood pressure, atherosclerosis, or the bursting of an arterial aneurysm (localized dilation of the blood vessel wall). The CF *aneurysm/o* means *a widening or a widened blood vessel.*

Use *aneurysm/o* to construct a medical word that means *excision of an aneurysm.*

_____ / _____

---

neur/o/glia
nū-RŎG-lē-ă

9–105   As discussed earlier, the entire nervous system is composed of two principal types of cells, neurons and neuroglia. The supporting cells in the CNS collectively are called neur/o/glia.

A term that literally means *nerve glue* is _____ / _____ / _____.

---

neur/o/cyte
NŪ-rō-sīt

9–106   A neur/o/cyte, commonly called a neuron, is a nerve cell. A term that literally means *nerve cell* is _____ / _____ / _____.

Mental Disorders

A **mental disorder**, also called **mental illness, psychiatric disorder,** or **emotional illness,** is a psychological pattern potentially reflected in behavior that is generally associated with distress or disability and that is not considered part of normal development. These disorders are generally defined by a combination of how a person feels, behaves, thinks, or perceives. The disorder may be associated with particular regions or functions of the brain or the rest of the nervous system, often in a social context. In most cases, mental illness symptoms can be managed with a combination of medications and counseling (psychotherapy). Examples of mental illness include depression, anxiety disorders, schizophrenia, eating disorders, and addictive behaviors.

---

carcin/o/phobia
KĂR-sĭn-ō-fō-bē-ă

9–107   Besides path/o/logical conditions, which were discussed earlier in this chapter, some CFs and suffixes are used to identify mental disorders. For example, phob/ic disorders are anxiety disorders characterized by extreme and irrational fear or social situations. The suffix *-phobia,* which means *fear,* is a general suffix used to describe all types of fears.

A person who has an extreme fear of cancer suffers from a phobia known as

_____ / _____ / _____.

Boldface indicates a word root or combining form. Blue indicates a suffix. Pink indicates a prefix.

xen/o/phobia zĕn-ō-FŌ-bē-ă	**9-108** The CF *xen/o* means *foreign or strange*. Combine *xen/o* and *-phobia* to identify the disorder of a person who has a fear of strangers. _____ / ____ / _____
necr/o/phobia nĕk-rō-FŌ-bē-ă	**9-109** The CF *necr/o* means *death* or *necrosis*. A person who has a fear of corpses or death suffers from the phobia known as _____ / ____ / _____.
fear	**9-110** Whenever you see *-phobia* in a term, you will know it means _____ and refers to an anxiety disorder.
neur/osis nū-RŌ-sĭs **neur/oses** nū-RŌ-sēz	**9-111** Earlier in this chapter, you learned that *neur/o* refers to a nerve. The CF *neur/o* is also used to form words that refer to mental disorders. For example, neur/osis is an emotional disorder that involves an ineffective way of coping with anxiety or inner conflict. Build a word that means *abnormal condition of nerves:* _____ / _____ The plural form of *neur/osis* is _____ / _____.
psych/iatry sī-KĪ-ă-trē	**9-112** The CF *psych/o* means *mind;* the suffix *-iatry* means *physician, treatment.* The medical specialty concerned with diagnosis and treatment of mental disorders is _____ / _____.
psych/o/therapy sī-kō-THĔR-ă-pē	**9-113** *Psych/o* is used to form words about a mental condition that represents a marked distortion of or sharp break from reality and is a serious cognitive disorder. Combine *psych/o* and *-therapy* to form a word that means *treatment of the mind (mental condition).* _____ / ____ / _____
psych/o/ses sī-KŌ-sēz	**9-114** What is the plural form of psych/osis? _____ / ____ / _____
	9-115 Some psychoses are identified with the suffix *-mania,* which means a *state of mental disorder or frenzy.* Examples include klept/o/mania (the urge to steal items you don't need and that usually have little value) and pyr/o/mania (the urge to start fires).
schiz/o/phren/ia skĭz-ō-FRĔN-ē-ă	**9-116** Schiz/o/phren/ia is a psych/osis that commonly involves delusions, such as believing that someone or something is controlling your thoughts. Another of its manifestations is hallucinations, most commonly "hearing" voices or other sounds. Use the CF *schiz/o,* meaning *split,* and *phren/o,* meaning *mind,* along with the suffix *-ia* to build the term for a *psychiatric disorder characterized by delusions, hallucinations, or both.* _____ / ____ / _____ / _____

Pronunciation Help	Long sound	ā in rāte	ē in rēbirth	ī in īsle	ō in ōver	ū in ūnite
	Short sound	ă in ălone	ĕ in ĕver	ĭ in ĭt	ŏ in nŏt	ŭ in cŭt

SECTION REVIEW 9-5

Using the following table, write the CF, suffix, or prefix that matches its definition in the space provided to the left of the definition. There may be more than one word element that matches a definition.

Combining Forms

cerebr/o	myel/o
encephal/o	neur/o
gli/o	scler/o
meningi/o	thromb/o
mening/o	vascul/o

Suffixes

-glia	-rrhagia
-malacia	
-osis	
-phasia	
-rrhage	

Prefixes

a-
dys-

1. _____ abnormal condition; increase (used primarily with blood cells)

2. _____ bad; painful; difficult

3. _____ blood clot

4. _____ vessel

5. _____ brain

6. _____ bursting forth (of)

7. _____ glue; neuroglial tissue

8. _____ hardening; sclera (white of the eye)

9. _____ meninges (membranes covering the brain and spinal cord)

10. _____ nerve

11. _____ cerebrum

12. _____ softening

13. _____ speech

14. _____ bone marrow; spinal cord

15. _____ without, not

Competency Verification: Check your answers in Appendix B: Answer Key, page 592. If you are not satisfied with your level of comprehension, go back to Frame 9–81 and rework the frames.

Correct Answers _____ × 6.67 = _____ % Score

ABBREVIATIONS

This section introduces endocrine and nervous system–related abbreviations and their meanings.

Abbreviation	Meaning	Abbreviation	Meaning
Endocrine System			
ADH	antidiuretic hormone	GTT	glucose tolerance test
ACTH	adenocorticotropic hormone	HRT	hormone replacement therapy
ALS	amyotrophic lateral sclerosis	LH	luteinizing hormone
BMI	body mass index	OGTT	oral glucose tolerance test
BG	blood glucose	PGH	pituitary growth hormone
DM	diabetes mellitus	PTH	parathyroid hormone
FBG	fasting blood glucose	RAIU	radioactive iodine uptake
GH	growth hormone	TSH	thyroid-stimulating hormone
Nervous System			
C1, C2, and so on	first cervical vertebra, second cervical vertebra, and so on	L1, L2, and so on	first lumbar vertebra, second lumbar vertebra, and so on
CNS	central nervous system	LP	lumbar puncture
CP	cerebral palsy	MS	mitral stenosis; musculoskeletal; multiple sclerosis; mental status; magnesium sulfate
CSF	cerebrospinal fluid	S1, S2, and so on	first sacral vertebra, second sacral vertebra, and so on
CVA	cerebrovascular accident; costovertebral angle	T1, T2, and so on	first thoracic vertebra, second thoracic vertebra, and so on
EEG	electroencephalogram	TIA	transient ischemic attack
Radiographic Procedures			
AP	anteroposterior	MRI	magnetic resonance imaging
CT	computed tomography	MSI	magnetic source imaging
IV	intravenous	PA	posteroanterior
MEG	magnetoencephalography	PET	positron emission tomography

ADDITIONAL MEDICAL TERMS

The following are additional terms related to the endocrine and nervous systems. Recognizing and learning these terms will help you understand the connection between a pathological condition, its diagnosis, and the rationale behind the method of treatment selected for a particular disorder.

Diseases and Conditions

Endocrine System

Addison disease
Ă-dĭ-sŭn

Rare chronic disorder caused by a deficiency of cortical hormones that results when the adrenal cortex is damaged or atrophied and can be life threatening

Atrophy of adrenal glands is usually the result of an autoimmune process in which circulating adrenal antibodies slowly destroy the gland.

Cushing syndrome
KOOSH-ing

Cluster of symptoms caused by excessive amounts of cortisol or adrenocorticotropic hormone (ACTH) circulating in the blood

Most cases of Cushing syndrome are caused by administration of glucocorticoids in the treatment of immune disorders, such as asthma, rheumatoid arthritis, and lupus erythematosus.

diabetes mellitus (DM) dī-ă-BĒ-tēz MĔ-lĭ-tŭs	Chronic metabolic disorder of impaired carbohydrate, protein, and fat metabolism due to insufficient production of insulin or the body's inability to use insulin properly *When used alone, the term diabetes refers to diabetes mellitus. Hyperglycemia and ketosis are responsible for its host of troubling and commonly life-threatening symptoms. Diabetes mellitus occurs in two primary forms: type 1 diabetes and type 2 diabetes.*
type 1 diabetes	Form of diabetes mellitus that is abrupt in onset and due to the failure of the pancreas to produce insulin, making this type of disease difficult to regulate *Type 1 diabetes is usually diagnosed in children and young adults. Treatment includes insulin injections to maintain a normal level of glucose in the blood.*
type 2 diabetes	Form of diabetes mellitus that is gradual in onset and results from the body's deficiency in producing enough insulin or resistance to the action of insulin by the body's cells *Type 2 is the most common form of diabetes. It is usually diagnosed in adults older than age 40. Management of this disease is less problematic than that of type 1. Treatment includes diet, weight loss, and exercise. It may also include insulin or oral antidiabetic agents, which activate the release of pancreatic insulin and improve the body's sensitivity to insulin.*
Graves disease grāvz	Multisystem autoimmune disorder that involves growth of the thyroid (hyperthyroidism) associated with hypersecretion of thyroxine; also called *exophthalmic goiter,* *thyrotoxicosis,* or *toxic goiter* *Graves disease is characterized by an enlarged thyroid gland and exophthalmos (bulging of the eyes), which develops because of edema in the tissues of the eye sockets and swelling of the extrinsic eye muscles. (See Fig. 9–4.)*

insulinoma
ĭn-sū-lĭn-Ō-mă
  insulin: insulin
  -oma: tumor
	Tumor of the islets of Langerhans; also called *pancreatic tumor*
	
	Insulinoma is a rare tumor that secretes insulin and causes hypoglycemia.

myxedema
mĭks-ĕ-DĒ-mă
  myx: mucus
  -edema: swelling
	Advanced form of hypothyroidism in adults that results from hypofunction of the thyroid gland and affects body fluids, causing edema
	
	Myxedema also increases blood volume and blood pressure.

pancreatitis
păn-krē-I-tĭs
  pancreat: pancreas
  -itis: inflammation
	Inflammation of the pancreas that occurs when pancreatic enzymes that digest food are activated in the pancreas instead of the duodenum and attack pancreatic tissue, causing damage to the gland
	
	The two most common causes of pancreatitis are alcoholism and biliary tract disease, such as a gallstone that blocks the lower common bile duct and causes pancreatic enzymes to back up into the pancreas. Treatment includes abstaining from alcohol, maintaining fluid volume, taking medication to decrease pancreatic secretions, relieving pain, treating infection, and undergoing choledocholithotomy to remove the gallstone.

panhypopituitarism păn-hī-pō-pĭ-TŪ-ĭ-tăr-ĭzm *pan-:* all *hyp/o:* under, below, deficient *pituitar:* pituitary gland *-ism:* condition	Total pituitary impairment that brings about a progressive and general loss of hormone activity
pheochromocytoma fē-ō-krō-mō-sī-TŌ-mă	Rare adrenal gland tumor that causes excessive release of epinephrine (adrenaline) and norepinephrine (hormones that regulate heart rate and blood pressure) and induces severe blood pressure elevation

Nervous System

Alzheimer disease ĂLTS-hī-měr	Chronic, organic mental disorder that is a progressive form of presenile dementia caused by atrophy of the frontal and occipital lobes of the brain *The onset of Alzheimer disease usually occurs between ages 40 and 60. It involves progressive irreversible loss of memory, deterioration of intellectual functions, apathy, speech and gait disturbances, and disorientation. The course may take from a few months to 4 or 5 years to progress to complete loss of intellectual function.*
amyotrophic lateral sclerosis (ALS) ă-mī-ō-TRŌ-fĭk, sklĕ-RŌ-sĭs	Degenerative disorder in which the progressive loss of motor neurons in the spinal cord and brainstem leads to muscle weakness and paralysis; also called Lou Gehrig disease (named after the baseball player who became afflicted with ALS) *ALS manifests in adulthood with symptoms of weakness and atrophy of muscles in the hands, forearms, and legs; difficulty in swallowing and talking; and dyspnea as the throat and respiratory muscles become affected. The cause of and cure for ALS are unknown.*
epilepsy ĔP-ĭ-lĕp-sē	Neurological disorder in which the nerve cell activity in the brain is disturbed, causing a seizure, including loss of consciousness *Epilepsy has many possible causes, including illness, brain injury, and abnormal brain development. Seizure symptoms vary. Some people with epilepsy simply stare blankly for a few seconds during a seizure, while others repeatedly twitch their arms or legs.*
Huntington chorea HŬN-tĭng-tŭn kō-RĒ-ă	Hereditary nervous disorder caused by the progressive loss of brain cells, leading to bizarre, involuntary, dancelike movements

multiple sclerosis (MS) MŬL-tĭ-pl sklĕ-RŌ-sĭs *scler:* hardening; sclera (white of the eye) *-osis:* abnormal condition; increase (used primarily with blood cells)	Progressive degenerative disease of the central nervous system characterized by inflammation, hardening, and loss of myelin throughout the spinal cord and brain, which produces weakness and other muscle symptoms
neuroblastoma nū-rō-blăs-TŌ-mă *neur/o:* nerve *blast:* embryonic cell *-oma:* tumor	Malignant tumor composed principally of cells resembling neuroblasts *Neuroblastoma occurs most commonly in infants and children.*
palsy PAWL-zē	Partial or complete loss of motor function
Bell palsy	Facial paralysis on one side of the face because of inflammation of a facial nerve (cranial nerve VII), most likely caused by a viral infection *Bell palsy commonly results in grotesque facial disfigurement and facial spasms. Treatment includes corticosteroid drugs to decrease nerve swelling. Ordinarily, the condition lasts a month and resolves by itself.*
cerebral palsy (CP) SĔR-ĕ-brăl *cerebr:* cerebrum *-al:* pertaining to	Bilateral, symmetrical, nonprogressive motor dysfunction and partial paralysis, which is usually caused by damage to the cerebrum during gestation or birth trauma but can also be hereditary
paralysis pă-RĂL-ĭ-sĭs	Loss of voluntary motion due to an inability to contract one or more muscles *Paralysis may be caused by a variety of problems, such as head trauma, spinal cord injury, and stroke. Paralysis may be classified according to the cause, muscle tone, distribution, or body part affected. (See Fig. 9–10.)*
paraplegia păr-ă-PLĒ-jē-ă *para:* near, beside; beyond *-plegia:* paralysis	Paralysis of the lower portion of the body and both legs *Paraplegia results in loss of sensory and motor control below the level of injury. Other common problems occurring with spinal cord injury to the lumbar and thoracic regions include loss of bladder, bowel, and sexual control.*
quadriplegia kwŏd-rĭ-PLĒ-jē-ă *quadri:* four *-plegia:* paralysis	Paralysis of all four extremities and, usually, the trunk *Quadriplegia generally results in loss of motor and sensory function below the level of injury. Paralysis includes the trunk, legs, and pelvic organs with partial or total paralysis in the upper extremities. The higher the trauma, the more debilitating the motor and sensory impairments will be.*

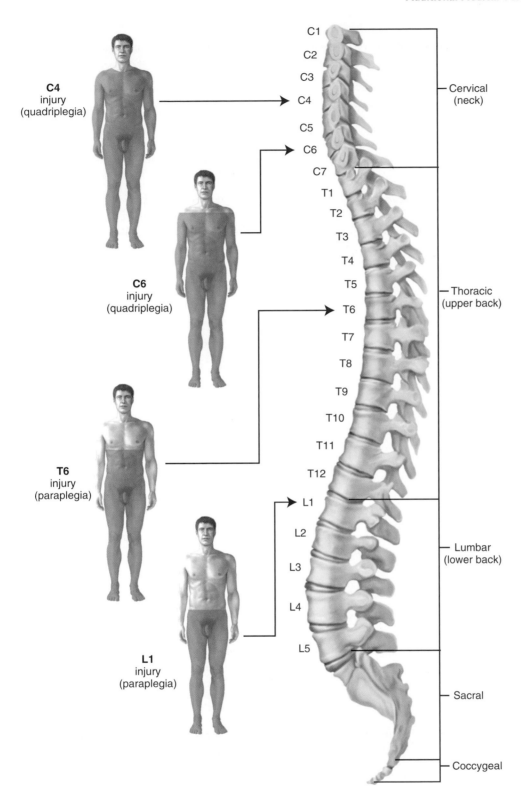

C4 injury (quadriplegia)

C6 injury (quadriplegia)

T6 injury (paraplegia)

L1 injury (paraplegia)

C1
C2
C3
C4
C5
C6
C7

Cervical (neck)

T1
T2
T3
T4
T5
T6
T7
T8
T9
T10
T11
T12

Thoracic (upper back)

L1
L2
L3
L4
L5

Lumbar (lower back)

Sacral

Coccygeal

Figure 9-10 Spinal cord injuries showing the extent of paralysis.

Parkinson disease PĂR-kĭn-sŭn	Progressive, degenerative neurological disorder affecting the portion of the brain responsible for controlling movement *The unnecessary skeletal muscle movements of Parkinson disease commonly interfere with voluntary movement—for example, causing the hand to shake (called tremor), the most common symptom of Parkinson disease.*
poliomyelitis pō-lē-ō-mī-ĕl-Ī-tĭs *poli/o:* gray; gray matter (of the brain or spinal cord) *myel:* bone marrow; spinal cord *-itis:* inflammation	Disease in which the gray matter of the spinal cord is destroyed by a slow-acting virus, eventually leading to paralysis and muscular atrophy *Vaccines have made poliomyelitis, commonly known as polio, relatively uncommon in the United States. Nevertheless, postpolio syndrome is a complication that develops in some patients, usually 30 or more years after they are first infected. Muscles that were already weak may get weaker. Weakness may also develop in muscles that were not affected before.*
sciatica sī-ĂT-ĭ-kă	Severe pain in the leg along the course of the sciatic nerve, which travels from the hip to the foot
seizure SĒ-zhŭr	Abnormal, uncontrolled discharge of electrical activity in the brain, which is commonly a symptom of underlying brain pathology; also called *convulsion* *Chronic, recurrent seizures are a characteristic symptom of epilepsy.*
tonic-clonic (grand mal)	Seizure characterized by unconsciousness with excessive motor activity and the body alternating between excessive muscle tone with rigidity (tonic) and involuntary muscular contractions (clonic) in the extremities *Tonic-clonic seizures last about 1 to 2 minutes. Other symptoms include tongue biting, difficulty breathing, and incontinence. The recovery after a seizure is known as the postictal period.*
absence (petit mal)	Seizure characterized by a brief, sudden, loss of consciousness lasting only a few seconds *A person can have many absence seizures during the course of the day.*
shingles SHĬNG-lz	Eruption of acute, inflammatory, herpetic vesicles on the trunk of the body along a peripheral nerve *Shingles is caused by the herpes zoster virus.*
spina bifida SPĪ-nă BĬF-ĭ-dă	Congenital neural tube defect characterized by incomplete closure of the spinal canal through which the spinal cord and meninges may or may not protrude *Spina bifida usually occurs in the lumbosacral area and has several forms. (See Fig. 9–11.)*
spina bifida occulta SPĪ-nă BĬF-ĭ-dă ŏ-KŬL-tă	Most common and least severe form of spina bifida without protrusion of the spinal cord or meninges
spina bifida cystica SPĪ-nă BĬF-ĭ-dă SĬS-tĭk-ă	More severe type of spina bifida that involves protrusion of the meninges (meningocele), spinal cord (myelocele), or both (meningomyelocele). *The severity of neurological dysfunction in spina bifida cystica depends directly on the degree of nerve involvement.*

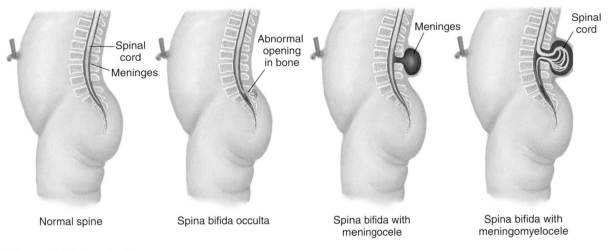

Figure 9-11 Spina bifida.

| transient ischemic attack (TIA)
TRĂN-zhĕnt ĭs-KĒ-mĭk
ischem: to hold back; block
-ic: pertaining to | Short episodes of neurological dysfunction due to temporary interference with blood supply to the brain, lasting a few minutes to a few hours; also called *ministroke*

TIAs may recur, and each TIA increases the risk of a subsequent stroke. The neurological symptoms range according to the amount of ischemia and the location of the vessels involved, but it does not destroy brain cells or cause permanent disability. |

Diagnostic Procedures

Endocrine System

fasting blood glucose (FBG)	Test that measures glucose levels in the blood after the patient has fasted (not eaten) for at least 8 hours; also called *fasting blood sugar (FBS)* *FBG helps determine if the pancreas is secreting a normal amount of insulin and diagnose other pancreatic disorders, such as diabetes and hypoglycemia.*
glucose tolerance test (GTT)	Screening test in which a patient fasts for 8 to 12 hours, ingests glucose, and then undergoes blood draws to determine how quickly the glucose is cleared from the blood; also called *oral glucose tolerance test (OGTT)* *GTT helps diagnose diabetes with higher accuracy than other blood glucose tests. It also helps diagnose gestational diabetes or rarer disorders of carbohydrate metabolism.*
radioactive iodine uptake (RAIU) test	Imaging procedure that measures levels of radioactivity in the thyroid after oral or IV administration of radioactive iodine *RAIU is used to determine thyroid function by monitoring the thyroid's ability to take up (uptake) iodine from the blood.*

Nervous System

cerebrospinal fluid (CSF) analysis sĕr-ĕ-brō-SPĪ-năl *cerebr/o:* cerebrum *spin:* spine *-al:* pertaining to	Laboratory test in which CSF obtained from a lumbar puncture is evaluated macroscopically for clarity and color, microscopically for cells, and chemically for proteins and other substances *CSF analysis helps detect bacteria, viruses, and tumor cells. The analysis also helps diagnose tumors, infection, or multiple sclerosis (MS).*
electroencephalography (EEG)	Diagnostic procedure in which electrodes on the scalp record patterns of electrical activity within the brain *EEG helps evaluate seizure disorders, periods of unconsciousness, and sleep disorders; monitors the brain during brain surgery; and determines if a person is in a coma or brain dead.*
lumbar puncture (LP) LŬM-băr *lumb:* loins (lower back) *-ar:* pertaining to	Insertion of a needle into the subarachnoid space of the spinal column at the level of the fourth intervertebral space to withdraw cerebral spinal fluid (CSF) in order to perform various diagnostic and therapeutic procedures; also called spinal tap or spinal puncture *In lumbar puncture, CSF flows through the needle and is collected and sent to the laboratory for analysis. Therapeutic procedures include withdrawing CSF to reduce intracranial pressure, introducing a local anesthetic to induce spinal anesthesia, and administering intrathecal medications. (See Fig. 9–12.)*
magnetoencephalography (MEG) măg-nĕt-ō-ĕn-cĕf-ă-LŎG-ră-fē	Noninvasive functional imaging technique in which magnetic forces associated with the electrical activity of the brain are recorded externally on the scalp *When the data from an MEG are superimposed on an anatomical image of the brain, typically an MRI scan, it produces a functional, anatomical image of the brain called magnetic source imaging (MSI). MSI aids in presurgical evaluation of patients with epilepsy to identify and localize areas of epileptic activity. MSI results in a high-resolution image that is a direct measure of brain function.*

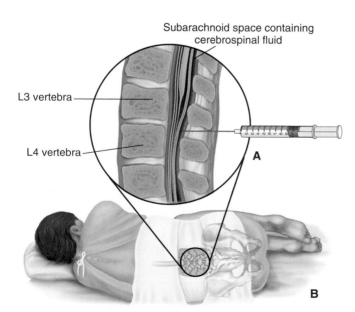

Subarachnoid space containing
cerebrospinal fluid

L3 vertebra

L4 vertebra

A

B

Figure 9-12 Lumbar puncture. (**A**) Collection of cerebrospinal fluid. (**B**) Position for lumbar puncture.

magnetic resonance imaging (MRI) măg-NĔT-ĭc RĔZ-ĕn-ăns ĬM-ĭj-ĭng	Radiographic technique that uses electromagnetic energy to produce multiplanar cross-sectional images of the body *MRI of the brain produces cross-sectional, frontal, and sagittal plane views of the brain. It is regarded as superior to CT for most CNS abnormalities, particularly those of the brainstem and spinal cord. A contrast medium is not required but may be used to enhance internal structure visualization.*
positron emission tomography (PET) PŎZ-ĭ-trŏn ē-MĬSH-ŭn tō-MŎG-ră-fē *tom/o:* to cut *-graphy:* process of recording	Radiographic technique that combines computed tomography with radiopharmaceuticals to produce a cross-sectional (transverse) image of the dispersement of radioactivity (through emission of positrons) in a section of the body, revealing areas where the radiopharmaceutical is metabolized and where metabolism is deficient *PET scanning aids in diagnosis of such neurological disorders as brain tumors, epilepsy, stroke, Alzheimer disease, and abdominal and pulmonary disorders.*

Medical and Surgical Procedures

Endocrine System

transsphenoidal hypophysectomy trăns-sfē-NOY-dăl hī-pō-fĭ-SĔK-tō-mē	Minimally invasive endoscopic surgery that removes pituitary tumors through the nasal cavity via the sphenoid sinus (transsphenoidal) without affecting brain tissue (See Fig. 9–13.) *Although most tumors can be removed via transsphenoidal hypophysectomy, some large tumors may need to be removed via transfrontal craniotomy (entry through the frontal bone of the skull).*

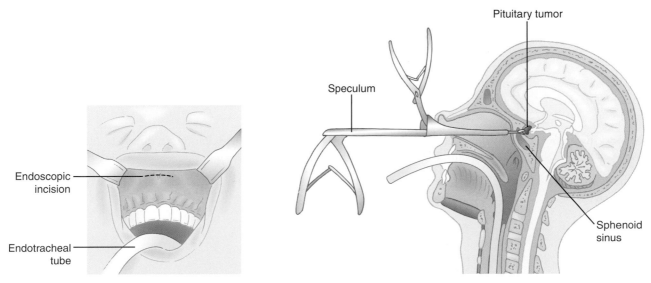

Figure 9-13 Transsphenoidal hypophysectomy. (**A**) Incision beneath the upper lip to enter the nasal cavity and gain access to the pituitary gland. (**B**) Insertion of a speculum and special forceps to remove the pituitary tumor.

Nervous System

craniotomy krā-nē-ŎT-ō-mē *crani/o:* cranium (skull) *-tomy:* incision	Surgical procedure that creates an opening in the skull to gain access to the brain during neurosurgical procedures *A craniotomy is also performed to relieve intracranial pressure, control bleeding, or remove a tumor.*
thalamotomy thăl-ă-MŎT-ō-mē *thalam/o:* thalamus *-tomy:* incision	Partial destruction of the thalamus to treat psychosis, intractable pain, or involuntary movements, including tremors in Parkinson disease
trephination trĕf-ĭn-Ā-shŭn	Excision of a circular disk of bone using a specialized saw called a trephine to reveal brain tissue during neurosurgery or to relieve intracranial pressure

PHARMACOLOGY

The following table lists common drug categories used to treat reproductive disorders, as well as their therapeutic actions.

Drug Category	Action
Endocrine System	
hormone replacement therapy (HRT)	Correct a deficiency in such hormones as estrogen, testosterone, or thyroid hormone *HRT may include oral administration or injection of synthetic hormones.*
oral hypoglycemics hī-pō-glī-SĒ-mĭcs	Stimulate insulin secretion from pancreatic cells in non–insulin-dependent diabetics with some pancreatic function
Nervous System	
anesthetics ăn-ĕs-THĔT-ĭks	Produce partial or complete loss of sensation, with or without loss of consciousness *General anesthetics act on the brain to produce complete loss of feeling with loss of consciousness. Local anesthetics act on nerves or nerve tracts to affect only a local area.*
anticonvulsants ăn-tĭ-kŏn-VŬL-sănts	Prevent or reduce the severity of epileptic or other convulsive seizures; also called *antiepileptics*
antiparkinsonian agents ăn-tĭ-păr-kĭn-SŌN-ē-ăn	Control tremors and muscle rigidity associated with Parkinson disease by increasing dopamine levels in the brain
antipsychotics ăn-tĭ-sī-KŎT-ĭkz	Alter neurotransmitters in the brain to alleviate symptoms of psychosis, paranoia, and schizophrenia

ADDITIONAL MEDICAL TERMS REVIEW

Match the medical terms below with the definitions in the numbered list.

Alzheimer disease	Huntington chorea	panhypopituitarism	sciatica
antipsychotics	hypophysectomy	Parkinson disease	shingles
Bell palsy	lumbar puncture	PET	spina bifida
EEG	MRI	pheochromocytoma	TIA
epilepsy	myxedema	poliomyelitis	thalamotomy
exophthalmos	neuroblastoma	quadriplegia	Type 1 diabetes
Graves disease			

1. _____ is facial paralysis on one side of the face because of inflammation of a facial nerve.

2. _____ describes short episodes of neurological dysfunction due to temporary interference with blood supply to the brain.

3. _____ are used to alter symptoms of psychosis and schizophrenia.

4. _____ is abnormal protrusion of eyeball, possibly due to thyrotoxicosis.

5. _____ means hyperthyroidism and is also called toxic goiter, which is characterized by exophthalmos.

6. _____ is a surgical procedure to remove a pituitary tumor.

7. _____ is advanced hypothyroidism in adults resulting from hypofunction of the thyroid gland and causes edema and increased blood pressure.

8. _____ is a small chromaffin cell tumor, usually located in the adrenal medulla.

9. _____ is a progressive degenerative neurological disorder that causes hand tremors.

10. _____ refers to inflammation of the gray matter caused by a virus, commonly resulting in spinal and muscle deformity and paralysis.

11. _____ refers to severe pain in the leg along the course of the sciatic nerve.

12. _____ is a congenital defect characterized by incomplete closure of the spinal canal through which the spinal cord and meninges may or may not protrude.

13. _____ is a diagnostic procedure in which electrodes placed on the scalp record electrical activity within the brain.

14. _____ is a malignant tumor composed principally of cells resembling neuroblasts and occurs chiefly in infants and children.

15. _____ is a brain disorder marked by deterioration of mental capacity (dementia) that begins in middle age and leads to total disability and death.

16. _____ is a radiographic technique that uses electromagnetic energy to produce cross sectional, frontal, and sagittal views of the brain.

17. _____ is a chronic disease due to insufficient production of insulin or the body's inability to use insulin properly.

18. _____ refers to eruption of acute, inflammatory, herpetic vesicles on the trunk of the body along a peripheral nerve.

19. _____ is a paralysis of four extremities and usually the trunk.

20. _____ refers to total pituitary impairment that brings about progressive and general loss of hormone activity.

21. _____ is a hereditary nervous disorder caused by progressive loss of brain cells that leads to bizarre, involuntary, dancelike movements.

22. _____ is the withdrawal of spinal fluid for diagnostic or therapeutic purposes.

23. _____ is a neurological disorder in which the nerve cell activity in the brain is disturbed, causing a seizure.

24. _____ refers to partial destruction of the thalamus to treat psychosis or intractable pain.

25. _____ produces a cross-sectional image of radioactivity in a section of the body to reveal areas where the radiopharmaceutical is metabolized and where metabolism is deficient.

Competency Verification: Check your answers in Appendix B: Answer Key, page 592. If you are not satisfied with your level of comprehension, review the additional medical terms and retake the review.

Correct Answers _____ × 4 = _____ % Score

MEDICAL RECORD ACTIVITIES

Medical reports included in the following activities reflect common, real-life clinical scenarios using medical terminology to document patient care.

MEDICAL RECORD ACTIVITY 9-1

DIABETES MELLITUS

Terminology

Terms listed in the table below come from the medical report Diabetes Mellitus *that follows. Use a medical dictionary such as* Taber's Cyclopedic Medical Dictionary, *the appendices of this book, or other resources to define each term. Then practice reading the pronunciations aloud for each term.*

Term	Definition
acidosis ăs-ĭ-DŌ-sĭs	
ADA	
BG	
diabetes mellitus dī-ă-BĒ-tēz MĚ-lĭ-tŭs	
electrolytes ē-LĔK-trō-līts	
glycemic glī-SĒ-mĭk	

Term	Definition
glycosuria glĭ-kō-SŪ-rē-ă	
Humulin L HŬ-mū-lĭn	
Humulin R HŬ-mū-lĭn	
ketones KĒ-tōnz	
metabolically mĕt-ă-BŎL-ĭk-ă-lē	
polydipsia pŏl-ē-DĬP-sē-ă	
polyuria pŏl-ē-Ū-rē-ă	
type 1 diabetes mellitus dī-ă-BĒ-tēz MĔ-lĭ-tŭs	
WNL	

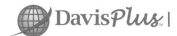 Davis*Plus* | Visit the *Medical Terminology Simplified* online resource center at Davis*Plus* to hear pronunciation and meanings of selected terms in this medical report.

Reading

Practice pronunciation of medical terms by reading the following medical report aloud.

Diabetes Mellitus

ADMITTING DIAGNOSIS: Diabetes mellitus, new onset.

DISCHARGE DIAGNOSIS: Type 1 diabetes mellitus, new onset.

HISTORY OF PRESENT ILLNESS: Patient is a 15-year-old white boy who presented in the office complaining of increased appetite, polydipsia, and polyuria and was found to have elevated blood glucose of 400 and glycosuria. He was sent to the hospital for further evaluation and treatment.

HOSPITAL COURSE: On admission, laboratory tests showed electrolytes, WNL, and ketones were negative. Urinalysis showed a trace of glucose, BG 380, and there was no evidence of acidosis. Metabolically the patient was stable. Patient was started on split-mixed insulin dosing. The patient and his family received full diabetic instruction during his hospitalization and seemed to understand this well. The patient picked up on all of this information quickly, asked appropriate questions, and appeared to be coping well with his new condition. By the 5th day, his polyuria and polydipsia resolved. When the patient was able to draw up and give his own insulin and perform his own fingersticks, he was discharged.

DISCHARGE INSTRUCTIONS: The patient was discharged to home with parents on a mixture of Humulin L 12 units and Humulin R 6 units each morning, with Humulin L 5 units and Humulin R 6 units each afternoon. He will continue with fingerstick BG 4 times daily at home until seen in the office for follow-up. I warned him of all glycemic symptoms to watch for, and he is to call the office with any problems that may occur. He is to follow an ADA 2,000-calorie diet.

DISCHARGE CONDITION: The patient's overall condition was much improved, and at the time of discharge BG levels were stabilized and he was doing well.

Evaluation

Review the medical record to answer the following questions. Use a medical dictionary such as Taber's Cyclopedic Medical Dictionary *and other resources if needed.*

1. What symptoms of DM did the patient experience before his office visit?

   _____

   _____

2. What confirmed the patient's new diagnosis of DM?

   _____

   _____

3. What conditions had to be met before the patient could be discharged from the hospital?

   _____

   _____

4. How many times a day does the patient have to take insulin?

   _____

   _____

5. Why does the patient have to perform fingersticks four times a day?

   _____

   _____

6. What is an ADA 2,000-calorie diet? Why is it important?

   _____

   _____

MEDICAL RECORD ACTIVITY 9-2

STROKE

Terminology

Terms listed in the table below come from the medical report Stroke *that follows. Use a medical dictionary such as* Taber's Cyclopedic Medical Dictionary, *the appendices of this book, or other resources to define each term. Then practice reading the pronunciations aloud for each term.*

Term	Definition
adenocarcinoma ăd-ĕ-nō-kăr-sĭn-Ō-mă	
anorexia ăn-ō-RĔK-sē-ă	
aphasia ă-FĀ-zē-ă	
biliary BĬL-ē-ār-ē	
cholecystojejunostomy kō-lē-sĭs-tō-jĕ-jū-NŎS-tō-mē	
deglutition dē-gloo-TĬSH-ŭn	
diplopia dĭp-LŌ-pē-ă	
jaundice JAWN-dĭs	
jejunojejunostomy jĕ-jū-nō-jĕ-jū-NŎS-tō-mē	
metastasis mĕ-TĂS-tă-sis	

Term	Definition
pruritus proo-RĪ-tŭs	
stroke STRŌK	
vertigo VĔR-tĭ-gō	

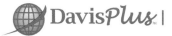 **DavisPlus** | Visit the *Medical Terminology Simplified* online resource center at Davis*Plus* to hear pronunciation and meanings of selected terms in this medical report.

Reading

Practice pronunciation of medical terms by reading the following medical report aloud.

Stroke

The patient is a moderately obese white woman who was admitted to Riverside Hospital because of a sudden episode of stroke. She recalls an episode of vertigo 3 days ago. The patient is being nursed at home by her daughter because of terminal adenocarcinoma of the head of the pancreas with metastasis to the liver, which was diagnosed in December. The patient fell to the floor with paralysis of the right arm and right leg and aphasia. She has not noticed any difficulty with deglutition. Apparently with the onset of the stroke, she also experienced diplopia. She denies any difficulty with her cardiovascular system in the past. The patient was in the hospital 5 years ago because of generalized biliary-type disease with jaundice, pruritus, weight loss, and anorexia. Subsequently, she was seen in consultation, and cholecysto-jejunostomy and jejunojejunostomy were performed.

Diagnosis: 1. Stroke, probably secondary to metastatic lesion of the brain or cerebrovascular disease.
2. Evidence of the previously described deterioration secondary to carcinoma of the pancreas with metastases to the liver.

Evaluation

Review the medical record to answer the following questions. Use a medical dictionary such as Taber's Cyclopedic Medical Dictionary *and other resources if needed.*

1. Did the patient have a history of cardiovascular problems before her stroke?

   _____

   _____

2. What symptoms did the patient experience just before her stroke?

   _____

   _____

3. What is the primary site of this patient's cancer?

   _____

   _____

4. What is cerebrovascular disease?

   _____

   _____

5. What is the probable cause of the patient's stroke?

   _____

   _____

ENDOCRINE AND NERVOUS SYSTEMS CHAPTER REVIEW

WORD ELEMENTS SUMMARY

The following table summarizes CFs, suffixes, and prefixes related to the endocrine and nervous systems. Study the word elements and their meanings before completing the Word Elements Chapter Review that follows.

Word Element	Meaning	Word Element	Meaning
Combining Forms			
Endocrine System			
aden/o	gland	pituitar/o	pituitary gland
adren/o, adrenal/o	adrenal glands	thym/o	thymus gland
pancreat/o	pancreas	thyroid/o	thyroid gland
parathyroid/o	parathyroid glands		
Nervous System			
cephal/o	brain	mening/o, meningi/o	meninges (membranes covering the brain and spinal cord)
cerebr/o	cerebrum	myel/o	bone marrow; spinal cord
encephal/o	brain	neur/o	nerve
gli/o	glue; neuroglial tissue	spin/o	spine
Other			
cyst/o	bladder	orchid/o, orchi/o, orch/o	testis (plural, testes)
enter/o	intestine (usually small intestine)	scler/o	hardening; sclera (white of eye)
gluc/o, glyc/o	sugar, sweetness	thromb/o	blood clot
hem/o	blood	toxic/o	poison
nephr/o, ren/o	kidney	vascul/o	blood vessel
Suffixes			
-algia, -dynia	pain	-oid	resembling
-dipsia	thirst	-osis	abnormal condition; increase (used primarily with blood cells)
-emia	blood condition	-pathy	disease
-gen, -genesis	forming, producing, origin	-penia	decrease, deficiency
-glia	glue; neuroglial tissue	-phagia	swallowing, eating
-iasis	abnormal condition (produced by something specified)	-phasia	speech
-ism	condition	-plegia	paralysis
-lith	stone, calculus	-rrhagia	bursting forth (of)
-logist	specialist in the study of	-rrhea	discharge, flow

Word Element	Meaning	Word Element	Meaning
-logy	study of	-tome	instrument to cut
-malacia	softening	-tomy	incision
-megaly	enlargement	-uria	urine
Prefixes			
a-	without, not	hyper-	excessive, above normal
dys-	bad; painful; difficult	hypo-	under, below, deficient
endo-	within	para-	near, beside; beyond

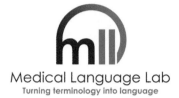

Medical Language Lab
Turning terminology into language

Visit the *Medical Language Lab* at *medicallanguagelab.com*. Use the flash-card–word elements exercise to reinforce your study of word elements. We recommend you complete the flash-card activity before starting the Word Elements Chapter Review that follows.

WORD ELEMENTS CHAPTER REVIEW

This review provides a verification of your knowledge of the word elements covered in this chapter. Write the meaning of the word element in the space provided. To reinforce your understanding of the word parts that comprise a medical term, each word element is identified as a prefix (P), word root (WR), combining form (CF), or suffix (S). The first word is completed for you.

Medical Term	Word Elements	Meaning
1. hyper/calc/emia	hyper- (P)	excessive, above normal
	calc: (WR)	calcium
	-emia: (S)	blood
2. aden/o/carcin/oma		
3. adrenal/ectomy		
4. cerebr/o/spin/al		

Medical Term	Word Elements	Meaning
5. encephal/itis		
6. gli/oma		
7. gluc/o/genesis		
8. hemi/paresis		
9. hydr/o/cephal/us		

Continued

Medical Term	Word Elements	Meaning
10. hypo/pituitar/ism		
11. hyper/trophy		
12. mening/o/cele		
13. myel/algia		
14. neur/o/lysis		
15. poly/dipsia		

Medical Term	Word Elements	Meaning
16. poli/o/myel/itis		
17. quadri/plegia		
18. thalam/o/tomy		
19. thromb/o/cyte		
20. thyr/o/megaly		

Competency Verification: Check your answers in Appendix B: Answer Key page 593. If you are not satisfied with your level of comprehension, review the chapter's flash-card exercise at *medicallanguagelab.com* and retake the review.

Correct Answers _____ × 5 = _____ % Score

VOCABULARY REVIEW

Match the medical term(s) below with the definitions in the numbered list.

acromegaly	deglutition	hyperglycemia	neurohypophysis	polydipsia
adenohypophysis	diabetes mellitus	insulin	neuromalacia	polyphagia
adrenalectomy	glycogenesis	jaundice	pancreatolith	pruritus
adrenaline	hormone	meningocele	pancreatolysis	thyrotoxicosis
cerebral palsy	hypercalcemia	metastasis	pancreatopathy	vertigo

1. _____ is an enlargement of the extremities.

2. _____ is the destruction of the pancreatic tissue due to a pathological condition.

3. _____ is the anterior lobe of the pituitary gland, composed of glandular tissue.

4. _____ refers to partial paralysis and lack of muscular coordination caused by damage to the cerebrum before or during the birth process.

5. _____ refers to excessive amounts of calcium in the blood.

6. _____ is a pancreatic hormone that decreases blood glucose level.

7. _____ is the posterior lobe of the pituitary, composed primarily of nerve tissue.

8. _____ is a disease of the pancreas.

9. _____ refers to excessive consumption of food.

10. _____ is a chronic metabolic disorder marked by hyperglycemia.

11. _____ is an increase of blood glucose, as in diabetes.

12. _____ is a calculus or stone in the pancreas.

13. _____ refers to excessive thirst.

14. _____ is a toxic condition due to hyperactivity of the thyroid gland.

15. _____ is the excision of an adrenal gland.

16. _____ is a hormone secreted by the adrenal medulla that causes some of the physiological expressions of fear and anxiety and is also called epinephrine.

17. _____ is the production or formation of sugar.

18. _____ refers to protrusion of the membranes of the brain or spinal cord through a defect in the skull or spinal column.

19. _____ is a softening of nerve tissue.

20. _____ refers to severe itching.

21. _____ refers to the act of swallowing.

22. _____ is an illusion of movement.

23. _____ is a yellowish discoloration of the skin and eyes.

24. _____ refers to the spread of a malignant tumor beyond its primary site to a secondary organ or location.

25. _____ is a chemical substance produced by specialized cells of the body and released slowly into the bloodstream.

Competency Verification: Check your answers in Appendix B: Answer Key, page 595. If you are not satisfied with your level of comprehension, review the chapter vocabulary and retake the review.

Musculoskeletal System

OBJECTIVES

Upon completion of this chapter, you will be able to:

- Describe the type of medical treatment orthopedists, osteopathic physicians, and chiropractors provide.
- Identify skeletal structures by labeling them on anatomical illustrations.
- Describe the primary functions of the musculoskeletal system.
- Describe diseases, conditions, and procedures related to the musculoskeletal system.
- Apply your word-building skills by constructing medical terms related to the musculoskeletal system.
- Describe common abbreviations and symbols related to the musculoskeletal system.
- Recognize, define, pronounce, and spell terms correctly.
- Demonstrate your knowledge of this chapter by successfully completing the frames, reviews, and medical report evaluations.

MEDICAL SPECIALTIES

Orthopedics

Orthopedics is the branch of medicine concerned with prevention, diagnosis, care, and treatment of musculoskeletal disorders. These disorders include injury to or disease of the body's bones, joints, ligaments, muscles, and tendons. **Orthopedists** are surgeons who specialize in orthopedics. They employ medical, physical, and surgical methods to restore function that is lost as a result of injury or disease to the musculoskeletal system. Orthopedists coordinate their treatments with other health-care providers, such as physical therapists, occupational therapists, and sports medicine physicians. In addition to the orthopedist who treats bone and joint diseases, the **rheumatologist** (also a medical doctor) specializes in treatment of arthritis and other diseases of joints, muscles, and bones.

Osteopathy

The **osteopathic physician (DO)** may also provide medical treatment for musculoskeletal disorders. The osteopathic philosophy maintains that good health requires a holistic approach that includes proper alignment of bones, muscles, ligaments, and nerves. Like a medical doctor (MD), osteopathic physicians provide state-of-the-art methods of medical treatment, including prescribing drugs and performing surgeries, and may specialize in such areas as orthopedics, cardiology, and pulmonology.

Chiropractic

Another health-care provider who treats musculoskeletal disorders is the **chiropractor.** Unlike medical doctors and osteopaths, chiropractors are not physicians. They do not employ drugs or surgery, the primary basis of treatment used by medical physicians. **Chiropractic medicine** is a system of therapy based on the theory that disease is caused by pressure on nerves. Nevertheless, chiropractors employ the use of radiographic images to diagnose pathological disorders and determine the most effective type of treatment. In most instances, chiropractic treatment involves physical manipulation of the spinal column.

ANATOMY AND PHYSIOLOGY OVERVIEW

The musculoskeletal system includes muscles, bones, joints, and related structures, such as tendons and connective tissue, that function in the movement of body parts and organs.

Muscles have four key functions: producing body movements, stabilizing body positions, storing and moving substances within the body, and generating heat. Through contraction, muscles cause motion and help maintain body posture. Less apparent motions that muscles are responsible for include the passage and elimination of food through the digestive system, propulsion of blood through the arteries, and contraction of the bladder to eliminate urine. In addition, muscles function in body movements in several different ways to allow a range of motion for the contraction and relaxation of muscle fibers. (See Fig. 10–1.)

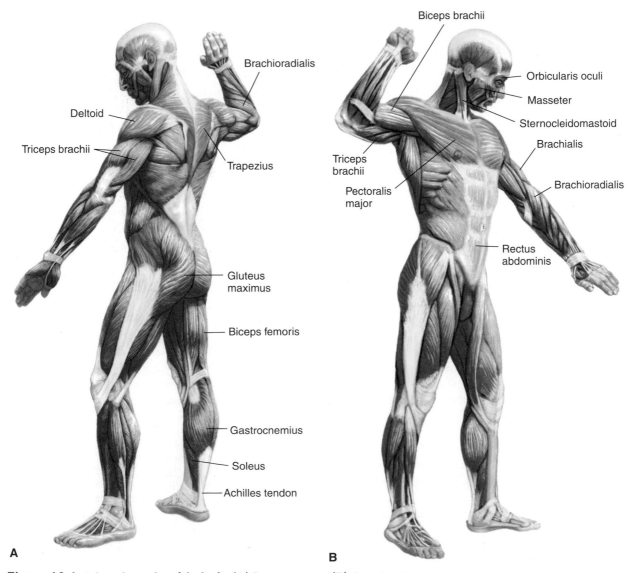

Figure 10-1 Selected muscles of the body. (**A**) Posterior view. (**B**) Anterior view.

The main function of bones is to form a skeleton to support and protect the body and serve as storage areas for mineral salts, especially calcium and phosphorus. Joints, also called **articulations,** are the places where two bones connect. Joints vary widely in the degree of movement they afford. Some joints are constructed in such a way that no movement is possible, such as suture joints between the skull bones. Most joints, however, allow a wide range of motion, such as finger, elbow, and knee joints. Because bones cannot move without the help of muscles, muscle tissue must provide contraction.

WORD ELEMENTS

This section introduces combining forms (CFs) related to the muscles of the body. Included are key suffixes; prefixes are defined in the right-hand column as needed. Review the following table and pronounce each word in the word analysis column aloud before you begin to work the frames.

Word Element	Meaning	Word Analysis
Combining Forms Muscles and Related Structures		
fasci/o	band, fascia (fibrous membrane supporting and separating muscles)	**fasci/o/plasty** (FĂSH-ē-ō-plăs-tē): surgical repair of fascia *-plasty:* surgical repair
fibr/o	fiber, fibrous tissue	**fibr/oma** (fĭ-BRŌ-mă): tumor of fibrous tissue *-oma:* tumor
leiomy/o	smooth muscle (visceral)	**leiomy/oma** (lī-ō-mī-Ō-mă): tumor of smooth muscle *-oma:* tumor
lumb/o	loins (lower back)	**lumb/o/cost/al** (lŭm-bō-KŎS-tăl): pertaining to the lumbar region and the ribs *cost:* ribs *-al:* pertaining to
muscul/o **my/o**	muscle	**muscul/ar** (MŬS-kū-lăr): pertaining to muscles *-ar:* pertaining to **my/o/rrhexis** (mī-or-ĔK-sĭs): rupture of a muscle *-rrhexis:* rupture
ten/o **tend/o** **tendin/o**	tendon	**ten/o/tomy** (tĕn-ŎT-ō-mē): incision of a tendon *-tomy:* incision Tenotomy is performed to correct muscle imbalance, such as in the correction of strabismus of the eye or clubfoot. **tend/o/plasty** (TĔN-dō-plăs-tē): surgical repair of a tendon *-plasty:* surgical repair **tendin/itis** (tĕn-dĭn-Ī-tĭs): inflammation of a tendon, usually resulting from strain; also called tendonitis *-itis:* inflammation *Tendinitis usually results from a strain.*

Continued

Word Element	Meaning	Word Analysis
Suffixes		
-algia	pain	my/**algia** (mī-ĂL-jē-ă): pain or tenderness in muscles *my:* muscle
-asthenia	weakness, debility	my/**asthenia** (mī-ăs-THĒ-nē-ă): weakness of muscle (and abnormal fatigue) *my:* muscle
-pathy	disease	my/o/**pathy** (mī-ŎP-ă-thē): disease of muscle tissue *my/o:* muscle *Myopathy is a disease that commonly indicates a skeletal muscle disorder.*
-plegia	paralysis	hemi/**plegia** (hĕm-ē-PLĒ-jē-ă): paralysis of one side of the body *hemi-:* one half *Types of hemiplegia include cerebral hemiplegia and facial hemiplegia.*
-rrhaphy	suture	my/o/**rrhaphy** (mī-OR-ă-fē): suture of muscle, usually due to a muscle wound *my/o:* muscle
-sarcoma	malignant tumor of connective tissue	my/o/**sarcoma** (mī-ō-sar-KŌ-mă): malignant tumor of muscle tissue *my/o:* muscle
-tomy	incision	chondr/o/**tomy** (kŏn-DRŎT-ō-mē): incision of cartilage *chondr/o:* cartilage

Pronunciation Help	Long sound	ā in rāte	ē in rēbirth	ī in īsle	ō in ōver	ū in ūnite
	Short sound	ă in ălone	ĕ in ĕver	ĭ in ĭt	ŏ in nŏt	ŭ in cŭt

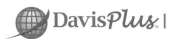

Visit the *Medical Terminology Simplified* online resource center at Davis*Plus* for an audio exercise of the terms in this table. It will help you master pronunciations and meanings of medical terms.

SECTION REVIEW 10-1

For the following medical terms, first write the suffix and its meaning. Then translate the meaning of the remaining elements starting with the first part of the word. The first word is completed for you.

Term	Meaning
1. my/o/sarcoma	-sarcoma: malignant tumor of connective tissue; muscle
2. my/o/rrhaphy	
3. hemi/plegia	
4. ten/o/tomy	
5. cost/o/chondr/itis	
6. tend/o/lysis	
7. my/o/pathy	
8. lumb/o/cost/al	
9. tendin/itis	
10. my/algia	

Competency Verification: Check your answers in Appendix B: Answer Key, page 595. If you are not satisfied with your level of comprehension, review the vocabulary and retake the review.

Correct Answers _____ × 10 = _____ % Score

MUSCLES

Types of Muscle Fibers

There are three types of muscular fibers or tissue:

- **Skeletal muscle fibers** are composed of striations that move bones of the skeleton and work mainly in a voluntary manner. Muscle fibers contract in response to stimulation and then relax when the stimulation ends. Their activity can be consciously controlled by neurons that are part of the somatic (voluntary) division of the nervous system. To some extent, skeletal muscles are also controlled subconsciously. For example, the diaphragm continues to alternately contract and relax without conscious control so that breathing does not stop.
- **Cardiac muscle fibers,** also composed of striations, are found only in the heart and form most of the heart wall. The alternating contraction and relaxation of the heart is involuntary and is not consciously controlled. Rather, the heart beats because it has a pacemaker that initiates each contraction. This built-in rhythm is called **autorhythmicity.** Several hormones and neurotransmitters can adjust heart rate by speeding or slowing the pacemaker.
- **Smooth muscle fibers** are shorter and lack the striations of skeletal and cardiac muscle tissue. For this reason, the tissue has a smooth appearance, which gives it its name. The action of smooth muscle is usually involuntary and some smooth muscle tissue, such as the muscles that propel food through the gastrointestinal tract, has autorhythmicity. Smooth muscle and cardiac muscle are regulated by neurons that are part of the autonomic (involuntary) division of the nervous system and hormones released by endocrine glands.

muscle(s)	**10-1** Fibers within each muscle are characteristically arranged into specific patterns that provide specific functional capabilities. Most skeletal muscles lie between the skin and the skeleton. My/o/genesis is the embryonic formation of _____.
my/o/plasty MĪ-ō-plăs-tē **my/o/rrhaphy** mī-OR-ă-fē **my/o/tomy** mī-ŎT-ō-mē	**10-2** Practice building medical words that mean *surgical repair of muscle:* _____ / _____ / _____ *suture of muscle:* _____ / _____ / _____ *incision of muscle:* _____ / _____ / _____
my/o/rrhexis mī-or-ĔK-sĭs	**10-3** Sports-related injuries are commonly caused by the tremendous stress exerted on certain parts of musculoskeletal structures. In many instances, these types of athletic injuries may result in a torn muscle. Form a word that means *rupture (tear) of a muscle.* _____ / _____ / _____
my/algia mī-ĂL-jē-ă	**10-4** My/o/dynia refers to muscle pain. Form another word that means *muscle pain.* _____ / _____
my/o/pathy mī-ŎP-ă-thē	**10-5** Form a medical term that means *disease of muscle.* _____ / _____ / _____
muscle	**10-6** My/o/genesis refers to forming, producing, or origin of _____.
hardening, sclera	**10-7** The CF *scler/o* refers to _____; _____ (white of the eye).
scler/osis sklĕ-RŌ-sĭs **my/o/scler/osis** mī-ō-sklĕr-Ō-sĭs	**10-8** An abnormal condition of hardening is called _____ / _____. An abnormal condition of muscle hardening is called _____ / _____ / _____ / _____.
anterior **posterior**	**10-9** To become familiar with the names of the major muscles of the body, study Figure 10–1 and identify words in the caption that mean *in front of:* _____ *back (of body), behind:* _____

Boldface indicates a word root or combining form. Blue indicates a suffix. Pink indicates a prefix.

tendon	**10-10** The CF *tend/o* means *tendon,* which is fibrous connective tissue that attaches muscles to bone. Tend/o/plasty is a surgical repair of a _____.
tend/o/tome TĔN-dō-tōm **tend/o/tomy** tĕn-DŎT-ō-mē **tend/o/plasty** TĔN-dō-plăs-tē	**10-11** Use *tend/o* to form words that mean *instrument to cut a tendon:* _____ / _____ / _____ *incision of a tendon:* _____ / _____ / _____ *surgical repair of a tendon:* _____ / _____ / _____
inferior	**10-12** The Achilles tendon is attached to a muscle in the lower leg. Locate the Achilles tendon in Figure 10–1A. It is located (superior, inferior) _____ to the gastrocnemius muscle.
paralysis pă-RĂL-ĭ-sĭs	**10-13** The prefix *quadri-* refers to *four.* Quadri/plegia is a _____ of all four extremities.
paralysis pă-RĂL-ĭ-sĭs	**10-14** The prefix *hemi-* means *one half.* Hemi/plegia is a _____ of half the body.
	10-15 With the exception of rotations of the body, other types of body movements occur in pairs, as summarized in Figure 10–2.

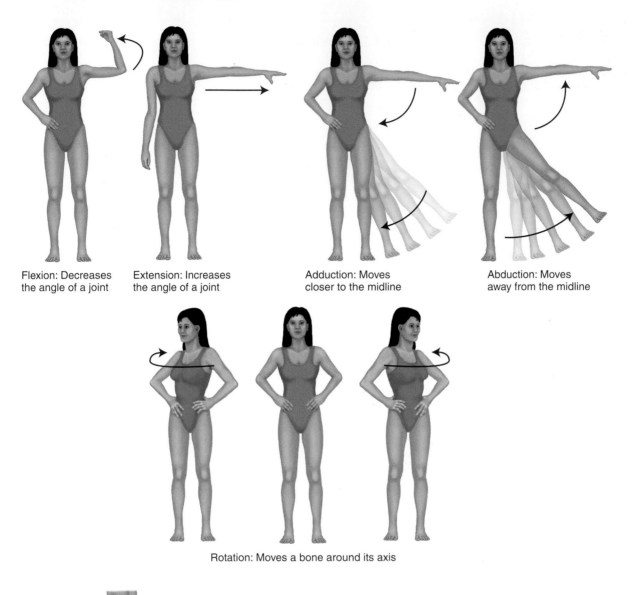

Flexion: Decreases the angle of a joint

Extension: Increases the angle of a joint

Adduction: Moves closer to the midline

Abduction: Moves away from the midline

Rotation: Moves a bone around its axis

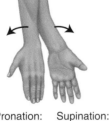

Pronation: Turns the palm down   Supination: Turns the palm up

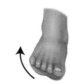

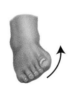

Eversion: Moves the sole of the foot inward   Inversion: Moves the sole of the foot outward

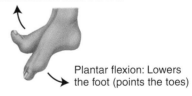

Dorsiflexion: Elevates the foot

Plantar flexion: Lowers the foot (points the toes)

Figure 10-2 Body movements generated by muscles.

SECTION REVIEW 10-2

Using the table below, write the combining form, suffix, or prefix that matches its definition in the space provided to the left of the definition. There may be more than one word element that matches a definition.

Combining Forms		Suffixes		Prefixes
chondr/o	tendin/o	-cyte	-rrhaphy	hemi-
cyst/o	tend/o	-genesis	-rrhexis	quadri-
enter/o	ten/o	-lysis	-sarcoma	
hepat/o		-osis	-tome	
my/o		-plasty	-tomy	
scler/o		-plegia		

1. _____ abnormal condition; increase (used primarily with blood cells)

2. _____ bladder

3. _____ cell

4. _____ four

5. _____ one half

6. _____ hardening; sclera (white of eye)

7. _____ incision

8. _____ intestine (usually small intestine)

9. _____ liver

10. _____ muscle

11. _____ paralysis

12. _____ forming, producing, origin

13. _____ rupture

14. _____ surgical repair

15. _____ suture

16. _____ tendon

17. _____ instrument to cut

18. _____ cartilage

19. _____ malignant tumor of connective tissue

20. _____ separation; destruction; loosening

Competency Verification: Check your answers in Appendix B: Answer Key, page 595. If you are not satisfied with your level of comprehension, go back to Frame 10–1 and rework the frames.

Correct Answers _____ × 5 = _____ % Score

SKELETAL SYSTEM

The skeleton of a human adult consists of 206 individual bones, but this chapter covers only the major bones. For anatomical purposes, the human skeleton is divided into the axial skeleton (distinguished with bone color in Figure 10–3) and the appendicular skeleton (distinguished with blue color in Figure 10–3). The axial skeleton protects internal organs and provides central support of the body around which other parts move. It consists of the bones of the head, chest, and spine. The appendicular skeleton enables the body to move. It consists of the bones of the shoulders, arms, hips, and legs. The ability to walk, run, or catch a ball is possible due to the movable joints of the limbs.

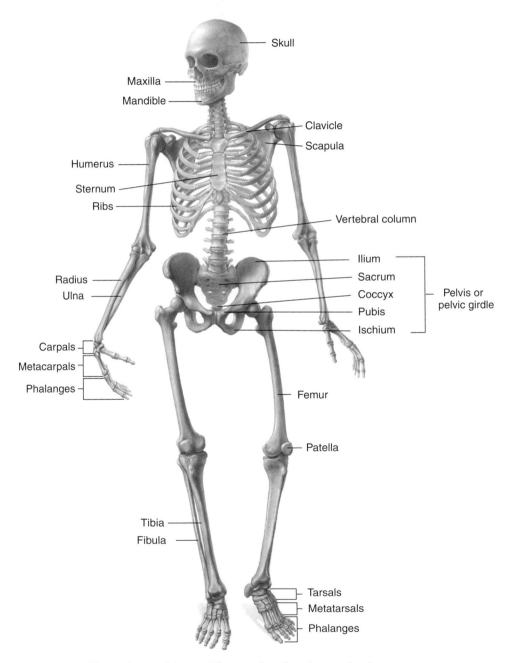

Figure 10-3 Anterior view of the skeleton of the axial (bone-colored) and appendicular (blue) skeleton.

WORD ELEMENTS

This section introduces CFs related to the bones. Included are key suffixes; prefixes are defined in the right-hand column as needed. Review the following table, and pronounce each word in the word analysis column aloud before you begin to work the frames.

Word Element	Meaning	Word Analysis
Combining Forms		
Specific Bones of the Upper Extremities		
carp/o	carpus (wrist bones)	**carp/o/ptosis** (kăr-pŏp-TŌ-sĭs): downward displacement of the wrist; also called *dropped wrist* *-ptosis:* prolapse, downward displacement
cervic/o	neck; cervix uteri (neck of the uterus)	**cervic/al** (SĔR-vĭ-kăl): pertaining to the neck *-al:* pertaining to *The term cervical is also used to denote the region of the neck or a constricted area of a necklike structure, such as the neck of a tooth or the cervix uteri.*
cost/o	ribs	**sub/cost/al** (sŭb-KŎS-tăl): beneath the ribs *sub-:* under, below *-al:* pertaining to
crani/o	cranium (skull)	**crani/o/tomy** (krā-nē-ŎT-ō-mē): incision through the cranium, usually to gain access to the brain during neurosurgical procedures *-tomy:* incision *Craniotomy is performed to relieve intracranial pressure, control bleeding, or remove a tumor.*
humer/o	humerus (upper arm bone)	**humer/al** (HŪ-měr-ăl): pertaining to the humerus *-al:* pertaining to
metacarp/o	metacarpus (hand bones)	**metacarp/ectomy** (mĕt-ă-kăr-PĔK-tō-mē): excision of one or more metacarpal bones *-ectomy:* excision, removal
phalang/o	phalanges (bones of the fingers and toes)	**phalang/itis** (făl-ăn-JĪ-tĭs): inflammation of one or more phalanges *-itis:* inflammation
spondyl/o*	vertebra (backbone)	**spondyl/itis** (spŏn-dĭl-Ī-tĭs): inflammation of any of the vertebrae (plural), usually characterized by stiffness and pain *-itis:* inflammation *Ankylosing spondylitis is a form of arthritis that may eventually cause the spine to fuse in a fixed, immobile position. Spondylitis may result from a traumatic injury to the spine, infection, or rheumatoid disease.*
vertebr/o*		**vertebr/al** (VĔR-tĕ-brăl): pertaining to a vertebra or the vertebral column *-al:* pertaining to
stern/o	sternum (breastbone)	**stern/o/cost/al** (stĕr-nō-KŎS-tăl): pertaining to the sternum and ribs *cost:* ribs *-al:* pertaining to
Specific Bones of the Lower Extremities		
calcane/o	calcaneum (heel bone)	**calcane/o/dynia** (kăl-kăn-ē-ō-DĬN-ē-ă): painful condition of the heel *-dynia:* pain
femor/o	femur (thigh bone)	**femor/al** (FĔM-or-ăl): pertaining to the femur *-al:* pertaining to

Continued

Word Element	Meaning	Word Analysis
fibul/o	fibula (smaller, outer bone of the lower leg)	**fibul**/ar (FĬB-ū-lăr): pertaining to the fibula *-ar:* pertaining to
patell/o	patella (kneecap)	**patell**/ectomy (păt-ĕ-LĔK-tō-mē): excision of the patella *-ectomy:* excision, removal
pelv/i† **pelv/o**	pelvis	**pelv/i**/metry (pĕl-VĬM-ĕ-trē): measurement of the pelvic dimensions or proportions *-metry:* act of measuring *Pelvimetry helps determine whether or not it will be possible to deliver a fetus through the normal route.* **pelv**/is (PĔL-vĭs): pertaining to the pelvis *-is:* noun ending *A woman's pelvis is usually less massive but wider and more circular than a man's pelvis.*
radi/o	radiation, x-ray; radius (lower arm bone on the thumb side)	**radi/o**/graph (RĀ-dē-ō-grăf): x-ray image *-graph:* instrument for recording
tibi/o	tibia (larger bone of the lower leg)	**tibi**/al (TĬB-ē-ăl): pertaining to the tibia (shin bone) *-al:* pertaining to

Other Related Structures

Word Element	Meaning	Word Analysis
ankyl/o	stiffness; bent, crooked	**ankyl**/osis (ăng-kĭ-LŌ-sĭs): immobility of a joint *-osis:* abnormal condition; increase (used primarily with blood cells) *Ankylosis may be congenital or it may be due to disease, trauma, surgery, or contractures resulting from immobility.*
arthr/o	joint	**arthr**/itis (ăr-THRĪ-tĭs): inflammation of a joint *-itis:* inflammation *Arthritis is commonly accompanied by pain, swelling, stiffness, and deformity.*
chondr/o	cartilage	**cost/o**/chondr/itis (kŏs-tō-kŏn-DRĪ-tĭs): inflammation of cartilage of the anterior chest wall (ribs) *cost/o:* ribs *-itis:* inflammation *Costochondritis is characterized by pain and tenderness that may radiate from the initial site of inflammation.*
lamin/o	lamina (part of the vertebral arch)	**lamin**/ectomy (lăm-ĭ-NĔK-tŏ-mē): excision of the lamina (bony arches of one or more vertebrae) *-ectomy:* excision, removal
myel/o	bone marrow; spinal cord	**myel/o**/cele (MĪ-ĕ-lō-sēi): herniation of the spinal cord *-cele:* hernia, swelling *Myelocele is a sacklike protrusion of the spinal cord through a congenital defect in the vertebral column.*

Word Element	Meaning	Word Analysis
orth/o	straight	**orth/o/ped/ics** (or-thō-PĒ-dĭks): branch of medicine concerned with prevention and correction of musculoskeletal system disorders *ped:* foot; child *-ics:* pertaining to
oste/o	bone	**oste/itis** (ŏs-tē-Ī-tĭs): inflammation of bone *-itis:* inflammation
Suffixes		
-clast	to break; surgical fracture	oste/o/**clast** (ŎS-tē-ō-klăst): (mononucleated cell that) breaks down bone *oste/o:* bone *An osteoclast destroys the matrix of bone. An osteoclast also refers to an instrument used to surgically fracture a bone (osteoclasis).*
-cyte	cell	oste/o/**cyte** (ŎS-tē-ō-sīt): bone cell *oste/o:* bone
-desis	binding, fixation (of a bone or joint)	arthr/o/**desis** (ăr-thrō-DĒ-sĭs): surgical immobilization of a joint *arthr/o:* joint
-malacia	softening	oste/o/**malacia** (ŏs-tē-ō-mă-LĀ-shē-ă): softening and bending of the bones *oste/o:* bone *Osteomalacia is caused by a deficiency in vitamin D that results in a shortage or loss of calcium salts, causing bones to become increasingly soft, flexible, brittle, and deformed.*
-physis	growth	dia/**physis** (dī-ĂF-ĭ-sĭs): shaft or middle region of a long bone *dia-:* through, across
-porosis	porous	oste/o/**porosis** (ŏs-tē-ō-por-Ō-sĭs): porous bones *oste/o:* bone *Osteoporosis is characterized by a decrease in bone density with an increase in porosity, causing bones to become brittle and increasing the risk of fractures.*

Pronunciation Help	Long sound	ā in rāte	ē in rēbirth	ī in īsle	ō in ōver	ū in ūnite
	Short sound	ă in ălone	ĕ in ĕver	ĭ in ĭt	ŏ in nŏt	ŭ in cŭt

*The CF **spondyl/o** is used to form words about the condition of a structure. The CF **vertebr/o** is used to form words that describe a structure.
†Using the combining vowel *i* instead of *o* is an exception to the rule.

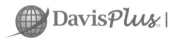

Visit the *Medical Terminology Simplified* online resource center at Davis*Plus* for an audio exercise of the terms in this table. It will help you master pronunciations and meanings of medical terms.

SECTION REVIEW 10-3

For the following medical terms, first write the suffix and its meaning. Then translate the meaning of the remaining elements starting with the first part of the word. The first word is completed for you.

Term	Meaning
1. dia/physis	-physis: growth; through, across
2. sub/cost/al	
3. oste/o/malacia	
4. lamin/ectomy	
5. pelv/i/metry	
6. myel/o/cele	
7. oste/o/porosis	
8. ankyl/osis	
9. carp/o/ptosis	
10. crani/o/tomy	

Competency Verification: Check your answers in Appendix B: Answer Key, page 595. If you are not satisfied with your level of comprehension, review the vocabulary and retake the review.

Correct Answers _____ × 10 = _____ % Score

Structure and Function of Bones

oste/o

10-16 To understand the skeletal system, it is important to know the types and names of major bones, their functions, and where they are located. Regardless of the size or shape of a bone, the CF used to designate bone is _____ / _____.

10-17 There are four basic types of bones: long, short, flat, and irregular. **Long bones** are longer than they are wide and are slightly curved for strength. Long bones vary tremendously in size and include those in the thigh (femur), leg (tibia and fibula), arm (humerus), and fingers and toes (phalanges). **Short bones** are somewhat cube-shaped and are nearly equal in length and width. Examples of short bones are the carpal (wrist) bones and the tarsal (ankle) bones. **Flat bones** are broad and thin. They cover and protect soft body parts, such as the cranial bones, which protect the brain, and the sternum and ribs, which protect organs in the thorax. **Irregular bones** have varied shapes and sizes and are commonly clustered, such as the bones of the vertebrae and certain bones of the ears and face.

Refer to Figure 10–3 to review the different types of bones.

Boldface indicates a word root or combining form. Blue indicates a suffix. Pink indicates a prefix.

10-18   Identify the four types of bones described in Frame 10–17.

Cube-shaped bones of the wrists, and ankles are the

_____ _____.

Broad bones in the shoulders and ribs are the

_____ _____.

Certain bones of the ears and the bones of the vertebrae are the

_____ _____.

Type of bones that are longer than they are wide and slightly curved are known as

_____ _____.

short bones

flat bones

irregular bones

long bones

10-19   Typically, long bones are found in the extremities of the body. The main elongated portion of such a bone, the (1) **diaphysis,** is composed of several tissue layers: the thin fibrous outer membrane, the (2) **periosteum,** the thick layer of hard (3) **compact bone,** and the inner (4) **medullary cavity.** Label the parts of the long bone in Figure 10–4.

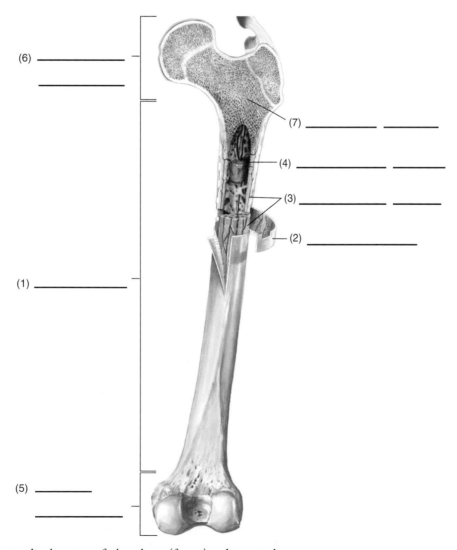

(6) _____

_____

(7) _____ _____

(4) _____ _____

(3) _____ _____

(2) _____

(1) _____

(5) _____

_____

Figure 10-4 Longitudinal section of a long bone (femur) and interior bone structure.

10–20   The two ends of bones, the (5) **distal epiphysis** and (6) **proximal epiphysis**, have a bulbous shape to provide space for muscle and ligament attachments near the joints. Label these structures in Figure 10–4.

10–21   There are two kinds of bone tissue based on porosity, and most bones have both types. Compact (dense) bone tissue is the hard, outer layer; (7) **spongy (cancellous) bone** tissue is the porous, highly vascular inner portion. Compact bone tissue is covered by periosteum that serves as a place of attachment for muscles, provides protection, and gives durable strength to the bone. The spongy bone tissue makes the bone lighter and provides a space for bone marrow, where blood cells are produced. Label the spongy bone in Figure 10–4, and note the position and structure of compact and spongy bone.

10–22   In Figure 10–4, observe how the diaphysis forms a cylinder that surrounds the medullary cavity. In adults, the medullary cavity contains fat yellow marrow, so named because of the large amounts of fat it contains.

oste/o/blasts
ŎS-tē-ō-blăstz

peri/oste/um
pĕr-ē-ŎS-tē-ŭm

10–23   The peri/oste/um, as illustrated in Figure 10–4, covers the entire surface of the bone. Its blood vessels supply nutrients, and its nerves signal pain. In growing bones, the inner layer contains bone-forming cells known as oste/o/blasts. Because blood vessels and oste/o/blasts are located in the peri/oste/um, this site provides a means for bone repair and general bone nutrition. Bones that lose peri/oste/um through injury or disease usually scale or die. As discussed earlier, the peri/oste/um also provides a point of attachment for muscles.

Identify terms in this frame that mean

embryonic cell (that develops into) bone: _____ / _____ / _____

structure around bone: _____ / _____ / _____

-genesis

oste/o

oste/o/cytes
ŎS-tē-ō-sītz

10–24   Oste/o/genesis is the formation or development of bones.

Identify elements in this frame that mean

forming, producing, origin: _____

bone: _____ / _____

When we are talking about bone cells, the medical term to use is

_____ / _____ / _____.

leuk/o/poiesis
loo-kō-poy-Ē-sĭs

erythr/o/poiesis
ĕ-rĭth-rō-poy-Ē-sĭs

10–25   In an adult, production of red blood cells (erythr/o/poiesis) occurs in red bone marrow. Red bone marrow is also responsible for formation of white blood cells (leuk/o/poiesis) and platelets.

Identify terms in this frame that mean

formation or production of white blood cells:

_____ / _____ / _____

formation or production of red blood cells:

_____ / _____ / _____

Boldface indicates a word root or combining form. Blue indicates a suffix. Pink indicates a prefix.

chondr/itis kŏn-DRĪ-tĭs **chondr/oma** kŏn-DRŌ-mă **chondr/o/genesis** kŏn-drō-JĔN-ĕ-sĭs	**10–26** Cartilage, which is more elastic than bone, composes parts of the skeleton. It is found chiefly in the joints, thorax, trachea, and nose. Use ***chondr/o*** (cartilage) to form words that mean *inflammation of cartilage:* _____ / _____ *tumor composed of cartilage:* _____ / _____ *producing or forming cartilage:* _____ / _____ / _____
chondr/o/cyte KŎN-drō-sīt	**10–27** Use *-cyte* to build a word that means *cartilage cell.* _____ / _____ / _____

Competency Verification: Check your labeling of Figure 10–4 in Appendix B: Answer Key, page 596.

oste/o/dynia ŏs-tē-ō-DĬN-ē-ă	**10–28** Oste/algia means *pain in a bone.* Form another term that means *pain in a bone.* _____ / _____ / _____
oste/o/cytes ŎS-tē-ō-sīts	**10–29** Bone is living tissue composed of oste/o/cytes, blood vessels, and nerves. Determine the medical term for bone cells. _____ / _____ / _____
oste/itis ŏs-tē-Ī-tĭs **oste/o/pathy** ŏs-tē-ŎP-ă-thē **oste/o/tomy** ŏs-tē-ŎT-ō-mē **oste/o/rrhaphy** ŏs-tē-OR-ă-fē **oste/o/scler/osis** ŏs-tē-ō-sklĕ-RŌ-sĭs	**10–30** Practice developing medical words that mean *inflammation of bone:* _____ / _____ *disease of bone:* _____ / _____ / _____ *incision of bone:* _____ / _____ / _____ *suture of bone (wiring of bone fragments):* _____ / _____ / _____ *abnormal condition of bone hardening:* _____ / _____ / _____ / _____
dist/o	**10–31** Dist/al is a directional word that means *pertaining to (a structure) farthest from the point of attachment to the trunk, or far from the beginning of a structure.* From dist/al, build the CF that means *far or farthest.* _____ / _____

proxim/o	**10–32** Proxim/al is a directional word that means *pertaining to (a structure) near the point of attachment to the trunk, or near the beginning of a structure.* From proxim/al, build the CF that means *near or nearest.* _____ / _____
farthest from **nearest to**	**10–33** To complete this frame, use the words *farthest from* or *nearest to.* The dist/al epiphysis is located _____ _____ the trunk. The proxim/al epiphysis is located _____ _____ the trunk.
oste/o/malacia ŏs-tē-ō-mă-LĀ-shē-ă **oste/o/genesis** ŏs-tē-ō-JĔN-ĕ-sĭs	**10–34** Milk is a good source of vitamin D. Deficiency of this vitamin results in a softening and weakening of the skeleton, causing pain and bowing of the bones. Construct medical terms that mean *softening of bones:* _____ / _____ / _____ *producing or forming bone:* _____ / _____ / _____
oste/o/malacia ŏs-tē-ō-mă-LĀ-shē-ă	**10–35** Oste/o/malacia is the result of inadequate amounts of phosphorus and calcium in blood for mineralization of the bones. It may be caused by a diet lacking these minerals, deficiency in vitamin D, or a metabolic disorder that causes malabsorption of minerals. The medical term that means softening of bones is _____ / _____ / _____.
oste/o/malacia ŏs-tē-ō-mă-LĀ-shē-ă	**10–36** A form of oste/o/malacia known as rickets is seen in infants and children in many underdeveloped countries. It is a result of vitamin D deficiency. Symptoms of rickets include soft, pliable bones that cause such deformities as bowlegs and knock-knees. Rickets is another name for _____ / _____ / _____.
rickets RĬK-ĕts	**10–37** Calcium provides bone strength that is needed for its supportive functions. Many children in underdeveloped countries develop rickets because of an inadequate milk supply. When oste/o/malacia occurs in children, it is called _____.
calc/emia kăl-SĒ-mē-ă	**10–38** Combine *calc/o* and *-emia* to form a word that means *calcium in the blood.* _____ / _____
under, below, deficient	**10–39** Recall that *hypo-* means _____, _____, _____.

hyper/calc/emia hī-pĕr-kăl-SĒ-mē-ă	**10–40** Hypo/calc/emia is a deficiency of calcium in the blood. The term that means *excessive amount of calcium in the blood* is _____ / _____ / _____.
radi/o/logist rā-dē-ŎL-ō-jĭst	**10–41** Radi/o/logy, initially widely called roentgen/o/logy, was developed after discovery of an unknown ray in 1895 by Wilhelm Roentgen, who called his discovery a *roentgen* (x-ray). Occasionally you still may see words with **roentgen/o**, but **radi/o** is the preferred term used in the context of medical imaging today. Radi/o/logy is the branch of medicine concerned with radioactive substances. It is used to diagnose path/o/log/ical conditions of the skeletal system. A physician who specializes in the study of x-rays is called a _____ / _____ / _____.
radi/o/therapy rā-dē-ō-THĔR-ă-pē	**10–42** Radiation is used for diagnostic and therapeutic purposes. Radiation therapy, also called radi/o/therapy, is treatment of diseases using an external source of high-energy rays or internally implanted radioactive substances. These rays and substances are effective in damaging cancer cells and halting their growth. Treatment of disease using radiation is called _____ / _____ / _____.
radi/o/logist rā-dē-ŎL-ō-jĭst	**10–43** Combine **radi/o** + *-logist* to build a word that means *specialist in the study of x-rays*. _____ / _____ / _____.
muscle, bone marrow, spinal cord	**10–44** Although **my/o** and **myel/o** sound alike, they have different meanings. *My/o* refers to _____. *Myel/o* refers to _____ _____ or the _____ _____.
myel/o	**10–45** A myel/o/gram is a radi/o/graph of the spin/al cord after injection of a contrast medium. The CF for *bone marrow and spinal cord* is _____ / _____.
myel/o/genesis mī-ĕ-lō-JĔN-ĕ-sĭs	**10–46** Use *-genesis* to build a word that means *formation of bone marrow*. _____ / _____ / _____
myel/o/malacia mī-ĕl-ō-mă-LĀ-shē-ă **myel/o/gram** MĪ-ĕl-ō-grăm	**10–47** Develop medical words that mean *softening of the spinal cord:* _____ / _____ / _____ *record of the spinal cord:* _____ / _____ / _____

myel/o/gram MĪ-ĕl-ō-grăm	**10–48** A myel/o/gram, a radiograph of the spinal canal after injection of a contrast medium, is used to identify and study spinal lesions caused by trauma or disease. To identify any distortions of the spinal cord, the physician may order a radiograph called a _____ / _____ / _____ .
oste/o/myel/itis ŏs-tē-ō-mī-ĕ-LĪ-tĭs	**10–49** Oste/o/myel/itis is an inflammation of the bone and bone marrow, most commonly due to infection. (See Fig. 10–5.) Localized or generalized infection of the bone and bone marrow is charted as _____ / _____ / _____ / _____ .
bone **bone marrow, spinal cord** **inflammation**	**10–50** Oste/o/myel/itis is usually caused by bacteria introduced through trauma or surgery, by direct extension from a nearby infection, or via the bloodstream. Staphylococci are the most common causative agents. Analyze the elements of the term oste/o/myelitis: *oste/o:* _____ *myel:* _____ _____ ; _____ _____ *-itis:* _____

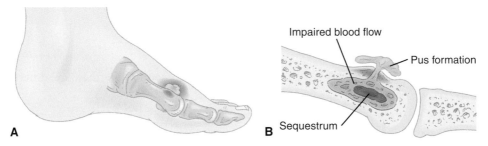

Figure 10-5 Osteomyelitis. (**A**) Bone infection in the toe. (**B**) Blocked blood flow in the area of infection with sequestrum (bone death) and pus formation at the infection site.

SECTION REVIEW 10-4

Using the following table, write the CF, suffix, or prefix that matches its definition in the space provided to the left of the definition. There may be more than one word element that matches a definition.

Combining Forms

calc/o	radi/o
chondr/o	scler/o
dist/o	
my/o	
myel/o	
oste/o	
proxim/o	

Suffixes

-algia	-graphy
-cele	-itis
-cyte	-logist
-dynia	-malacia
-emia	-oma
-genesis	-rrhaphy
-gram	-tomy

Prefixes

hyper-
hypo-
peri-

1. _____ excessive, above normal

2. _____ around

3. _____ blood condition

4. _____ bone

5. _____ cartilage

6. _____ calcium

7. _____ cell

8. _____ far, farthest

9. _____ hardening; sclera (white of eye)

10. _____ hernia, swelling

11. _____ incision

12. _____ inflammation

13. _____ near, nearest

14. _____ muscle

15. _____ pain

16. _____ process of recording

17. _____ forming, producing, origin

18. _____ record, writing

19. _____ softening

20. _____ specialist in study of

21. _____ bone marrow; spinal cord

22. _____ suture

23. _____ tumor

24. _____ under, below, deficient

25. _____ radiation, x-ray; radius (lower arm bone on thumb side)

Competency Verification: Check your answers in Appendix B: Answer Key, page 596. If you are not satisfied with your level of comprehension, go back to Frame 10–16 and rework the frames.

Correct Answers _____ × 4 = _____ % Score

Joints

synarthroses
sĭn-ăr-THRŌ-sēz

diarthroses
dī-ăr-THRŌ-sēz

amphiarthroses
ăm-fē-ăr-THRŌ-sēz

10–51   To allow for body movements, bones must have points where they meet (articulate). These articulating points form joints that have various degrees of mobility. Some are freely movable (diarthroses); others are only slightly movable (amphiarthroses), and the remaining are totally immovable (synarthroses). All three types are necessary for smooth, coordinated body movements.

Use the information above to identify the term that means

totally immovable joints: _____

freely movable joints: _____

slightly movable joints: _____

arthr/o/pathy
ăr-THRŎP-ă-thē

arthr/itis
ăr-THRĪ-tĭs

arthr/o/centesis
ăr-thrō-sĕn-TĒ-sĭs

10–52   Use *arthr/o* (joint) to develop medical words that mean

disease of a joint: _____ / _____ / _____

inflammation of a joint: _____ / _____

surgical puncture of a joint:

_____ / _____ / _____

arthr/o/scope
ĂR-thrō-skōp

10–53   Arthr/o/scopy is the visual examination of the interior of a joint performed by inserting an endo/scope through a small incision. Arthr/o/scopy is performed to repair and remove joint tissue, especially of the knee, ankle, and shoulder. (See Fig. 10–6.)

The endo/scope used to perform arthr/o/scopy is called an

_____ / _____ / _____.

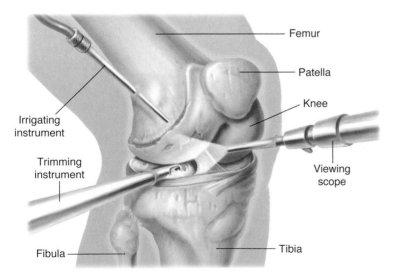

Figure 10-6 Arthroscopy.

Boldface indicates a word root or combining form. Blue indicates a suffix. Pink indicates a prefix.

arthr/o/plasty ĂR-thrō-plăs-tē	**10–54** A total hip replacement (THR), or total hip arthr/o/plasty, is a surgical procedure that replaces the upper end of the thighbone (femur) with a metal ball and resurfaces the hip socket (acetabulum) with a metal shell and plastic liner. The acetabulum is plastic coated to avoid metal-to-metal articulating surfaces. (See Fig. 10–7.) Use arthr/o to build a term that means *surgical repair of a joint.* _____ / _____ / _____ .
THR	**10–55** The surgical procedure to replace a hip joint that has been destroyed by disease or osteoarthritis is known as total hip arthroplasty, or _____ (abbreviation).
joints	**10–56** Just as a piece of machinery is lubricated by oil, joints are lubricated by synovial fluid. The fluid is secreted within the synovial membranes. Synovial fluid allows free movement of the _____ .
arthr/o/centesis ăr-thrō-sĕn-TĒ-sĭs	**10–57** To aspirate or remove accumulated fluid from a joint, a surgical puncture of a joint is performed. This surgical procedure is called _____ / _____ / _____ .
arthr/o/dynia ăr-thrō-DĬN-ē-ă	**10–58** A person with arthr/itis suffers, not only from an inflammation of the joints, but also from arthr/algia. Construct another medical word that means *pain in a joint.* _____ / _____ / _____

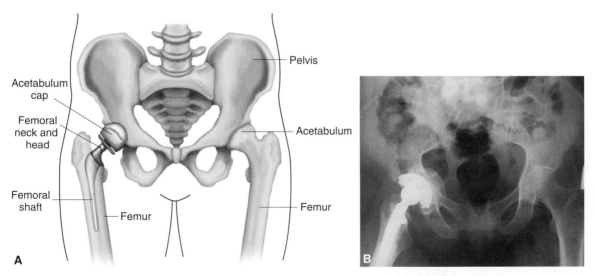

Figure 10-7 Total hip replacement. **(A)** Right total hip replacement. **(B)** Radiograph showing total hip replacement of an arthritic hip.

arthr/itis ăr-THRĪ-tĭs **oste/o/arthr/itis** ŏs-tē-ō-ăr-THRĪ-tĭs	**10-59** Although there are various forms of arthr/itis, all of them result in an inflammation of the joints. This condition is accompanied by pain and swelling. Form medical words that mean *inflammation of joints:* _____ / _____ *inflammation of bones and joints:* _____ / _____ / _____ / _____
oste/o/arthr/o/pathy ŏs-tē-ō-ăr-THRŎP-ă-thē	**10-60** A disease of the bones and joints is called _____ / _____ / _____ / _____ / _____.
oste/o/arthr/o/sis ŏs-tē-ō-ăr-THRŌ-sĭs	**10-61** Select element(s) from oste/o/arthr/o/pathy to build a word that means an *abnormal condition of the bones and joints.* _____ / _____ / _____ / _____ / _____

Combining Forms Related to Specific Bones

The CF:

- *crani/o* refers to the (1) cranium (skull).
- *stern/o* refers to the (2) sternum (breastbone).
- *cost/o* refers to the (3) ribs, which are attached to the sternum.
- *vertebr/o* refers to the (4) vertebra (backbone). The vertebral column, also called the spinal column, is composed of 26 bones called vertebr/ae.
- *humer/o* refers to the (5) humerus (upper arm bone). The humerus articulates with the scapula at the shoulder and with the radius and ulna at the elbow.
- *carp/o* refers to the (6) carpus (wrist bones). There are eight wrist bones.
- *metacarp/o* refers to the (7) metacarpus (hand bone). The metacarpals (plural) radiate from the wrist like spokes and form the palm of the hand.
- *phalang/o* refers to the (8) phalanges (bones of the fingers and toes).
- *pelv/i* and *pelv/o* refer to the (9) pelvis. The pelvis, also called the pelvic girdle, is composed of three pairs of fused bones (the ilium, pubis, and ischium), the sacrum, and the coccyx. The pelvis provides attachment for the legs and supports the soft organs of the abdominal cavity.
- *femor/o* refers to the (10) femur (thigh bone). The femur is the longest and strongest bone in the body. It articulates with the hip bone and the bones of the lower leg.
- *patell/o* refers to the (11) patella (kneecap). The patella articulates with the femur but is, essentially, a floating bone. The main function of this bone is to protect the knee joint, but its exposed position makes it vulnerable to dislocation and fracture.
- *tibi/o* refers to the (12) tibia (larger bone of the lower leg). The tibia is the weight-bearing bone of the lower leg.
- *fibul/o* refers to the (13) fibula (smaller bone of the lower leg). The fibula is not a weight-bearing bone but is important because muscles are attached and anchored to it.
- *calcane/o* refers to the (14) calcaneum (heel bone).

10-62   The word roots of bones are derived from the specific anatomical names of the bones. Learn the CFs for the bones as you label them in Figure 10–8.

Boldface indicates a word root or combining form. Blue indicates a suffix. Pink indicates a prefix.

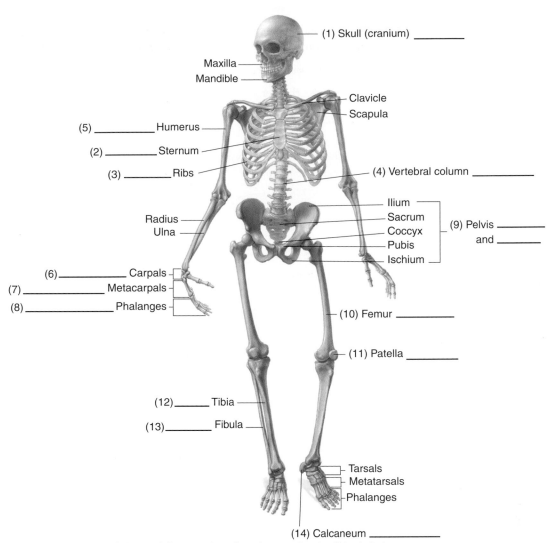

(1) Skull (cranium) _____

Maxilla

Mandible

Clavicle

Scapula

(5) _____ Humerus

(2) _____ Sternum

(3) _____ Ribs

(4) Vertebral column _____

Ilium

Sacrum

Coccyx

Pubis

Ischium

(9) Pelvis _____
and _____

Radius

Ulna

(6) _____ Carpals

(7) _____ Metacarpals

(8) _____ Phalanges

(10) Femur _____

(11) Patella _____

(12) _____ Tibia

(13) _____ Fibula

Tarsals

Metatarsals

Phalanges

(14) Calcaneum _____

Figure 10-8 Anterior view of the axial (bone-colored) and appendicular (blue) skeleton.

Competency Verification: Check your labeling of Figure 10–8 with Appendix B: Answer Key, page 596.

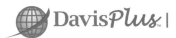 Davis*Plus* | You are not expected to know the CFs and the names of bones from memory. If needed, you can always refer to Figure 10–8, Appendix A: Glossary of Medical Word Elements, or a medical dictionary to obtain information about a bone or its CF.

pain, head	**10–63** Words that contain *cephal/o* refer to the head. Cephal/o/dynia is a _____ in the _____.
cephal/algia sĕf-ă-LĂL-gē-ă	**10–64** Cephal/o/dynia is the medical term for a headache. Construct another word that means *pain in the head*. _____ / _____

head **-meter**	**10–65** A meter is a metric unit of length equal to 39.37 inches. However, when used as a suffix *-meter* means *instrument for measuring*. Thus, a cephal/o/meter is an instrument for measuring the _____. In cephal/o/meter, the element that means *instrument for measuring* is _____.
encephal/o	**10–66** The prefix *en-* means *in, within*. Combine *en-* + *cephal/o* to create a new CF that refers to the brain. _____ / _____
encephal/oma ĕn-sĕf-ă-LŌ-mă **encephal/itis** ĕn-sĕf-ă-LĪ-tĭs **encephal/o/malacia** ĕn-sĕf-ă-lō-mă-LĀ-sē-ă	**10–67** Use *encephal/o* to build words that mean *tumor of the brain:* _____ / _____ *inflammation of the brain:* _____ / _____ *softening of the brain (tissue):* _____ / _____ / _____
encephal/itis ĕn-sĕf-ă-LĪ-tĭs	**10–68** Encephal/itis is usually caused by viruses (such as arbovirus and herpes virus). Less commonly, it may occur as a component of rabies and acquired immuno-deficiency syndrome (AIDS). It may also occur as a result of systemic viral diseases, such as influenza, rubella, and chickenpox. The medical term for an inflammatory condition of the brain is _____ / _____.
disease, brain	**10–69** Encephal/o/pathy is a _____ of the _____.
brain	**10–70** An encephal/o/cele is a protrusion of _____ substance through an opening of the skull.
inter- **cost** **-al**	**10–71** Inter/cost/al muscles, located between the ribs, move the ribs during the breathing process. Write the elements in this frame that mean *between:* _____ *ribs:* _____ *pertaining to:* _____

Boldface indicates a word root or combining form. Blue indicates a suffix. Pink indicates a prefix.

under *or* **below, ribs**	**10–72** Sub/cost/al refers to the area _____ the _____.

pain, rib	**10–73** Cost/algia is a _____ in a _____.

Fractures and Repairs

10–74   A fracture is a break or crack in the bone. Fractures are defined according to the type and extent of the break. A (1) **closed fracture** means the bone is broken with no open wound, and surrounding tissue damage is minimal. An (2) **open fracture**, also called a **compound fracture**, means the broken end of a bone pierces the skin, creating an open wound. In such a fracture, there may be extensive damage to surrounding blood vessels, nerves, and muscles. Label the closed and open fractures in Figure 10–9.

10–75   In addition to determining the extent of a break in a fracture, there are many different types of bone fractures, some of which are discussed here. A (3) **greenstick fracture** is an incomplete break of a soft bone, which means the bone is partially bent and partially broken. These fractures usually occur in children because their growing bones are soft and tend to splinter, rather than break completely. A (4) **comminuted fracture** occurs when the bone is broken into pieces. In an (5) **impacted fracture**, the broken ends of a bone are forced into one another; many bone fragments may be created by such a fracture. A (6) **complicated fracture** involves extensive soft tissue injury, such as when a broken rib pierces a lung. A (7) **Colles fracture** is a break of the lower end of the radius, which occurs just above the wrist. It causes displacement of the hand and usually occurs as a result of flexing a hand to cushion a fall. An (8) **incomplete fracture** is when the line of fracture does not include the whole bone. Label and study the different types of fractures in Figure 10–9.

Competency Verification: Check your labeling of Figure 10–9 in Appendix B: Answer Key, page 596.

open fracture, compound fracture **closed fracture**	**10–76** Identify the fractures that describe the following statements. (Refer to Figure. 10–9.) A bone pierces the skin and causes extensive damage to surrounding blood vessels: _____ _____, also called _____ _____ A bone is broken with no external wound present: _____ _____

greenstick fracture **impacted fracture** ĭm-PĂK-tĕd	**10–77** Identify the fractures that describe the following statements. (Refer to Fig. 10–9.) A bone is partially bent and partially broken (found more commonly in children): _____ _____ The broken ends of bone segments are wedged into one another: _____ _____

Vertebral Column

spin/al column SPĪ-năl **spin/o**	**10–78** The vertebr/al or spin/al column supports the body and provides a protective bony canal for the spinal cord. Another name for the vertebr/al column is _____ / _____ _____. From the word spin/al, construct the CF for *spine*. _____ / _____
vertebra VĔR-tĕ-bră	**10–79** *Spondyl/o* and *vertebr/o* are CFs that refer to the vertebrae (backbone). The singular form of vertebrae is _____.
vertebra VĔR-tĕ-bră **vertebra** VĔR-tĕ-bră	**10–80** Vertebr/ectomy is an excision of a _____. Spondyl/o/dynia is a painful condition of a _____.

10–81   Change the following words from singular to plural form by retaining the *a* and adding an *e*.

vertebrae VĔR-tĕ-brē **bursae** BĔR-sē **pleurae** PLOO-rē	**Singular** **Plural** vertebra _____ bursa _____ pleura _____
spondyl/itis spŏn-dĭl-Ī-tĭs **spondyl/o/pathy** spŏn-dĭl-ŎP-ă-thē **spondyl/o/malacia** spŏn-dĭl-ō-mă-LĀ-shē-ă	**10–82** Whereas *vertebr/o* is used to form words that describe the vertebra, *spondyl/o* is used to form words about the condition of the vertebra. Build medical words that mean *inflammation of vertebrae:* _____ / _____ *disease of vertebrae:* _____ / _____ / _____ *softening of vertebrae:* _____ / _____ / _____
vertebra, vertebra VĔR-tĕ-bră	**10–83** As discussed previously, *vertebr/o* is used to form words that describe the vertebral structure. For example, vertebr/o/cost/al means *pertaining to a* _____ *and a rib.* Vertebr/o/stern/al means *pertaining to a* _____ *and the sternum, or chest plate.*

Boldface indicates a word root or combining form. Blue indicates a suffix. Pink indicates a prefix.

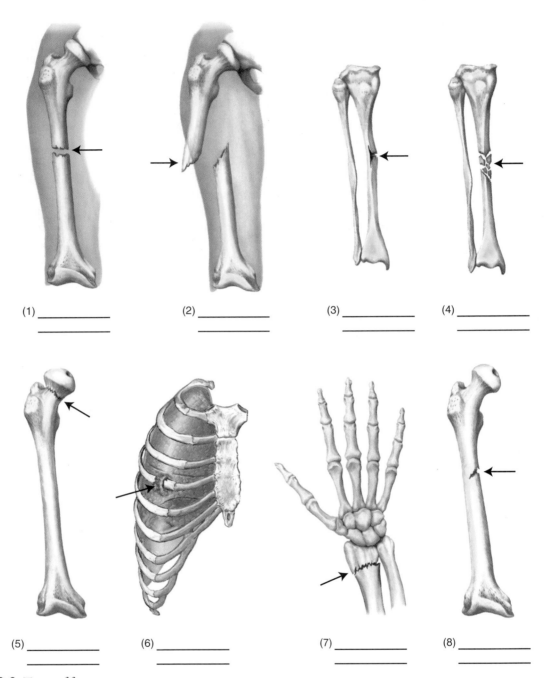

(1) _____
_____

(2) _____
_____

(3) _____
_____

(4) _____
_____

(5) _____
_____

(6) _____
_____

(7) _____
_____

(8) _____
_____

Figure 10-9 Types of fractures.

10-84 Vertebrae are separated and cushioned from each other by (1) **interverte-bral disks** composed of cartilage. Label Figure 10–10 as you learn about the vertebr/al or spin/al column.

inter- vertebr/o -al	**10–85** Determine the elements in inter/vertebr/al that mean *between:* _____ *vertebra (backbone):* _____ / _____ *pertaining to:* _____

10–86   The vertebr/al column, also called the spin/al column or backbone, is composed of 26 bones known as vertebrae (singular, vertebra). There are five regions of these bones in the vertebr/al column, each of which derives its name from its location along the length of the spin/al column. Seven (2) **cervical vertebrae** form the skeletal framework of the neck. The first cervic/al vertebra is called the (3) **atlas** and supports the skull. The second, the (4) **axis,** enables the skull to rotate on the neck. Label these structures in Figure 10–10.

neck	**10–87** The CF *cervic/o* means *neck; cervix uteri (neck of the uterus).* Cervic/o/facial refers to the face and _____.

atlas ĂT-lăs **cervic/al** SĔR-vĭ-kăl	**10–88** The name of the first cervic/al vertebra is the _____. A term that means pertaining to the neck is _____ / _____.

C5	**10–89** In medical reports, the first cervical vertebra is designated as C1. The fifth cervical vertebra is designated as _____.

C5	**10–90** A diagnosis of C4 to C5 herniation means the cervic/al disk between C4 and _____ is ruptured or herniated.

C2	**10–91** The second vertebra is identified as _____.

seven	**10–92** There are a total of _____ cervic/al vertebrae.

10–93   Twelve (5) **thoracic vertebrae** support the chest and serve as a point of articulation (joining together to allow motion between parts) for the ribs. The next five vertebrae are the (6) **lumbar vertebrae.** These are situated in the lower back and carry most of the weight of the torso. Label these structures in Figure 10–10.

Boldface indicates a word root or combining form. Blue indicates a suffix. Pink indicates a prefix.

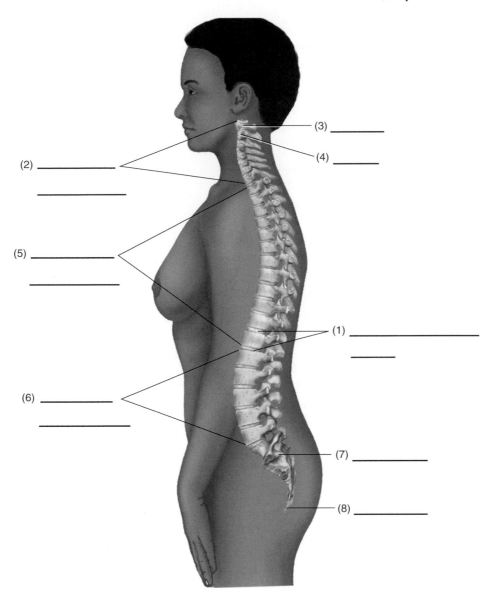

Figure 10-10 Vertebral column, lateral view, with regions of the spine shown with normal curves.

articulation ăr-tĭk-ū-LĀ-shŭn **thorac/ic** thō-RĂS-ĭk	**10–94** Identify the terms in Frame 10–93 that mean *a place where two bones meet:* _____ *pertaining to the chest:* _____ / _____

pertaining to, back	**10–95** The CF *lumb/o* refers to the *loins (lower back).* Lumb/ar means _____ _____ *the loins or* *lower* _____.

pain	**10-96** Lumb/o/dynia is a _____ in the lower back.

lumbar, five LŬM-băr	**10-97** Examine the position of the five lumbar vertebrae in Figure 10–10, designated as L1 to L5 in medical reports. An obese person with weak abdominal muscles tends to experience pain in the lower back area, or L1 to L5. L5 refers to _____ vertebra _____.

	10-98 Below the lumbar vertebrae are five **sacral vertebrae** that are fused into a single bone in the adult. The single bone is known as the (7) **sacrum** and the tail of the vertebral column, the (8) **coccyx**. Label the sacrum and coccyx in Figure 10–10.

pain **sacr/um, spine** SĀ-krŭm	**10-99** The CF *sacr/o* means *sacr/um*. The suffix in the term *sacr/um* means structure, thing. Sacr/o/dynia is a _____ in the sacrum. Sacr/o/spin/al refers to the _____ / _____ and _____.

S5	**10-100** Although the sacral vertebrae are fused into a single bone, to designate the exact position of abnormalities on the sacrum, the labels S1 to S5 are used. The first vertebra of the sacrum is designated as S1. The fifth vertebra of the sacrum is designated as _____.

lumbar, sacrum LŬM-băr, SĀ-krŭm	**10-101** A ruptured disk can cause severe pain, muscle weakness, or numbness in either leg. The disk that most commonly ruptures is the L5 to S1 disk. L5 refers to _____ *five*. S1 refers to _____ *one*.

Competency Verification: Check your labeling of Figure 10–10 in Appendix B: Answer Key, page 596.

Boldface indicates a word root or combining form. Blue indicates a suffix. Pink indicates a prefix.

SECTION REVIEW 10-5

Using the following table, write the CF or suffix that matches its definition in the space provided to the left of the definition. There may be more than one word element that matches a definition.

Combining Forms

arthr/o	oste/o
cephal/o	sacr/o
cervic/o	spondyl/o
cost/o	thorac/o
encephal/o	vertebr/o
lumb/o	

Suffixes

-centesis
-ectomy
-osis
-pathy
-um

1. _____ abnormal condition; increase (used primarily with blood cells)

2. _____ bone

3. _____ brain

4. _____ chest

5. _____ disease

6. _____ excision, removal

7. _____ head

8. _____ joint

9. _____ loins (lower back)

10. _____ neck; cervix uteri (neck of the uterus)

11. _____ structure, thing

12. _____ ribs

13. _____ sacrum

14. _____ surgical puncture

15. _____ vertebra (backbone)

Competency Verification: Check your answers in Appendix B: Answer Key, page 597. If you are not satisfied with your level of comprehension, go back to Frame 10–51 and rework the frames.

Correct Answers _____ × 6.67 = _____ % Score

ABBREVIATIONS

This section introduces musculoskeletal system–related abbreviations and their meanings.

Abbreviation	Meaning	Abbreviation	Meaning
AIDS	acquired immunodeficiency syndrome	HNP	herniated nucleus pulposus (herniated disk)
AP	anteroposterior	L1, L2, to L5	first lumbar vertebra, second lumbar vertebra, and so on
C1, C2, to C7	first cervical vertebra, second cervical vertebra, and so on	MG	myasthenia gravis
D.O., DO	Doctor of Osteopathy	RA	rheumatoid arthritis
CT	computed tomography	S1, S2, to S5	first sacral vertebra, second sacral vertebra, and so on
CTS	carpal tunnel syndrome	THR	total hip replacement
Fx	fracture	T1, T2, to T12	first thoracic vertebra, second thoracic vertebra, and so on

ADDITIONAL MEDICAL TERMS

The following are additional terms related to the musculoskeletal system. Recognizing and learning these terms will help you understand the connection between a pathological condition, its diagnosis, and the rationale behind the method of treatment selected for a particular disorder.

Diseases and Conditions

Muscular Disorders

muscular dystrophy MŬS-kū-lăr DĬS-trō-fē *muscul:* muscle *-ar:* pertaining to *dys-:* bad; painful; difficult *-trophy:* development, nourishment	Group of hereditary diseases characterized by gradual atrophy and weakness of muscle tissue *There is no cure for muscular dystrophy. Duchenne muscular dystrophy is the most common form with an average life span of 20 years.*
myasthenia gravis (MG) mī-ăs-THĒ-nē-ă GRĂV-ĭs	Autoimmune neuromuscular disorder characterized by severe muscular weakness and progressive fatigue
sprain	Trauma to a joint that causes injury to the surrounding ligament, accompanied by pain and disability

strain	Trauma to a muscle from overuse or excessive forcible stretch in which great toe is angled laterally toward the other toes.
tendinitis těn-dĭn-Ī-tĭs	Inflammation of a tendon, usually caused by injury or overuse; also called *tendonitis*
torticollis tōr-tĭ-KŎL-ĭs	Spasmodic contraction of the neck muscles, causing stiffness and twisting of the neck; also called wryneck *Torticollis may be congenital or acquired.*

Bones and Joints

bunion BŬN-yŭn	Deformity characterized by lateral deviation of the great toe as it turns in toward the second toe (angulation), which may cause the tissues surrounding the metatarsophalangeal joint to become swollen and tender; also called *hallux valgus* (See Fig. 10–11.) *Bunion is associated with rheumatoid arthritis, chronic irritation and pressure from tight-fitting shoes, or heredity. Treatment includes proper footwear, wearing padding around the toes to relieve pressure, medication for pain and swelling, or bunionectomy and arthroplasty.*
carpal tunnel syndrome (CTS) KĂR-păl TŬN-ĕl SĬN-drōm	Pain or numbness resulting from compression of the median nerve within the carpal tunnel (wrist canal through which the flexor tendons and median nerve pass)
contracture kŏn-TRĂK-chŭr	Fibrosis of connective tissue in the skin, fascia, muscle, or joint capsule that prevents normal mobility of the related tissue or joint
crepitation krĕp-ĭ-TĀ-shŭn	Grating sound made by movement of bone ends rubbing together, indicating a fracture or joint destruction

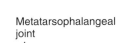
Metatarsophalangeal joint

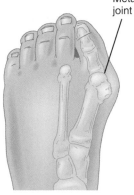

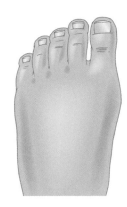

Figure 10-11 Bunion. **(A)** Preoperative. **(B)** Postoperative.

Ewing sarcoma Ū-ĭng săr-KŌ-mă	Malignant tumor that develops from bone marrow, usually in long bones or the pelvis *Ewing sarcoma occurs most commonly in adolescent boys.*
ganglion cyst GĂNG-lē-ŏn SĬST	Fluid-filled tumor that most commonly develops along the tendons or joint of the wrists or hands but may also occur in the ankles and feet *In most instances, ganglion cysts cause no pain, require no treatment, and go away on their own. Reasons for treatment are cosmetic or when the cyst causes pain (presses on a nearby nerve) or interferes with joint movement. Treatment involves removing the fluid or excising the cyst. (See Fig. 10–12.)*
gout GOWT	Hereditary metabolic disease that is a form of acute arthritis, characterized by excessive uric acid in the blood and around the joints
herniated disk HĔR-nē-āt-ĕd	Herniation or rupture of the nucleus pulposus (center gelatinous material within an intervetebral disk) between two vertebrae; also called *prolapsed disk* (See Fig. 10–13.) *A herniated disk places pressure on a spinal root nerve or the spinal cord. Displacement of the disk irritates the spinal nerves, causing muscle spasms and pain. It occurs most commonly in the lower spine.*

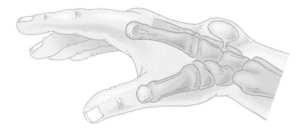

Figure 10-12 Ganglion cyst of the wrist

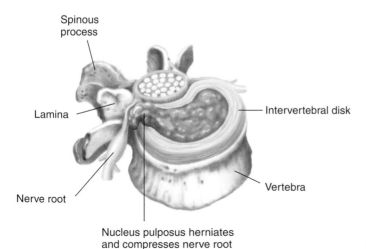

Spinous process

Lamina

Nerve root

Nucleus pulposus herniates and compresses nerve root

Intervertebral disk

Vertebra

Figure 10-13 Herniated disk.

osteoporosis ŏs-tē-ō-pōr-Ō-sĭs *oste/o:* bone *-porosis:* porous	Decrease in bone density with an increase in porosity, causing bones to become brittle and increasing the risk of fractures
Paget disease PĂJ-ĕt	Skeletal disease affecting elderly people that causes chronic inflammation of bones, resulting in thickening and softening of bones and bowing of long bones; also called *osteitis deformans*
rheumatoid arthritis (RA) ROO-mă-toyd ăr-THRĪ-tĭs *arthr:* joint *-itis:* inflammation	Chronic, systemic, inflammatory disease affecting the synovial membranes of multiple joints, eventually resulting in crippling deformities (See Fig. 10–14.) *As RA develops, congestion and edema of the synovial membrane and joint occur, causing formation of a thick layer of granulation tissue. This tissue invades cartilage, destroying the joint and bone. Eventually, a fibrous immobility of joints (ankylosis) occurs, causing visible deformities and total immobility.*
rotator cuff injury	Trauma to the capsule of the shoulder joint, which is reinforced by muscles and tendons; also called musculotendinous rotator cuff injury *Rotator cuff injuries occur in sports in which there is a complete abduction of the shoulder, followed by a rapid and forceful rotation and flexion of the shoulder. This type of injury occurs most commonly in baseball when the player throws a baseball.*
subluxation sŭb-lŭk-SĀ-shŭn	Partial or complete dislocation

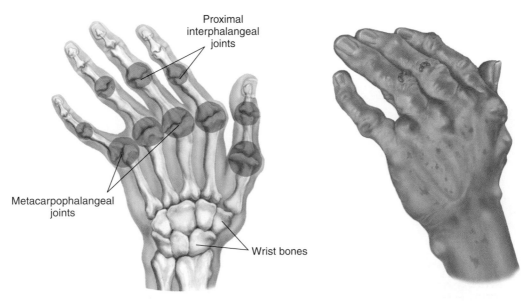

Proximal interphalangeal joints

Metacarpophalangeal joints

Wrist bones

Figure 10-14 Rheumatoid arthritis.

sequestrum sē-KWĔS-trŭm	Fragment of a necrosed bone that has become separated from surrounding tissue

talipes equinovarus TĂL-ĭ-pēz ē-kwī-nō- VĀR-ŭs	Congenital deformity of the foot; also called *clubfoot* (See Fig. 10–15.) *In talipes, the heel never rests on the ground. Treatment consists of applying casts to progressively straighten the foot and surgical correction for severe cases.*

Spinal Disorders

ankylosing spondylitis
ĂNG-kĭ-lōs-ĭng spŏn-
dĭl-Ī-tĭs
   spondyl/o: vertebra
          (backbone)
   -itis: inflamma-
          tion
	Chronic inflammatory disease of unknown origin that first affects the spine and is characterized by fusion and loss of mobility of two or more vertebrae; also called *rheumatoid spondylitis*
	
	Treatment includes nonsteroidal anti-inflammatory drugs and, in advanced cases of a badly deformed spine, surgery.

kyphosis
kī-FŌ-sĭs
   kyph: humpback
   -osis: abnormal condi-
          tion; increase
          (used primarily
          with blood cells)
	Increased curvature of the thoracic region of the vertebral column, leading to a humpback posture; also called *hunchback*
	
	Kyphosis may be caused by poor posture, arthritis, or osteomalacia. (See Fig. 10–16.)

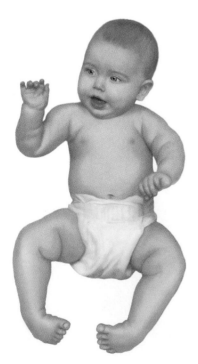

Figure 10-15 Talipes equinovarus

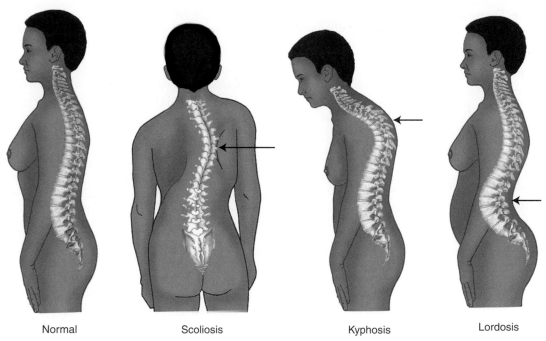

Normal Scoliosis Kyphosis Lordosis

Figure 10-16 Spinal curvatures.

lordosis lōr-DŌ-sĭs *lord:* curve, swayback *-osis:* abnormal condition; increase (used primarily with blood cells)	Forward curvature of the lumbar region of the vertebral column, leading to a swayback posture *Lordosis may be caused by increased weight in the abdomen, such as during pregnancy. (See Fig. 10-16.)*
scoliosis skō-lē-Ō-sĭs *scoli:* crooked, bent *-osis:* abnormal condition; increase (used primarily with blood cells)	Abnormal sideward curvature of the spine to the left or right *Scoliosis eventually causes back pain, disk disease, or arthritis. It is commonly a congenital disease, but may result from poor posture. (See Fig. 10–16.)*
spondylolisthesis spŏn-dĭ-lō-lĭs-THĒ-sĭs *spondyl/o:* vertebra (backbone) *-listhesis:* slipping	Partial forward dislocation of one vertebra over the one below it, most commonly the fifth lumbar vertebra over the first sacral vertebra; also called spinal cord compression

Diagnostic Procedures

arthrocentesis
ăr-thrō-sĕn-TĒ-sĭs
  arthr/o: joint
  -centesis: surgical
      puncture

Puncture of a joint space with a needle to remove fluid

Arthrocentesis is performed to obtain samples of synovial fluid for diagnostic purposes. It may also be used to instill medications and remove accumulated fluid from joints to relieve pain.

---

bone density test (bone densitometry)

Low energy x-ray absorption of the wrist, pelvis, and spinal column to measure bone density for purposes of diagnosis and management of osteoporosis; also called *dual-energy x-ray absorptiometry (DEXA)*

---

bone scan

Nuclear medicine procedure that visualizes bone(s) after the intravenous injection of a radiopharmaceutical

A special scanning device detects areas of increased uptake of the radiopharmaceutical to indicate abnormalities of bone such as infection, inflamamtion, fractures, and tumors.

---

rheumatoid factor
ROO-mă-toyd

Blood test to detect the presence of rheumatoid factor, a substance present in patients with rheumatoid arthritis

Medical and Surgical Procedures

arthroplasty
ĂR-thrō-plăs-tē
  arthr/o: joint
  -plasty: surgical repair

Surgical reconstruction or replacement of a painful, degenerated joint to restore mobility in rheumatoid arthritis or osteoarthritis or to correct a congenital deformity

---

sequestrectomy
sē-kwĕs-TRĔK-tō-mē
  sequestr: separation
  -ectomy: excision,
      removal

Excision of a sequestrum (segment of necrosed bone)

PHARMACOLOGY

The following table lists common drug categories used to treat musculoskeletal disorders, as well as their therapeutic actions.

Drug Category	Action
bone reabsorption inhibitors	Reduce reabsorption of bone in the treatment of weak and fragile bones, as seen in osteoporosis and Paget disease
gold salts	Treat rheumatoid arthritis by inhibiting activity within the immune system to prevent further disease progression
nonsteroidal anti-inflammatory drugs (NSAIDs) nŏn-STĔR-oyd-ăl ăn-tē-ĭn-FLĂM-ă-tō-rē	Relieve mild to moderate pain and reduce inflammation in the treatment of musculoskeletal conditions, such as sprains and strains, and inflammatory disorders, such as rheumatoid arthritis, osteoarthritis, bursitis, gout, and tendinitis

Pronunciation Help Long sound ā in rāte ē in rēbirth ī in īsle ō in ōver ū in ūnite
Short sound ă in ălone ĕ in ĕver ĭ in ĭt ŏ in nŏt ŭ in cŭt

ADDITIONAL MEDICAL TERMS REVIEW

Match the medical terms below with the definitions in the numbered list.

ankylosis	crepitation	kyphosis	RA	sprain
arthroplasty	CTS	lordosis	rheumatoid factor	strain
arthroscopy	Ewing sarcoma	muscular dystrophy	scoliosis	talipes
bunion	gout	myasthenia gravis	sequestrectomy	tendinitis
contracture	herniated disk	Paget disease	sequestrum	torticollis

1. _____ is a deformity characterized by lateral deviation of the great toe.

2. _____ is an inflammation of a tendon.

3. _____ refers to trauma to a joint, causing injury to the surrounding ligament.

4. _____ refers to trauma to a muscle that results from overuse or excessive, forcible stretch.

5. _____ refers to a hunchback or humpback.

6. _____ is a malignant tumor that develops from bone marrow, usually in long bones or the pelvis, and occurs most commonly in adolescent boys.

7. _____ is characterized by spasmodic contraction of the neck muscles and is also called *wryneck.*

8. _____ is a disease characterized by excessive uric acid in the blood and around the joints.

9. _____ is a disease characterized by inflammatory changes in joints and related structures that result in crippling deformities.

10. _____ is a skeletal disease of the elderly with chronic inflammation of bones, resulting in thickening and softening of bones and bowing of long bones, and is also called osteitis deformans.

11. _____ is a fragment of necrosed bone that has become separated from surrounding tissue.

12. _____ is the replacement of a joint.

13. _____ is a grating sound made by the ends of bone rubbing together.

14. _____ is a neuromuscular disorder characterized by muscular weakness and progressive fatigue.

15. _____ refers to a forward curvature of the lumbar spine, also called *swayback.*

16. _____ refers to a group of hereditary diseases characterized by gradual atrophy and weakness of muscle, with the most common form called Duchenne.

17. _____ is connective tissue fibrosis that prevents normal mobility of the related tissue or joint.

18. _____ is an immobility of a joint.

19. _____ refers to rupture of the nucleus pulposus between two vertebrae.

20. _____ is pain or numbness resulting from compression of the median nerve within the carpal tunnel.

21. _____ is excision of a necrosed piece of bone.

22. _____ is a blood test to detect a substance present in the blood of patients with rheumatoid arthritis.

23. _____ is a congenital foot deformity that is also called clubfoot.

24. _____ is the visual examination of a joint.

25. _____ is an abnormal sideward curvature of the spine to the left or right.

Competency Verification: Check your answers in Appendix B: Answer Key, page 597. If you are not satisfied with your level of comprehension, review the additional medical terms and retake the review.

Correct Answers _____ × 4 = _____ % Score

MEDICAL RECORD ACTIVITIES

Medical reports included in the following activities reflect common, real-life clinical scenarios using medical terminology to document patient care.

MEDICAL RECORD ACTIVITY 10-1

DEGENERATIVE, INTERVERTEBRAL DISK DISEASE

Terminology

Terms listed in the table below come from the medical report Degenerative, Intervertebral Disk Disease *that follows. Use a medical dictionary such as* Taber's Cyclopedic Medical Dictionary, *the appendices of this book, or other resources to define each term. Then practice reading the pronunciations aloud for each term.*

Term	Definition
bilateral bī-LĂT-ĕr-ăl	
degenerative dĕ-JĔN-ĕr-ă-tĭv	
hypertrophic hī-pĕr-TRŌF-ĭk	
intervertebral ĭn-tĕr-VĔRT-ĕ-brăl	
L5	

Continued

Term	Definition
laminectomies lăm-ĭ-NĔK-tō-mēz	
lipping LĬP-ĭng	
lumbar LŬM-băr	
S1	
sacroiliac sā-krō-ĬL-ē-ăk	
sacrum SĀ-krŭm	

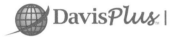 **DavisPlus** | Visit the *Medical Terminology Simplified* online resource center at Davis*Plus* to hear pronunciation and meanings of selected terms in this medical report.

Reading

Practice pronunciation of medical terms by reading the following medical report aloud.

Degenerative, Intervertebral Disk Disease

Anteroposterior and lateral views of the lumbar spine and an AP view of the sacrum show a displacement of L5 on S1. The L5–S1 intervertebral disk space contains a slight shadow of decreased density. There is now slight narrowing of the L3–L4 and L4–L5. Bilateral laminectomies appear to have been done at L5–S1. Slight hypertrophic lipping of the upper lumbar vertebral bodies is now seen, as is slight lipping of the upper margin of the body of L4. The sacroiliac joint spaces are well preserved. Lateral views of the lumbosacral spine taken with the spine in flexion and extension show slight motion at all of the lumbar and lumbosacral levels.

IMPRESSION: 1. Degenerative, intervertebral disk disease at L5–S1, now also accompanied by slight narrowing of the L3–L4 and L4–L5.
2. Slight motion at all of the lumbar and lumbosacral levels.

Evaluation

Review the medical report above to answer the following questions. Use a medical dictionary such as Taber's Cyclopedic Medical Dictionary *and other resources if needed.*

1. Why does the x-ray show a decreased density at L5–S1?

   _____

   _____

2. What is the most common cause of degenerative intervertebral disk disease?

   _____

   _____

3. What happens to the gelatinous material of the disk as aging occurs?

   _____

   _____

4. What is the probable cause of the narrowing of the L3–L4 and L4–L5?

   _____

   _____

MEDICAL RECORD ACTIVITY 10-2

ROTATOR CUFF TEAR, RIGHT SHOULDER

Terminology

Terms listed in the table below come from the medical report Rotator Cuff Tear, Right Shoulder *that follows. Use a medical dictionary such as* Taber's Cyclopedic Medical Dictionary, *the appendices of this book, or other resources to define each term. Then practice reading the pronunciations aloud for each term.*

Term	Definition
AC joint	
acromial ăk-RŌ-mē-ăl	
acromioclavicular ă-krō-mē-ō-klă-VĬK-ū-lăr	
arthroscopy ăr-THRŎS-kō-pē	
biceps BĪ-sĕps	

Continued

Term	Definition
bursectomy bŭr-SĔK-tō-mē	
calcification kăl-sĭ-fĭ-KĀ-shŭn	
degenerative dĕ-JĔN-ĕr-ă-tĭv	
glenohumeral glē-nō-HŪ-mĕr-ăl	
glenoid GLĒ-noyd	
gouty GOW-tē	
intra-articular ĭn-tră-ăr-TĬK-ū-lăr	
labra (singular, *labrum*) LĂ-bră	
osteophyte ŎS-tē-ō-fīt	
spur SPĔR	
tuberosity tū-bĕr-ŎS-ĭ-tē	

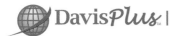

Visit the *Medical Terminology Simplified* online resource center at Davis*Plus* to hear pronunciation and meanings of selected terms in this medical report.

Reading

Practice pronunciation of medical terms by reading the following medical report aloud.

Rotator Cuff Tear, Right Shoulder

PREOPERATIVE DIAGNOSIS: Rotator cuff tear, right shoulder. Degenerative arthritis, right acromioclavicular joint. Calcific tendinitis at the level of the superior glenoid tuberosity, right shoulder. Early degenerative osteoarthritis of the right shoulder. History of gouty arthritis.

POSTOPERATIVE DIAGNOSIS: Rotator cuff tear, right shoulder. Degenerative arthritis, right acromioclavicular joint. Calcific tendinitis at the level of the superior glenoid tuberosity, right shoulder. Early degenerative osteoarthritis of the right shoulder. History of gouty arthritis.

OPERATION: Open repair of rotator cuff, open incision outer end of clavicle, anterior acromioplasty, glenohumeral and subacromial arthroscopy with arthroscopic bursectomy.

FINDINGS: A glenohumeral arthroscopy revealed the superior, anterior, inferior, and posterior glenoid labra were intact. There was some fraying of the anterior glenoid labrum. The long head of the biceps was intact. We were unable to visualize any intra-articular calcification. We observed the takeoff of the long head of the biceps from the posterior-superior edge of the glenoid labrum and the glenoid tuberosity. There was an osteophyte inferiorly on the humeral head. There was a deep surface tear of the rotator cuff at the posterior-superior corner of the greater tuberosity of the humerus at the infraspinatus insertion. There was an extremely dense subacromial bursal scar. There was prominence of the inferior edge of the AC joint, with inferior AC joint and anterior acromial spurs.

Evaluation

Review the medical report above to answer the following questions. Use a medical dictionary such as Taber's Cyclopedic Medical Dictionary *and other resources if needed.*

1. What type of arthritis did the patient have?

   _____

   _____

2. Did the patient have calcium deposits in the right shoulder?

   _____

   _____

3. What type of instrument did the physician use to visualize the glenoid labra?

   _____

   _____

4. What are labra?

   _____

   _____

5. Did the patient have any outgrowths of bone? If so, where?

   _____

   _____

6. Did they find any deposits of calcium salts within the shoulder joint?

   _____

   _____

MUSCULOSKELETAL SYSTEM CHAPTER REVIEW

WORD ELEMENTS SUMMARY

The following table summarizes CFs, suffixes, and prefixes related to the musculoskeletal system. Study the word elements and their meanings before completing the Word Elements Chapter Review that follows.

Word Element	Meaning	Word Element	Meaning
Combining Forms			
arthr/o	joint	**metacarp/o**	metacarpus (hand bones)
calc/o	calcium	**myel/o**	bone marrow; spinal cord
calcane/o	calcaneum (heel bone)	**my/o**	muscle
carp/o	carpus (wrist bones)	**oste/o**	bone
cephal/o	head	**patell/o**	patella (kneecap)
cervic/o	neck; cervix uteri (neck of the uterus)	**proxim/o**	near
chondr/o	cartilage	**radi/o**	radiation, x-ray; radius (lower arm bone on the thumb side)
cost/o	ribs	**roentgen/o**	x-ray
crani/o	cranium (skull)	**sacr/o**	sacrum
cyt/o	cell	**scler/o**	hardening; sclera (white of the eye)
dist/o	far, farthest	**spin/o**	spine
encephal/o	brain	**spondyl/o, vertebr/o**	vertebra (backbone)
femor/o	femur (thigh bone)	**stern/o**	sternum (breastbone)
humer/o	humerus (upper arm bone)	**tend/o**	tendon
lumb/o	loin (lower back)	**tibi/o**	tibia (larger inner bone of the lower leg)
Suffixes			
-algia, -dynia	pain	**-logist**	specialist in the study of
-cele	hernia, swelling	**-malacia**	softening
-centesis	surgical puncture	**-meter**	instrument for measuring
-cyte	cell	**-oma**	tumor
-ectomy	excision, removal	**-osis**	abnormal condition
-emia	blood condition	**-pathy**	disease
-genesis	forming, producing, origin	**-plasty**	surgical repair
-gram	record, writing	**-plegia**	paralysis
-graphy	process of recording	**-rrhaphy**	suture
-ist	specialist	**-rrhexis**	rupture
-itis	inflammation	**-tomy**	incision

Word Element	Meaning	Word Element	Meaning
Prefixes			
en-	in, within	inter-	between
hemi-	one half	peri-	around
hypo-	under, below, deficient	quadri-	four

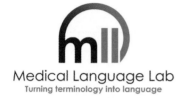

Medical Language Lab
Turning terminology into language

Visit the *Medical Language Lab* at *medicallanguagelab.com.* Use the flash-card–word elements exercise to reinforce your study of word elements. We recommend you complete the flash-card activity before starting the Word Elements Chapter Review that follows.

WORD ELEMENTS CHAPTER REVIEW

This review provides a verification of your knowledge of the word elements covered in this chapter. Write the meaning of the word element in the space provided. To reinforce your understanding of the word parts that comprise a medical term, each word element is identified as a prefix (P), word root (WR), combining form (CF), or suffix (S). The first word is completed for you.

Medical Term	Word Element	Meaning
1. arthr/o/desis	*arthr/o (CF)*	*joint*
	-desis (S)	*binding; fixation (of a bone or joint)*
2. calcane/o/dynia		
3. chondr/oma		
4. cost/o/chondr/itis		
5. dia/physis		

Medical Term	Word Element	Meaning
6. fasci/o/plasty		
7. hemi/plegia		
8. lamin/ectomy		
9. leiomy/oma		
10. my/algia		
11. myel/o/cele		

Continued

Medical Term	Word Element	Meaning
12. my/esthenia		
13. my/o/sarc/oma		
14. orth/o/ped/ics		
15. oste/o/clast		
16. oste/o/malacia		

Medical Term	Word Element	Meaning
17. oste/o/porosis		
18. patell/ectomy		
19. pelv/i/metry		
20. radi/o/graph		

Competency Verification: Check your answers in Appendix B: Answer Key, page 598. If you are not satisfied with your level of comprehension, review the chapter's flash-card activity at the website *medicallanguagelab.com* and retake the review.

Correct Answers _____ × 5 = _____ % Score

VOCABULARY REVIEW

Match the medical terms below with the definitions in the numbered list.

AP	bone marrow	distal	proximal
arthrocentesis	cephalometer	intervertebral	quadriplegia
articulation	cervical vertebrae	myelogram	radiologist
atlas	closed fracture	myorrhexis	radiology
bilateral	diaphysis	open fracture	spondylomalacia

1. _____ is the study of x-rays and radioactive substances used for diagnosing and treating diseases.

2. _____ is the shaft, or main part, of a bone.

3. _____ refers to passing from the front to the rear.

4. _____ is a fracture in which the bone is broken, but there is no external wound and surrounding tissue damage is minimal.

5. _____ means *pertaining to or affecting two sides.*

6. _____ means *near the point of attachment to the trunk.*

7. _____ is the place of union between two or more bones and is also called a joint.

8. _____ is a fracture in which the broken end of a bone has moved so that it pierces the skin, with possibly extensive damage to surrounding blood vessels, nerves, and muscles.

9. _____ is the first cervical vertebra, which supports the skull.

10. _____ is a surgical puncture of a joint to remove fluid.

11. _____ is soft tissue that fills the medullary cavities of long bones.

12. _____ is an instrument used to measure the head.

13. _____ refers to a radiograph of the spinal canal after injection of a contrast medium.

14. _____ means *rupture of a muscle.*

15. _____ means *softening of vertebrae.*

16. _____ is a directional term that means *farthest from the point of attachment to the trunk.*

17. _____ is a physician who specializes in the use of x-rays for the diagnosis and treatment of disease.

18. _____ are bones that form the skeletal framework of the neck.

19. _____ is situated between two adjacent vertebrae.

20. _____ means *paralysis of all four extremities.*

Competency Verification: Check your answers in Appendix B: Answer Key, page 599. If you are not satisfied with your level of comprehension, review the chapter vocabulary and retake the review.

Correct Answers:_____ × 5 = _____ % Score

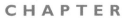
Special Senses: Eyes and Ears

OBJECTIVES

Upon completion of this chapter, you will be able to:

• Describe the type of medical treatment the ophthalmologist and otolaryngologist provide.

• Identify the structures of the eye and ear by labeling them on the anatomical illustrations.

• Describe the primary functions of the eye and ear.

• Describe diseases, conditions, and procedures related to the eye and ear.

• Apply your word-building skills by constructing medical terms related to the eye and ear.

• Describe common abbreviations and symbols related to the eye and ear.

• Recognize, define, pronounce, and spell terms correctly.

• Demonstrate your knowledge of this chapter by successfully completing the frames, reviews, and medical report evaluations.

MEDICAL SPECIALTIES

Ophthalmology

Ophthalmology is the branch of medicine concerned with diagnosis and treatment of eye disorders. The medical specialist in ophthalmology is called an **ophthalmologist.**

Although ophthalmologists specialize in the treatment of the eyes only, it is important for them to be cognizant of other abnormalities that may be revealed during an eye examination. The importance of an eye examination cannot be overestimated, because it commonly reveals the first signs of systemic illnesses (such as diabetes) that may be taking place in other parts of the body. The medical practice of ophthalmology includes prescribing corrective lenses and performing various types of corrective eye surgeries. Specialized surgeries involve techniques that are as delicate and precise as that of neurosurgery and are commonly performed using magnifying glasses and laser beams. Corrective eye surgeries include cornea transplantation, cataract removal, repair of ocular muscle dysfunction, glaucoma treatment, lens removal, and radial keratotomy.

Two other health-care providers, the **optometrist** and **optician,** specialize in providing corrective lenses for the eyes. They are not medical doctors, but are licensed to examine and test the eyes. They also diagnose and treat visual defects by prescribing corrective lenses.

Otolaryngology

Otolaryngology is the medical and surgical management of patients with disorders of the ear, nose, and throat (ENT) and related structures of the head and neck. **Otolaryngologists,** also known as **ENT physicians**, commonly treat disorders related to the sinuses, including allergies and disorders of the sense of smell. Their diagnostic techniques are used to detect the causes of such symptoms as hoarseness, hearing and breathing difficulty, and swelling around the head or neck. Another important part of the ENT physician's practice is treatment of sleep disorders, most commonly sleep apnea. Various types of procedures, including but not limited to surgery, may be performed to treat sleep apnea or snoring disorders. ENT physicians are also involved in introducing rehabilitative programs for children and adults who have suffered hearing loss. Such programs commonly include collaborations with community agencies to identify hearing-impaired individuals (through public screenings) and provide them with needed medical treatment. Another health-care provider, the audiologist (not a medical doctor), detects, evaluates, and treats hearing loss.

ANATOMY AND PHYSIOLOGY OVERVIEW

The major senses of the body are sight, hearing, smell, taste, touch, and balance. These sensations are identified with specific body organs. Senses of smell, taste, and touch were discussed in previous chapters. This chapter focuses on the eyes and ears, which include the senses of sight, hearing, and balance.

EYES

The eyes and their accessory structures are receptor organs that provide vision. As one of the most important sense organs of the body, the eyes not only provide most of the information about what we see, but also of what we learn from printed material. Similar to other sensory organs, the eyes are constructed to detect stimuli in the environment and to transmit those observations to the brain for interpretation.

WORD ELEMENTS

This section introduces combining forms (CFs) related to the eye. Included are key suffixes; prefixes are defined in the right-hand column as needed. Review the following table, and pronounce each word in the word analysis column aloud before you begin to work the frames.

Word Element	Meaning	Word Analysis
Combining Forms		
blephar/o	eyelid	**blephar/o/spasm** (BLĔF-ă-rō-spăzm): involuntary contraction of eyelid muscles *-spasm:* involuntary contraction, twitching *Blepharospasm may be due to eye strain or nervous irritability.*
conjunctiv/o	conjunctiva	**conjunctiv/itis** (kŏn-jŭnk-tĭ-VĪ-tĭs): inflammation of the conjunctiva; also called *pinkeye* *-itis:* inflammation *Conjunctivitis can be caused by bacteria, allergy, irritation, or a foreign body.*
choroid/o	choroid	**choroid/o/pathy** (kō-roy-DŎP-ă-thē): noninflammatory degeneration of the choroid *-pathy:* disease *The choroid is a thin, highly vascular layer of the eye between the retina and sclera.*
corne/o	cornea	**corne/itis** (kŏr-nē-Ī-tĭs): inflammation of the cornea; also called *keratitis* *-itis:* inflammation

cor/o	pupil	**aniso/cor/ia** (ăn-ī-sō-KŌ-rē-ă): inequality of pupil size
		   aniso-: unequal, dissimilar
		      -ia: condition
		Anisocoria may be congenital or associated with a neurological injury or disease.

core/o		**core/o/meter** (kō-rē-ŎM-ĕ-tĕr): instrument for measuring the pupil *-meter:* instrument for measuring
pupill/o		**pupill/ary** (PŪ-pĭ-lăr-ē): pertaining to the pupil *-ary:* pertaining to

Word Element	Meaning	Word Analysis
dacry/o	tear; lacrimal apparatus (duct, sac, or gland)	**dacry/o/rrhea** (dăk-rē-ō-RĒ-ă): excessive secretion of tears *-rrhea:* discharge, flow
lacrim/o		**lacrim/ation** (lăk-rĭ-MĀ-shŭn): secretion and discharge of tears *-ation:* process (of)
dipl/o	double	**dipl/opia** (dĭp-LŌ-pē-ă): two images of an object seen at the same time; also called *double vision* *-opia:* vision
irid/o	iris	**irid/o/plegia** (ĭr-ĭd-ō-PLĒ-jē-ă): paralysis of the sphincter of the iris *-plegia:* paralysis
kerat/o	horny tissue; hard; cornea	**kerat/o/plasty** (KĔR-ă-tō-plăs-tē): replacement of a cloudy cornea with a transparent one, typically derived from an organ donor; also called *corneal transplant* *-plasty:* surgical repair
ocul/o	eye	**intra/ocul/ar** (ĭn-tră-ŎK-ū-lăr): within the eyeball *intra-:* in, within *-ar:* pertaining to
ophthalm/o		**ophthalm/o/scope** (ŏf-THĂL-mō-skōp): instrument for examining the interior of the eye, especially the retina *-scope:* instrument for examining
opt/o	eye, vision	**opt/ic** (ŎP-tĭk): pertaining to the eye or vision *-ic:* pertaining to
retin/o	retina	**retin/o/pathy** (rĕt-ĭn-ŎP-ă-thē): disease of the retina *-pathy:* disease
scler/o	hardening; sclera (white of the eye)	**scler/itis** (sklĕ-RĪ-tĭs): inflammation of the sclera *-itis:* inflammation
Suffixes		
-opia	vision	**ambly/opia** (ăm-blē-Ō-pē-ă): reduction or dimness of vision, usually in one eye, with no apparent pathological condition; also called *lazy eye* *ambly:* dull, dim
-opsia		**heter/opsia** (hĕt-ĕr-ŎP-sē-ă): inequality of vision in the two eyes *heter-:* different
-ptosis	prolapse, downward displacement	**blephar/o/ptosis** (blĕf-ă-rō-TŌ-sĭs): drooping of the upper eyelid *blephar/o:* eyelid
-tropia	turning	**hyper/tropia** (hī-pĕr-TRŌ-pē-ă): ocular deviation (strabismus) with one eye located higher than the other *hyper-:* excessive, above normal *Upward deviation of the eye is usually due to paresis of one of the muscles that either elevate or depress the eye. This condition is congenital or acquired.*

Pronunciation Help	Long sound	ā in rāte	ē in rēbirth	ī in īsle	ō in ōver	ū in ūnite
	Short sound	ă in ălone	ĕ in ĕver	ĭ in ĭt	ŏ in nŏt	ŭ in cŭt

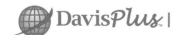 DavisPlus |

Visit the *Medical Terminology Simplified* online resource center at DavisPlus for an audio exercise of the terms in this table. It will help you master pronunciations and meanings of the selected medical terms.

SECTION REVIEW 11-1

For the following medical terms, first write the suffix and its meaning. Then translate the meaning of the remaining elements starting with the first part of the word. The first word is completed for you.

Term	Meaning
1. conjunctiv/itis	-itis: inflammation; conjunctiva
2. blephar/o/ptosis	
3. ambly/opia	
4. retin/o/pathy	
5. scler/itis	
6. ophthalm/o/scope	
7. intra/ocul/ar	
8. dacry/o/rrhea	
9. dipl/opia	
10. blephar/o/spasm	

Competency Verification: Check your answers in Appendix B: Answer Key, page 599. If you are not satisfied with your level of comprehension, review the vocabulary and retake the review.

Correct Answers _____ × 10 = _____ % Score

---

eye

11-1   The eye is a globe-shaped, hollow structure set within a bony cavity. The bony cavity, or orbit, houses the eyeball and associated structures, such as the eye muscles, nerves, and blood vessels. Most of the eyeball is protected from trauma by the orbit's bony cavity. The eyeball consists of three basic layers: the fibrous tunic, the vascular tunic, and the sensory tunic, or retina.

The CFs *ocul/o* and *ophthalm/o* refer to the _____.

Boldface indicates a word root or combining form. Blue indicates a suffix. Pink indicates a prefix.

Fibrous Tunic

11–2   The **fibrous tunic** is the outer layer of the eyeball. It consists of the posterior opaque (1) **sclera** and the anterior transparent (2) **cornea.** The sclera is the white part of the eyeball. It is composed of tightly bound elastic and collagenous fibers, which give shape to the eyeball and protect its inner structures. The sclera is avascular but does contain sensory receptors for pain. At the junction of the sclera and cornea is an opening known as the **canal of Schlemm.** A fluid called aqueous humor drains into this sinus. The cornea is transparent and convex to permit the passage and cause refraction (bending) of incoming lightwaves. The **optic nerve** exits through the sclera at the posterior portion of the eyeball.

Observe the location of the outer layer of the eyeball (fibrous tunic) as you label the sclera and cornea in Figure 11–1.

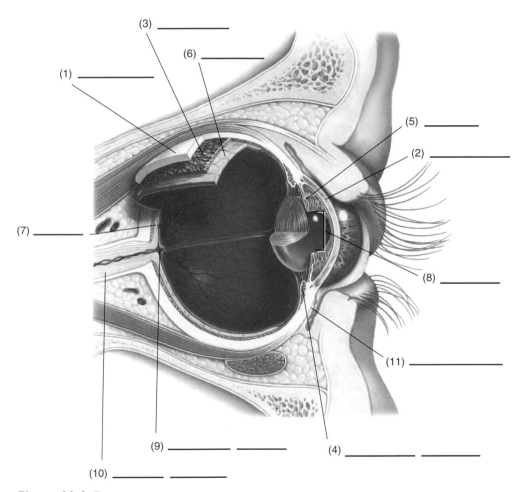

Figure 11-1 Eye structures.

Vascular Tunic

11–3   The **vascular tunic,** or **uvea,** is the middle layer of the eyeball. It is composed of the choroid, ciliary body, and iris. The (3) **choroid** layer lies below the sclera and contains blood vessels. It also contains a dark, pigmented tissue that prevents glare within the eyeball because of its ability to absorb light. The anterior portion of the choroid is modified and forms the (4) **ciliary body** (or muscle) and the (5) **iris,** the colored portion of the eye. Observe the location of the middle layer of the eyeball (vascular tunic) as you label the choroid, ciliary body, and iris in Figure 11–1.

Sensory Tunic

11–4   The innermost layer, the **sensory tunic,** is the delicate, double layered (6) **retina.** This structure lines the posterior two-thirds of the eyeball and is the beginning of the visual pathway. It contains rods and cones, the sensory receptors for vision and image formation. Rods perceive the presence of light only, whereas cones perceive different wavelengths of light as colors. Cones are concentrated in the depression near the center of the retina called the (7) **fovea,** which is the area of sharpest vision. Surrounding the fovea is the yellowish macula, which also has an abundance of cones. In addition, the retina is the only place in the body where blood vessels can be seen directly. Label Figure 11–1 as you observe the location of the structures responsible for image formation.

scler/itis
sklĕ-RĪ-tĭs

choroid/itis
kō-royd-Ī-tĭs

retin/itis
rĕt-ĭ-NĪ-tĭs

11–5   The CF **scler/o** refers to hardening; sclera (white of the eye); **choroid/o** refers to the choroid; and **retin/o** refers to the retina.

Use these CFs to build medical terms that mean *inflammation of the*

sclera: _____ / _____

choroid: _____ / _____

retina: _____ / _____

choroid/o/pathy
kō-roy-DŎP-ă-thē

retin/o/pathy
rĕt-ĭn-ŎP-ă-thē

11–6   Practice building medical words that mean *disease of the*

choroid: _____ / _____ / _____

retina: _____ / _____ / _____

kerat/o/rrhexis
kĕr-ă-tō-RĔK-sĭs

irid/o/cele
ĭ-RĬD-ō-sēl

11–7   The CF **kerat/o** refers to horny tissue; hard; cornea. The CF **irid/o** refers to the iris.

Use these CFs to build medical terms that mean

rupture of the cornea: _____ / _____ / _____

herniation of the iris: _____ / _____ / _____

Boldface indicates a word root or combining form. Blue indicates a suffix. Pink indicates a prefix.

kerat/o	**11–8** Kerat/itis, a vision-threatening infection, can occur if contact lenses are not cleaned and disinfected properly. From kerat/itis, construct the CF for cornea. _____ / _____
scler/itis sklĕ-RĪ-tĭs **scler/o/malacia** sklĕ-rō-mă-LĀ-shē-ă	**11–9** Form medical words that mean *inflammation of the sclera:* _____ / _____ *softening of the sclera:* _____ / _____ / _____
kerat/o/tomy kĕr-ă-TŎT-ō-mē	**11–10** In some cases, laser kerat/o/tomy can be used to correct vision. Doing so eliminates the need for contact lenses or glasses. Shallow, bloodless, hairline, radial incisions are made using a laser in the outer portion of the cornea, where they will not interfere with vision. This allows the cornea to flatten and helps to correct nearsightedness. About two-thirds of patients are able to eliminate the use of glasses or contact lenses by undergoing the surgical procedure called *laser* _____ / _____ / _____.
	11–11 The opening in the center of the iris is called the (8) **pupil.** The amount of light entering the eye is controlled by contractions and dilations of the pupil. Constriction of the pupil permits a sharper near vision. It is also a reflex that protects the retina from intense light. Label the pupil in Figure 11–1.
ŏf-THĂL-mō	**11–12** Words with **ophthalm/o** (eye) may be difficult to pronounce when you first encounter them. To avoid confusion, write the pronunciation ŏf-THĂL-mō and practice saying it aloud. _____
instrument	**11–13** An ophthalm/o/scope is an _____ for examining the interior of the eye.
ophthalm/o/scopy ŏf-thăl-MŎS-kō-pē	**11–14** The diagnostic term that describes visual examination of the eye is _____ / _____ / _____.
	11–15 Nerve fibers unite at the (9) **optic disc** and form the (10) **optic nerve.** Because the optic disk has no rods or cones for vision, it is known as the blind spot. The optic nerve transmits impulses to the brain for processing visual information. Label the two structures in Figure 11-1.
eye(s)	**11–16** An ophthalm/o/logist is a physician who specializes in disorders and treatment of the _____.

ophthalm/ectomy ŏf-thăl-MĔK-tō-mē **ophthalm/o/malacia** ŏf-thăl-mō-mă-LĀ-shē-ă **ophthalm/o/plegia** ŏf-thăl-mō-PLĒ-jē-ă	**I I–I 7** Use **ophthalm/o** to build words that mean *surgical excision of the eye:* _____ / _____ *softening of the eye:* _____ / _____ / _____ *paralysis of the eye:* _____ / _____ / _____
ophthalm/o/plegia ŏf-thăl-mō-PLĒ-jē-ă	**I I–I 8** A stroke can prevent eye movement and cause paralysis of eye muscles. A person with paralysis of eye (muscles) has a condition called _____ / _____ / _____.
conjuctiv/itis kŏn-jŭnk-tĭ-VĪ-tĭs	**I I–I 9** The (11) **conjunctiva** is a thin, mucus-secreting membrane that lines the interior surface of the eyelids and the exposed anterior surface of the eyeballs. Conjuctiv/itis is commonly caused by an allergy and manifests as itchy, watery, red eyes. The medical term for inflammation of the conjunctiva is _____ / _____.

Competency Verification: Check your labeling of Figure 11–1 in Appendix B: Answer Key, page 600.

blephar/o/plasty BLĔF-ă-rō-plăs-tē	**I I–20** The surgical procedure to remove wrinkles from the eyelids is known as blephar/o/plasty. This procedure is performed for functional and cosmetic reasons. Surgical repair of the eyelid(s) is known as _____ / _____ / _____.
blephar/o/plasty BLĔF-ă-rō-plăs-tē	**I I–2 I** Excessive skin around the upper eyelids may cause a decrease or lack of peripheral vision. To improve vision, the surgical procedure to remove the excessive skin is performed. This procedure is known as _____ / _____ / _____.
blephar/ectomy blĕf-ă-RĔK-tō-mē **blephar/o/tomy** blĕf-ă-RŎT-ō-mē **blephar/o/spasm** BLĔF-ă-rō-spăzm **blephar/o/plegia** blĕf-ă-rō-PLĒ-jē-ă	**I I–22** Form medical words that mean *excision of part or all of the eyelid:* _____ / _____ *surgical incision of eyelid:* _____ / _____ / _____ *twitching or spasm of eyelid:* _____ / _____ / _____ *paralysis of an eyelid:* _____ / _____ / _____

Boldface indicates a word root or combining form. Blue indicates a suffix. Pink indicates a prefix.

red **yellow**	**11–23** The suffix *-opia* is used in words to mean *vision*. Erythr/opia is a condition in which objects that are not red appear to be _____. Xanth/opia is a condition in which objects that are not yellow appear to be _____.
dipl/opia dĭp-LŌ-pē-ă	**11–24** Elements *dipl-* and *dipl/o* mean *double*. Dipl/opia occurs when both eyes are used but are not in focus. A person with double vision has a condition called _____ / _____.
dipl/opia dĭp-LŌ-pē-ă	**11–25** Dipl/opia can occur with brain tumors, strokes, head trauma, and migraine headaches. Write the word in this frame that means *double vision*. _____ / _____
hyper- **-opia** **my/o**	**11–26** Two common vision defects are my/opia (nearsightedness) and hyper/opia (farsightedness). See Figure 11–2 to compare a normal eye (emmetropia) with my/opia and hyper/opia. Write the element in this frame that means *excessive, above normal:* _____ *vision:* _____ *muscle:* _____ / _____
hyper/opia hī-pĕr-Ō-pē-ă	**11–27** In normal vision, the lens focuses the visual image on the retina. Hyper/opia, also called farsightedness, occurs when the lens focuses the visual image beyond the retina (see Fig. 11–2), causing difficulty in seeing objects that are close. This is a condition common in people over 40 years of age, but can be corrected with "reading" glasses. The medical term for farsightedness is _____ / _____.
close	**11–28** People with hyper/opia (farsightedness) have difficulty seeing objects that are _____.
my/opia mī-Ō-pē-ă	**11–29** If the eyeball is too long, the visual image falls in front of the retina (see Fig. 11–2), causing difficulty seeing objects that are far away. The medical term for nearsightedness is _____ / _____.
hyper/opia hī-pĕr-Ō-pē-ă	**11–30** The opposite of my/opia, or nearsightedness, is _____ / _____, or farsightedness.

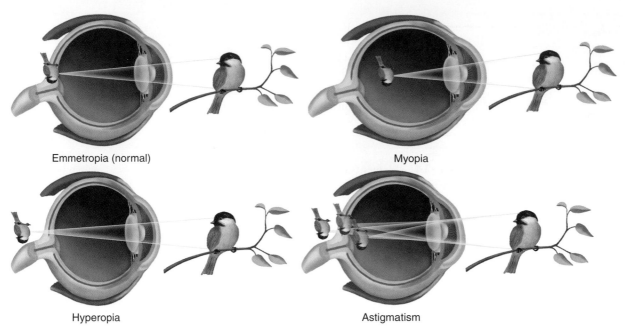

Emmetropia (normal)   Myopia

Hyperopia   Astigmatism

Figure 11-2 Refraction of the eye.

---

blephar/o/plasty
BLĔF-ă-rō-plăs-tē

blephar/o/spasm
BLĔF-ă-rō-spăzm

blephar/o/ptosis
blĕf-ă-rō-TŌ-sĭs

11–31 Eyelids shade the eyes during sleep, protect them from excessive light and foreign objects, and spread lubricating secretions over the eyeballs.

Use **blephar/o** (eyelid) to construct medical words that mean

surgical repair of eyelid: _____ / _____ / _____

twitching of an eyelid: _____ / _____ / _____

prolapse of an eyelid: _____ / _____ / _____

---

blephar/o

-ptosis

11–32 Blephar/o/ptosis is commonly seen after a stroke, because the muscles leading to the eyelids become paralyzed.

Indicate the elements in this frame that mean

eyelid: _____ / _____

prolapse, downward displacement: _____

---

tears

11–33 The (1) **lacrimal gland** is located above the outer corner of each eye. These glands produce tears, which keep the eyeballs moist. The (2) **lacrimal sac** collects and drains tears into the (3) **nasolacrimal duct.** Label the lacrimal structures in Figure 11–3.

---

tears

11–34 The CF *dacry/o* is used in words to mean *tear; lacrimal sac.* Dacry/o/rrhea is an excessive flow of _____.

Boldface indicates a word root or combining form. Blue indicates a suffix. Pink indicates a prefix.

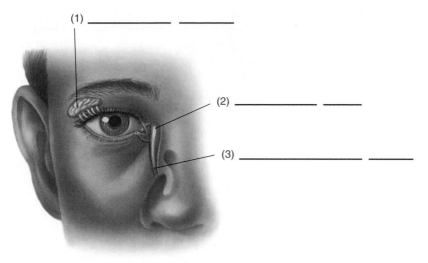

(1) _____ _____

(2) _____ _____

(3) _____ _____

Figure 11-3 Lacrimal apparatus.

pain	**11-35** Dacry/aden/algia is _____ in a tear gland.

tear gland	**11-36** Dacry/aden/itis is an inflammation of a _____ _____.

Competency Verification: Check your labeling of Figure 11–3 in Appendix B: Answer Key, page 600.

EARS

The ears and their accessory structures are receptor organs that enable us to hear and maintain balance. Each ear consists of three divisions: the external ear, middle ear, and inner ear. The external and middle ear conduct sound waves through the ear. The inner ear contains auditory structures that receive sound waves and transmit them to the brain for interpretation. The inner ear also contains specialized receptors that maintain balance and equilibrium in response to fluctuations in body position and motion.

WORD ELEMENTS

This section introduces CFs related to the ear. Included are key suffixes; prefixes are defined in the right-hand column as needed. Review the following table and pronounce each word in the word analysis column aloud before you begin to work the frames.

Word Elements	Meaning	Word Analysis
Combining Forms		
acous/o	hearing	**acous**/tic (ă-KOOS-tĭk): pertaining to sound or the sense of hearing -*tic:* pertaining to
audi/o		**audi**/o/meter (aw-dē-ŎM-ĕ-tĕr): instrument for testing hearing -*meter:* instrument for measuring
audit/o		**audit**/ory (AW-dĭ-tō-rē): pertaining to the sense of hearing -*ory:* pertaining to
myring/o	tympanic membrane (eardrum)	**myring**/o/tomy (mĭr-ĭn-GŎT-ō-mē): incision of the tympanic membrane -*tomy:* incision
tympan/o		**tympan**/o/plasty (tĭm-păn-ō-PLĂS-tē): surgical repair of the tympanic membrane; also called *myringoplasty* -*plasty:* surgical repair *A tympanoplasty is any of several surgical procedures designed to cure a chronic in-flammatory process in the middle ear or restore function to the sound-transmitting mechanism of the middle ear.*
ot/o	ear	**ot**/o/rrhea (ō-tō-RĒ-ă): inflammation of the ear with purulent discharge -*rrhea:* discharge, flow
salping/o	tube (usually fallopian or eustachian [auditory] tubes)	**salping**/o/pharyng/eal (săl-pĭng-gō-fă-RĬN-jē-ăl): concerning the eustachian tube and pharynx *pharyng:* pharynx (throat) -*eal:* pertaining to
Suffix		
-acusis	hearing	an/**acusis** (ăn-ă-KŪ-sĭs): total deafness *an-:* without, not

Pronunciation Help						
	Long sound	ā in rāte	ē in rēbirth	ī in īsle	ō in ōver	ū in ūnite
	Short sound	ă in ălone	ĕ in ĕver	ĭ in ĭt	ŏ in nŏt	ŭ in cŭt

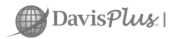

Visit the *Medical Terminology Simplified* online resource center at Davis*Plus* for an audio exercise of the terms in this table. It will help you master pronunciations and meanings of the selected medical terms.

SECTION REVIEW 11-2

For the following medical terms, first write the suffix and its meaning. Then translate the meaning of the remaining elements starting with the first part of the word. The first word is completed for you.

Term	Meaning
1. tympan/o/centesis	-centesis: surgical puncture; tympanic membrane (eardrum)
2. acous/tic	
3. hyper/tropia	
4. ot/o/rrhea	
5. an/acusis	
6. myring/o/tomy	
7. tympan/o/plasty	
8. audi/o/meter	
9. ot/o/scope	
10. salping/o/pharyng/eal	

Competency Verification: Check your answers in Appendix B: Answer Key, page 600. If you are not satisfied with your level of comprehension, review the vocabulary and retake the review.

Correct Answers _____ × 10 = _____ % Score

11-37 The ear can be divided into three anatomical sections: external, middle, and inner. The external ear includes the (1) **auricle,** which directs sound waves to the (2) **ear canal.** Eventually, the sound waves hit the (3) **tympanic membrane** (eardrum) and make the eardrum vibrate. Transmission of sound waves ultimately generates impulses that are transmitted to and interpreted by the brain as sound. Label Figure 11–4 as you learn about the ear.

---

ot/algia
ō-TĂL-jē-ă

11-38 Swimmer's ear, resulting from an infection transmitted in the water of a swimming pool, may cause severe ot/o/dynia or

_____ / _____.

---

eardrum

11-39 The CFs *tympan/o* and *myring/o* refer to the tympanic membrane (eardrum). Tympan/itis is an inflammation of the tympanic membrane, or

_____.

---

tympan/o, myring/o	**11–40** The tympan/ic membrane is stretched across the end of the ear canal and vibrates when sound waves strike it. The CFs for the tympanic membrane (eardrum) are _____ / _____ and _____ / _____.
	11–41 Vibrations of the tympanic membrane are transmitted to the three auditory bones in the middle ear: the (4) **malleus,** the (5) **incus,** and the (6) **stapes.** The (7) **eustachian (auditory) tube** leads from the middle ear to the nasopharynx and permits air to enter or leave the middle ear cavity. Label and review the position of the middle ear structures in Figure 11–4.
salping/itis săl-pĭn-JĪ-tĭs	**11–42** The CF *salping/o* means *tube (usually fallopian or eustachian [auditory] tubes).* Inflammation of the eustachian tube would be diagnosed as _____ / _____.
salping/o/scope săl-PĬNG-gō-skōp **salping/o/scopy** săl-pĭng-GŎS-kō-pē **salping/o/stenosis** săl-pĭng-gō-stĕn-NŌ-sĭs	**11–43** The eustachian tube equalizes air pressure in the middle ear with that of the outside atmosphere. Air pressure must be equalized for the eardrum to vibrate properly. Build medical words that mean *instrument for examining the eustachian tube:* _____ / _____ / _____ *visual examination of the eustachian tube:* _____ / _____ / _____ *narrowing or stricture of the eustachian tube:* _____ / _____ / _____
	11–44 Components of the inner ear include the (8) **cochlea** for hearing, the (9) **semicircular canals** for equilibrium, and the (10) **vestibule,** which is a chamber that joins the cochlea and semicircular canals. Label inner ear structures in Figure 11–4.
	11–45 The inner ear, also called the labyrinth, consists of complicated, mazelike structures, all of which contain the functional organs for hearing and equilibrium. (See Fig. 11–5.) Use your medical dictionary to define labyrinth and list two types of inner ear labyrinths. _____ _____
ot/o	**11–46** The CF *ot/o* refers to the ear. From ot/o/sclero/sis, determine the CF for ear. _____ / _____

Boldface indicates a word root or combining form. Blue indicates a suffix. Pink indicates a prefix.

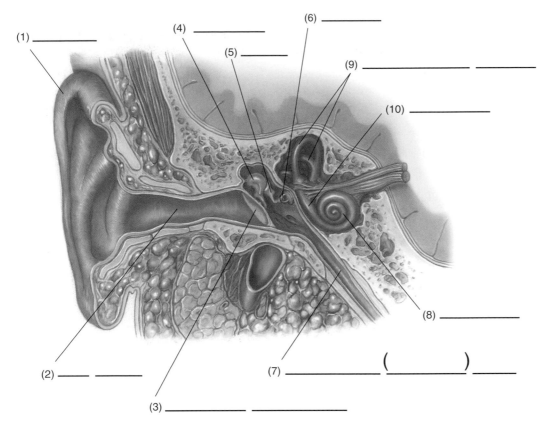

(1) _____

(4) _____

(5) _____

(6) _____

(9) _____ _____

(10) _____

(8) _____

(2) _____ _____

(7) _____ _____ (_____) _____

(3) _____ _____

Figure 11-4 Ear structures.

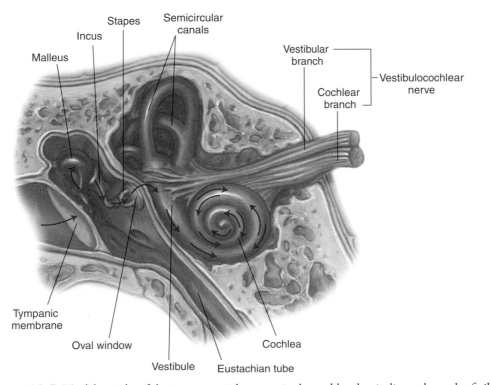

Malleus

Incus

Stapes

Semicircular canals

Vestibular branch

Cochlear branch

Vestibulocochlear nerve

Tympanic membrane

Oval window

Vestibule

Eustachian tube

Cochlea

Figure 11-5 The labyrinths of the inner ear with arrows in the cochlea that indicate the path of vibrations.

ot/o/sclerosis ō-tō-sklĕ-RŌ-sĭs	**I I–47** Ot/o/sclerosis is a hereditary condition of unknown cause in which irregular ossification occurs in the ossicles of the middle ear, especially of the stapes, causing hearing loss. Chronic progressive deafness, especially for low tones, may be caused by a hereditary condition called _____ / _____ / _____.
staped/ectomy stā-pē-DĔK-tō-mē	**I I–48** A patient diagnosed with ot/o/scler/osis may have hearing restored with a surgical procedure called staped/ectomy. To improve hearing, especially in cases of ot/o/scler/osis, the surgeon may excise the stapes using a surgical procedure called _____ / _____.
staped/ectomy stā-pē-DĔK-tō-mē	**I I–49** Staped/ectomy involves removal of the stapes and replacement by a prosthesis to restore hearing loss. When the surgeon excises the stapes, the surgery performed is called _____ / _____.
hearing	**I I–50** The inner ear contains the receptors for two senses: hearing and equilibrium. The CFs *acous/o, audi/o,* and *audit/o* refer to _____.
audi/o/logist aw-dē-ŎL-ō-jĭst	**I I–51** The branch of science that studies hearing, balance, and related disorders is known as audi/o/logy. It encompasses rehabilitation of persons with hearing impairments. The specialist in the study of hearing is called an _____ / _____ / _____.
ot/o/scopy ō-TŎS-kŏ-pē	**I I–52** Ear infections can be diagnosed with an ot/o/scope. Visual examination of the ear is known as _____ / _____ / _____.
URI	**I I–53** Ot/itis media, infection of the middle ear, usually occurs following upper respiratory infection (URI). Upon ot/o/scopy, redness and stiffness of the tympanic membrane is observed, indicating inflammation. The abbreviation for upper respiratory infection is _____.
myring/o/tomy mĭr-ĭn-GŎT-ō-mē	**I I–54** Ot/itis media caused by bacteria is commonly treated with antibiotics. When the condition persists and becomes chronic, a myring/o/tomy may be required. During this surgical procedure, a pressure-equalizing (PE) tube is inserted into the eardrum to relieve pressure and promote drainage. (See Fig. 11–6.) Build the medical word that means *incision into the eardrum.* _____ / _____ / _____

Boldface indicates a word root or combining form. Blue indicates a suffix. Pink indicates a prefix.

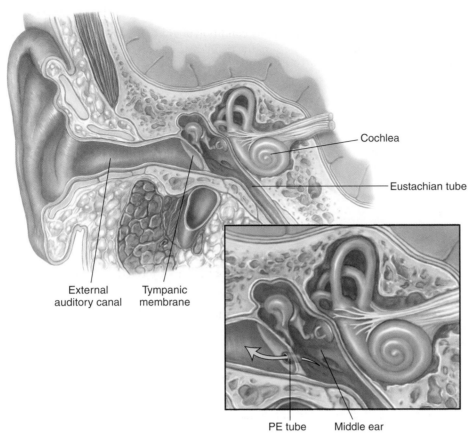

Figure 11-6 Placement of pressure-equalizing (PE) tubes.

ot/o/plasty Ō-tō-plăs-tē	**11–55** Plastic surgery of the ear (to correct defects and deformities) is called _____ / _____ / _____.

Competency Verification: Check your labeling of Figure 11–4 in Appendix B: Answer Key, page 600.

SECTION REVIEW 11-3

Using the following table, write the CF, suffix, or prefix that matches its definition in the space provided to the left of the definition. There may be more than one word element that matches a definition.

Combining Forms

aden/o	myring/o
audi/o	ophthalm/o
blephar/o	ot/o
choroid/o	retin/o
corne/o	salping/o
dacry/o	scler/o
dipl/o	tympan/o
irid/o	xanth/o
kerat/o	

Suffixes

-acusis	-spasm
-edema	-stenosis
-logist	
-malacia	
-opia	
-opsia	
-ptosis	
-rrhexis	
-salpinx	

Prefixes

dipl-
hyper-

1. _____ excessive, above normal

2. _____ choroid

3. _____ horny tissue; hard; cornea

4. _____ double

5. _____ ear

6. _____ tube (usually fallopian or eustachian [auditory] tubes)

7. _____ eye

8. _____ eyelid

9. _____ gland

10. _____ hardening; sclera (white of the eye)

11. _____ involuntary contraction, twitching

12. _____ iris

13. _____ prolapse, downward displacement

14. _____ specialist in the study of

15. _____ retina

16. _____ rupture

17. _____ softening

18. _____ hearing

19. _____ narrowing, stricture

20. _____ swelling

21. _____ tear; lacrimal apparatus (duct, sac, or gland)

22. _____ tympanic membrane (eardrum)

23. _____ cornea

24. _____ vision

25. _____ yellow

Competency Verification: Check your answers in Appendix B: Answer Key, page 600. If you are not satisfied with your level of comprehension, go back to Frame 11–1 and rework the frames.

Correct Answers _____ × 4 = _____ % Score

ABBREVIATIONS

This section introduces abbreviations related to the eyes and ears and their meanings.

Abbreviation	Meaning	Abbreviation	Meaning
Eyes			
ARMD, AMD	age-related macular degeneration	LASIK	laser-assisted in situ keratomileusis
ECCE	extracapsular cataract extraction	O.D.	Doctor of Optometry
IOL	intraocular lens	RK	radial keratotomy
IOP	intraocular pressure	VA	visual acuity
Ears			
AC	air conduction	NIHL	noise-induced hearing loss
BC	bone conduction	OM	otitis media
ENT	ear, nose, and throat	PE	physical examination; pulmonary embolism; pressure-equalizing (tube)
IVFA	intravenous fluorescein angiography	URI	upper respiratory infection

ADDITIONAL MEDICAL TERMS

The following are additional terms related to the eyes and ears. Recognizing and learning these terms will help you understand the connection between a pathological condition, its diagnosis, and the rationale behind the method of treatment selected for a particular disorder.

Diseases and Conditions

Eye

achromatopsia
ă-krō-mă-TŎP-sē-ă
  a-: without, not
chromat: color
  -opsia: vision

Congenital deficiency in color perception; also called color blindness

Achromatopsia is more common in men.

astigmatism (Ast)
ă-STĬG-mă-tĭzm
  a-: without, not
stigmat: point, mark
  -ism: condition

Defective curvature of the cornea and lens, which causes light rays to focus unevenly over the retina rather than being focused on a single point, resulting in a distorted image (See Fig. 11–2.)

cataract KĂT-ă-răkt	Degenerative disease in which the lens of the eye becomes progressively cloudy, causing decreased vision *Cataracts are usually a result of the aging process, caused by protein deposits on the surface of the lens that slowly build up until vision is lost. Treatment includes surgical intervention to remove the cataract.*
diabetic retinopathy dī-ă-BĔT-ĭk rĕt-ĭn-ŎP-ă-thē *retin/o:* retina *-pathy:* disease	Retinal damage marked by aneurysmal dilation and bleeding of blood vessels or the formation of new blood vessels, causing visual changes *Diabetic retinopathy occurs in people with diabetes, manifested by small hemorrhages, edema, and formation of new vessels leading to scarring and eventual loss of vision.*
glaucoma glaw-KŌ-mă *glauc:* gray *-oma:* tumor	Condition in which aqueous humor fails to drain properly and accumulates in the anterior chamber of the eye, causing elevated intraocular pressure (IOP) (See Fig. 11–7.) *Glaucoma eventually leads to loss of vision and, commonly, blindness. Treatment for glaucoma includes miotics (eyedrops) that cause the pupils to constrict, permitting aqueous humor to escape from the eye, thereby relieving pressure. If miotics are ineffective, surgery may be necessary.*
open-angle	Most common form of glaucoma that results from degenerative changes that cause congestion and reduce flow of aqueous humor through the canal of Schlemm *Open-angle glaucoma is painless but destroys peripheral vision, causing tunnel vision.*
closed-angle	Type of glaucoma caused by an anatomically narrow angle between the iris and the cornea, which prevents outflow of aqueous humor from the eye into the lymphatic system, causing a sudden increase in IOP *Closed-angle glaucoma constitutes an emergency situation. Symptoms include severe pain, blurred vision, and photophobia.*
hordeolum hor-DĒ-ō-lŭm	Small, purulent inflammatory infection of a sebaceous gland of the eyelid; also called sty (See Fig. 11–8.)
macular degeneration (MD) MĂK-ū-lăr	Breakdown of the tissues in the macula, resulting in loss of central vision *Macular degeneration is the most common cause of visual impairment in persons over age 50. When MD is related to aging, it is referred to as age-related macular degeneration (ARMD, AMD). (See Fig. 11–9).*
photophobia fō-tō-FŌ-bē-ă *phot/o:* light *-phobia:* fear	Unusual intolerance and sensitivity to light *Photophobia occurs in such disorders as meningitis, eye inflammation, measles, and rubella.*

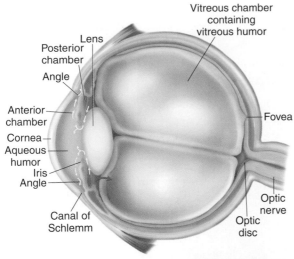

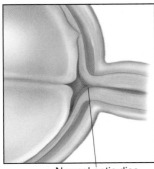
Normal optic disc

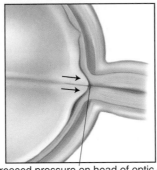
Increased pressure on head of optic disc causing destruction of the nerve fiber

Figure 11-7 Glaucoma.

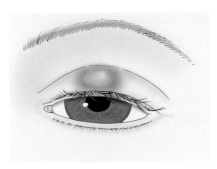

Figure 11-8 Hordeolum.

retinal detachment
RĔT-ĭ-năl
 	
  retin: retina
  -al: pertaining to
	Separation of the retina from the choroid, which disrupts vision and results in blindness if not repaired
	
	Retinal detachment may follow trauma, choroidal hemorrhages, or tumors and may be associated with diabetes mellitus.

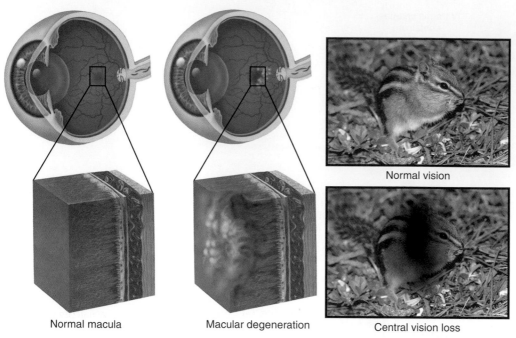

Normal macula   Macular degeneration   Central vision loss

Normal vision

Figure 11-9 Macular degeneration.

strabismus stră-BĬZ-mŭs	Muscular eye disorder in which the eyes turn from the normal position so that they deviate in different directions
	Various forms of strabismus are referred to as tropias, their direction being indicated by the appropriate prefix, such as esotropia and exotropia. (See Fig. 11–10.)

esotropia
ĕs-ō-TRŌ-pē-ă
   eso-: inward
   -tropia: turning
	Strabismus in which there is deviation of the visual axis of one eye toward that of the other eye, resulting in diplopia; also called cross-eye and convergent strabismus

exotropia
ĕks-ō-TRŌ-pē-ă
   exo-: outside,
        outward
   -tropia: turning
	Strabismus in which there is deviation of the visual axis of one eye away from that of the other eye, resulting in diplopia; also called wall-eye and divergent strabismus

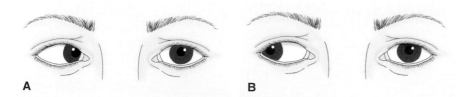

A   B

Figure 11-10 Types of strabismus. **(A)** Esotropia. **(B)** Exotropia.

Ear

acoustic neuroma
a-KOOS-tĭk nū-RŌ-mă
acous: hearing
  -tic: pertaining to
neur: nerve
  -oma: tumor
	Benign tumor that develops from the eighth cranial (vestibulocochlear) nerve and grows within the auditory canal
	
	Depending on the location and size of the tumor, progressive hearing loss, headache, facial numbness, dizziness, and an unsteady gait may result.

hearing loss	Decreased ability to perceive sounds compared to what the individual or examiner would regard as normal
anacusis ăn-ă-KŪ-sĭs *an-:* without, not *-acusis:* hearing	Total deafness (complete hearing loss)
conductive kŏn-DŬK-tĭv	Hearing loss resulting from any condition that prevents sound waves from being transmitted to the auditory receptors *Conductive hearing loss may result from wax obstructing the external auditory canal, inflammation of the middle ear, ankylosis of the ear bones, or fixation of the footplate of the stirrup.*
noise-induced	Hearing loss that results from exposure to very loud sounds *Working with noisy machinery, listening to loud music, or discharging rifles, guns, or explosives may cause noise-induced hearing loss.*

sensorineural
sĕn-sō-rē-NŪ-răl
sensori: to feel
  neur: nerve
    -al: pertaining to
	Hearing loss caused by permanent or temporary damage to the sensory cells or nerve fibers of the inner ear

Ménière disease mĕn-ē-ĀR	Rare disorder of unknown etiology within the labyrinth of the inner ear that can lead to a progressive loss of hearing *Symptoms of Ménière disease include vertigo, hearing loss, tinnitus, and a sensation of pressure in the ear.*

otitis externa
ō-TĪ-tĭs
  ot: ear
  -itis: inflammation
	Infection of the external auditory canal
	
	Otitis externa can develop when water remains in the outer ear canal, most commonly after swimming (swimmer's ear). Other causes include allergies, eczema, and a foreign object lodged in the ear.

otitis media (OM)
ō-TĪ-tĭs MĒ-dē-ă
    ot: ear
    -itis: inflammation
  med: middle
    -ia: condition
	Inflammation of the middle ear, which is commonly the result of an upper respiratory infection (URI)

serous	Noninfectious inflammation of the middle ear with accumulation of serum (clear fluid) *Treatment for serous OM may include myringotomy to aspirate fluid and the surgical insertion of pressure-equalizing (PE) tubes. (See Fig. 11–6.)*
suppurative	Inflammation of the middle ear with pus formation *Suppurative OM is a common affliction in infants and young children, due to the horizontal orientation and small diameter of the eustachian tube in such patients, which predisposes them to infection. If left untreated, complications include ruptured tympanic membrane, mastoiditis, labyrinthitis, hearing loss, and meningitis.*

presbycusis
prĕz-bĭ-KŪ-sĭs
  presby: old age
    -cusis: hearing
	Impairment of hearing that results from the aging process

tinnitus tĭn-Ī-tĭs	Ringing or tinkling noise heard constantly or intermittently in one or both ears, even in a quiet environment *Tinnitus may be a sign of injury to the ear, some disease process, or toxic levels of some medications (such as aspirin).*
vertigo VĔR-tĭ-gō	Sensation of moving around in space or a feeling of spinning or dizziness *Vertigo usually results from inner ear structure damage associated with balance and equilibrium.*

Diagnostic Procedures

Eye

slit-lamp examination	Eye evaluation that provides a stereoscopic (three-dimensional) view of the eye's interior using a binocular microscope (slit lamp) of a high-intensity light source to accentuate the anatomical structure of the eye, allowing close inspection *The slit lamp provides greater magnification (10 to 25 times) and illumination than most handheld devices. (See Fig. 11–11.)*

tonometry
tōn-ŎM-ĕ-trē
  ton/o: tension
    -metry: act of measuring
	Test to measure increased intraocular pressure (IOP) to detect glaucoma
	
	Tonometry is performed with the slit lamp, but also uses a small, flat disk pressed against the cornea or a short burst of air directed at the cornea to measure IOP. (See Fig. 11–11.)

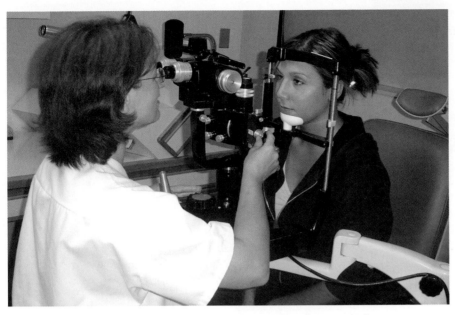

Figure 11-11 Slit-lamp examination measuring intraocular pressure by tonometry.

intravenous fluorescein angiography (IVFA) *intra-:* in, within *ven:* vein *-ous:* pertaining to *angi/o:* vessel (usually blood or lymph) *-graphy:* process of recording	Imaging technique used to study retinal blood vessels and circulation of blood in the retina using photographs of the retina after injection of a fluorescent dye *IVFA produces images that show retinal blood flow and an angiogram that helps detect vascular changes in diabetic retinopathy, macular degeneration, and retinal vascular disease, as well as other types of macular disease.*
visual acuity (VA) test ă-KŪ-ĭ-tē	Examination that identifies the smallest letters that can be correctly read on a standardized Snellen vision chart from a distance of 20 feet *VA is expressed as a ratio. The first number is the distance at which a person reads the chart, and the second number is the distance at which a person with normal vision can read the same chart. For example, 20/20 indicates that the person correctly read letters at 20 feet that could be read by a person with normal vision at 20 feet. Normal vision is 20/20. (See Fig. 11–12.)*

Ear

audiometry ăw-dē-ŎM-ĕ-trē *audi/o:* hearing *-metry:* act of measuring	Test that measures hearing acuity at various sound frequencies *In audiometry, an instrument called an audiometer delivers acoustic stimuli at different frequencies, and results are plotted on a graph called an audiogram.*

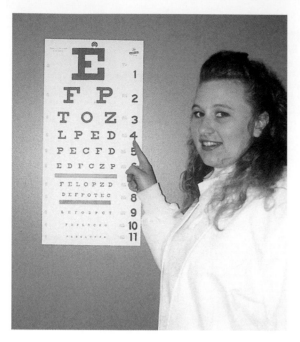

Figure 11-12 Snellen chart with letters. *From Med/Surg, 4 ed by Williams, p. 1233, Fig 51.3.*

otoscopy
ō-TŎS-kŏ-pē
   ot/o: ear
   -scopy: visual
         examination
	Visual examination of the external auditory canal and the tympanic membrane using an otoscope

pneumatic nū-MĂT-ĭk	Otoscopic procedure that assesses the ability of the tympanic membrane to move in response to a change in air pressure *In pneumatic otoscopy, the increase and decrease in pressure causes the healthy tympanic membrane to move in and out. Lack of movement indicates increased impedance or eardrum perforation.*

tuning fork test	Hearing test that uses a turning fork (instrument that produces constant pitch when struck) that is struck and then placed against or near the bones on the side of the head to assess nerve and bone conduction of sound *There are two types of tuning fork tests: the Rinne test and the Weber test.*
Rinne RĬN-nē	Tuning fork test that evaluates bone conduction of sound in one ear at a time (See Fig. 11–13.) *The Rinne test is useful for differentiating between conductive and sensorineural hearing loss.*
Weber	Tuning fork test that evaluates bone conduction of sound in both ears at the same time *During the Weber test, hearing sound equally in both ears indicates normal hearing.*

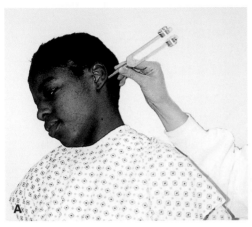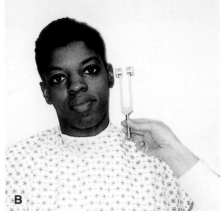

Figure 11-13 Rinne test. **(A)** Bone conduction. **(B)** Air conduction.

Medical and Surgical Procedures

Eye

cataract surgery KĂT-ă-răkt	Excision of a lens affected by a cataract *Extracapsular cataract extraction (ECCE) and phacoemulsification are the two primary ways to remove a cataract. In both surgeries, the central part of the lens is removed and replaced with an artificial intraocular lens (IOL) implant.*
extracapsular cataract extraction (ECCE) ĕks-tră-KĂP-sū-lăr KĂT-ă-răkt	Excision of the anterior segment of the lens capsule along with the lens, allowing for the insertion of an IOL implant
phacoemulsification făk-ō-ē-mŭl-sĭ-fĭ-KĀ-shŭn	Excision of the lens by inserting an ultrasonic probe whose sound waves break the lens into tiny particles which are suctioned out of the eye and the IOL is implanted (See Fig. 11–14.)
corneal transplant KŎR-nē-ăl *corne:* cornea *-al:* pertaining to	Surgical transplantation of a donor cornea (from a cadaver) into the eye of a recipient; also called keratoplasty
iridectomy ĭr-ĭ-DĔK-tŏ-mē *irid:* iris *-ectomy:* excision, removal	Excision of a portion of the iris used to relieve intraocular pressure in patients with glaucoma *Iridectomy is usually performed to create an opening through which aqueous humor can drain.*

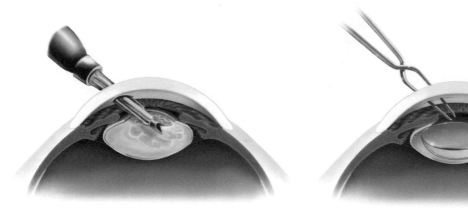

Cataract removal   Artificial lens insertion

Figure 11-14 Phacoemulsification.

laser photocoagulation	Use of an argon laser to treat diabetic retinopathy by sealing leaking blood vessels in the retina *The laser uses the gas argon to produce blue-green wavelengths that are absorbed by the cells that lie under the retina and the red hemoglobin in blood but pass through fluid in the eye without damaging structures. Laser photocoagulation is also used to treat macular degeneration and attach a detached retina.*
laser-assisted in situ keratomileusis (LASIK)	Use of an excimer laser to correct errors of refraction, such as myopia, hyperopia, and astigmatism, by reshaping the cornea and improving visual acuity *LASIK provides a permanent alternative to wearing corrective lenses or contact lenses. Many patients who are treated with LASIK find an improvement of up to 20/20 vision.*

Ear

cochlear implant KŎK-lē-ăr 　*cochle:* cochlea 　　*-ar:* pertaining to	Electronic transmitter surgically implanted into the cochlea of a deaf person to restore hearing
ear irrigation	Process of flushing the external ear canal with sterile water or sterile saline solution to treat patients who complain of foreign body or cerumen (ear wax) impaction (See Fig. 11–15.)

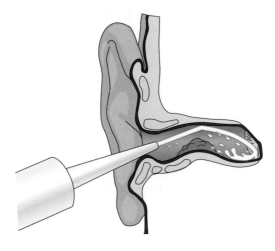

Figure 11-15 Ear irrigation.

myringotomy mĭr-ĭn-GŎT-ō-mē *myring/o:* tympanic membrane (eardrum) *-tomy:* incision	Incision of the eardrum to relieve pressure and release pus or serous fluid from the middle ear or to insert PE tubes (tympanostomy tubes) in the eardrum via surgery (See Fig. 11–6.) *PE tubes provide ventilation and drainage of the middle ear when repeated ear infections do not respond to antibiotic treatment. They are used when persistent, severely negative middle ear pressure is present.*

Pronunciation Help	Long sound	ā in rāte	ē in rēbirth	ī in īsle	ō in ōver	ū in ūnite
	Short sound	ă in ălone	ĕ in ĕver	ĭ in ĭt	ŏ in nŏt	ŭ in cŭt

PHARMACOLOGY

The table below lists common drug categories used to treat urinary disorders, as well as their therapeutic actions.

Drug Category	Action
antiglaucoma agents ăn-tĭ-glaw-KŌ-mă	Reduce intraocular pressure by lowering the amount of aqueous humor in the eyeball, reducing its production, or increasing its outflow
miotics mī-ŎT-ĭks	Cause the pupil to constrict *Miotics are used to treat glaucoma.*
mydriatics mĭd-rē-ĂT-ĭks	Cause the pupil to dilate and prepare the eye for an internal examination *Mydriatics provide accurate measurements for prescribing corrective lenses.*
vertigo and motion sickness drugs VĔR-tĭ-gō	Decrease sensitivity of the inner ear to motion and prevent nerve impulses from the inner ear from reaching the vomiting center of the brain
wax emulsifiers ē-MŬL-sĭ-fī-ĕrs	Loosen and help remove impacted cerumen (ear wax)

Pronunciation Help	Long sound	ā in rāte	ē in rēbirth	ī in īsle	ō in ōver	ū in ūnite
	Short sound	ă in ălone	ĕ in ĕver	ĭ in ĭt	ŏ in nŏt	ŭ in cŭt

ADDITIONAL MEDICAL TERMS REVIEW

Match the medical terms below with the definitions in the numbered list.

achromatopsia   conductive hearing loss   iridectomy   otosclerosis   Rinne test
acoustic neuroma   conjunctivitis   macular degeneration   phacoemulsification   strabismus
anacusis   diabetic retinopathy   Ménière disease   photophobia   tinnitus
astigmatism   glaucoma   myringotomy   presbycusis   tonometry
cataract   hordeolum   otitis media   retinal detachment   vertigo

1. _____ means *ringing in the ears.*

2. _____ is progressive deafness due to ossification in the bony labyrinth of the inner ear.

3. _____ means *color blindness.*

4. _____ is a rare disorder characterized by progressive deafness, vertigo, and tinnitus.

5. _____ is a disorder in which both eyes cannot focus on the same point, resulting in looking in different directions at the same time.

6. _____ means *total deafness.*

7. _____ refers to middle ear infection that is most commonly seen in young children.

8. _____ refers to pinkeye.

9. _____ means *intolerance or unusual sensitivity to light.*

10. _____ is hearing loss due to old age.

11. _____ refers to IOP caused by the failure of the aqueous humor to drain.

12. _____ refers to a feeling of spinning or dizziness.

13. _____ refers to separation of the retina from the choroid.

14. _____ is another term for sty.

15. _____ is abnormal curvature of the cornea, which causes light rays to focus unevenly over the retina, resulting in a distorted image.

16. _____ is a benign tumor of the eighth cranial nerve.

17. _____ measures intraocular pressure and is used to diagnose glaucoma.

18. _____ refers to excision of a portion of the iris.

19. _____ is caused by an impairment in sound transmission because of damage to the eardrum or ossicles or ear canal obstruction.

20. _____ refers to opacity (cloudiness) of the lens as a result of protein deposits on its surface.

21. _____ is a type of cataract surgery.

22. _____ is a hearing acuity test that is performed with a vibrating tuning fork.

23. _____ refers to retinal damage marked by aneurysmal dilation of blood vessels.

24. _____ is a loss of central vision due to the aging process.

25. _____ is an incision of the eardrum to relieve pressure and release pus or serous fluid from the middle ear.

Competency Verification: Check your answers in Appendix B: Answer Key, page 601. If you are not satisfied with your level of comprehension, review the additional medical terms and retake the review.

Correct Answers _____ × 4 = _____ % Score

MEDICAL RECORD ACTIVITIES

Medical reports included in the following activities reflect common, real-life clinical scenarios using medical terminology to document patient care.

MEDICAL RECORD ACTIVITY 11-1

RETINAL DETACHMENT

Terminology

Terms listed in the table below come from the medical report Retinal Detachment *that follows. Use a medical dictionary such as* Taber's Cyclopedic Medical Dictionary, *the appendices of this book, or other resources to define each term. Then practice reading the pronunciations aloud for each term.*

Term	Definition
akinesia ă-kĭ-NĒ-zē-ă	
cannula KĂN-ū-lă	
conjunctival kŏn-jŭnk-TĪ-văl	
limbus LĬM-bŭs	
mm	
retinal detachment RĔT-ĭ-năl	

Continued

Term	Definition
retrobulbar rĕt-rō-BŬL-băr	
sclerotomy sklĕ-RŎT-ō-mē	
vitrectomy vĭ-TRĔK-tō-mē	

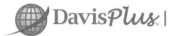 Visit the *Medical Terminology Simplified* online resource center at Davis*Plus* to practice pronunciation and reinforce the meanings of selected terms in this medical report.

Reading

Practice pronunciation of medical terms by reading the following medical report aloud.

Retinal Detachment

DIAGNOSIS: Total retinal detachment, left eye, secondary to complications of retinitis.

PROCEDURE: Patient was taken to the operating room, placed on the operating table, IV infusion begun, EKG lead monitor attached, and retrobulbar anesthetic given, achieving good anesthesia and akinesia. The patient was scrubbed, prepped, and draped in a standard sterile fashion for retinal surgery. A 360-degree conjunctival opening was made and 2-0 silk sutures were placed around each rectus muscle. Four millimeters from the limbus, a mark in the sclera was made and preplaced 5-0 Mersiline suture was passed. A mitrovitreoretinal stab incision was made, and a 4-mm infusion cannula was slipped into position and visualized inside the eye. Similar sclerotomy sites were made superior nasally and superior temporally. Trans pars plana vitrectomy was undertaken. Dense vitreous hemorrhage and debris were found, which were removed. There was incomplete posterior vitreous attachment. The retina was almost totally detached, and a small amount of nasal retina was still attached. A linear retinal break was seen just above the disk along a vessel. Gradually, all peripheral vitreous was removed.

Air-fluid exchange was performed with some difficulty because some sort of vitreous was found anteriorly, which loculated the bubble. It gave me a peculiar view, but slowly the retina became totally flat, and we treated the retinal break with the diode laser. A 240 band was wrapped around the eye and fixed with the Watke's sleeve superior temporally. The sclerotomies were all sewn closed. Before the last sclerotomy was closed, the air was exchanged for silicone. The eye was left soft because the patient had poor perfusion.

Evaluation

Review the medical report above to answer the following questions. Use a medical dictionary such as Taber's Cyclopedic Medical Dictionary *and other resources if needed.*

1. Where is the retina located?

   _____

   _____

2. Was the anesthetic administered behind or in front of the eyeball?

_____

_____

3. How much movement remained in the eye following anesthesia?

_____

_____

4. Where was the hemorrhage located?

_____

_____

5. What type of vitrectomy was undertaken?

_____

_____

6. Why was the eye left soft?

_____

_____

MEDICAL RECORD ACTIVITY 11-2

OTITIS MEDIA

Terminology

Terms listed in the table below come from the medical report Otitis Media *that follows. Use a medical dictionary such as* Taber's Cyclopedic Medical Dictionary, *the appendices of this book, or other resources to define each term. Then practice reading the pronunciations aloud for each term.*

Term	Definition
cholesteatoma kō-lē-stē-ă-TŌ-mă	
ENT	
general anesthesia ăn-ĕs-THĒ-zē-ă	
mucoserous mū-kō-SĒR-ŭs	
otitis media ō-TĪ-tĭs MĒ-dē-ă	

Continued

Term	Definition
postoperatively pōst-ŎP-ĕr-ă-tĭv-lē	
tympanoplasty tĭm-păn-ō-PLĂS-tē	

DavisPlus | Visit the *Medical Terminology Simplified* online resource center at DavisPlus to practice pronunciation and reinforce the meanings of selected terms in this medical report.

Reading

Practice pronunciation of medical terms by reading the following medical report aloud.

Otitis Media

A 25-year-old white woman with a diagnosis of mucoserous otitis media in the right ear was seen by the ENT specialist. The patient was admitted to the hospital and developed cholesteatoma. A tube was inserted for the chronic adhesive otitis media with secondary cholesteatoma. The patient progressed favorably postoperatively, but the cholesteatoma continued to enlarge in size. Currently, she has been admitted to the hospital for a right tympanoplasty performed under general anesthesia.

Evaluation

Review the medical record above to answer the following questions. Use a medical dictionary such as Taber's Cyclopedic Medical Dictionary *and other resources if needed.*

1. Where was the patient's infection located?

   _____

   _____

2. What complication developed while the patient was hospitalized?

   _____

   _____

3. What is the purpose of the tube placement?

   _____

   _____

4. What surgery is being performed to resolve the cholesteatoma?

   _____

   _____

5. Will the patient be asleep during the surgery?

   _____

   _____

SPECIAL SENSES: EYES AND EARS CHAPTER REVIEW

WORD ELEMENTS SUMMARY

The table below summarizes CFs, suffixes, and prefixes related to the special senses. Study the word elements and their meanings before completing the Word Elements Chapter Review that follows.

Word Element	Meaning	Word Element	Meaning
Combining Forms			
acous/o, audi/o, audit/o	hearing	**my/o**	muscle
blephar/o	eyelid	**myring/o, tympan/o**	tympanic membrane (eardrum)
choroid/o	choroid	**neur/o**	nerve
chromat/o	color	**ocul/o, ophthalm/o**	eye
cochle/o	cochlea	**ot/o**	ear
corne/o	cornea	**presby/o**	old age
dacry/o, lacrim/o	tear; lacrimal apparatus (duct, sac, or gland)	**retin/o**	retina
dipl/o	double	**salping/o**	tube (usually fallopian or eustachian [auditory] tubes)
erythr/o	red	**scler/o**	hardening; sclera (white of the eye)
irid/o	iris	**ton/o**	tension
kerat/o	horny tissue; hard; cornea	**xanth/o**	yellow
Suffixes			
-acusis	hearing	**-pathy**	disease
-algia, -dynia	pain	**-plasty**	surgical repair
-ectomy	excision, removal	**-ptosis**	prolapse, downward displacement
-edema	swelling	**-rrhexis**	rupture
-logist	specialist in the study of	**-salpinx**	tube (usually fallopian or eustachian [auditory] tubes)
-logy	study of	**-scope**	instrument for examining
-malacia	softening	**-scopy**	visual examination
-metry	act of measuring	**-spasm**	involuntary contraction, twitching
-oma	tumor	**-stenosis**	narrowing, stricture
-opia, -opsia	vision	**-tomy**	incision
-osis	abnormal condition; increase (used primarily with blood cells)	**-tropia**	turning

Continued

Word Element	Meaning	Word Element	Meaning
Prefixes			
a-	without, not	eso-	inward
ana-	against; up; back	exo-	outside, outward
dipl-	double	hyper-	excessive, above normal

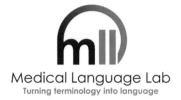

Medical Language Lab
Turning terminology into language

Visit the *Medical Language Lab* at the website *medicallanguagelab.com*. Use the flash-card exercise to reinforce your study of word elements. We recommend you complete the flash-card exercise before starting the Word Elements Chapter Review that follows.

WORD ELEMENTS CHAPTER REVIEW

This review provides a verification of your knowledge of the word elements covered in this chapter. Write the meaning of the word element in the space provided. To reinforce your understanding of the word parts that make up a medical term, identify each word element as a prefix (P), word root (WR), combining form (CF), or suffix (S). The first word is completed for you.

Medical Term	Word Element	Meaning
1. acoustic	*acous (WR)*	*hearing*
	-tic (S)	*pertaining to*
2. anisocoria		
3. audiometer		
4. blepharoptosis		
5. conjunctivitis		

Continued

Medical Term	Word Element	Meaning
6. choroidopathy		
7. dacryorrhea		
8. esotropia		
9. iridectomy		
10. keratitis		
11. myopia		

Medical Term	Word Element	Meaning
12. myringotomy		
13. ophthalmoscope		
14. otoscopy		
15. photophobia		
16. presbycusis		
17. salpingostenosis		

Continued

Medical Term	Word Element	Meaning
18. scleromalacia		
19. stapedectomy		
20. tympanoplasty		

Competency Verification: Check your answers in Appendix B: Answer Key, page 602. If you are not satisfied with your level of comprehension, review the chapter's flash-card exercise at *medicallanguagelab.com* and retake the review.

Correct Answers _____ × 5 = _____ % Score

VOCABULARY REVIEW

Match the medical terms below with the definitions in the numbered list.

blepharoptosis	diplopia	labyrinth	otitis media
cholesteatoma	eustachian tube	mastoid surgery	postoperatively
chronic	general anesthetic	mucoserous	salpingostenosis
dacryorrhea	hyperopia	myopia	sclera
diagnosis	keratitis	ophthalmologist	tympanic membrane

1. _____ means *double vision.*

2. _____ refers to the white of the eye.

3. _____ is the eardrum; it vibrates when soundwaves strike it.

4. _____ means *excessive flow of tears.*

5. _____ equalizes the air pressure in the middle ear with that of the outside atmosphere.

6. _____ refers to inflammation of the cornea due to a vision-threatening infection and sometimes occurs when contact lenses are not disinfected properly.

7. _____ is a process of determining the cause and nature of a pathological condition.

8. _____ means *composed of mucus and serum.*

9. _____ is inflammation of the middle ear.

10. _____ is a tumorlike sac filled with keratin debris most commonly found in the middle ear.

11. _____ is an operation on the mastoid process of the temporal bone.

12. _____ is anesthesia that affects the entire body with loss of consciousness.

13. _____ is a physician who specializes in the treatment of eye disorders.

14. _____ means *of long duration,* designating a disease showing little change or slow progression.

15. _____ means *farsightedness.*

16. _____ means *occurring after surgery.*

17. _____ is a system of intercommunicating canals, especially of the inner ear.

18. _____ is prolapse of an eyelid.

19. _____ is a narrowing or stricture of the eustachian tube.

20. _____ means *nearsightedness.*

Competency Verification: Check your answers in Appendix B: Answer Key, page 603. If you are not satisfied with your level of comprehension, review the chapter vocabulary and retake the review.

Correct Answers _____ × 5 = _____ % Score

A

Glossary of Medical Word Elements

Medical Word Element	Meaning	Medical Word Element	Meaning
A		alveol/o	alveolus; air sac
a-	without, not	ambly/o	dull, dim
ab-	from, away from	amni/o	amnion (amniotic sac)
abdomin/o	abdomen	an-	without, not
abort/o	to miscarry	an/o	anus
-ac	pertaining to	ana-	against; up; back
acid/o	acid	andr/o	male
acous/o	hearing	aneurysm/o	widened blood vessel
acr/o	extremity	angi/o	vessel (usually blood or lymph)
acromi/o	acromion (projection of the scapula)	aniso-	unequal, dissimilar
		ankyl/o	stiffness; bent, crooked
-acusis	hearing	ante-	before, in front of
-ad	toward	anter/o	anterior, front
ad-	toward	anthrac/o	coal, coal dust
aden/o	gland	anti-	against
adenoid/o	adenoids	aort/o	aorta
adip/o	fat	append/o	appendix
adren/o	adrenal glands	appendic/o	appendix
adrenal/o	adrenal glands	aque/o	water
aer/o	air	-ar	pertaining to
af-	toward	-arche	beginning
agglutin/o	clumping, gluing	arteri/o	artery
agora-	marketplace	arteriol/o	arteriole
-al	pertaining to	arthr/o	joint
albin/o	white	-ary	pertaining to
albumin/o	albumin (protein)	asbest/o	asbestos
-algesia	pain	-asthenia	weakness, debility
-algia	pain	astr/o	star
allo-	other, differing from the normal		

Medical Word Element	Meaning	Medical Word Element	Meaning
-ate	having the form of, possessing	cephal/o	head
atel/o	incomplete; imperfect	-ceps	head
ather/o	fatty plaque	-ception	conceiving
-ation	process (of)	cerebell/o	cerebellum
atri/o	atrium	cerebr/o	cerebrum
audi/o	hearing	cervic/o	neck; cervix uteri (neck of the uterus)
audit/o	hearing		
aur/o	ear	chalic/o	limestone
auricul/o	ear	cheil/o	lip
auto-	self, own	chem/o	chemical; drug
ax/o	axis, axon	chlor/o	green
azot/o	nitrogenous compounds	chol/e	bile, gall
		cholangi/o	bile vessel
B		cholecyst/o	gallbladder
bacteri/o	bacteria (singular, *bacterium*)	choledoch/o	bile duct
balan/o	glans penis	chondr/o	cartilage
bas/o	base (alkaline, opposite of acid)	chori/o	chorion
bi-	two	choroid/o	choroid
bi/o	life	chrom/o	color
bil/i	bile, gall	chromat/o	color
-blast	embryonic cell	-cide	killing
blast/o	embryonic cell	cine-	movement
blephar/o	eyelid	circum-	around
brachi/o	arm	cirrh/o	yellow
brachy-	short	-cision	a cutting
brady-	slow	-clasia	to break; surgical fracture
bronch/o	bronchus (plural, *bronchi*)	-clasis	to break; surgical fracture
bronchi/o	bronchus (plural, *bronchi*)	-clast	to break; surgical fracture
bronchiol/o	bronchiole	clavicul/o	clavicle (collar bone)
bucc/o	cheek	-cleisis	closure
		clon/o	clonus (turmoil)
C		-clysis	irrigation, washing
calc/o	calcium	coccyg/o	coccyx (tailbone)
calcane/o	calcaneum (heel bone)	cochle/o	cochlea
-capnia	carbon dioxide (CO_2)	col/o	colon
carcin/o	cancer	colon/o	colon
cardi/o	heart	colp/o	vagina
-cardia	heart condition	condyl/o	condyle
carp/o	carpus (wrist bones)	coni/o	dust
cata-	down	conjunctiv/o	conjunctiva
caud/o	tail	-continence	to hold back
cauter/o	heat, burn	contra-	against, opposite
cec/o	cecum	cor/o	pupil
-cele	hernia, swelling		
-centesis	surgical puncture		

Continued

Medical Word Element	Meaning	Medical Word Element	Meaning
core/o	pupil	dors/o	back (of the body)
corne/o	cornea	duct/o	to lead; carry
coron/o	heart	-duction	act of leading, bringing, conducting
corp/o	body	duoden/o	duodenum (first part of the small intestine)
corpor/o	body		
cortic/o	cortex	dur/o	dura mater; hard
cost/o	ribs	-dynia	pain
crani/o	cranium (skull)	dys-	bad; painful; difficult
crin/o	secrete	**E**	
-crine	secrete	-eal	pertaining to
cruci/o	cross	ec-	out, out from
cry/o	cold	echo-	a repeated sound
crypt/o	hidden	-ectasis	dilation, expansion
culd/o	cul-de-sac	ecto-	outside, outward
-cusia	hearing	-ectomy	excision, removal
-cusis	hearing	-edema	swelling
cutane/o	skin	ef-	away from
cyan/o	blue	electr/o	electricity
cycl/o	ciliary body of the eye; circular; cycle	-ema	state of; condition
		embol/o	embolus (plug)
-cyesis	pregnancy	-emesis	vomiting
cyst/o	bladder	-emia	blood condition
cyt/o	cell	emphys/o	to inflate
-cyte	cell	en-	in, within
D		encephal/o	brain
dacry/o	tear; lacrimal apparatus (duct, sac, or gland)	end-	in, within
		endo-	in, within
dacryocyst/o	lacrimal sac	enter/o	intestine (usually small intestine)
dactyl/o	fingers; toes	eosin/o	dawn (rose-colored)
de-	cessation	epi-	above, upon
dendr/o	tree	epididym/o	epididymis
dent/o	teeth	epiglott/o	epiglottis
derm/o	skin	episi/o	vulva
-derma	skin	erythem/o	red
dermat/o	skin	erythemat/o	red
-desis	binding, fixation (of a bone or joint)	erythr/o	red
		eschar/o	scab
di-	double	-esis	condition
dia-	through, across	eso-	inward
dipl-	double	esophag/o	esophagus
dipl/o	double	esthes/o	feeling
dips/o	thirst	-esthesia	feeling
-dipsia	thirst		
dist/o	far, farthest		

Medical Word Element	Meaning	Medical Word Element	Meaning
eti/o	cause	granul/o	granule
eu-	good; normal	-graph	instrument for recording
ex-	out, out from	-graphy	process of recording
exo-	outside, outward	-gravida	pregnant woman
extra-	outside	gyn/o	woman, female
F		gynec/o	woman, female
faci/o	face	**H**	
fasci/o	band, fascia (fibrous membrane supporting and separating muscles)	hallucin/o	hallucination
		hedon/o	pleasure
femor/o	femur (thigh bone)	hem/o	blood
-ferent	to carry	hemangi/o	blood vessel
fibr/o	fiber, fibrous tissue	hemat/o	blood
fibul/o	fibula (smaller bone of the lower leg)	hemi-	one half
		hepat/o	liver
fluor/o	luminous, fluorescence	hetero-	different
G		hidr/o	sweat
galact/o	milk	hist/o	tissue
gangli/o	ganglion (knot or knotlike mass)	histi/o	tissue
gastr/o	stomach	home/o	same, alike
-gen	forming, producing, origin	homeo-	same, alike
gen/o	forming, producing, origin	homo-	same
-genesis	forming, producing, origin	humer/o	humerus (upper arm bone)
genit/o	genitalia	hydr/o	water
gest/o	pregnancy	hyp-	under, below, deficient
gingiv/o	gum(s)	hyp/o	under, below, deficient
glauc/o	gray	hyper-	excessive, above normal
gli/o	glue; neuroglial tissue	hypn/o	sleep
-glia	glue; neuroglial tissue	hypo-	under, below, deficient
-globin	protein	hyster/o	uterus (womb)
glomerul/o	glomerulus	**I**	
gloss/o	tongue	-ia	condition
glott/o	glottis	-iac	pertaining to
gluc/o	sugar, sweetness	-iasis	abnormal condition (produced by something specified)
glucos/o	sugar, sweetness		
glyc/o	sugar, sweetness	iatr/o	physician; medicine; treatment
glycos/o	sugar, sweetness	-iatry	medicine; treatment
gnos/o	knowing	-ic	pertaining to
-gnosis	knowing	-ical	pertaining to
gon/o	seed (ovum or spermatozoon)	-ice	noun ending
gonad/o	gonads, sex glands	ichthy/o	dry, scaly
-grade	to go	-ician	specialist
-graft	transplantation	-icle	small, minute
-gram	record, writing	-icterus	jaundice

Continued

Medical Word Element	Meaning	Medical Word Element	Meaning
idi/o	unknown; peculiar	kinet/o	movement
-ile	pertaining to	kyph/o	humpback
ile/o	ileum (third part of the small intestine)	**L**	
ili/o	ilium (lateral, flaring portion of the hip bone)	labi/o	lip
im-	not	labyrinth/o	labyrinth (inner ear)
immun/o	immune, immunity, safe	lacrim/o	tear; lacrimal apparatus (duct, sac, or gland)
in-	in; not	lact/o	milk
-ine	pertaining to	-lalia	speech, babble
infer/o	lower, below	lamin/o	lamina (part of vertebral arch)
infra-	below, under	lapar/o	abdomen
inguin/o	groin	laryng/o	larynx (voice box)
insulin/o	insulin	later/o	side, to one side
inter-	between	lei/o	smooth
intra-	in, within	leiomy/o	smooth muscle (visceral)
-ion	the act of	-lepsy	seizure
-ior	pertaining to	lept/o	thin, slender
irid/o	iris	leuk/o	white
-is	noun ending	lingu/o	tongue
isch/o	to hold back; block	lip/o	fat
ischi/o	ischium (lower portion of the hip bone)	lipid/o	fat
-ism	condition	-listhesis	slipping
iso-	same, equal	-lith	stone, calculus
-ist	specialist	lith/o	stone, calculus
-isy	state of; condition	lob/o	lobe
-itic	pertaining to	log/o	study of
-itis	inflammation	-logist	specialist in the study of
-ive	pertaining to	-logy	study of
-ization	process (of)	lord/o	curve, swayback
		-lucent	to shine; clear
J		lumb/o	loins (lower back)
jaund/o	yellow	lymph/o	lymph
jejun/o	jejunum (second part of the small intestine)	lymphaden/o	lymph gland (node)
		lymphangi/o	lymph vessel
		-lysis	separation; destruction; loosening
K		**M**	
kal/i	potassium (an electrolyte)	macro-	large
kary/o	nucleus	mal-	bad
kerat/o	horny tissue; hard; cornea	-malacia	softening
ket/o	ketone bodies (acids and acetones)	mamm/o	breast
keton/o	ketone bodies (acids and acetones)	-mania	state of mental disorder, frenzy
kinesi/o	movement	mast/o	breast
-kinesia	movement		

Medical Word Element	Meaning	Medical Word Element	Meaning
mastoid/o	mastoid process	nat/o	birth
maxill/o	maxilla (upper jaw bone)	natr/o	sodium (an electrolyte)
meat/o	opening, meatus	necr/o	death, necrosis
medi-	middle	neo-	new
medi/o	middle	nephr/o	kidney
mediastin/o	mediastinum	neur/o	nerve
medull/o	medulla	neutr/o	neutral; neither
mega-	enlargement	nid/o	nest
megal/o	enlargement	noct/o	night
-megaly	enlargement	nucle/o	nucleus
melan/o	black	nulli-	none
men/o	menses, menstruation	nyctal/o	night
mening/o	meninges (membranes covering the brain and spinal cord)	**O**	
meningi/o	meninges (membranes covering the brain and spinal cord)	obstetr/o	midwife
ment/o	mind	ocul/o	eye
meso-	middle	odont/o	teeth
meta-	change, beyond	-oid	resembling
metacarp/o	metacarpus (hand bones)	-ole	small, minute
metatars/o	metatarsus (foot bones)	olig/o	scanty
-meter	instrument for measuring	-oma	tumor
metr/o	uterus (womb); measure	omphal/o	navel (umbilicus)
metri/o	uterus (womb)	onc/o	tumor
-metry	act of measuring	onych/o	nail
mi/o	smaller, less	oophor/o	ovary
micr/o	small	-opaque	obscure
micro-	small	ophthalm/o	eye
mono-	one	-opia	vision
morph/o	form, shape, structure	-opsia	vision
muc/o	mucus	-opsy	view of
multi-	many, much	opt/o	eye, vision
muscul/o	muscle	optic/o	eye, vision
mut/a	genetic change	or/o	mouth
my/o	muscle	orch/o	testis (plural, *testes*)
myc/o	fungus (plural, *fungi*)	orchi/o	testis (plural, *testes*)
mydr/o	widen, enlarge	orchid/o	testis (plural, *testes*)
myel/o	bone marrow; spinal cord	-orexia	appetite
myos/o	muscle	orth/o	straight
myring/o	tympanic membrane (eardrum)	-ory	pertaining to
myx/o	mucus	-ose	pertaining to; sugar
N		-osis	abnormal condition; increase (used primarily with blood cells)
narc/o	stupor; numbness; sleep	-osmia	smell
nas/o	nose	oste/o	bone

Continued

Medical Word Element	Meaning	Medical Word Element	Meaning
ot/o	ear	phleb/o	vein
-ous	pertaining to	-phobia	fear
ovari/o	ovary	-phonia	voice
ox/i	oxygen	-phoresis	carrying, transmission
ox/o	oxygen	-phoria	feeling (mental state)
-oxia	oxygen	phot/o	light
P		phren/o	diaphragm; mind
palat/o	palate (roof of mouth)	-phylaxis	protection
pan-	all	-physis	growth
pancreat/o	pancreas	pil/o	hair
para-	near, beside; beyond	pituitar/o	pituitary gland
-para	to bear (offspring)	-plakia	plaque
parathyroid/o	parathyroid glands	plas/o	formation, growth
-paresis	partial paralysis	-plasia	formation, growth
patell/o	patella (kneecap)	-plasm	formation, growth
path/o	disease	-plasty	surgical repair
-pathy	disease	-plegia	paralysis
pector/o	chest	pleur/o	pleura
ped/i	foot; child	-plexy	stroke
ped/o	foot; child	-pnea	breathing
pedicul/o	lice	pneum/o	air; lung
pelv/i	pelvis	pneumon/o	air; lung
pelv/o	pelvis	pod/o	foot
pen/o	penis	-poiesis	formation, production
-penia	decrease, deficiency	poikil/o	varied, irregular
-pepsia	digestion	poli/o	gray; gray matter (of the brain or spinal cord)
peri-	around		
perine/o	perineum (area between the scrotum [or vulva in the female] and anus)	poly-	many, much
		polyp/o	small growth
		-porosis	porous
peritone/o	peritoneum	post-	after, behind
-pexy	fixation (of an organ)	poster/o	back (of the body), behind, posterior
phac/o	lens		
phag/o	swallowing, eating	-potence	power
-phage	swallowing, eating	-prandial	meal
-phagia	swallowing, eating	pre-	before, in front of
phalang/o	phalanges (bones of the fingers and toes)	presby/o	old age
		primi-	first
pharmaceutic/o	drug, medicine	pro-	before, in front of
pharyng/o	pharynx (throat)	proct/o	anus, rectum
-phasia	speech	prostat/o	prostate gland
-phil	attraction for	proxim/o	near, nearest
phil/o	attraction for	pseudo-	false
-philia	attraction for	psych/o	mind

Medical Word Element	Meaning	Medical Word Element	Meaning
-ptosis	prolapse, downward displacement	-schisis	a splitting
ptyal/o	saliva	schiz/o	split
-ptysis	spitting	scler/o	hardening; sclera (white of the eye)
pub/o	pelvis bone (anterior part of the pelvic bone)	scoli/o	crooked, bent
pulmon/o	lung	-scope	instrument for examining
pupill/o	pupil	-scopy	visual examination
py/o	pus	scot/o	darkness
pyel/o	renal pelvis	seb/o	sebum, sebaceous
pylor/o	pylorus	semi-	one half
pyr/o	fire	semin/i	semen; seed
		semin/o	semen; seed
Q, R		sept/o	septum
quadri-	four	septic/o	infection
rachi/o	spine	sequestr/o	separation
radi/o	radiation, x-ray; radius (lower arm bone on the thumb side)	ser/o	serum
radicul/o	nerve root	sial/o	saliva, salivary gland
rect/o	rectum	sider/o	iron
ren/o	kidney	sigmoid/o	sigmoid colon
reticul/o	net, mesh	sin/o	sinus, cavity
retin/o	retina	sinus/o	sinus, cavity
retro-	backward, behind	-sis	state of; condition
rhabd/o	rod-shaped (striated)	somat/o	body
rhabdomy/o	rod-shaped (striated) muscle	somn/o	sleep
rhin/o	nose	son/o	sound
rhytid/o	wrinkle	-spadias	slit, fissure
roentgen/o	x-ray	-spasm	involuntary contraction, twitching
-rrhage	bursting forth (of)	sperm/i	spermatozoa, sperm cells
-rrhagia	bursting forth (of)	sperm/o	spermatozoa, sperm cells
-rrhaphy	suture	spermat/o	spermatozoa, sperm cells
-rrhea	discharge, flow	sphygm/o	pulse
-rrhexis	rupture	-sphyxia	pulse
-rrhythm/o	rhythm	spin/o	spine
rube/o	red	spir/o	breathe
		splen/o	spleen
S		spondyl/o	vertebra (backbone)
sacr/o	sacrum	squam/o	scale
salping/o	tube (usually fallopian or eustachian [auditory] tubes)	staped/o	stapes
-salpinx	tube (usually fallopian or eustachian [auditory] tubes)	-stasis	standing still
		steat/o	fat
sarc/o	flesh (connective tissue)	sten/o	narrowing, stricture
-sarcoma	malignant tumor of connective tissue	-stenosis	narrowing, stricture
		stern/o	sternum (breastbone)
scapul/o	scapula (shoulder blade)		

Continued

Medical Word Element	Meaning	Medical Word Element	Meaning
steth/o	chest	-tomy	incision
sthen/o	strength	ton/o	tension
stigmat/o	point, mark	tonsill/o	tonsils
stomat/o	mouth	tox/o	poison
-stomy	forming an opening (mouth)	-toxic	pertaining to poison
sub-	under, below	toxic/o	poison
sudor/o	sweat	trabecul/o	trabecula (supporting bundles of fibers)
super-	upper, above		
super/o	upper, above	trache/o	trachea (windpipe)
supra-	above; excessive; superior	trans-	across, through
sym-	union, together, joined	tri-	three
syn-	union, together, joined	trich/o	hair
synapt/o	synapsis, point of contact	trigon/o	trigone (triangular region at the base of the bladder)
synov/o	synovial membrane, synovial fluid		
T		-tripsy	crushing
		-trophy	development, nourishment
tachy-	rapid	-tropia	turning
tax/o	order, coordination	-tropin	stimulate
-taxia	order, coordination	tubercul/o	a little swelling
ten/o	tendon	tympan/o	tympanic membrane (eardrum)
tend/o	tendon	**U**	
tendin/o	tendon	-ula	small, minute
-tension	to stretch	-ule	small, minute
test/o	testis (plural, testes)	uln/o	ulna (lower arm bone on the opposite side of the thumb)
thalam/o	thalamus		
thalass/o	sea	ultra-	excess, beyond
thec/o	sheath (usually referring to the meninges)	-um	structure, thing
		umbilic/o	umbilicus, navel
thel/o	nipple	ungu/o	nail
therapeut/o	treatment	uni-	one
-therapy	treatment	ur/o	urine, urinary tract
therm/o	heat	ureter/o	ureter
thorac/o	chest	urethr/o	urethra
-thorax	chest	-uria	urine
thromb/o	blood clot	urin/o	urine, urinary tract
thym/o	thymus gland	-us	condition; structure
-thymia	mind; emotion	uter/o	uterus (womb)
thyr/o	thyroid gland	uvul/o	uvula
thyroid/o	thyroid gland	**V**	
tibi/o	tibia (larger bone of the lower leg)	vagin/o	vagina
-tic	pertaining to	valv/o	valve
-tocia	childbirth, labor	varic/o	dilated vein
tom/o	to cut, slice	vas/o	vessel; vas deferens; duct
-tome	instrument to cut		

Medical Word Element	Meaning	Medical Word Element	Meaning
vascul/o	vessel (usually blood or lymph)	vitre/o	glassy
ven/o	vein	vol/o	volume
ventr/o	belly, belly side	vulv/o	vulva
ventricul/o	ventricle (of the heart or brain)	**X, Y, Z**	
-version	turning	xanth/o	yellow
vertebr/o	vertebra (backbone)	xen/o	foreign, strange
vesic/o	bladder	xer/o	dry
vesicul/o	seminal vesicle	xiph/o	sword
vest/o	clothes	-y	condition; process
viscer/o	internal organs		
vitr/o	vitreous body (of the eye)		

Answer Key

CHAPTER 1: INTRODUCTION TO PROGRAMMED LEARNING AND MEDICAL WORD BUILDING

Frame 1–51

Medical Term	Combining Form (Root + o)	Word Root	Suffix
arthr/o/scop/ic ăr-thrōs-KŎP-ĭk	*arthr/o*	*scop*	*-ic*
erythr/o/cyt/osis ĕ-rĭth-rō-sī-TŌ-sĭs	erythr/o	cyt	-osis
append/ix ă-PĔN-dĭks		append	-ix
dermat/itis dĕr-mă-TĪ-tĭs		dermat	-itis
gastr/o/enter/itis găs-trō-ĕn-tĕr-Ī-tĭs	gastr/o	enter	-itis
orth/o/ped/ic or-thō-PĒ-dĭk	orth/o	ped	-ic
oste/o/arthr/itis ŏs-tē-ō-ăr-THRĪ-tĭs	oste/o	arthr	-itis
vagin/itis văj-ĭn-Ī-tĭs		vagin	-itis

Section Review 1–1

1. breve	3. long	5. pn	7. n	9. second
2. macron	4. short	6. hard	8. eye	10. separate

Surgical Suffixes

Term	Meaning
arthr/o/**centesis** ăr-thrō-sĕn-TĒ-sĭs *arthr/o:* joint	*surgical puncture of a joint*
arthr/o/**desis** ăr-thrō-DĒ-sĭs *arthr/o:* joint	binding or fixation of a joint
append/**ectomy** ăp-ĕn-DĔK-tō-mē *append:* appendix	excision or removal of the appendix
thromb/o/**lysis** thrŏm-BŎL-ĭ-sĭs *thromb/o:* blood clot	separation, destruction, or loosening of a blood clot
mast/o/**pexy** MĂS-tō-pĕks-ē *mast/o:* breast	fixation of the breast(s)
rhin/o/**plasty** RĪ-nō-plăs-tē *rhin/o:* nose	surgical repair of the nose (to change the shape or size)
my/o/**rrhaphy** mī-OR-ă-fē *my/o:* muscle	suture of a muscle
trache/o/**stomy** trā-kē-ŎS-tō-mē *trache/o:* trachea (windpipe)	forming an opening (mouth) into the trachea
oste/o/**tome** ŎS-tē-ō-tōm *oste/o:* bone	instrument to cut bone
trache/o/**tomy** trā-kē–ŎT-ō–mē *trache/o:* trachea (windpipe)	incision into the trachea
lith/o/**tripsy** LĬTH-ō-trĭp-sē *lith/o:* stone, calculus	crushing a stone or calculus

Diagnostic Suffixes

Term	Meaning
electr/o/cardi/o/**gram** ē-lĕk-trō-KĂR-dē-ō-grăm *electr/o:* electricity *cardi/o:* heart	record of electrical activity of the heart
cardi/o/**graph** KĂR-dē-ō-grăf *cardi/o:* heart	instrument to record electrical activity of the heart
angi/o/**graphy** ăn-jē-ŎG-ră-fē *angi/o:* vessel (usually blood or lymph)	process of recording images of blood vessels (recording images of blood vessels after injection of a contrast medium)
pelv/i/**meter** pĕl-VĬM-ĕ-tĕr *pelv/i:* pelvis	instrument for measuring the pelvis
pelv/i/**metry** pĕl-VĬM-ĕ-trē *pelv/i:* pelvis	act of measuring the pelvis
endo/**scope** ĔN-dō-skōp *endo-:* in, within	instrument for examining within (or inside a hollow organ or cavity)
endo/**scopy** ĕn-DŎS-kō-pē *endo-:* in, within	visual examination within (a cavity or canal using a specialized lighted instrument called an endoscope)

Pathologic Suffixes

Term	Meaning
neur/**algia** nū-RĂL-jē-ă *neur:* nerve	pain of a nerve (or pain along the path of a nerve)
ot/o/**dynia** ō-tō-DĬN-ē-ă *ot/o:* ear	pain in the ear (earache)
hepat/o/**cele** hĕ-PĂT-ō-sēl *hepat/o:* liver	hernia or swelling of the liver
bronchi/**ectasis** brŏng-kē-ĔK-tă-sĭs *bronchi:* bronchus (plural, bronchi)	abnormal dilation or expansion of a bronchus or bronchi
lymph/**edema** lĭmf-ĕ-DĒ-mă *lymph:* lymph	swelling of lymph tissue (swelling resulting from accumulation of tissue fluid)
hyper/**emesis** hī-pĕr-ĔM-ĕ-sĭs *hyper-:* excessive, above normal	excessive or above normal vomiting

Term	Meaning
an/**emia** ă-NĒ-mē-ă *an-:* without, not	literally means without blood (blood condition caused by iron deficiency or a decrease in red blood cells)
chol/e/**lith/iasis** kō-lē-lĭ-THĪ-ă-sĭs *chol/e:* bile, gall *lith:* stone, calculus	presence or formation of gallstones (in the gallbladder or common bile duct)
gastr/**itis** găs-TRĪ-tĭs *gastr:* stomach	inflammation of the stomach
chol/e/**lith** KŌ-lē-lĭth *cho/e:* bile, gall	gallstone
chondr/o/**malacia** kŏn-drō-mă-LĀ-shē-ă *chondr/o:* cartilage	softening of cartilage
cardi/o/**megaly** kăr-dē-ō-MĔG-ă–lē *cardi/o:* heart	enlargement of the heart
neur/**oma** nū-RŌ-mă *neur:* nerve	tumor composed of nerve cells
cyan/**osis** sī-ă-NŌ-sĭs *cyan:* blue	abnormal condition of dark blue (bluish or purple discoloration of the skin and mucous membrane)
my/o/**pathy** mī-ŎP-ă-thē *my/o:* muscle	any disease of muscle
erythr/o/**penia** ĕ-rĭth-rō-PĒ-nē-ă *erythr/o:* red	abnormal decrease or deficiency in red (blood cells)
hem/o/**phobia** hē-mō-FŌ-bē-ă *hem/o:* blood	fear of blood
hemi/**plegia** hĕm-ē-PLĒ-jē-ă *hemi-:* one half	paralysis of one half (paralysis of one side of the body)
hem/o/**rrhage** HĔM-ĕ-rĭj *hem/o:* blood	bursting forth of blood (loss of large amounts of blood within a short period, externally or internally)
men/o/**rrhagia** mĕn-ō-RĀ-jē-ă *men/o:* menses, menstruation	bursting forth of menses (profuse discharge of blood during menstruation)

Continued

Term	Meaning
dia/**rrhea** dī-ă-RĒ-ă *dia-*: through, across	discharge or flow through (abnormally frequent discharge or flow of fluid fecal matter from the bowel)
arteri/o/**rrhexis** ăr-tē-rē-ō-RĔK-sĭs *arteri/o*: artery	rupture of an artery
arteri/o/**stenosis** ăr-tē-rē-ō-stě-NŌ-sĭs *arteri/o*: artery	narrowing or stricture of an artery
hepat/o/**toxic** HĔP-ă-tō-tŏk-sĭk *hepat/o*: liver	potentially destructive to the liver
dys/**trophy** DĬS-trō-fē *dys-*: bad; painful; difficult	bad development or nourishment (abnormal condition caused by defective nutrition or metabolism)

Section Review 1–2

Singular	Plural	Rule
1. sarcoma	*sarcomata*	*Retain the* ma *and add* ta.
2. thrombus	thrombi	Drop *us* and add *i*.
3. appendix	appendices	Drop *ix* and add *ices*.
4. diverticulum	diverticula	Drop *um* and add *a*.
5. ovary	ovaries	Drop *y* and add *ies*.
6. diagnosis	diagnoses	Drop *is* and add *es*.
7. lumen	lumina	Drop *en* and add *ina*.
8. vertebra	vertebrae	Retain the *a* and add *e*.
9. thorax	thoraces	Drop the *x* and add *ces*.
10. spermatozoon	spermatozoa	Drop *on* and add *a*.

Common Prefixes

Term	Meaning
a/mast/ia ă-MĂS-tē-ă *mast*: breast *-ia*: condition	without a breast
an/esthesia ăn-ěs-THĒ-zē-ă *-esthesia*: feeling	without feeling (partial or complete loss of sensation with or without loss of consciousness)

Term	Meaning
circum/duction sĕr-kŭm-DŬK-shŭn *-duction:* act of leading, bringing, conducting	act of leading around (movement of a part, such as an extremity, in a circular direction)

peri/odont/al
pĕr-ē-ō-DŎN-tăl
   odont: teeth
     -al: pertaining to
	pertaining to around a tooth

dia/rrhea dī-ă-RĒ-ă *-rrhea:* discharge, flow	flow through

trans/vagin/al
trăns-VĂJ-ĭn-ăl
   vagin: vagina
     -al: pertaining to
	pertaining to across the vagina

dipl/opia dĭp-LŌ-pē-ă *-opia:* vision	double vision

diplo/bacteri/al
dĭp-lō-băk-TĒR-ē-ăl
   bacteri: bacteria
     -al: pertaining to
	pertaining to bacteria linked together in pairs

endo/crine ĔN-dō-krīn *-crine:* secrete	secrete within

intra/muscul/ar
ĭn-tră-MŬS-kū-lăr
   muscul: muscle
     -ar: pertaining to
	pertaining to within the muscle

homo/graft HŌ-mō-grăft *-graft:* transplantation	literally means transplantation of same (transplantation of tissue between the same species)
homeo/plasia hō-mē-ō-PLĀ-zē-ă *-plasia:* formation, growth	formation or growth of new tissue similar to that already existing in a part

hypo/derm/ic
hī-pō-DĔR-mĭk
   derm: skin
     -ic: pertaining to
	pertaining to under the skin (under or inserted under the skin, as in a hypodermic injection)

macro/cyte MĂK-rō-sīt *-cyte:* cell	abnormally large cell (usually erythrocyte), such as those found in pernicious anemia
micro/scope MĪ-krō-skōp *-scope:* instrument for examining	instrument for examining minute objects

Continued

Term	Meaning
mono/cyte MŎN-ō-sīt *-cyte:* cell	large mononuclear leukocyte
uni/nucle/ar ū-nĭ-NŪ-klē-ăr *nucle:* nucleus *-ar:* pertaining to	pertaining to one nucleus
post/nat/al pōst-NĀ-tăl *nat:* birth *-al:* pertaining to	pertaining to (the period) after birth
pre/nat/al prē-NĀ-tăl *nat:* birth *-al:* pertaining to	pertaining to (the period) before birth
pro/gnosis prŏg-NŌ-sĭs *-gnosis:* knowing	before knowing; knowing beforehand (prediction of the course and end of a disease, and the estimated chance of recovery)
primi/gravida prī-mĭ-GRĂV-ĭ-dă *-gravida:* pregnant woman	woman during her first pregnancy
retro/version rĕt-rō-VĔR-shŭn *-version:* turning	literally means turning backward (tipping backward of an organ, such as the uterus, from its normal position)
super/ior soo-PĒ-rē-or *-ior:* pertaining to	pertaining to upper or above (toward the head or upper portion of a structure)

CHAPTER 2: BODY STRUCTURE

Section Review 2–1

Term	Meaning
1. dist/al	*-al: pertaining to; far, farthest*
2. poster/ior	-ior: pertaining to; back (of body), behind, posterior
3. hist/o/logist	-logist: specialist in study of; tissue
4. dors/al	-al: pertaining to; back (of body)
5. anter/ior	-ior: pertaining to; anterior, front
6. later/al	-al: pertaining to; side, to one side
7. medi/ad	-ad: toward; middle
8. chondr/oma	-oma: tumor
9. proxim/al	-al: pertaining to; near, nearest
10. ventr/al	-al: pertaining to; belly, belly side

Section Review 2–2

1. hist/o	4. proxim/o	7. ventr/o	10. caud/o	13. infer/o
2. -al, -ior	5. -logy	8. -toxic	11. -logist	14. -lysis
3. medi/o	6. cyt/o	9. -ad	12. dist/o	15. later/o

Section Review 2–3

Term	Meaning
1. ili/ac	*-ac: pertaining to; ilium (lateral, flaring portion of hip bone)*
2. abdomin/al	-al: pertaining to; abdomen
3. inguin/al	-al: pertaining to; groin
4. spin/al	-al: pertaining to; spine
5. peri/umbilic/al	-al: pertaining to; around; umbilicus, navel
6. cephal/ad	-ad: toward; head
7. gastr/ic	-ic: pertaining to; stomach
8. thorac/ic	-ic: pertaining to; chest
9. cervic/al	-al: pertaining to; neck, cervix uteri (neck of the uterus)
10. lumb/ar	-ar: pertaining to; loins (lower back)

Section Review 2–4

1. -ad	4. pelv/o	7. -ac, -al, -ic, -ior	10. hypo-	13. umbilic/o
2. inguin/o	5. chondr/o	8. lumb/o	11. crani/o	14. poster/o
3. gastr/o	6. epi-	9. thorac/o	12. spin/o	15. abdomin/o

Additional Medical Terms Review

1. CT	4. MRI	7. anastomosis	10. radiopharmaceutical	13. adhesion
2. fluoroscopy	5. C&S	8. inflammation	11. endoscopy	14. radiography
3. US	6. endoscope	9. tomography	12. cauterize	15. septicemia

Word Elements Chapter Review

Medical Term	Word Element	Meaning
1. anterior	*anter (WR)*	*anterior, front*
	-ior (S)	*pertaining to*
2. cephalad	cephal (WR)	head
	-ad (S)	toward
3. cervical	cervic (WR)	neck; cervix uteri (neck of uterus)
	-al (S)	pertaining to
4. chondroma	chondr/o (CF)	cartilage
	-oma (S)	tumor

Continued

Medical Term	Word Element	Meaning
5. craniometer	crani/o (CF)	cranium (skull)
	-meter (S)	instrument for measuring
6. cutaneous	cutane/o (WR)	skin
	-ous (S)	pertaining to
7. cytology	cyt/o (CF)	cell
	-logy (S)	study of
8. cytolysis	cyt/o (CF)	cell
	-lysis (S)	separation; destruction; loosening
9. distal	dist (WR)	far, farthest
	-al (S)	pertaining to
10. dorsal	dors (WR)	back (of body)
	-al (S)	pertaining to
11. endoscopy	endo- (PR)	in, within
	-scopy (S)	instrument for examining
12. epigastric	epi- (PR)	above, upon
	gastr (WR)	stomach
	-ic (S)	pertaining to
13. histologist	hist/o (CF)	tissue
	-logist (S)	specialist in the study of
14. hypochondriac	hypo- (P)	under, below, deficient
	chondr (WR)	cartilage
	-iac (S)	pertaining to
15. inferior	infer (WR)	lower, below
	-ior (S)	pertaining to
16. lumbar	lumb (WR)	loins (lower back)
	-ar (S)	pertaining to
17. periumbilical	peri- (PR)	around
	umbilic (WR)	umbilicus, navel
	-al (S)	pertaining to
18. proximal	proxim (WR)	near, nearest
	-al (S)	pertaining to
19. radiography	radi/o (CF)	radiation, x-ray, radius (lower arm bone on thumb side)
	-graphy (S)	process of recording
20. transverse	trans- (P)	across, through
	-verse (S)	to turn

CHAPTER 3: INTEGUMENTARY SYSTEM

Section Review 3–1

Term	Meaning
1. hypo/derm/ic	*-ic: pertaining to; under, below, deficient; skin*
2. melan/oma	-oma: tumor; black
3. kerat/osis	-osis: abnormal condition, increase (used primarily with blood cells); horny tissue; hard; cornea
4. cutane/ous	-ous: pertaining to; skin
5. lip/o/cyte	-cyte: cell; fat
6. onych/o/malacia	-malacia: softening; nail
7. scler/o/derma	-derma: skin; hardening; sclera (white of the eye)
8. dia/phoresis	-phoresis: carrying, transmission; through, across
9. dermat/o/myc/osis	-osis: abnormal condition, increase (used primarily with blood cells); skin; fungus
10. cry/o/therapy	-therapy: treatment; cold

Competency Verification, Figure 3–2

Identifying integumentary structures, page 69.

1. epidermis
2. dermis
3. stratum corneum
4. basal layer
5. hair follicle
6. sebaceous (oil) gland
7. sudoriferous (sweat) gland
8. subcutaneous tissue

Competency Verification, Figure 3–3

Structure of a fingernail, page 75.

1. nail root
2. matrix
3. cuticle
4. nail bed
5. nail body
6. lunula

Section Review 3–2

1. -pathy
2. xer/o
3. lip/o, adip/o, steat/o
4. -rrhea
5. trich/o, pil/o
6. scler/o
7. -cele
8. onych/o
9. derm/o, dermat/o, cutane/o, -derma
10. -malacia
11. -logist
12. epi-
13. -osis
14. hidr/o
15. hypo-

Section Review 3–3

1. melan/o
2. cyan/o
3. -emia
4. cyt/o, -cyte
5. -penia
6. -pathy
7. -rrhea
8. erythr/o
9. auto-
10. -derma
11. -oma
12. leuk/o
13. xanth/o
14. necr/o
15. -osis

Additional Medical Terms Review

1. verruca
2. vitiligo
3. tinea
4. furuncle
5. eczema
6. urticaria
7. biopsy
8. dermabrasion
9. fulguration
10. cryosurgery
11. débridement
12. scabies
13. alopecia
14. comedo
15. petechia

Medical Record Activity 3–1: Compound Nevus

Evaluation

1. What is a nevus?

   A mole; a type of skin tumor

2. Locate the vermilion border on your lip. Where is it located?

   It is the edge of the red portion of the upper or lower lip.

3. Was the lesion limited to a certain area?

   Yes, the right side of the lower lip

4. In the impression, the pathologist has ruled out melanoma. What does this mean?

   The nevus is not cancerous.

5. Is melanoma a dangerous condition? If so, explain why.

   Yes, it metastasizes rapidly.

Medical Record Activity 3–2: Psoriasis

Evaluation

1. What causes psoriasis?

   The etiology is unknown, but heredity is a significant determining factor.

2. On what parts of the body does psoriasis typically occur?

   Scalp, elbows, knees, sacrum, and around the nails, arms, legs, and abdomen

3. How is psoriasis treated?

   Mild to moderate psoriasis is treated with corticosteroids and phototherapy.

4. What is a histiocytoma?

   A tumor containing histiocytes, which are macrophages present in all loose connective tissue

Word Elements Chapter Review

Medical Term	Word Elements	Meaning
1. adipocele	*adip/o (CF)*	*fat*
	-cele (S)	*hernia, swelling*
2. anhidrosis	an- (P)	without, not
	hidr (WR)	sweat
	-osis (S)	abnormal condition; increase (used primarily with blood cells)
3. cryotherapy	cry/o (CF)	cold
	-therapy (S)	treatment
4. dermatomycosis	dermat/o (CF)	skin
	myc (WR)	fungus (plural, fungi)
	-osis (S)	abnormal condition; increase (used primarily with blood cells)

Medical Term	Word Elements	Meaning
5. diaphoresis	dia- (P)	through, across
	-phoresis (S)	carrying, transmission
6. epidermis	epi- (P)	above, upon
	derm (WR)	skin
	-is (S)	noun ending
7. erythrocyte	erythr/o (CF)	red
	-cyte (S)	cell
8. hidradenitis	hidr (WR)	sweat
	aden (WR)	gland
	-itis (S)	inflammation
9. hypodermic	hypo- (P)	under, below, deficient
	derm (WR)	skin
	-ic (S)	pertaining to
10. ichthyosis	ichthy (WR)	dry, scaly
	-osis (S)	abnormal condition; increase (used primarily with blood cells)
11. keratosis	kerat (WR)	horny tissue; hard; cornea
	-osis (S)	abnormal condition; increase (used primarily with blood cells)
12. lipocele	lip/o (CF)	fat
	-cele (S)	hernia, swelling
13. onychomalacia	onych/o (CF)	nail
	-malacia (S)	softening
14. pyoderma	py/o (CF)	pus
	-derma (S)	skin
15. scleroderma	scler/o (CF)	hardening; sclera (white of the eye)
	-derma (S)	skin
16. seborrhea	seb/o (CF)	sebum, sebaceous
	-rrhea (S)	discharge, flow
17. subcutaneous	sub- (P)	under, below
	cutane (WR)	skin
	-ous (S)	pertaining to
18. trichopathy	trich/o (CF)	hair
	-pathy (S)	disease
19. xanthoma	xanth (WR)	yellow
	-oma (S)	tumor
20. xeroderma	xer/o (CF)	dry
	-derma (S)	skin

Vocabulary Review

1. subcutaneous
2. diaphoresis
3. trichopathy
4. autograft
5. Kaposi sarcoma
6. suction lipectomy
7. onychomycosis
8. pressure ulcers
9. leukemia
10. ecchymosis
11. onychoma
12. hirsutism
13. pustule
14. papules
15. erythrocyte
16. xeroderma
17. melanoma
18. lipocele
19. xanthoma
20. onychomalacia

CHAPTER 4: RESPIRATORY SYSTEM

Section Review 4–1

Term	Meaning
1. laryng/o/scope	-scope: instrument for examining; larynx (voice box)
2. py/o/thorax	-thorax: chest; pus
3. hyp/oxia	-oxia: oxygen; under, below, deficient
4. trache/o/stomy	-stomy: forming an opening (mouth); trachea (windpipe)
5. a/pnea	-pnea: breathing; without, not
6. pulmon/o/logist	-logist: specialist in the study of; lung
7. pneumon/ia	-ia: condition; air; lung
8. rhin/o/rrhea	-rrhea: discharge, flow; nose
9. an/osmia	-osmia: smell; without, not
10. pneum/ectomy	-ectomy: excision, removal; air; lung

Section Review 4–2

1. aer/o
2. para-
3. myc/o
4. -ectasis
5. -stomy
6. -tomy
7. -tome
8. laryng/o
9. -cele
10. neo-
11. nas/o, rhin/o
12. -plegia
13. pharyng/o
14. -stenosis
15. -phagia
16. trache/o
17. -therapy
18. a-, an-
19. -scopy
20. hydr/o

Competency Verification, Figure 4–2

Identifying upper and lower respiratory tracts, page 113.

1. nasal cavity
2. pharynx (throat)
3. larynx (voice box)
4. epiglottis
5. trachea (windpipe)
6. right and left primary bronchi
7. bronchioles
8. left lung
9. alveoli
10. pulmonary capillaries
11. pleura
12. diaphragm

Section Review 4–3

1. -osis
2. brady-
3. dys-
4. melan/o
5. -pnea
6. bronch/o, bronchi/o
7. hem/o
8. thorac/o
9. -ectasis
10. -phobia
11. myc/o
12. eu-
13. -cele
14. -scope
15. -spasm
16. macro-
17. tachy-
18. pneum/o, pneumon/o
19. pleur/o
20. micro-
21. orth/o
22. -stenosis
23. -centesis
24. a-
25. chondr/o

Additional Medical Terms Review

1. stridor	5. coryza	9. pneumothorax	13. MRI	17. hypoxemia
2. epistaxis	6. cystic fibrosis	10. rales	14. atelectasis	18. SIDS
3. influenza	7. lung cancer	11. bronchodilators	15. epiglottitis	19. hypoxia
4. acidosis	8. pleural effusion	12. ARDS	16. pertussis	20. rhonchi

Medical Record Activity 4–1: Papillary Carcinoma

Evaluation

1. What types of patients are at risk for nasal polyps?

   Patients with chronic inflammation of the nasal cavity and sinus mucosa that is usually due to allergies

2. When is a polypectomy indicated?

   When the patient fails to respond to medical treatment or if there is severe nasal obstruction

3. Were the patient's nasal polyps cancerous?

   No, polyps are benign

4. What contributed to the patient's death?

   Papillary carcinoma that metastasized to the lymph node

5. Why was a biopsy of the liver performed?

   Enlarged liver nodes; to check for metastasis

6. What does "patient expired at home" mean?

   Patient died at home

Medical Record Activity 4–2: Bronchoscopy

Evaluation

1. What does "bronchoscope was inserted transnasally" mean?

   It was inserted through the nose.

2. What was seen in the left lower bronchus?

   Endobronchial friable mucosal lesion, partially occluding the entire left lower lobe bronchus

3. What kinds of biopsies were obtained during the bronchoscopy?

   Transbronchial biopsies of the left lower lung area, transbronchial needle aspiration, bronchial brush biopsies, and bronchial brush washings

4. What type of radiographic procedure was used to enhance visualization to obtain biopsies for cytology evaluation?

   Fluoroscopic

5. What condition results from the bacterium *Legionella*?

   Legionnaire disease

Word Elements Chapter Review

Medical Term	Word Elements	Meaning
1. anoxia	*an- (P)*	*without, not*
	-oxia (S)	*oxygen*
2. apnea	a- (P)	without, not
	-pnea (S)	breathing
3. atelectasis	atel (WR)	incomplete; imperfect
	-ectasis (S)	dilation, expansion
4. bronchiole	bronch/i* (CF)	bronchus (plural, bronchi)
	-ole (S)	small, minute
5. bronchoscopy	bronch/o (CF)	bronchus (plural, bronchi)
	-scopy (S)	visual examination
6. cyanosis	cyan (WR)	blue
	-osis (S)	abnormal condition; increase (used primarily with blood cells)
7. endotracheal	endo- (P)	in, within
	trache (WR)	trachea
	-al (S)	pertaining to
8. epiglottitis	epiglott (WR)	epiglottis
	-itis (S)	inflammation
9. hypoxemia	hyp- (P)	under, below, deficient
	ox (WR)	oxygen
	-emia (S)	blood
10. laryngoscope	laryng/o (WR)	larynx
	-scope (S)	instrument for examining
11. pleurodynia	pleur/o (CF)	pleura
	-dynia (S)	pain
12. pneumectomy	pneum (WR)	air; lung
	-ectomy (S)	excision, removal
13. pneumothorax	pneum/o (CF)	air; lung
	-thorax (S)	chest
14. pulmonologist	pulmon/o (CF)	lung
	-logist (S)	specialist in the study of
15. polysomnography	poly- (P)	many, much
	somn/o (CF)	sleep
	-graphy (S)	instrument for recording
16. pyothorax	py/o (CF)	pus
	-thorax (S)	chest

Medical Term	Word Elements	Meaning
17. rhinorrhea	rhin/o (CF)	nose
	-rrhea (S)	discharge, flow
18. spirometry	spir/o (CF)	to breathe
	-metry (S)	act of measuring
19. thoracopathy	thorac/o (CF)	chest
	-pathy (S)	disease
20. tracheostomy	trache/o (CF)	trachea
	-stomy (S)	forming an opening (mouth)

*The *i* in *bronch/i* in the term *bronchiole* is an exception to the rule of using the connecting vowel *o*.

Vocabulary Review

1. pyothorax	6. diagnosis	11. atelectasis	16. catheter
2. thoracentesis	7. apnea	12. anosmia	17. rhinoplasty
3. asthma	8. aerophagia	13. pharyngoplegia	18. TB
4. croup	9. aspirate	14. pleurisy	19. COPD
5. tracheostomy	10. chondroma	15. *Pneumocystis*	20. pneumothorax

CHAPTER 5: CARDIOVASCULAR AND LYMPHATIC SYSTEMS

Section Review 5–1

Term	Meaning
1. endo/cardi/um	-um: *structure, thing; in, within; heart*
2. cardi/o/megaly	-megaly: enlargement; heart
3. aort/o/stenosis	-stenosis: narrowing, stricture; aorta
4. tachy/cardia	-cardia: heart condition; rapid
5. phleb/itis	-itis: inflammation; vein
6. thromb/o/lysis	-lysis: separation; destruction; loosening; blood clot
7. vas/o/spasm	-spasm: involuntary contraction, twitching; vessel; vas deferens; duct
8. ather/oma	-oma: tumor; fatty plaque
9. electr/o/cardi/o/graphy	-graphy: process of recording; electricity; heart
10. atri/o/ventricul/ar	-ar: pertaining to; atrium; ventricle (of the heart or brain)

Competency Verification, Figure 5–2

Heart structures, page 161.

1. endocardium
2. myocardium
3. pericardium
4. aorta
5. right atrium
6. superior vena cava
7. inferior vena cava
8. pulmonary trunk
9. right lung
10. left lung
11. left atrium
12. right pulmonary veins
13. left pulmonary veins

Competency Verification, Figure 5–3

Internal structures of the heart, page 163.

1. right atrium (RA)
2. left atrium (LA)
3. right ventricle (RV)
4. left ventricle (LV)
5. interventricular septum (IVS)
6. superior vena cava (SVC)
7. inferior vena cava (IVC)
8. tricuspid valve
9. pulmonary valve
10. right pulmonary artery
11. left pulmonary artery
12. right pulmonary veins
13. left pulmonary veins
14. mitral valve
15. aortic valve
16. aorta
17. branches of the aorta
18. descending aorta

Competency Verification, Figure 5–5

Heart structures depicting valves and cusps, page 172.

1. tricuspid valve
2. mitral valve
3. chordae tendineae
4. pulmonary valve
5. aortic valve
6. three cusps
7. two cusps

Section Review 5–2

1. -osis
2. epi-
3. aort/o
4. peri-
5. arteri/o
6. atri/o
7. hem/o, hemat/o
8. -pnea
9. -pathy
10. -ectasis
11. scler/o
12. cardi/o
13. -spasm
14. my/o
15. tachy-
16. -rrhexis
17. brady-
18. -ole, -ule
19. -rrhaphy
20. -stenosis
21. -phagia
22. tri-
23. bi-
24. phleb/o, ven/o
25. ventricul/o

Competency Verification, Figure 5–6

Conduction pathway of the heart, page 175.

1. sinoatrial (SA) node
2. right atrium (RA)
3. atrioventricular (AV) node
4. bundle of His
5. bundle branches
6. Purkinje fibers

Section Review 5–3

Term	Meaning
1. agglutin/ation	*-ation: process (of); clumping, gluing*
2. thym/oma	-oma: tumor; thymus gland
3. phag/o/cyte	-cyte: cell; swallowing, eating
4. lymphaden/itis	-itis: inflammation; lymph gland (node)
5. splen/o/megaly	-megaly: enlargement; spleen
6. aden/o/pathy	-pathy: disease; gland
7. ana/phylaxis	-phylaxis: protection; against; up; back
8. lymphangi/oma	oma: tumor; lymph vessel
9. lymph/o/poiesis	-poiesis: formation, production; lymph
10. immun/o/gen	-gen: forming, producing, origin; immune, immunity, safe

Competency Verification, Figure 5–10

Lymphatic system, page 185.

1. lymph capillaries
2. lymph vessels
3. thoracic duct
4. right lymphatic duct
5. cervical nodes
6. axillary nodes
7. inguinal nodes
8. tonsil
9. spleen
10. thymus

Section Review 5–4

1. aort/o
2. hem/o
3. thromb/o
4. -cyte
5. cerebr/o
6. necr/o
7. -pathy
8. electr/o
9. -megaly
10. cardi/o
11. lymph/o
12. my/o
13. -graphy
14. -gram
15. -al, -ic
16. -rrhexis
17. -lysis
18. -stenosis
19. -plasty
20. angi/o

Additional Medical Terms Review

1. varicose veins
2. mononucleosis
3. thrombolytics
4. embolus
5. lymphadenitis
6. DVT
7. hypertension
8. arrhythmia
9. statins
10. bruit
11. Doppler US
12. rheumatic heart disease
13. atherosclerosis
14. Holter monitor
15. Raynaud phenomenon
16. ischemia
17. Hodgkin disease
18. AIDS
19. HF
20. fibrillation
21. valvuloplasty
22. lymphangiography
23. tissue typing
24. troponin I
25. CABG

Medical Record Activity 5–1: Myocardial Infarction

Evaluation

1. What symptoms did the patient experience before admission to the hospital?

    Generalized malaise, increased shortness of breath (SOB) while at rest, and dyspnea followed by periods of apnea and syncope

2. What was found during clinical examination?

    Irregular radial pulse, uncontrolled atrial fibrillation with evidence of a recent myocardial infarction (MI)

3. What is the danger of atrial fibrillation?

   A decrease in cardiac output and promotion of thrombus formation in the upper chambers, syncope, angina, palpitations, and HF

4. Did the patient have a prior history of heart problems? If so, describe them.

   Yes, sinus tachycardia attributed to preoperative anxiety and thyroiditis

5. Was the patient's prior heart problem related to her current one?

   No

Medical Record Activity 5–2: Cardiac Catheterization

Evaluation

1. What coronary arteries were under examination?

   The left and right coronary arteries

2. Which surgical procedure was used to clear the stenosis?

   Balloon angioplasty

3. What symptoms did the patient exhibit before balloon inflation?

   The patient had significant ST elevations in the inferior leads and severe throat tightness and shortness of breath.

4. Why was the patient put on heparin?

   To prevent postsurgical clots from forming

Word Elements Chapter Review

Medical Term	Word Elements	Meaning
1. agglutin/ation	*agglutin (WR)*	*clumping, gluing*
	-ation (S)	*process of*
2. ana/phylaxis	ana- (P)	against; up; back
	-phylaxis (S)	protection
3. aneurysm/o/rrhaphy	aneurysm/o (CF)	widening, widened blood vessel
	-rrhaphy (S)	suture
4. a/rrhythm/ia	a- (P)	without, not
	rrhythm (WR)	rhythm
	-ia (S)	condition
5. arteri/o/scler/osis	arteri/o (CF)	artery
	scler (WR)	hardening, sclera (white of the eye)
	-osis (S)	abnormal condition; increase (used primarily with blood cells)
6. ather/oma	ather (WR)	fatty plaque
	-oma (S)	tumor
7. atri/o/ventricul/ar	atri/o (CF)	atrium
	ventricul (WR)	ventricle (of the heart or brain)
	-ar (S)	pertaining to

Medical Term	Word Elements	Meaning
8. echo/cardi/o/graphy	echo- (P)	a repeated sound
	cardi/o (CF)	heart
	-graphy (S)	process of recording
9. electr/o/cardi/o/gram	electr/o (CF)	electricity
	cardi/o (CF)	heart
	-gram (S)	record, writing
10. embol/us	embol (WR)	embolus (plug)
	-us (S)	condition; structure
11. hem/o/rrhage	hem/o (CF)	blood
	-rrhage	bursting forth (of)
12. hyper/tension	hyper- (P)	excessive, above normal
	-tension (S)	to stretch
13. immun/o/gen	immun/o (CF)	immune, immunity, safe
	-gen (S)	forming, producing, origin
14. isch/emia	isch (WR)	to hold back; block
	-emia (S)	blood
15. lymph/aden/itis	lymph (WR)	lymph
	aden (WR)	gland
	-itis (S)	inflammation
16. lymph/angi/oma	lymph (WR)	lymph
	angi (WR)	vessel (usually blood or lymph)
	-oma (S)	tumor
17. phag/o/cyte	phag/o (CF)	swallowing, eating
	-cyte (S)	cell
18. phleb/o/stenosis	phleb/o	vein
	-stenosis	narrowing, stricture
19. splen/o/megaly	splen/o (CF)	spleen
	-megaly (S)	enlargement
20. tachy/cardia	tachy- (P)	rapid
	-cardia (S)	heart condition
21. thromb/o/genesis	thromb/o (CF)	blood clot
	-genesis (S)	forming, producing, origin
22. thyroid/ectomy	thyroid (WR)	thyroid gland
	-ectomy (S)	excision, removal
23. ultra/son/o/graphy	ultra- (P)	excess, beyond
	son/o (CF)	sound
	-graphy (S)	process of recording

Continued

Medical Term	Word Elements	Meaning
24. valv/o/tomy	valv/o (CF)	valve
	-tomy (S)	incision
25. varic/ose	varic (WR)	dilated vein
	-ose (S)	pertaining to; sugar

Vocabulary Review

1. myocardium
2. tachypnea
3. arteriosclerosis
4. phagocyte
5. systole
6. diastole
7. ECG
8. malaise
9. desiccated
10. cardiomegaly
11. aneurysm
12. angina pectoris
13. MI
14. agglutination
15. statins
16. anaphylaxis
17. capillaries
18. hemangioma
19. arterioles
20. pacemaker

CHAPTER 6: DIGESTIVE SYSTEM

Section Review 6–1

Term	Meaning
1. gingiv/itis	-itis: inflammation; gum(s)
2. dys/pepsia	-pepsia: digestion; bad, painful, difficult
3. pylor/o/tomy	-tomy: incision; pylorus
4. dent/ist	-ist: specialist; teeth
5. esophag/o/scope	-scope: instrument for examining; esophagus
6. gastr/o/scopy	-scopy: visual examination; stomach
7. dia/rrhea	-rrhea: discharge, flow; through, across
8. hyper/emesis	-emesis: vomiting; excessive, above normal
9. an/orexia	-orexia: appetite; without, not
10. sub/lingu/al	-al: pertaining to; under, below; tongue

Competency Verification, Figure 6–2

Oral cavity, esophagus, pharynx, and stomach, page 223.

1. oral cavity
2. sublingual gland
3. submandibular gland
4. parotid gland
5. bolus
6. pharynx (throat)
7. esophagus
8. stomach

Section Review 6–2

1. -oma
2. -al, -ary, -ic
3. peri-
4. hypo-
5. -rrhea
6. myc/o
7. gingiv/o
8. pylor/o
9. dys-
10. hyper-
11. sial/o
12. gastr/o
13. -ist
14. orth/o
15. dent/o, odont/o
16. dia-
17. lingu/o, gloss/o
18. -scope
19. -tomy
20. -orexia
21. stomat/o, or/o
22. -algia, -dynia
23. -phagia
24. an-
25. -pepsia

Section Review 6–3

Term	Meaning
1. duoden/o/scopy	*-scopy: visual examination; duodenum (first part of the small intestine)*
2. appendic/itis	-itis: inflammation; appendix
3. enter/o/pathy	-pathy: disease; intestine (usually small intestine)
4. col/o/stomy	-stomy: forming an opening (mouth); colon
5. rect/o/cele	-cele: hernia, swelling; rectum
6. sigmoid/o/tomy	-tomy: incision; sigmoid colon
7. proct/o/logist	-logist: specialist in the study of; anus, rectum
8. jejun/o/rrhaphy	-rrhaphy: suture; jejunum (second part of the small intestine)
9. append/ectomy	-ectomy: excision, removal; appendix
10. ile/o/stomy	-stomy: forming an opening (mouth); ileum (third part of the small intestine)

Competency Verification, Figure 6–3

Small intestine and colon, page 235.

1. duodenum	4. ascending colon	7. sigmoid colon
2. jejunum	5. transverse colon	8. rectum
3. ileum	6. descending colon	9. anus

Section Review 6–4

1. enter/o	4. -spasm	7. jejun/o	10. -stomy	13. -rrhaphy
2. -tome	5. ile/o	8. col/o, colon/o	11. proct/o	14. -tomy
3. rect/o	6. -scopy	9. duoden/o	12. -stenosis	15. sigmoid/o

Section Review 6–5

Term	Meaning
1. hepat/itis	*-itis: inflammation; liver*
2. hepat/o/megaly	-megaly: enlargement; liver
3. chol/e/lith	-lith: stone, calculus; bile, gall
4. cholangi/ole	-ole: small, minute; bile vessel
5. cholecyst/ectomy	-ectomy: excision, removal; gallbladder
6. post/prandial	-prandial: meal; after, behind
7. chol/e/lith/iasis	-iasis: abnormal condition (produced by something specified); bile, gall; stone, calculus
8. choledoch/o/tomy	-tomy: incision; bile duct
9. pancreat/o/lith	-lith: stone, calculus; pancreas
10. pancreat/itis	-itis: inflammation; pancreas

Competency Verification, Figure 6–6

Liver, gallbladder, pancreas, and duodenum with associated ducts and blood vessels, page 247.

1. liver
2. gallbladder
3. pancreas
4. duodenum
5. common bile duct

6. right hepatic duct
7. left hepatic duct
8. hepatic duct
9. cystic duct
10. pancreatic duct

Section Review 6–6

1. -oma
2. -iasis
3. choledoch/o
4. chol/e

5. cyst/o
6. -megaly
7. -ectomy
8. -stomy

9. cholecyst/o
10. therm/o
11. hepat/o
12. -algia, -dynia

13. pancreat/o
14. toxic/o, tox/o, -toxic
15. -graphy
16. -gram

17. -lith
18. -plasty
19. -rrhaphy
20. -emesis

Additional Medical Terms Review

1. hemoccult
2. NG intubation
3. polyp

4. ascites
5. Crohn disease
6. lithotripsy

7. fistula
8. jaundice
9. barium enema

10. IBD
11. hematochezia
12. volvulus

13. cirrhosis
14. barium swallow
15. IBS

Medical Record Activity 6–1: Rectal Bleeding

Evaluation

1. What is the patient's symptom that made him seek medical help?

   Weight loss of 40 pounds since his last examination

2. What surgical procedures were performed on the patient for regional enteritis?

   Ileostomy and appendectomy

3. What abnormality was found with the sigmoidoscopy?

   Dark blood and rectal bleeding

4. What is causing the rectal bleeding?

   It could be due to a polyp, bleeding, diverticulum, or rectal carcinoma.

5. Write the plural form of *diverticulum.*

   Diverticula

Medical Record Activity 6–2: Carcinosarcoma of the Esophagus

Evaluation

1. What surgery was performed on this patient?

   Resection of the esophagus with anastomosis of the stomach; mediastinal lymph node excision

2. What diagnostic testing confirmed malignancy?

   Pathology tests on the biopsy specimen from esophagoscopy

3. Where was the carcinosarcoma located?

   Middle third of the esophagus

4. Why was the adjacent lymph node excised?

   Metastasis was suspected.

Word Elements Chapter Review

Medical Term	Word Elements	Meaning
1. anorexia	*an- (P)*	*without, not*
	-orexia (S)	*appetite*
2. appendicitis	appendic (WR)	appendix
	-itis (S)	inflammation
3. cholangiography	cholangi/o (CF)	bile vessel
	-graphy (S)	process of recording
4. cholecystectomy	cholecyst (WR)	gallbladder
	-ectomy (S)	excision, removal
5. choledochotomy	choledoch/o (CF)	bile duct
	-tomy (S)	incision
6. cirrhosis	cirrh (WR)	yellow
	-osis (S)	abnormal condition; increase (used primarily with blood cells)
7. colonoscopy	colon/o (CF)	colon
	-scopy (S)	visual examination
8. colostomy	col/o (CF)	colon
	-stomy (S)	forming an opening (mouth)
9. duodenorrhaphy	duoden/o (CF)	duodenum
	-rrhaphy (S)	suture
10. enteropathy	enter/o (CF)	intestine (usually small intestine)
	-pathy (S)	disease
11. gastroenterologist	gastr/o (CF)	stomach
	enter/o (CF)	intestine (usually small intestine)
	-logist (S)	specialist in the study of
12. gingivitis	gingiv (WR)	gum(s)
	-itis (S)	inflammation
13. hematemesis	hemat (WR)	blood
	-emesis (S)	vomiting
14. hepatomegaly	hepat/o (CF)	liver
	-megaly (S)	enlargement
15. ileostomy	ile/o (CF)	ileum
	-stomy (S)	forming an opening (mouth)
16. jejunorrhaphy	jejun/o (CF)	jejunum
	-rrhaphy (S)	suture

Continued

Medical Term	Word Elements	Meaning
17. lithotripsy	lith/o (CF)	stone, calculus
	-tripsy (S)	crushing
18. pancreatolysis	pancreat/o (CF)	pancreas
	-lysis (S)	separation; destruction; loosening
19. peritonitis	periton (WR)	peritoneum
	-itis (S)	inflammation
20. postprandial	post- (P)	after, behind
	-prandial	meal
21. proctologist	proct/o (CF)	anus, rectum
	-logist (S)	specialist in the study of
22. rectostenosis	rect/o (CF)	rectum
	-stenosis (S)	narrowing, stricture
23. sigmoidotomy	sigmoid/o (CF)	sigmoid colon
	-tomy (S)	incision
24. sublingual	sub- (P)	under, below
	lingu (WR)	tongue
	-al (S)	pertaining to
25. toxicology	toxic/o (CF)	poison
	-logy (S)	study of

Vocabulary Review

1. gastroscopy
2. dyspepsia
3. hematemesis
4. ultrasound
5. antiemetics

6. celiac disease
7. stomatalgia
8. duodenotomy
9. hepatomegaly
10. dysphagia

11. cholecystectomy
12. anastomosis
13. sigmoidotomy
14. rectoplasty
15. GERD

16. ileostomy
17. cholelithiasis
18. friable
19. peritonitis
20. bariatric

CHAPTER 7: URINARY SYSTEM

Section Review 7–1

Term	Meaning
1. glomerul/o/scler/osis	-osis: abnormal condition, increase (used primarily with blood cells); glomerulus; hardening; sclera (white of the eye)
2. cyst/o/scopy	-scopy: visual examination; bladder
3. poly/uria	-uria: urine; many, much
4. lith/o/tripsy	-tripsy: crushing; stone, calculus
5. dia/lysis	-lysis: separation; destruction; loosening; through, across
6. ureter/o/stenosis	-stenosis: narrowing, stricture; ureter

Term	Meaning
7. meat/us	-us: condition, structure; opening, meatus
8. ur/emia	-emia: blood condition; urine
9. nephr/oma	-oma: tumor; kidney
10. azot/emia	-emia: blood; nitrogenous compounds

Section Review 7–2

1. -osis
2. -iasis
3. supra-
4. -pathy
5. -megaly
6. dia-
7. -pexy
8. scler/o
9. -tome
10. -tomy
11. nephr/o, ren/o
12. -ptosis
13. lith/o
14. -rrhaphy
15. poly-

Competency Verification, Figure 7–2

Urinary structures, page 283.

1. right kidney
2. renal cortex
3. renal medulla
4. renal artery
5. renal vein
6. nephron
7. ureters
8. urinary bladder
9. urethra
10. urinary meatus

Section Review 7–3

1. -iasis
2. cyst/o, vesic/o
3. carcin/o
4. -pathy
5. -megaly
6. -ectomy
7. -ectasis
8. aden/o
9. -tomy
10. -itis
11. -scope
12. enter/o
13. pyel/o
14. rect/o
15. -lith
16. -plasty
17. -rrhaphy
18. -oma
19. ureter/o
20. urethr/o

Competency Verification, Figure 7–7

Structure of a nephron, page 297.

1. renal cortex
2. renal medulla
3. glomerular capsule
4. glomerulus
5. renal tubule
6. collecting tubule

Section Review 7–4

1. cyst/o, vesic/o
2. hemat/o
3. -logist
4. glomerul/o
5. scler/o
6. -ist
7. nephr/o, ren/o
8. py/o
9. azot/o
10. pyel/o
11. olig/o
12. ureter/o
13. urethr/o
14. ur/o
15. noct/o
16. -cele
17. poly-
18. -ptosis
19. intra-
20. a-, an-

Additional Medical Terms Review

1. urinalysis
2. Wilms tumor
3. azoturia
4. US
5. diuresis
6. retrograde pyelography
7. hypospadias
8. interstitial nephritis
9. BUN
10. enuresis
11. catheterization
12. VCUG
13. uremia
14. renal hypertension
15. dialysis

Medical Record Activity 7–1: Cystitis

Evaluation

1. What was found when the patient had a cystoscopy?

   Cystitis

2. What are the symptoms of cystitis?

   Nocturia, urinary frequency, pelvic pain, and hematuria, in this case

3. What is the patient's past surgical history?

   Cholecystectomy, choledocholithotomy, and incidental appendectomy

4. What is the treatment for cystitis?

   Antibiotics and consumption of a lot of fluids

5. What are the dangers of untreated cystitis?

   The spreading of infection to the kidneys or to the bloodstream (sepsis)

6. What instrument is used to perform a cystoscopy?

   A cystoscope

Medical Record Activity 7–2: Dysuria with Benign Prostatic Hypertrophy

Evaluation

1. What prompted the consultation with the urologist, Dr. Mori?

   Preoperative catheterization was not possible.

2. What abnormality did the urologist discover?

   Mild to moderate benign prostatic hypertrophy

3. Did the patient have any previous surgery on his prostate?

   No

4. Where was the patient's hernia?

   In the groin and scrotum (hydrocele)

5. What in the patient's past medical history contributed to his present urological problem?

   Nothing in his past history contributed to his benign prostatic hypertrophy; he had a previous colon resection for carcinoma of the colon.

Word Elements Chapter Review

Medical Term	Word Elements	Meaning
1. anuria	*an- (P)*	*without, not*
	-uria (S)	*urine*
2. azotemia	azot/o (CF)	nitrogenous compounds
	-emia (S)	blood condition
3. dialysis	dia- (P)	through, across
	-lysis (S)	separation; destruction; loosening
4. dysuria	dys- (P)	bad; painful; difficult
	-uria (S)	urine
5. glomeropathy	glomerul/o (CF)	glomerulus
	-pathy (S)	disease
6. hypertension	hyper- (P)	excessive, above normal
	-tension (S)	to stretch
7. hypospadias	hypo- (P)	under, below, deficient
	-spadias (S)	slit, fissure
8. lithotripsy	lith/o (CF)	stone, calculus
	-tripsy (S)	crushing
9. meatus	meat (WR)	opening, meatus
	-us (S)	condition, structure
10. nephralgia	nephr (WR)	kidney
	-algia (S)	pain
11. nephrolithotomy	nephr/o (CF)	kidney
	lith/o (CF)	stone, calculus
	-tomy (S)	incision
12. nephromegaly	nephr/o (CF)	kidney
	-megaly (S)	enlargement
13. nephropexy	nephr/o (CF)	kidney
	-pexy (S)	fixation (of an organ)
14. nephroptosis	nephr/o (CF)	kidney
	-ptosis (S)	prolapse, downward displacement
15. nocturia	noct (WR)	night
	-uria (S)	urine
16. polyuria	poly- (P)	many, much
	-uria (S)	urine

Continued

Medical Term	Word Elements	Meaning
17. pyeloplasty	pyel/o (CF)	renal pelvis
	-plasty (S)	surgical repair
18. pyelostomy	pyel/o (CF)	renal pelvis
	-stomy (S)	forming an opening (mouth)
19. suprarenal	supra- (P)	above; excessive; superior
	ren (WR)	kidney
	-al (S)	pertaining to
20. ureterolithiasis	ureter/o (CF)	ureter
	lith (WR)	stone, calculus
	-iasis (S)	abnormal condition (produced by something specified)
21. ureterocystoscopy	ureter/o (CF)	ureter
	cyst/o (CF)	bladder
	-scopy (S)	visual examination
22. urography	ur/o (CF)	urine, urinary tract
	-graphy (S)	process of recording
23. urethrocele	urethr/o (CF)	urethra
	-cele (S)	hernia, swelling
24. urologist	ur/o (CF)	urine
	-logist (S)	specialist
25. vesicocele	vesic/o (CF)	bladder
	-cele (S)	hernia, swelling

Vocabulary Review

1. malignant
2. nephrons
3. cholelithiasis
4. renal pelvis
5. IVP
6. diuretics
7. edema
8. benign
9. nephrolithotomy
10. acute renal failure
11. nephroptosis
12. ureteropyeloplasty
13. bilateral
14. nocturia
15. urinary incontinence
16. hematuria
17. polyuria
18. oliguria
19. anuria
20. cystocele

CHAPTER 8: REPRODUCTIVE SYSTEMS

Section Review 8–1

Term	Definition
1. primi/gravida	*-gravida: pregnant woman; first*
2. colp/o/scopy	-scopy: visual examination; vagina
3. gynec/o/logist	-logist: specialist in the study of; woman, female
4. perine/o/rrhaphy	-rrhaphy: suture; perineum
5. hyster/ectomy	-ectomy: excision, removal; uterus (womb)
6. oophor/oma	-oma: tumor; ovary
7. dys/tocia	-tocia: childbirth, labor; bad, painful, difficult
8. endo/metr/itis	-itis: inflammation; in, within; uterus (womb); measure
9. mamm/o/gram	-gram: record, writing; breast
10. amni/o/centesis	-centesis: surgical puncture; amnion (amniotic sac)

Section Review 8–2

1. cyst/o
2. hemat/o, hem/o
3. -rrhage, -rrhagia
4. hyster/o, uter/o, metr/o

5. -cele
6. -tomy
7. -tome
8. -scope

9. salping/o, -salpinx
10. -pexy
11. muc/o
12. oophor/o, ovari/o

13. -arche
14. metr/o
15. -ptosis
16. -oid

17. -logist
18. -logy
19. -plasty
20. colp/o, vagin/o

Competency Verification, Figures 8–2 and 8–3

Lateral view of the female reproductive system, page 335.

1. ovary (singular)
2. fallopian tube (singular)
3. uterus

4. vagina
5. labia majora
6. labia minora

7. clitoris
8. Bartholin gland
9. cervix

Anterior view of the female reproductive system, page 335.

1. ovary (singular)
2. fallopian tube (singular)
3. uterus

4. vagina
5. labia majora (Shown in lateral view only.)
6. labia minora (Shown in lateral view only.)

7. clitoris (Shown in lateral view only.)
8. Bartholin gland
9. cervix

Competency Verification, Figure 8–7

Structure of mammary glands, page 349.

1. adipose tissue
2. glandular tissue

3. lobe
4. lactiferous duct

5. nipple
6. areola

Section Review 8–3

1. post-
2. gynec/o
3. pre-
4. mamm/o, mast/o

5. -pathy
6. -ectomy
7. -rrhea
8. -itis

9. -tome
10. -scope
11. -scopy
12. men/o

13. cervic/o
14. -algia, -dynia
15. -ary, -ous
16. -logist

17. salping/o
18. colp/o, vagin/o
19. vulv/o, episi/o
20. dys-

Section Review 8–4

Term	Meaning
1. vas/ectomy	-ectomy: excision, removal; vessel; vas deferens; duct
2. balan/itis	-itis: inflammation; glans penis
3. spermi/cide	-cide: killing; spermatozoa, sperm cells
4. gonad/o/tropin	-tropin: stimulate; gonads, sex glands
5. orchi/o/pexy	-pexy: fixation (of an organ); testis (plural, testes)
6. a/sperm/ia	-ia: condition; without, not; spermatozoa, sperm cells
7. vesicul/itis	-itis: inflammation; seminal vesicle
8. orchid/ectomy	-ectomy: excision, removal; testis (plural, testes)
9. andr/o/gen	-gen: forming, producing, origin; male
10. crypt/orch/ism	-ism: condition; hidden; testis (plural, testes)

Competency Verification, Figure 8–10

Lateral view of the male reproductive system, page 357.

1. testis (singular) or testicle (singular)
2. scrotum
3. epididymis
4. vas deferens
5. seminal vesicle
6. prostate gland
7. bulbourethral gland
8. penis
9. glans penis
10. foreskin

Section Review 8–5

1. -rrhaphy
2. dys-
3. cyst/o
4. carcin/o
5. -cyte
6. -pathy
7. -megaly
8. -cele
9. -itis
10. -tome
11. vas/o
12. muc/o
13. neo-
14. -genesis
15. prostat/o
16. test/o, orchi/o, orchid/o
17. olig/o
18. spermat/o, sperm/o
19. -pexy
20. hyper-

Additional Medical Terms Review

1. cryptorchidism
2. fibroid
3. sterility
4. anorchism
5. candidiasis
6. chlamydia
7. circumcision
8. cerclage
9. leukorrhea
10. endometriosis
11. mammography
12. gonorrhea
13. syphilis
14. toxic shock
15. trichomoniasis
16. D&C
17. phimosis
18. impotence
19. oligomenorrhea
20. gonadotropins

Medical Record Activity 8–1: Postmenopausal Bleeding

Evaluation

1. How many times has the patient been pregnant? How many children has the patient given birth to?

   Four; four

2. Why is the patient being admitted to the hospital?

   To have a gynecological laparoscopy and diagnostic D&C to rule out the neoplastic process

3. What is a D&C?

   Dilatation and curettage; a surgical procedure that expands the cervical canal of the uterus so that the surface lining of the uterine wall can be scraped

4. What is the patient's past surgical history?

Simple mastectomy a year ago

5. At what sites did the patient have malignant growth?

Left breast with metastases to the axilla, liver, and bone

Medical Record Activity 8–2: Bilateral Vasectomy

Evaluation

1. What is the end result of a bilateral vasectomy?

Sterilization

2. Was the patient awake during the surgery? What type of anesthesia was used?

Yes; 1% Xylocaine

3. What was used to prevent bleeding?

Hemostats, cautery, and sutures

4. What type of suture material was used to close the incision?

2-0 chromic

5. What was the patient given for pain relief at home?

Darvocet-N 100

6. Why is it important for the patient to go for a follow-up visit?

To analyze his semen and confirm sterilization

Word Elements Chapter Review

Medical Term	Word Elements	Meaning
1. hyster/ectomy	hyster (WR)	uterus (womb)
	-ectomy (S)	excision, removal
2. amni/o/centesis	amni/o (CF)	amnion (amniotic sac)
	-centesis (S)	surgical puncture
3. andr/o/gen	andr/o (CF)	male
	-gen (S)	forming, producing, origin
4. balan/itis	balan (WR)	glans penis
	-itis (S)	inflammation
5. dys/tocia	dys- (P)	bad; painful; difficult
	-tocia (S)	childbirth, labor
6. episi/o/tomy	episi/o (CF)	vulva
	-tomy (S)	incision
7. galact/o/rrhea	galact/o (CF)	milk
	-rrhea (S)	discharge, flow

Continued

Medical Term	Word Elements	Meaning
8. gynec/o/logist	gynec/o (CF)	woman, female
	-logist (S)	specialist in the study of
9. mamm/o/gram	mamm/o (CF)	breast
	-gram (S)	record, writing
10. men/o/rrhagia	men/o (CF)	menses, menstruation
	-rrhagia (S)	bursting forth (of)
11. multi/para	multi- (P)	many, much
	-para (S)	to bear (offspring)
12. oophor/oma	oophor/o (CF)	ovary
	-oma (S)	tumor
13. orchi/o/rrhaphy	orchi/o (CF)	testis (plural, testes)
	-rrhaphy (S)	suture
14. primi/gravida	primi- (P)	first
	-gravida (S)	pregnant woman
15. prostat/o/megaly	prostat/o (CF)	prostate gland
	-megaly	enlargement
16. rect/o/scope	rect/o (CF)	rectum
	-scope (S)	instrument for examining
17. salping/ectomy	salping (WR)	tube (usually fallopian or eustachian [auditory] tubes)
	-ectomy (S)	excision, removal
18. vagin/o/cele	vagin/o (CF)	vagina
	-cele (S)	hernia; swelling
19. vas/ectomy	vas (WR)	vessel; vas deferens; duct
	-ectomy (S)	excision, removal
20. vas/o/vas/o/stomy	vas/o (CF)	vessel; vas deferens; duct
	vas/o (CF)	vessel; vas deferens; duct
	-stomy (S)	forming an opening (mouth)

Vocabulary Review

1. prostatomegaly
2. testopathy
3. testosterone
4. amenorrhea
5. estrogen, progesterone
6. oophoritis
7. aspermatism
8. gravida 4
9. uterus
10. prostatic cancer
11. epididymis
12. hydrocele
13. vas deferens
14. para 4
15. cervix uteri
16. dysmenorrhea
17. postmenopausal
18. aplasia
19. vasectomy
20. PID

CHAPTER 9: ENDOCRINE AND NERVOUS SYSTEMS

Section Review 9–1

Term	Definition
1. toxic/o/logist	-logist: specialist in the study of; poison
2. pancreat/itis	-itis: inflammation; pancreas
3. thyr/o/megaly	-megaly: enlargement; thyroid gland
4. hyper/trophy	-trophy: development, nourishment; excessive, above normal
5. gluc/o/genesis	-genesis: forming, producing, origin; sugar, sweetness
6. hypo/calc/emia	-emia: blood condition; under, below, deficient; calcium
7. adrenal/ectomy	-ectomy: excision, removal; adrenal glands
8. poly/dipsia	-dipsia: thirst; many, much
9. aden/oma	-oma: tumor; gland
10. thyroid/ectomy	-ectomy: excision, removal; thyroid gland

Section Review 9–2

1. -osis	5. -emia	9. acr/o	13. -tome	17. -logist
2. hyper-	6. calc/o	10. anter/o	14. neur/o	18. poly-
3. poster/o	7. -pathy	11. aden/o	15. toxic/o	19. thyroid/o, thyr/o
4. dys-	8. -megaly	12. -tomy	16. radi/o	20. hypo

Competency Verification, Figure 9–3

Locations of major endocrine glands, page 401.

1. pituitary gland	4. adrenal glands	7. thymus gland
2. thyroid gland	5. pancreas	8. ovaries
3. parathyroid glands	6. pineal gland	9. testes

Section Review 9–3

1. -iasis	5. -pexy	9. pancreat/o	13. gluc/o, glyc/o	17. thym/o
2. supra-	6. -rrhea	10. -gen, -genesis	14. -phagia	18. hypo-
3. adrenal/o, adren/o	7. poly-	11. -lysis	15. orch/o, orchi/o, orchid/o	19. -uria
4. -pathy	8. para-	12. -lith	16. -dipsia	20. toxic/o

Section Review 9–4

Term	Meaning
1. meningi/oma	-oma: tumor; meninges
2. neur/o/lysis	-lysis: separation, destruction, loosening; nerve
3. hemi/paresis	-paresis: partial paralysis; one half
4. myel/algia	-algia: pain; bone marrow; spinal cord
5. cerebr/o/spin/al	-al: pertaining to; cerebrum; spine

Continued

Term	Meaning
6. a/phasia	-phasia: speech; without, not
7. mening/o/cele	-cele: hernia, swelling; meninges
8. encephal/itis	-itis: inflammation; brain
9. gli/oma	-oma: tumor; glue; neuroglial tissue
10. quadri/plegia	-plegia: paralysis; four

Competency Verification, Figure 9–8

Structures of the brain, page 421.

1. cerebrum
2. midbrain
3. pons
4. medulla

Competency Verification, Figure 9–9

Spinal nerves, page 423.

1. cervical nerves
2. thoracic nerves
3. lumbar nerves
4. sacral nerves
5. coccygeal nerves

Section Review 9–5

1. -osis
2. dys-
3. thromb/o
4. vascul/o
5. encephal/o
6. -rhage, -rrhagia
7. gli/o, -glia
8. scler/o
9. mening/o, meningi/o
10. neur/o
11. cerebr/o
12. -malacia
13. -phasia
14. myel/o
15. a-

Additional Medical Terms Review

1. Bell palsy
2. TIA
3. antipsychotics
4. exophthalmos
5. Graves disease
6. hypophysectomy
7. myxedema
8. pheochromocytoma
9. Parkinson disease
10. poliomyelitis
11. sciatica
12. spina bifida
13. EEG
14. neuroblastoma
15. Alzheimer disease
16. MRI
17. type 1 diabetes
18. shingles
19. quadriplegia
20. panhypopituitarism
21. Huntington chorea
22. lumbar puncture
23. epilepsy
24. thalamotomy
25. PET

Medical Record Activity 9–1: Diabetes Mellitus

Evaluation

1. What symptoms of DM did the patient experience before his office visit?

   Glycosuria, elevated blood glucose of 400, polydipsia, and increased appetite

2. What confirmed the patient's new diagnosis of DM?

   Elevated blood glucose and glycosuria

3. What conditions had to be met before the patient could be discharged from the hospital?

   He had to be able to draw up and give his own insulin and perform fingersticks.

4. How many times a day does the patient have to take insulin?

   Two times, once in the morning and once in the afternoon

5. Why does the patient have to perform fingersticks four times a day?

   To monitor his blood glucose levels closely and ensure they are within the normal range

6. What is an ADA 2,000-calorie diet? Why is it important?

   A 2,000-calorie diet designed by American Diabetic Association, which is important for maintaining the same number of calories each day to help control blood glucose levels

Medical Record Activity 9–2: Stroke

Evaluation

1. Did the patient have a history of cardiovascular problems before her stroke?

   No

2. What symptoms did the patient experience just before her stroke?

   Paralysis of the right arm and left leg, aphasia, and diplopia

3. What is the primary site of this patient's cancer?

   Head of the pancreas

4. What is cerebrovascular disease?

   A disorder resulting from a change within the blood vessel(s) of the brain

5. What is the probable cause of the patient's stroke?

   Metastatic lesion of the brain or cerebrovascular disease

Word Elements Chapter Review

Medical Term	Word Elements	Meaning
1. hyper/calc/emia	*hyper- (P)*	*excessive, above normal*
	calc (WR)	*calcium*
	-emia (S)	*blood*
2. aden/o/carcin/oma	aden/o (CF)	gland
	carcin (WR)	cancer
	-oma (S)	tumor
3. adrenal/ectomy	adrenal (WR)	adrenal glands
	-ectomy (S)	excision, removal
4. cerebr/o/spin/al	cerebr/o (CF)	cerebrum
	spin (WR)	spine
	-al (S)	pertaining to
5. encephal/itis	encephal (WR)	brain
	-itis (S)	inflammation
6. gli/oma	gli (WR)	glue; neuroglial tissue
	-oma (S)	tumor

Continued

Medical Term	Word Elements	Meaning
7. gluc/o/genesis	gluc/o (CF)	sugar, sweetness
	-genesis (S)	forming, producing, origin
8. hemi/paresis	hemi- (P)	one half
	-paresis (S)	partial paralysis
9. hydr/o/cephal/us	hydr/o (CF)	water
	cephal (WR)	head
	-us (S)	condition; structure
10. hypo/pituitar/ism	hypo- (P)	under, below, deficient
	pituitar (WR)	pituitary gland
	-ism (S)	condition
11. hyper/trophy	hyper- (P)	excessive, above normal
	-trophy (S)	development, nourishment
12. mening/o/cele	mening/o (CF)	meninges (membranes covering the brain and spinal cord)
	-cele (S)	hernia, swelling
13. myel/algia	myel (WR)	bone marrow, spinal cord
	-algia (S)	pain
14. neur/o/lysis	neur/o (CF)	nerve
	-lysis (S)	separation; destruction; loosening
15. poly/dipsia	poly (P)	many, much
	-dipsia (S)	thirst
16. poli/o/myel/itis	poli/o (CF)	gray; gray matter (of the brain or spinal cord)
	myel (WR)	bone marrow, spinal cord
	-itis (S)	inflammation
17. quadri/plegia	quadri- (P)	four
	-plegia (S)	paralysis
18. thalam/o/tomy	thalam/o (CF)	thalamus
	-tomy (S)	incision
19. thromb/ocyte	thromb/o (CF)	blood clot
	-cyte (S)	cell
20. thyr/o/megaly	thyr/o (CF)	thyroid gland
	-megaly (S)	enlargement

Vocabulary Review

1. acromegaly	6. insulin	11. hyperglycemia	16. adrenaline	21. deglutition
2. pancreatolysis	7. neurohypophysis	12. pancreatolith	17. glycogenesis	22. vertigo
3. adenohypophysis	8. pancreatopathy	13. polydipsia	18. meningocele	23. jaundice
4. cerebral palsy	9. polyphagia	14. thyrotoxicosis	19. neuromalacia	24. metastasis
5. hypercalcemia	10. diabetes mellitus	15. adrenalectomy	20. pruritus	25. hormone

CHAPTER 10: MUSCULOSKELETAL SYSTEM

Section Review 10–1

Term	Meaning
1. my/o/sarcoma	*-sarcoma: malignant tumor of connective tissue; muscle*
2. my/o/rrhaphy	-rrhaphy: suture; muscle
3. hemi/plegia	-plegia: paralysis; one half
4. ten/o/tomy	-tomy: incision; tendon
5. cost/o/chondr/itis	-itis: inflammation; ribs; cartilage
6. tend/o/lysis	-lysis: separation; destruction; loosening; tendon
7. my/o/pathy	-pathy: disease; muscle
8. lumb/o/cost/al	-al: pertaining to; loins (lower back); ribs
9. tendin/itis	-itis: inflammation; tendon
10. my/algia	-algia: pain; muscle

Section Review 10–2

1. -osis	5. hemi-	9. hepat/o	13. -rrhexis	17. -tome
2. cyst/o	6. scler/o	10. my/o	14. -plasty	18. chondr/o
3. -cyte	7. -tomy	11. -plegia	15. -rrhaphy	19. -sarcoma
4. quadri-	8. enter/o	12. -genesis	16. ten/o, tendin/o, tend/o	20. -lysis

Section Review 10–3

Term	Meaning
1. dia/physis	*-physis: growth; through, across*
2. sub/cost/al	-al: pertaining to; under, below; ribs
3. oste/o/malacia	-malacia: softening; bone
4. lamin/ectomy	-ectomy: excision, removal; lamina (part of the vertebral arch)
5. pelv/i/metry	-metry: act of measuring; pelvis

Continued

Term	Meaning
6. myel/o/cele	-cele: hernia, swelling; bone marrow; spinal cord
7. oste/o/porosis	-porosis: porous; bone
8. ankyl/osis	-osis: abnormal condition, increase (used primarily with blood cells); stiffness; bent, crooked
9. carp/o/ptosis	-ptosis: prolapse, downward displacement; carpus (wrist bones)
10. crani/o/tomy	-tomy: incision; cranium (skull)

Competency Verification, Figure 10–4

Longitudinal section of a long bone (femur) and interior bone structure, page 467.

1. diaphysis
2. periosteum
3. compact bone
4. medullary cavity
5. distal epiphysis
6. proximal epiphysis
7. spongy bone

Section Review 10–4

1. hyper-
2. peri-
3. -emia
4. oste/o
5. chondr/o
6. calc/o
7. -cyte
8. dist/o
9. scler/o
10. -cele
11. -tomy
12. -itis
13. proxim/o
14. my/o
15. -algia, -dynia
16. -graphy
17. -genesis
18. -gram
19. -malacia
20. -logist
21. myel/o
22. -rrhaphy
23. -oma
24. hypo-
25. radi/o

Competency Verification, Figure 10–8

Anterior view of the skeleton, page 477.

1. crani/o
2. stern/o
3. cost/o
4. vertebr/o
5. humer/o
6. carp/o
7. metacarp/o
8. phalang/o
9. pelv/i, pelv/o
10. femor/o
11. patell/o
12. tibi/o
13. fibul/o
14. calcane/o

Competency Verification, Figure 10–9

Types of fractures, page 481.

1. closed fracture
2. open fracture
3. greenstick fracture
4. comminuted fracture
5. impacted fracture
6. complicated fracture
7. Colles fracture
8. incomplete fracture

Competency Verification, Figure 10–10

Vertebral column, lateral view, page 483.

1. intervertebral disks
2. cervical vertebrae
3. atlas
4. axis
5. thoracic vertebrae
6. lumbar vertebrae
7. sacrum
8. coccyx

Section Review 10–5

1. -osis	4. thorac/o	7. cephal/o	10. cervic/o	13. sacr/o
2. oste/o	5. -pathy	8. arthr/o	11. -um	14. -centesis
3. encephal/o	6. -ectomy	9. lumb/o	12. cost/o	15. spondyl/o, vertebr/o

Additional Medical Terms Review

1. bunion	6. Ewing sarcoma	11. sequestrum	16. muscular dystrophy	21. sequestrectomy
2. tendinitis	7. torticollis	12. arthroplasty	17. contracture	22. rheumatoid factor
3. sprain	8. gout	13. crepitation	18. ankylosis	23. talipes
4. strain	9. RA	14. myasthenia gravis	19. herniated disk	24. arthroscopy
5. kyphosis	10. Paget disease	15. lordosis	20. CTS	25. scoliosis

Medical Record Activity 10–1: Degenerative, Intervertebral Disk Disease

Evaluation

1. Why does the x-ray show a decreased density at L5–S1?

   Appears that a bilateral laminectomy had been done

2. What is the most common cause of degenerative intervertebral disk disease?

   Aging, with degenerative intervertebral disk disease being a common finding in individuals ages 50 and older

3. What happens to the gelatinous material of the disk as aging occurs?

   The gelatinous material is replaced by harder fibrocartilage.

4. What is the probable cause of the narrowing of the L3–L4 and L4–L5?

   Narrowing commonly occurs as a result of degenerative intervertebral disk disease.

Medical Record Activity 10–2: Rotator Cuff Tear, Right Shoulder

Evaluation

1. What type of arthritis did the patient have?

   Degenerative

2. Did the patient have calcium deposits in the right shoulder?

   No

3. What type of instrument did the physician use to visualize the glenoid labra?

   Arthroscope

4. What are labra?

   Liplike structures; in this case, edges or rims of bones

5. Did the patient have any outgrowths of bone? If so, where?

   Yes, spurs were found at the inferior and anterior acromioclavicular joint.

6. Did they find any deposits of calcium salts within the shoulder joint?

   They were unable to visualize an intra-articular calcification.

Word Elements Chapter Review

Medical Term	Word Elements	Meaning
1. arthr/o/desis	*arthr/o (CF)*	*joint*
	-desis (S)	*binding; fixation (of a bone or joint)*
2. calcane/o/dynia	calcane/o (CF)	calcaneum (heel bone)
	-dynia (S)	pain
3. chondr/oma	chondr (WR)	cartilage
	-oma (S)	tumor
4. cost/o/chondr/itis	cost/o (CF)	ribs
	chondr (WR)	cartilage
	-itis (S)	inflammation
5. dia/physis	dia- (P)	through, across
	-physis (S)	growth
6. fasci/o/plasty	fasci/o (CF)	band, fascia (fibrous membrane supporting and separating muscles)
	-plasty (S)	surgical repair
7. hemi/plegia	hemi- (P)	one half
	-plegia (S)	paralysis
8. lamin/ectomy	lamin (WR)	lamina (part of the vertebral arch)
	-ectomy (S)	excision, removal
9. leiomy/oma	leiomy (WR)	smooth muscle (visceral)
	-oma (S)	tumor
10. my/algia	my (WR)	muscle
	-algia (S)	pain
11. myel/o/cele	myel/o (CF)	bone marrow; spinal cord
	-cele (S)	hernia, swelling
12. my/esthenia	my (WR)	muscle
	-esthenia (S)	weakness, debility
13. my/o/sarc/oma	my/o (CF)	muscle
	sarc (WR)	flesh (connective tissue)
	-oma (S)	tumor
14. orth/o/ped/ics	orth/o (CF)	straight
	ped (WR)	foot; child
	-ics (S)	pertaining to
15. oste/o/clast	oste/o (CF)	bone
	-clast (S)	to break; surgical fracture

Medical Term	Word Elements	Meaning
16. oste/o/malacia	oste/o (CF)	bone
	-malacia (S)	softening
17. oste/o/porosis	oste/o (CF)	bone
	-porosis (S)	porous
18. patell/ectomy	patell (WR)	patella (kneecap)
	-ectomy (S)	excision, removal
19. pelv/i/metry	pelv/i (CF)	pelvis
	-metry (S)	act of measuring
20. radi/o/graph	radi/o (CF)	radiation, x-ray; radius (lower arm bone on the thumb side)
	-graph (S)	instrument for recording

Vocabulary Review

1. radiology
2. diaphysis
3. AP
4. closed fracture
5. bilateral
6. proximal
7. articulation
8. open fracture
9. atlas
10. arthrocentesis
11. bone marrow
12. cephalometer
13. myelogram
14. myorrhexis
15. spondylomalacia
16. distal
17. radiologist
18. cervical vertebrae
19. intervertebral
20. quadriplegia

CHAPTER 11: SPECIAL SENSES: EYES AND EARS

Section Review 11–1

Term	Meaning
1. conjunctiv/itis	*-itis; inflammation; conjunctiva*
2. blephar/o/ptosis	-ptosis: prolapse, downward displacement; eyelid
3. ambly/opia	-opia: vision; dull, dim
4. retin/o/pathy	-pathy: disease; retina
5. scler/itis	-itis: inflammation; hardening; sclera (white of the eye)
6. ophthalm/o/scope	-scope: instrument for examining; eye
7. intra/ocul/ar	-ar: pertaining to; within, in; eye
8. dacry/o/rrhea	-rrhea: discharge, flow; tear; lacrimal apparatus (duct, sac, or gland)
9. dipl/opia	-opia: vision; double
10. blephar/o/spasm	-spasm: involuntary contraction, twitching; eyelid

Competency Verification, Figure 11–1

Eye structures, page 511.

1. sclera
2. cornea
3. choroid
4. ciliary body
5. iris
6. retina
7. fovea
8. pupil
9. optic disc
10. optic nerve
11. conjunctiva

Competency Verification, Figure 11–3

Lacrimal apparatus, page 517.

1. lacrimal gland
2. lacrimal sac
3. nasolacrimal duct

Section Review 11–2

Term	Meaning
1. tympan/o/centesis	*-centesis: surgical puncture; tympanic membrane (eardrum)*
2. acous/tic	-tic: pertaining to; hearing
3. hyper/tropia	-tropia: turning; excessive, above normal
4. ot/o/rrhea	-rrhea: discharge, flow; ear
5. an/acusis	-acusis: hearing; without, not
6. myring/o/tomy	-tomy: incision; tympanic membrane (eardrum)
7. tympan/o/plasty	-plasty: surgical repair; tympanic membrane (eardrum)
8. audi/o/meter	-meter: instrument for measuring; hearing
9. ot/o/scope	-scope: instrument for examining; ear
10. salping/o/pharyng/eal	-eal: pertaining to; tube (usually fallopian or eustachian [auditory] tubes); pharynx (throat)

Competency Verification, Figure 11–4

Ear structures, page 521.

1. auricle
2. ear canal
3. tympanic membrane
4. malleus
5. incus
6. stapes
7. eustachian (auditory) tube
8. cochlea
9. semicircular canals
10. vestibule

Section Review 11–3

1. hyper-
2. choroid/o
3. kerat/o
4. dipl/o, dipl-
5. ot/o
6. salping/o, -salpinx
7. ophthalm/o
8. blephar/o
9. aden/o
10. scler/o
11. -spasm
12. irid/o
13. -ptosis
14. -logist
15. retin/o
16. -rrhexis
17. -malacia
18. audi/o, -acusis
19. -stenosis
20. -edema
21. dacry/o
22. tympan/o, myring/o
23. corne/o
24. -opia, -opsia
25. xanth/o

Additional Medical Terms Review

1. tinnitus	6. anacusis	11. glaucoma	16. acoustic neuroma	21. phacoemulsification
2. otosclerosis	7. otitis media	12. vertigo	17. tonometry	22. Rinne test
3. achromatopsia	8. conjunctivitis	13. retinal detachment	18. iridectomy	23. diabetic retinopathy
4. Ménière disease	9. photophobia	14. hordeolum	19. conductive hearing loss	24. macular degeneration
5. strabismus	10. presbycusis	15. astigmatism	20. cataract	25. myringotomy

Medical Record Activity 11–1: Retinal Detachment

Evaluation

1. Where is the retina located?

   The retina is the innermost layer of the eye.

2. Was the anesthetic administered behind or in front of the eyeball?

   Behind the eyeball (retrobulbar)

3. How much movement remained in the eye following anesthesia?

   None; akinesia

4. Where was the hemorrhage located?

   In the orbit of the eye behind the lens, where the vitreous humor is located

5. What type of vitrectomy was undertaken?

   Trans pars plana vitrectomy

6. Why was the eye left soft?

   Because it had poor perfusion

Medical Record Activity 11–2: Otitis Media

Evaluation

1. Where was the patient's infection located?

   Right ear

2. What complication developed while the patient was hospitalized?

   Cholesteatoma

3. What is the purpose of the tube placement?

   It reduces the accumulation of fluid within the middle ear.

4. What surgery is being performed to resolve the cholesteatoma?

   Tympanoplasty, right ear

5. Will the patient be asleep during the surgery?

   Yes, under general anesthesia

Word Elements Chapter Review

Medical Term	Word Elements	Meaning
1. acoustic	*acous (WR)*	*hearing*
	-tic (S)	*pertaining to*
2. anisocoria	aniso- (P)	unequal, dissimilar
	cor (WR)	pupil
	-ia (S)	condition
3. audiometer	audi/o (CF)	hearing
	-meter (S)	instrument for measuring
4. blepharoptosis	blephar/o (CF)	eyelid
	-ptosis (S)	prolapse, downward displacement
5. conjunctivitis	conjunctiv (WR)	conjunctiva
	-itis (S)	inflammation
6. choroidopathy	choroid/o (CF)	choroid
	-pathy (S)	disease
7. dacryorrhea	dacry/o (CF)	tear; lacrimal apparatus
	-rrhea (S)	discharge, flow
8. esotropia	eso- (P)	inward
	-tropia (S)	turning
9. iridectomy	irid (WR)	iris
	-ectomy (S)	excision, removal
10. keratitis	kerat (WR)	horny tissue; hard; cornea
	-itis (S)	inflammation
11. myopia	my (WR)	muscle
	-opia (S)	vision
12. myringotomy	myring/o (CF)	tympanic membrane (eardrum)
	-tomy (S)	incision
13. ophthalmoscope	ophthalm/o (CF)	eye
	-scope (S)	instrument for examining
14. otoscopy	ot/o (CF)	ear
	-scopy (S)	visual examination
15. photophobia	phot/o (CF)	light
	-phobia (S)	fear
16. presbycusis	presby (WR)	old age
	-cusis (S)	hearing

Medical Term	Word Elements	Meaning
17. salpingostenosis	salping/o (CF)	tube (usually fallopian or eustachian [auditory] tubes)
	-stenosis (S)	narrowing, stricture
18. scleromalacia	scler/o (CF)	hardening; sclera (white of the eye)
	-malacia (S)	softening
19. stapedectomy	staped (WR)	stapes
	-ectomy (S)	excision, removal
20. tympanoplasty	tympan/o (CF)	tympanic membrane (eardrum)
	-plasty (S)	surgical repair

Vocabulary Review

1. diplopia
2. sclera
3. tympanic membrane
4. dacryorrhea
5. eustachian tube
6. keratitis
7. diagnosis
8. mucoserous
9. otitis media
10. cholesteatoma
11. mastoid surgery
12. general anesthetic
13. ophthalmologist
14. chronic
15. hyperopia
16. postoperatively
17. labyrinth
18. blepharoptosis
19. salpingostenosis
20. myopia

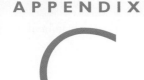

Index of Diagnostic, Medical, and Surgical Procedures

This section provides a list of the diagnostic, medical, and surgical procedures covered in the textbook along with page numbers. Diagnostic procedures help the physician determine a patient's health status, evaluate the factors influencing that status, and determine a method of treatment. Medical and surgical procedures are performed to treat a specific disorder that is diagnosed by the physician.

DIAGNOSTIC PROCEDURES

Amniocentesis, Chapter 8, Reproductive Systems, 372
Arterial blood gas (ABG), Chapter 4, Respiratory System, 136
Arthrocentesis, Chapter 10, Musculoskeletal System, 492
Audiometry, Chapter 11, Special Senses: Eyes and Ears, 532
Barium enema (BE), Chapter 6, Digestive System, 260
Barium swallow, Chapter 6, Digestive System, 260
Biopsy, Chapter 3, Integumentary System, 90
Blood urea nitrogen (BUN), Chapter 7, Urinary System, 307
Bone marrow aspiration biopsy, Chapter 5, Cardiovascular and Lymphatic Systems, 197
Bronchoscopy, Chapter 4, Respiratory System, 136
Cardiac catheterization (CC), Chapter 5, Cardiovascular and Lymphatic Systems, 194
Cardiac enzyme studies, Chapter 5, Cardiovascular and Lymphatic Systems, 194
Cerebrospinal fluid (CSF) analysis, Chapter 9, Endocrine and Nervous Systems, 436
Colposcopy, Chapter 8, Reproductive Systems, 372
Computed tomography (CT), Chapter 4, Respiratory System, 136
    Chapter 6, Digestive System, 260
    Chapter 7, Urinary System, 308
    Chapter 9, Endocrine and Nervous Systems, 437
Digital rectal examination (DRE), Chapter 8, Reproductive Systems, 374
Echocardiography, Chapter 5, Cardiovascular and Lymphatic Systems, 195
Electrocardiography (ECG), Chapter 5, Cardiovascular and Lymphatic Systems, 195
ELISA, Chapter 5, Cardiovascular and Lymphatic Systems, 197
Endoscopy, Chapter 2, Body Structure, 51
    Chapter 6, Digestive System, 261
Fluoroscopy, Chapter 2, Body Structure, 52
Holter monitor, Chapter 5, Cardiovascular and Lymphatic Systems, 195
Hysterosalpingo-oophorectomy, Chapter 8, Reproductive Systems, 376
Kidney, ureter, bladder (KUB), Chapter 7, Urinary System, 298

Laparoscopy, Chapter 8, Reproductive Systems, 372
Lumbar puncture, Chapter 9, Endocrine and Nervous Systems, 436
Lymphangiography, Chapter 5, Cardiovascular and Lymphatic Systems, 197
Magnetic resonance imaging (MRI), Chapter 2, Body Structure, 52
   Chapter 4, Respiratory System, 137
   Chapter 6, Digestive System, 261
   Chapter 9, Endocrine and Nervous Systems, 437
Mammography, Chapter 8, Reproductive Systems, 373
Nuclear scan, Chapter 2, Body Structure, 53
Otoscopy, Chapter 11, Special Senses: Eyes and Ears, 532
Papanicolaou (Pap) test, Chapter 8, Reproductive Systems, 374
Positron emission tomography (PET), Chapter 9, Endocrine and Nervous Systems, 437
Prostate-specific antigen (PSA) test, Chapter 8, Reproductive Systems, 361
Pulmonary function tests (PFTs), Chapter 4, Respiratory System, 137
Pyelography, Chapter 7, Urinary System, 308
Radioactive iodine uptake (RAIU) test, Chapter 9, Endocrine and Nervous Systems, 435
Radiography, Chapter 2, Body Structure, 43
Radiopharmaceutical, Chapter 2, Body Structure, 53
Renal scan, Chapter 7, Urinary System, 308
Rheumatoid factor, Chapter 10, Musculoskeletal System, 492
Rinne test, Chapter 11, Special Senses: Eyes and Ears, 532
Scan, Chapter 2, Body Structure, 53
Skin test, Chapter 3, Integumentary System, 90
Stool guaiac, Chapter 6, Digestive System, 261
Stress test, Chapter 5, Cardiovascular and Lymphatic Systems, 196
Tissue typing, Chapter 5, Cardiovascular and Lymphatic Systems, 198
Tomography, Chapter 2, Body Structure, 53
Tonometry, Chapter 11, Special Senses: Eyes and Ears, 531
Troponin I, Chapter 5, Cardiovascular and Lymphatic Systems, 196
Ultrasonography (US), Chapter 2, Body Structure, 53
   Chapter 5, Cardiovascular and Lymphatic Systems, 197
   Chapter 6, Digestive System, 261
   Chapter 8, Reproductive Systems, 374
Urinalysis, Chapter 7, Urinary System, 309
Visual acuity test, Chapter 11, Special Senses: Eyes and Ears, 531
Voiding cystourethrography (VCUG), Chapter 7, Urinary System, 309

MEDICAL AND SURGICAL PROCEDURES

Adrenalectomy, Chapter 9, Endocrine and Nervous Systems, 396
Anastomosis, Chapter 2, Body Structure, 54
Angioplasty, Chapter 5, Cardiovascular and Lymphatic Systems, 198
Arthroplasty, Chapter 10, Musculoskeletal System, 492
Bariatric surgery, Chapter 6, Digestive System, 262
Cardioversion, Chapter 5, Cardiovascular and Lymphatic Systems, 199
Cataract surgery, Chapter 11, Special Senses: Eyes and Ears, 533
Catheterization, Chapter 7, Urinary System, 309
Cauterize, Chapter 2, Body Structure, 54
Cerclage, Chapter 8, Reproductive Systems, 375
Circumcision, Chapter 8, Reproductive Systems, 377
Cochlear implant, Chapter 11, Special Senses: Eyes and Ears, 534
Corneal transplant, Chapter 11, Special Senses: Eyes and Ears, 533
Craniotomy, Chapter 9, Endocrine and Nervous Systems, 438
Cryosurgery, Chapter 3, Integumentary System, 91
Débridement, Chapter 3, Integumentary System, 91
Defibrillator, Chapter 5, Cardiovascular and Lymphatic Systems, 199

Dialysis, Chapter 7, Urinary System, 310
Dilatation and curettage (D&C), Chapter 8, Reproductive Systems, 375
Electrodesiccation, Chapter 3, Integumentary System, 91
Endarterectomy, Chapter 5, Cardiovascular and Lymphatic Systems, 200
Hysterosalpingo-oophorectomy, Chapter 8, Reproductive Systems, 376
Incision and drainage (I & D), Chapter 3, Integumentary System, 91
Iridectomy, Chapter 11, Special Senses: Eyes and Ears, 533
Lithotripsy, Chapter 6, Digestive Systems, 262
Lumpectomy, Chapter 8, Reproductive Systems, 376
Lymphangiectomy, Chapter 5, Cardiovascular and Lymphatic Systems, 201
Mastectomy, Chapter 8, Reproductive Systems, 376
Myringotomy, Chapter 11, Special Senses: Eyes and Ears, 535
Myringotomy, Chapter 11, Special Senses: Eyes and Ears, 535
Nasogastric intubation, Chapter 6, Digestive System, 263
Postural drainage, Chapter 4, Respiratory System, 139
Reconstructive breast surgery, Chapter 8, Reproductive Systems, 377
Renal transplantation, Chapter 7, Urinary System, 311
Sclerotherapy, Chapter 5, Cardiovascular and Lymphatic Systems, 200
Sequestrectomy, Chapter 10, Musculoskeletal System, 492
Skin graft, Chapter 3, Integumentary System, 91
Skin resurfacing, Chapter 3, Integumentary System, 92
Thalamotomy, Chapter 9, Endocrine and Nervous Systems, 438
Tubal ligation, Chapter 8, Reproductive Systems, 377
Transurethral resection of the prostate (TURP), Chapter 8, Reproductive Systems, 377
Valvuloplasty, Chapter 5, Cardiovascular and Lymphatic Systems, 200

Drug Classifications

This section provides a quick reference of common drug categories. They include prescription and over-the-counter drugs that are used to treat symptoms, signs, and diseases of the various body systems.

Drug Classification	Description
A	
alkylates	Treat certain types of malignancies
	Alkylates break deoxyribonucleic acid (DNA) strands in the cancerous cell by substituting an alkyl group for a hydrogen molecule in the DNA.
analgesics	Relieve minor to severe pain
	Analgesics include nonprescription drugs, such as aspirin and other nonsteroidal anti-inflammatory agents, and those classified as controlled substances that are available only by prescription.
angiotensin-converting enzyme inhibitors	Lower blood pressure by inhibiting conversion of angiotensin I (an inactive enzyme) to angiotensin II (a potent vasoconstrictor)
androgens	Increase testosterone levels
	Hyposecretion of testosterone may be due to surgical removal of the testes or decreased levels of luteinizing hormone (LH) from the anterior pituitary gland.
anesthetics	Produce partial or complete loss of sensation with or without loss of consciousness
	General anesthetics act on the brain to produce complete loss of feeling with loss of consciousness. Local anesthetics act on nerves or nerve tracts to affect a local area only without loss of consciousness.
antacids	Neutralize excess acid in the stomach and help relieve gastritis and ulcer pain
	Antacids are also used to relieve indigestion and reflux esophagitis (heartburn).
antianginals	Relieve angina pectoris by vasodilation
antianxiety drugs	Reduce anxiety and neurosis
	Antianxiety drugs are classified as minor tranquilizers and anxiolytics.
antiarrhythmics	Treat cardiac arrhythmias by stabilizing the electrical conduction of the heart
antibiotics	Inhibit growth of or destroy microorganisms
	Antibiotics are used extensively in treatment of infectious diseases.
anticoagulants	Prevent or delay blood coagulation
	Anticoagulants prevent deep vein thrombosis (DVT) and postoperative clot formation and decrease the risk of stroke.

Continued

Drug Classification	Description
anticonvulsants	Prevent or reduce the severity of epileptic or other convulsive seizures; also called antiepileptics
antidepressants	Regulate mood and reduce symptoms of depression by affecting the amount of neurotransmitters in the brain
antidiabetics	Stimulate the pancreas to produce more insulin and decrease peripheral resistance to insulin *Oral antidiabetics help treat type 2 diabetes mellitus.*
antidiarrheals	Control loose stools and relieve diarrhea by absorbing excess water in the bowel or slowing peristalsis in the intestinal tract
antidiuretics	Reduce the production of urine
antiemetics	Prevent or suppress vomiting *Antiemetics also help treat vertigo, motion sickness, and nausea.*
antifungals	Alter the cell wall of fungi or disrupt enzyme activity, resulting in cellular death
antihistamines	Counteract the effects of a histamine *Antihistamines inhibit allergic reactions of inflammation, redness, and itching, especially hay fever and other allergic disorders of the nasal passages.*
antihyperlipidemics	Lower lipid levels in the bloodstream *Antihyperlipidemics reduce the risk of heart attack by lowering lipid levels.*
antihypertensives	Lower blood pressure
anti-impotence agents	Treat erectile dysfunction (impotence) by increasing blood flow to the penis, resulting in an erection
anti-infectives, antibacterials, antifungals	Eliminate or inhibit bacterial or fungal infections *Anti-infectives, antibacterials, and antifungals can be administered topically or systemically.*
anti-inflammatories	Relieve the swelling, tenderness, redness, and pain of inflammation *Anti-inflammatories may be classified as steroidal (corticosteroids) or nonsteroidal.*
corticosteroids (glucocorticoids)	Relieve inflammation and replace hormones for adrenal insufficiency (Addison disease) *Corticosteroids are widely used to suppress the immune system's inflammatory response to tissue damage, control allergic reactions, reduce the rejection process in tissue and organ transplantation, and treat some cancers.*
nonsteroidals (nonsteroidal anti-inflammatory drugs [NSAIDs])	Relieve mild to moderate pain and reduce inflammation in the treatment of musculoskeletal conditions, such as sprains and strains, arthritis, and other related disorders
antimetabolites	Interfere with the use of enzymes required for cell division *Antimetabolites block folic acid, a B vitamin required for synthesis of some amino acids in the DNA of cancerous cells.*
antimicrobials	Destroy or inhibit the growth of bacteria, fungi, and protozoa, depending on the particular drug, generally by interfering with the functions of their cell membrane or their reproductive cycle
antiparkinsonians	Control tremors and muscle rigidity associated with Parkinson disease by increasing dopamine levels in the brain
antipruritics	Prevent or relieve itching

Drug Classification	Description
antipsychotics	Treat psychosis, paranoia, and schizophrenia by altering chemicals in the brain, including the limbic system (group of brain structures), which controls emotions
antiseptics	Topically applied agent that destroys or inhibits the growth of bacteria, preventing infection in cuts, scratches, and surgical incisions
antispasmodics	Act on the autonomic nervous system to reduce spasms in the bladder or gastrointestinal (GI) tract
antithyroids	Treat hyperthyroidism by impeding the formation of T_3 and T_4 hormone
antituberculars	Treat tuberculosis *Several antituberculars are used in combination to produce effective treatment.*
antitussives	Relieve or suppress coughing by blocking the cough reflex in the medulla of the brain
antivirals	Prevent replication of viruses within host cells *Antivirals treat HIV infection and AIDS.*
astringents	Shrink the blood vessels locally, dry up secretions from seeping lesions, and lessen skin sensitivity
B	
beta blockers	Decrease heart rate and dilate arteries by blocking beta receptors *Beta blockers treat angina pectoris, arrhythmias, and hypertension.*
bone resorption inhibitors	Inhibit breakdown of bone *Bone resorption inhibitors treat osteoporosis.*
bronchodilators	Stimulate bronchial muscles to relax, thereby expanding air passages and resulting in increased air flow to the lungs
C	
calcium channel blockers	Selectively block movement of calcium (required for blood vessel contraction) into myocardial cells and arterial walls, causing heart rate and blood pressure to decrease *Calcium channel blockers treat angina pectoris, arrhythmias, heart failure, and hypertension.*
contraceptives	Prevent conception or ovulation; also called birth control
birth control patch	Delivers two synthetic hormones, progestin and estrogen, through a transdermal patch, impeding pregnancy by preventing the ovaries from releasing eggs (ovulation) and thickening the cervical mucus *The patch is applied directly to the skin (buttocks, abdomen, upper torso, or upper outer arm) and has an effectiveness rate of 95%.*
injectable	Delivers a synthetic drug similar to progesterone (medroxyprogesterone acetate) through an injection administered four times per year that prevents the ovaries from releasing eggs (ovulation) and thickens the cervical mucus *When used as directed, an injectable contraceptive (Depo-Provera) may prevent pregnancy more than 99% of the time.*
oral	Inhibits ovulation and pituitary secretion of luteinizing hormone (LH), causing changes in cervical mucus that render it unfavorable to penetration by sperm and altering the nature of the endometrium; also called birth control pills *Oral contraceptives (OCs) contain mixtures of estrogen and progestin in various levels. When used as directed, OCs are nearly 100% effective.*

Continued

Drug Classification	Description
cycloplegics	Paralyze the ciliary muscles, resulting in pupil dilation *Cycloplegics dilate the pupils to facilitate certain eye examinations and surgical procedures.*
cytotoxics	Disrupt nucleic acid and protein synthesis, causing immunosuppression and cancer cell death *Cytotoxics treat cancer and autoimmune diseases, such as inflammatory bowel disease and systemic vasculitis. They also help prevent rejection in transplant recipients.*

D

Drug Classification	Description
decongestants	Decrease congestion of mucous membranes of the sinuses and nose *Decongestants are used for temporary relief of nasal congestion associated with the common cold, hay fever, other upper respiratory allergies, and sinusitis.*
diuretics	Act on the kidney to promote the excretion of sodium and water *Diuretics treat edema and hypertension.*

E

Drug Classification	Description
emetics	Induce vomiting, especially in cases of poisoning
estrogen hormone	Used in estrogen replacement therapy (ERT) during menopause to correct estrogen deficiency and as chemotherapy for some types of cancer, including tumors of the prostate
expectorants	Liquefy respiratory secretions so that they are more easily expelled during coughing episodes

F, G

Drug Classification	Description
fibrinolytics	Trigger the body to produce plasmin, an enzyme that dissolves clots *Fibrinolytics treat acute pulmonary embolism and, occasionally, deep vein thrombosis (DVT).*
gold compound drugs	Treat rheumatoid arthritis by inhibiting activity within the immune system to prevent further disease progression *Gold compound drugs actually contain gold.*
gonadotropins	Raise sperm count in infertility cases
growth hormone replacements	Increase skeletal growth in children and growth hormone deficiencies in adults

H

Drug Classification	Description
H_2 blockers	Block histamine-2 (H_2) receptors in the stomach to decrease the release of hydrochloric acid *H_2 blockers treat peptic ulcers.*
hemostatics	Prevent or control bleeding *Hemostatics treat blood disorders and certain bleeding problems associated with surgery.*
hypnotics	Depress the central nervous system (CNS) to induce or maintain sleep

I

Drug Classification	Description
inotropics, cardiotonics	Increase the efficiency of heart muscle contractions *Inotropics treat cardiac arrhythmias and cardiac failure.*
insulins	Lower glucose (sugar) level in the blood *Insulins are synthetic forms of the insulin hormone used to treat diabetes and administered by injection.*

Drug Classification	Description
K, L, M	
keratolytics	Destroy and soften the outer layer of skin so that it is sloughed off or shed
	Strong keratolytics are effective for removing warts and corns. Milder preparations promote the shedding of scales and crusts in eczema, psoriasis, and seborrheic dermatitis. Weak keratolytics irritate inflamed skin, acting as tonics that speed up the healing process.
laxatives (cathartics, purgatives)	Induce bowel movements or loosen stool
	When used in smaller doses, laxatives relieve constipation. When used in larger doses, they evacuate the entire gastrointestinal (GI) tract—for example, as preparation for surgery or intestinal radiologic examinations.
miotics	Constrict the pupil of the eye
	Miotics help treat glaucoma.
mucolytics	Liquefy sputum or reduce its viscosity so that it can be coughed up more easily
mydriatics	Dilate the pupil and paralyze the muscles of accommodation of the iris
	Mydriatics help prepare the eye for internal examination and treat inflammatory conditions of the iris.
N, O, P	
nitrates	Dilate arteries and increase blood flow to the myocardium
	Nitrates treat angina pectoris.
opiates	Relieve pain
	Opiates contain opium or its derivative. They are commonly prescribed on a short-term basis due to their strong addictive property.
parasiticides	Destroy systemic parasites, such as pinworm or tapeworm, in oral form or insect parasites, such as mites and lice, in topical form
potassium supplements	Increase the potassium level of the blood
	Potassium can be administered orally or intravenously (IV) when dangerously low levels occur. It is used as a replacement for potassium loss due to diuretics.
prostaglandins	Used to induce labor, terminate pregnancy, or treat erectile dysfunction, patent ductus arteriosus, or pulmonary hypertension
protectives	Function by covering, cooling, drying, or soothing inflamed skin
	Protectives do not penetrate or soften the skin but form a long-lasting film that protects the skin from air, water, and clothing during the natural healing process.
proton pump inhibitors	Block the final stage of hydrochloric acid production in the stomach
	Proton pump inhibitors treat peptic ulcers and gastroesophageal reflux disease (GERD).
psychotropics	Alter chemical balance in the brain, causing changes in perception, mood, and behavior
	Psychotropics are commonly employed in the management of psychiatric disorders.
R, S	
relaxants	Reduce tension, causing relaxation of muscles or bowel
salicylates	Relieve mild to moderate pain and reduce inflammation and fever
sedatives	Exert a calming or tranquilizing effect
skeletal muscle relaxants	Relieve muscle spasms and stiffness

Continued

Drug Classification	Description
spermicides	Chemically destroy sperm
	Spermicidals consist of jellies, creams, and foams and do not require a prescription. They are commonly used within the woman's vagina for contraceptive purposes.
statins	Lower cholesterol in the blood and reduce its production in the liver by blocking the enzyme that produces it

T

thrombolytics	Dissolve blood clots by destroying their fibrin strands
	Thrombolytics are used to break apart, or lyse, thrombi.
thyroid supplements	Replace or supplement thyroid hormones
topical anesthetics	Block sensation of pain by numbing the skin layers and mucous membranes
	Topical anesthetics are applied directly in sprays, creams, gargles, suppositories, and other preparations. They are also used to numb the skin to make the injection of medication more comfortable.
tranquilizers	Calm anxiousness or agitation without decreasing consciousness

U

uricosurics	Increase urinary excretion of uric acid, reducing the concentration of uric acid in the blood
	Uricosurics are used to treat gout.
uterine stimulants	Induce labor at term, control postpartum hemorrhage, and induce therapeutic abortion; also called oxytocic agents
	Oxytocin is a pharmaceutically prepared chemical that is similar to the pituitary hormone oxytocin. Uterine stimulants are also used to treat infertility in females.

V

vasoconstrictors	Narrow or constrict the diameter of blood vessels
	Vasoconstrictors decrease blood flow and increase blood pressure.
vasodilators	Dilate the diameter of blood vessels
	Vasodilators help treat angina pectoris and hypertension.
vitamin B_{12}	Treats pernicious anemia
	Vitamin B_{12} is delivered by nasal spray or intramuscular (IM) injection.
vertigo and motion sickness agents	Decrease sensitivity of the inner ear to motion and prevent nerve impulses in the inner ear from reaching the vomiting center of the brain

W, X, Y, Z

wax emulsifiers	Loosen and help remove impacted cerumen (ear wax)

Abbreviations and Symbols

ABBREVIATIONS

The table below lists common abbreviations used in health care and related fields along with their meanings.

Abbreviation	Meaning	Abbreviation	Meaning
A		AIDS	acquired immunodeficiency syndrome
A&P	anatomy and physiology; auscultation and percussion	AK	above the knee
A, B, AB, O	blood types in ABO blood group	ALL	acute lymphocytic leukemia
AAA	abdominal aortic aneurysm	ALS	amyotrophic lateral sclerosis (also called Lou Gehrig disease)
AB, Ab, ab	antibody; abortion		
ABC	aspiration, biopsy, cytology	ALT	alanine aminotransferase
ABG	arterial blood gas	AM, a.m	in the morning or before noon
a.c.*	before meals	AML	acute myelogenous leukemia
ACL	anterior cruciate ligament	ANS	autonomic nervous system
ACTH	adrenocorticotropic hormone	ant	anterior
AD*	right ear	AOM	acute otitis media
ad lib.	as desired	AP	anteroposterior
ADH	antidiuretic hormone (vasopressin)	ARDS	acute respiratory distress syndrome
ADHD	attention-deficit hyperactivity disorder	ARF	acute renal failure
ADLs	activities of daily living	ARMD, AMD	age-related macular degeneration
AE	above the elbow	AS	aortic stenosis
AED	automatic external defibrillator	AS*	left ear
AF	atrial fibrillation	ASD	atrial septal defect
AFB	acid-fast bacillus (TB organism)	ASHD	arteriosclerotic heart disease
AGN	acute glomerulonephritis	AST	angiotensin sensitivity test
AI	artificial insemination	Ast	astigmatism
AICD	automatic implantable cardioverter-defibrillator	AU*	both ears
		AV	atrioventricular; arteriovenous

Continued

Abbreviation	Meaning	Abbreviation	Meaning
B		CHF	congestive heart failure
Ba	barium	Chol	cholesterol
baso	basophil (type of white blood cell)	CLL	chronic lymphocytic leukemia
BBB	bundle branch block	CK	creatine kinase (cardiac enzyme); conductive keratoplasty
BC	bone conduction		
BCC	basal cell carcinoma	cm	centimeter (1/100 of a meter)
BE	barium enema; below the elbow	CML	chronic myelogenous leukemia
BG	blood glucose	CNS	central nervous system
b.i.d.*	twice a day	c/o	complains of, complaints
BK	below the knee	CO	cardiac output
BKA	below-knee amputation	CO₂	carbon dioxide
BM	bowel movement	COPD	chronic obstructive pulmonary disease
BMI	body mass index		
BMR	basal metabolic rate	CP	cerebral palsy
BNO	bladder neck obstruction	CPAP	continuous positive airway pressure
BP, B/P	blood pressure	CPD	cephalopelvic disproportion
BPH	benign prostatic hyperplasia; benign prostatic hypertrophy	CPK	creatine phosphokinase (enzyme released into the bloodstream after a heart attack)
BS	blood sugar		
BSE	breast self-examination	CPR	cardiopulmonary resuscitation
BSO	bilateral salpingo-oophorectomy	CRF	chronic renal failure
BUN	blood urea nitrogen	CRRT	continuous renal replacement therapy
Bx, bx	biopsy		
C		C&S	culture and sensitivity
C1, C2, and so on	first cervical vertebra, second cervical vertebra, and so on	CS, C-section	cesarean section
		CSF	cerebrospinal fluid
CA	cancer; chronological age; cardiac arrest	CT	computed tomography
		CTL	cytotoxic T lymphocytes
Ca	calcium; cancer	CTS	carpal tunnel syndrome
CABG	coronary artery bypass graft	CV	cardiovascular
CAD	coronary artery disease	CVA	cerebrovascular accident
CAH	chronic active hepatitis; congenital adrenal hyperplasia	CVD	cardiovascular disease
		CVS	chorionic villus sampling
CAT	computed axial tomography	CWP	childbirth without pain
Cath	catheterization; catheter	CXR	chest x-ray, chest radiograph
CBC	complete blood count	cysto	cystoscopy
CC	cardiac catheterization; chief complaint	D	
		D	diopter (lens strength)
cc*	cubic centimeters; same as milliliters (1/1,000 of a liter)	dc, DC, D/C*	discharge; discontinue
		D&C	dilation and curettage
CCU	coronary care unit	Decub.	decubitus (lying down)
CDH	congenital dislocation of the hip	derm	dermatology
CF	cystic fibrosis	DES	diffuse esophageal spasm; drug-eluting stent
CHD	coronary heart disease		
chemo	chemotherapy	DEXA, DXA	dual energy x-ray absorptiometry

Abbreviation	Meaning	Abbreviation	Meaning
DI	diabetes insipidus; diagnostic imaging	ESR	erythrocyte sedimentation rate
diff	differential count (white blood cells)	ESRD	end-stage renal disease
		ESWL	extracorporeal shock-wave lithotripsy
DJD	degenerative joint disease	ETT	exercise tolerance test
DKA	diabetic ketoacidosis	**F**	
DMARDs	disease-modifying antirheumatic drugs	FBS	fasting blood sugar
DM	diabetes mellitus	FECG, FEKG	fetal electrocardiogram
DNA	deoxyribonucleic acid	FH	family history
D.O., DO	Doctor of Osteopathy	FHR	fetal heart rate
DOE	dyspnea on exertion	FHT	fetal heart tone
DPI	dry powder inhaler	FS	frozen section
D.P.M.	Doctor of Podiatric Medicine	FSH	follicle-stimulating hormone
DPT	diphtheria, pertussis, tetanus	FTND	full-term normal delivery
DRE	digital rectal examination	FVC	forced vital capacity
DSA	digital subtraction angiography	Fx	fracture
DUB	dysfunctional uterine bleeding	**G**	
DVT	deep vein thrombosis; deep venous thrombosis	G	gravida (pregnant)
Dx	diagnosis	g, gm	gram
E		GB	gallbladder
		GBS	gallbladder series (x-ray studies)
EBV	Epstein-Barr virus	GC	gonococcus *(Neisseria gonorrhoeae)*
ECCE	extracapsular cataract extraction		
ECG, EKG	electrocardiogram; electrocardiography	G-CSF	granulocyte colony-stimulating factor
ECHO	echocardiogram; echocardiography; echoencephalogram; echoencephalography	GER	gastroesophageal reflux
		GERD	gastroesophageal reflux disease
		GH	growth hormone
ED	erectile dysfunction; emergency department	GI	gastrointestinal
		GTT	glucose tolerance test
EEG	electroencephalography; electroencephalogram	GU	genitourinary
		GVHD	graft-versus-host disease
EF	ejection fraction	GVHR	graft-versus-host reaction
EGD	esophagogastroduodenoscopy	GYN	gynecology
ELT	endovenous laser ablation; endoluminal laser ablation	**H**	
Em	emmetropia	HAV	hepatitis A virus
EMG	electromyography	Hb, Hgb, hgb	hemoglobin
ENT	ears, nose, and throat	HBV	hepatitis B virus
EOM	extraocular movement	HCG	human chorionic gonadotropin
eos	eosinophil (type of white blood cell)	HCl	hydrochloric acid
		HCT, Hct	hematocrit
ERCP	endoscopic retrograde cholangiopancreatography	HCV	hepatitis C virus

Continued

Abbreviation	Meaning	Abbreviation	Meaning
HD	hemodialysis; hip disarticulation; hearing distance	IRDS	infant respiratory distress syndrome
HDL	high-density lipoprotein	IT	intensive therapy
HDN	hemolytic disease of the newborn	IUD	intrauterine device
HDV	hepatitis D virus	IUGR	intrauterine growth rate; intrauterine growth retardation
HEV	hepatitis E virus	IV	intravenous
HF	heart failure	IVC	intravenous cholangiogram; intravenous cholangiography
HIV	human immunodeficiency virus		
HMD	hyaline membrane disease	IVF	in vitro fertilization
HNP	herniated nucleus pulposus (herniated disk)	IVF-ET	in vitro fertilization and embryo transfer
H₂O	water	IVP	intravenous pyelography
HP	hemipelvectomy	K	
HPV	human papillomavirus	K	potassium (an electrolyte)
HRT	hormone replacement therapy	KD	knee disarticulation
h.s.*	at bedtime	KUB	kidney, ureter, bladder
hs*	half strength	L	
HSG	hysterosalpingography	L	liter
HSV	herpes simplex virus	L1, L2, and so on	first lumbar vertebra, second lumbar vertebra, and so on
HTN	hypertension		
Hx	history	LA	left atrium
I, J		LASIK	laser-assisted in situ keratomileusis
IAS	interatrial septum	LAT, lat	lateral
I&D	incision and drainage; irrigation and débridement	LBBB	left bundle branch block
IBD	inflammatory bowel disease	LD	lactate dehydrogenase; lactic acid dehydrogenase (cardiac enzyme)
IBS	irritable bowel syndrome	LDL	low-density lipoprotein
ICD	implantable cardioverter-defibrillator	LES	lower esophageal sphincter
ICP	intracranial pressure	LFT	liver function test
ICU	intensive care unit	LH	luteinizing hormone
ID	intradermal	LLQ	left lower quadrant
IDDM	insulin-dependent diabetes mellitus	LMP	last menstrual period
Ig	immunoglobulin	LOC	loss of consciousness
IM	intramuscular; infectious mononucleosis	LP	lumbar puncture
		LPR	laryngopharyngeal reflux
IMP	impression (synonymous with diagnosis)	LS	lumbosacral spine
		LSO	left salpingo-oophorectomy
IOL	intraocular lens	lt	left
IT	intensive therapy	LUQ	left upper quadrant
IVP	intravenous pyelogram; intravenous pyelography	LV	left ventricle
		lymphos	lymphocytes
IOP	intraocular pressure	M	
IPPB	intermittent positive-pressure breathing	MCH	mean cell hemoglobin (average amount of hemoglobin per red cell)

Abbreviation	Meaning	Abbreviation	Meaning
MCHC	mean cell hemoglobin concentration (average concentration of hemoglobin per red cell)	**O**	
		O₂	oxygen
MCV	mean cell volume (average volume or size per red cell)	OB	obstetrics
		OCP	oral contraceptive pill
MDI	metered-dose inhaler	O.D.	Doctor of Optometry
MEG	magnetoencephalography	OD	overdose
MG	myasthenia gravis	OD*	right eye
mg	milligram (1/1,000 of a gram)	OM	otitis media
mg/dl, mg/dL	milligram per deciliter	OP	outpatient; operative procedure
MI	myocardial infarction	OR	operating room
mix astig	mixed astigmatism	ORTH, ortho	orthopedics
ml, mL	milliliter (1/1,000 of a liter)	OS*	left eye; by mouth (pharmacology)
mm	millimeter (1/1,000 of a meter)	OSA	obstructive sleep apnea
mm Hg	millimeters of mercury	OU*	both eyes
MR	mitral regurgitation	**P**	
MRA	magnetic resonance angiogram; magnetic resonance angiography	P	phosphorus; pulse
MRI	magnetic resonance imaging	PA	posteroanterior; pernicious anemia; pulmonary artery; physician assistant
MS	mitral stenosis; musculoskeletal; multiple sclerosis; mental status; magnesium sulfate	PAC	premature atrial contraction
		Pap	Papanicolaou (test)
MSH	melanocyte-stimulating hormone	para 1, 2, 3, and so on	unipara, bipara, tripara, and so on (number of viable births)
MUGA	multiple-gated acquisition (scan)	PAT	paroxysmal atrial tachycardia
MVP	mitral valve prolapse	PBI	protein-bound iodine
MVR	mitral valve replacement; massive vitreous retraction (blade); microvitreoretinal	pc, p.c.*	after meals
		PCL	posterior cruciate ligament
		PCNL	percutaneous nephrolithotomy
Myop	myopia (nearsightedness)	PCO₂	partial pressure of carbon dioxide
N		PCP	*Pneumocystis* pneumonia; primary care physician
Na	sodium (an electrolyte)		
NB	newborn	PE	physical examination; pulmonary embolism; pressure-equalizing (tube)
NCV	nerve conduction velocity		
NG	nasogastric	PERRLA	pupils equal, round, and reactive to light and accommodation
NIDDM	non–insulin-dependent diabetes mellitus		
NIHL	noise-induced hearing loss	PET	positron emission tomography
NK	natural killer cell	PFT	pulmonary function test
NMT	nebulized mist treatment	PGH	pituitary growth hormone
NPO, n.p.o.*	nothing by mouth	pH	symbol for degree of acidity or alkalinity
NSAID	nonsteroidal anti-inflammatory drug		
NSR	normal sinus rhythm	PID	pelvic inflammatory disease

Continued

Abbreviation	Meaning	Abbreviation	Meaning
PIH	pregnancy-induced hypertension	RLQ	right lower quadrant
PKD	polycystic kidney disease	R/O	rule out
PMH	past medical history	ROM	range of motion
PMI	point of maximum impulse	RP	retrograde pyelogram; retrograde pyelography
PMN, PMNL	polymorphonuclear leukocyte		
PMP	previous menstrual period	RSO	right salpingo-oophorectomy
PMS	premenstrual syndrome	rt	right
PND	paroxysmal nocturnal dyspnea	RUQ	right upper quadrant
PNS	peripheral nervous system	RV	residual volume; right ventricle
p.o.*	by mouth	S	
PO_2	partial pressure of oxygen	S1, S2, and so on	first sacral vertebra, second sacral vertebra, and so on
poly	polymorphonuclear leukocyte		
post	posterior	SA, S-A	sinoatrial
p.r.n.*	as required	SaO_2	arterial oxygen saturation
PSA	prostate-specific antigen	SD	shoulder disarticulation
pt	patient	SIADH	syndrome of inappropriate antidiuretic hormone
PT	prothrombin time; physical therapy		
PTCA	percutaneous transluminal coronary angioplasty	SICS	small incision cataract surgery
		SIDS	sudden infant death syndrome
PTH	parathyroid hormone (also called parathormone)	SLE	systemic lupus erythematosus; slit-lamp examination
PTHC	percutaneous transhepatic cholangeography	SMAS	superficial musculoaponeurotic system (flap)
PTT	partial thromboplastin time	SNS	sympathetic nervous system
PUD	peptic ulcer disease	SOB	shortness of breath
PVC	premature ventricular contraction	sono	sonogram
Q		SPECT	single-photon emission computed tomography
q.2h.*	every 2 hours	sp. gr.	specific gravity
qAM*	every morning	ST	esotropia
q.d.*	every day	stat., STAT	immediately
q.h.*	every hour	STD	sexually transmitted disease
q.i.d.*	four times a day	STI	sexually transmitted infection
q.o.d.*	every other day	subcu, Sub-Q, subQ*	subcutaneous (injection)
qPM*	every evening	Sx	symptom
R		T	
RA	right atrium; rheumatoid arthritis	T1, T2, and so on	first thoracic vertebra, second thoracic vertebra, and so on
RAI	radioactive iodine	T_3	triiodothyronine (thyroid hormone)
RAIU	radioactive iodine uptake		
RBC, rbc	red blood cell	T_4	thyroxine (thyroid hormone)
RD	respiratory distress	T&A	tonsillectomy and adenoidectomy
RDS	respiratory distress syndrome	TAH	total abdominal hysterectomy
RF	rheumatoid factor; radiofrequency	TB	tuberculosis
RGB	Roux-en-Y gastric bypass	TFT	thyroid function test
RK	radial keratotomy	THA	total hip arthroplasty

Abbreviation	Meaning	Abbreviation	Meaning
ther	therapy	U&L, U/L	upper and lower
THR	total hip replacement	ung	ointment
TIA	transient ischemic attack	UPP	uvulopalatopharyngoplasty
t.i.d.*	three times a day	URI	upper respiratory infection
TKA	total knee arthroplasty	US	ultrasound; ultrasonography
TKR	total knee replacement	UTI	urinary tract infection
TPPV	trans pars plana vitrectomy	V	
TPR	temperature, pulse, and respiration	VA	visual acuity
TRAM	transverse rectus abdominis muscle	VC	vital capacity
		VCUG	voiding cystourethrography
TRUS	transrectal ultrasonography	VD	venereal disease
TSE	testicular self-examination	VF	visual field
TSH	thyroid-stimulating hormone	VSD	ventricular septal defect
TSS	toxic shock syndrome	VT	ventricular tachycardia
TURP	transurethral resection of the prostate	VUR	vesicoureteral reflux
TVH	total vaginal hysterectomy	W	
TVH-BSO	total vaginal hysterectomy–bilateral salpingo-oophorectomy	WBC, wbc	white blood cell
		WD	well-developed
Tx	treatment	WN	well-nourished
U		WNL	within normal limits
UA	urinalysis	X, Y, Z	
UC	uterine contractions	XP, XDP	xeroderma pigmentosum
UGI	upper gastrointestinal	XT	exotropia
UGIS	upper gastrointestinal series		

*Although these abbreviations are currently found in medical records and clinical notes, they are easily misinterpreted. Thus, the Joint Commission (formerly JCAHO) requires their discontinuance. Instead, they recommend to write out their meanings. For a summary of these abbreviations, see the table that follows.

Discontinued Abbreviations

The Joint Commission (JC) and the Institute for Safe Medication Practices (ISMP) report that the following abbreviations are commonly misinterpreted and have resulted in harmful medical errors. Both organizations have compiled a comprehensive "Do Not Use" list (available on their websites) for health-care providers.

To prevent harmful medical errors, both organizations recommend discontinuance of these abbreviations. Instead the abbreviations should be written out. Nevertheless, some of the abbreviations on the "Do Not Use" list are still used by health-care providers. A selected number are listed below.

Abbreviation	Meaning
Medication and Therapy Time Schedule	
a.c.	before meals
b.i.d.	twice a day
hs	half strength
h.s.	at bedtime
NPO, n.p.o.	nothing by mouth
p.c.	after meals
p.o.	by mouth (orally)
p.r.n.	as required
qAM	every morning
q.d.	every day
q.h.	every hour
q.2h.	every 2 hours
q.i.d.	four times a day
q.o.d.	every other day
qPM	every evening
t.i.d.	three times a day
Other Related Abbreviations	
AD	right ear
AS	left ear
AU	both ears
cc	cubic centimeter; same as milliliter (1/1,000 of a liter) *Use* mL *for milliliters or write out the meaning.*
dc, DC, D/C	discharge; discontinue
OD	right eye
OS	left eye
OU	both eyes
subcu, Sub-Q, subQ	subcutaneous (injection)
U	unit

COMMON SYMBOLS

The table below lists some common symbols used in health care and related fields.

Symbol	Meaning	Symbol	Meaning
@	at	−	minus, negative
āā	of each	±	plus or minus; either positive or negative; indefinite
′	foot	∅	no
″	inch	#	number; following a number; pounds
c̄	with	÷	divided by
Δ	change; heat	/	divided by
p̄	after	×	multiplied by; magnification
pH	degree of acidity or alkalinity	=	equals
R	prescription, treatment, therapy	≈	approximately equal
s̄	without	°	degree
→	to, in the direction of	%	percent
↑	increase(d), up	♀	female
↓	decrease(d), down	♂	male
+	plus, positive		

Medical Specialties

Medical Specialty	Medical Specialist	Description of Medical Specialty
Allergy	Allergist	Diagnosis and treatment of allergic disorders caused by hypersensitivity to foods, pollens, dusts, and medicines
Anesthesiology	Anesthesiologist	Administration of agents capable of bringing about loss of sensation with or without loss of consciousness
Cardiology	Cardiologist	Diagnosis and treatment of heart and vascular disorders
General practice (GP)	General practitioner (GP)	Coordination of total health-care delivery to all members of the family, regardless of sex, including counseling; also known as family medicine *GP encompasses several branches of medicine, including internal medicine, preventive medicine, pediatrics, surgery, obstetrics, and gynecology.*
Geriatrics	Gerontologist, Geriatrician	Understanding of the physiological characteristics of aging and the diagnosis and treatment of diseases affecting elderly patients; also known as gerontology
Gynecology	Gynecologist	Diagnosis and treatment of diseases of the female reproductive organs
Hematology	Hematologist	Diagnosis and treatment of diseases of the blood and blood-forming tissues
Immunology	Immunologist	Study of various elements of the immune system and their functions *Immunology includes treatment of immunodeficiency diseases such as AIDS, autoimmune diseases such as lupus erythematosus, allergies, and various cancer types related to the immune system.*
Internal medicine	Internist	Study of the physiological and pathological characteristics of internal organs and the diagnosis and treatment of these organs
Neonatology	Neonatologist	Care and treatment of neonates
Nephrology	Nephrologist	Diagnosis and management of kidney disease, kidney transplantation, and dialysis therapies
Neurosurgery	Neurosurgeon	Surgery of the brain, spinal cord, and peripheral nerves
Obstetrics	Obstetrician	Care of women during pregnancy, childbirth, and postnatal care
Oncology	Oncologist	Diagnosis, treatment, and prevention of cancer *Oncologists are internal medicine physicians who specialize in the treatment of solid tumors (such as carcinomas and sarcomas) and liquid tumors (including hematologic malignancies such as leukemias).*
Ophthalmology	Ophthalmologist	Diagnosis and treatment of eye diseases, including prescribing corrective lenses

Medical Specialty	Medical Specialist	Description of Medical Specialty
Optometry	Optometrist	Primary eye care, including testing the eyes for visual acuity, diagnosing and managing eye health, prescribing corrective lenses, and recommending eye exercises *An optometrist, licensed by the state, is not a medical doctor but is known as a Doctor of Optometry (OD).*
Orthopedics	Orthopedist	Prevention, diagnosis, care, and treatment of musculoskeletal disorders *Musculoskeletal disorders include injury to or disease of bones, joints, ligaments, muscles, and tendons.*
Otolaryngology	Otolaryngologist	Medical and surgical management of disorders of the ear, nose, and throat (ENT) and related structures of the head and neck
Pathology	Pathologist	Study and cause of disease *A pathologist usually specializes in autopsy or clinical or surgical pathology.*
Pediatrics	Pediatrician	Diagnosis and treatment of disease in infants, children, and adolescents
Plastic surgery	Plastic surgeon	Surgery to alter, replace, or restore a body structure due to a defect or for cosmetic reasons
Physiatry	Physiatrist	Prevention, diagnosis, and treatment of disease or injury and the rehabilitation from resultant impairment and disability; also called physical medicine *Physiatrists are physicians who use physical agents, such as light, heat, cold water, therapeutic exercise, mechanical apparatus, and, sometimes, pharmaceutical agents.*
Pulmonology	Pulmonologist	Diagnosis and treatment of diseases involving the lungs, their airways and blood vessels, and the chest wall (thoracic cage); also called pulmonary medicine
Psychiatry	Psychiatrist	Diagnosis, treatment, and prevention of disorders of the mind *Psychiatry is different from others discussed in this book because it deals with pathological conditions of the mind, an entity that is not considered a body system.*
Radiology	Radiologist	Diagnosis using x-ray and other diagnostic procedures, such as ultrasound (US), computed tomography (CT), and magnetic resonance imaging (MRI) *Radiology also employs various radiation techniques to treat disease through other subspecialties of radiology, such as interventional radiology and nuclear medicine.*
Rheumatology	Rheumatologist	Diagnosis and treatment of inflammatory and degenerative diseases of the joints
Surgery	Surgeon	Use of operative procedures to treat deformity, injury, and disease
Thoracic surgery	Thoracic surgeon	Use of operative procedures to treat disease or injury of the thoracic area
Urology	Urologist	Diagnosis and treatment of the male urinary and reproductive systems and the female urinary system

Glossary of English-to-Spanish Translations

This appendix provides guidelines to help health-care practitioners communicate with their Spanish-speaking patients. The following information includes selected terms commonly used in various medical specialties.

SPANISH SOUNDS

Although the spelling of some Spanish terms resembles English terms, the terms are still pronounced with a Spanish accent. Because of these similarities, the practitioner should learn the meaning and pronunciations of certain Spanish words. The first step in communicating with Spanish-speaking patients is to learn the Spanish sound system. This section provides Spanish pronunciations of vowels and consonants. The table below lists vowels and their Spanish pronunciations. Practice the pronunciations before continuing with the other information in this appendix.

Letter	Spanish Pronunciation Sounds Like
Vowels	
a	*ah* as in father
e	*eh* as in net
i	*ee* as in keep
o	*oh* as in no
u	*oo* as in spoon; silent following *q* or *g*
y	*ee* as in bee
Consonants	
c	*k* as in kitten (before *a, o, u,* and any consonant except *h*); *s* as in sit (before *e* or *i*); *k* after *e* or *i*
g	*h* as in hit (when followed by *e* or *i*); otherwise, like *g* as in gold
h	silent; never pronounced unless preceded by *c*
j	*h* as in hot
ll	*y* as in yellow
ñ	*ni* as in onion

Letter	Spanish Pronunciation Sounds Like
qu*	*k* as in kite
r	trilled *r*
rr*	strongly trilled *r*
v	*v* as in void
z	*s* as in sun

*Note: *qu* and *rr* are not consonants but, rather, sounds. As such, they are not part of the Spanish alphabet. We include them here purely as an aid in pronunciation for non–Spanish-speaking health-care providers.

EMPHASIS IN SPANISH

In the tables that follow, capitalization is used to indicate primary emphasis of Spanish words. The capital letters in the Spanish pronunciation column indicate that emphasis is placed on the capitalized syllable. You will note that some Spanish terms, such as *perspiración* and *úlcera,* have a diacritical mark above a vowel. This mark indicates emphasis that falls on a syllable other than the one predicted by the rules of Spanish pronunciation.

Although there are some exceptions to these rules, the suggested guidelines here will help you learn Spanish terms and pronunciations of selected key terms in each chapter. Start by reviewing English and Spanish terms, and then practice Spanish pronunciations by applying the English system of phonetics.

ADJECTIVE ENDINGS

Many Spanish adjectives change the last letter of the word to denote the gender of the noun being modified. If the noun is feminine, the letter will be *a;* for a masculine noun, the letter used is *o.* For example, the adjective *lenta* (slow) modifies a feminine noun. The same adjective when modifying a masculine noun ends with the letter *o,* so it would be *lento.* To change the gender of an adjective to correspond with the noun it modifies, change the ending vowel. For example, if the noun is masculine, change the ending vowel to *o.* The table below clearly identifies Spanish adjectives that should receive a specific gender.

ENGLISH-TO-SPANISH TRANSLATIONS

The following selected terms are used in the medical environment to denote anatomical structures and their functions; signs, symptoms, and diseases; and other related terms.

English	Spanish	Spanish Pronunciation
abdomen	abdomen	ab-DOH-men
adrenal gland	glándula adrenal	GLAN-doo-lah ah-dreh-NAHL
adrenaline	adrenalina	ah-dreh-nah-LEE-nah
allergy	alergia	ah-LEHR-hee-ah
alveolus	alvéolo	ahl-VEH-oh-loh
aneurysm	aneurisma	a-neh-oo-REES-mah
ankle	tobillo	toh-BEE-yoh
antacid	antiácido	ahn-tee-AH-see-doh
appendix	apéndice	ah-PEHN-dee-seh
appetite	apetito	ah-peh-TEE-toh
arm	brazo	BRAH-soh

Continued

English	Spanish	Spanish Pronunciation
artery	arteria	ahr-TEH-ree-ah
arthritis	artritis	ahr-TREE-tees
asphyxia	asfixia	ahs-FEEK-see-ah
asthma	asma	AHS-mah
belch	eructar	eh-rook-TAHR
belly	barriga	bahr-REE-gah
benign	benigno	beh-NEEG-noh
birth	nacimiento	nah-see-mee-EHN-toh
black	negra (feminine)	NEH-grah
	negro (masculine)	NEH-groh
bladder	vejiga	beh-HEE-gah
blepharospasm	blefaroespasmo	bleh-fah-roh-ehs-PAHS-moh
blister	ampolla	am-PO-yah
blood	sangre	SAHN-greh
blood clot	coágulo de sangre	koh-AH-goo-loh deh SAHN-greh
blood pressure	presión sanguínea	preh-see-OHN san-GEE-neh-ah
blue	azul	ah-SOOL
bones	huesos	oo-EH-sohs
brain	cerebro	seh-REH-broh
breast	pecho	PEH-cho
breathe	respirar	rehs-pee-RAHR
breathing	respiración	rehs-pee-rah-see-OHN
bronchus	bronquios	BROHN-kee-ohs
brown	marrón	mahr-ROHN
	OR	
	café	cah-FAY
burn	quemar	keh-MAHR
calcium	calcio	KAHL-see-oh
calculus	cálculo	KAHL-coo-loh
capillary	capilar	kah-pee-LAHR
cartilage	cartílago	kahr-TEE-lah-goh
catheter	catéter	kah-TEH-tehr
catheterization	cateterización	kah-teh-teh-ree-sah-see-OHN
cerumen	cera de los oídos	CEH-rah deh lohs oh-EE-dohs
cervix	cervix	SERH-beex
cesarean section	cesárea	seh-SAH-reh-ah
chew	masticar	mahs-tee-KAHR
choroidopathy	coroidopatía	coh-roh-ee-doh-pah-TEE-ah

English	Spanish	Spanish Pronunciation
circumcision	circuncisión	seer-koon-see-see-OHN
clear	clara (feminine)	KLAH-rah
	claro (masculine)	KLAH-roh
cloudy	nublado	noo-BLAH-doh
collarbone	clavícula	klah-BEE-coo-lah
colon	colon	KOH-lohn
colonoscopy	colonoscopia	koh-loh-nohs-koh-PEE-ah
conception	concepción	khon-sehp-see-OHN
concussion	concusión	kohn-koo-see-OHN
condom	condón	kohn-DOHN
conscious	consciente	kohns-see-EHN-teh
constipation	estreñimiento	ehs-treh-nyee-mee-EHN-toh
cough	toser	toh-SEHR
cystoscopy	cistoscopia	sees-toh-scoh-PEE-ah
dark	obscuro	obs-COO-roh
deafness	sordera	sohr-DEH-rah
defecate	defecar	deh-feh-KAHR
dermatology	dermatologia	der-mah-to-lo-HEE-ah
diabetes	diabetes	dee-ah-BEH-tehs
dialysis	diálisis	dee-AH-lee-sees
diaphragm	diafragma	de-ah-FRAHG-mah
diarrhea	diarrea	dee-ah-RREH-ah
digestion	digestión	dee-hes-tee-OHN
diplopia	diplopia	dee-ploh-PEE-ah
diuretic	diurético	dee-oo-REH-tee-coh
dizzy	mareado	mah-reh-AH-doh
dyspepsia	dispepsia	dees-PEHP-see-ah
dysphagia	disfagia	dees-FAH-hee-ah
dysuria	disuria	dee-SOO-ree-ah
eardrum	tímpano del oído	TEEM-pah-noh dehl oh-EE-doh
ears	oídos	oh-EE-dohs
encephalopathy	encefalopatía	ehn-ceh-fah-loh-pah-TEE-ah
endometriosis	endometriosis	ehn-doh-meh-tree-OH-sees
epiglottis	epiglotis	eh-pee-GLOH-tees
epilepsy	epilepsia	eh-pee-LEHP-see-ah
erection	erección	eh-rek-see-OHN
esophagus	esófago	eh-SOH-fah-goh

Continued

English	Spanish	Spanish Pronunciation
excretion	excreción	ex-kreh-see-OHN
eyelid	párpado	PAHR-pah-doh
eyes	ojos	OH-hohs
fainting	desmayo	dehs-MAH-yoh
fracture	fractura	frahk-TOO-rah
gallbladder	vesícula biliar	beh-SEE-koo-lah bee-lee-AHR
gallstone	cálculo biliar	KAHL-koo-loh bee-lee-AHR
genitalia	genitalia	heh-nee-TAH-lee-ah
glucose	glucosa	gloo-KO-sah
goiter	bocio	BOH-see-oh
gums	encia	ehn-SEE-ah
hair	pelo	PEH-loh
hardening	endurecimiento	en-doo-reh-see-mee-EHN-toh
heart	corazón	koh-rah-SOHN
heart attack	ataque al corazón *OR* ataque cardíaco	ah-TAH-keh ahl koh-rah-SOHN ah-TAH-keh kar-DEE-ah-koh
heart rate	ritmo cardíaco	REET-moh kar-DEE-ah-koh
hematuria	hematuria	eh-mah-TOO-ree-ah
hernia	hernia	EHR-nee-ah
herniated disk	disco herniado	DEES-coh ehr-nee-AH-doh
hip	cadera	kah-DEH-rah
hormone replacement	reemplazo de hormonas	reh-ehm-PLAH-soh deh or-MOH-nahs
hyperopia	hiperopía	ee-pehr-oh-PEE-ah
hysterectomy	histerectomía	ees-teh-rek-toh-MEE-ah
impotency	impotencia	eem-poh-TEHN-see-ah
influenza	influenza	een-floo-EHN-sah
inner ear	oído interior	oh-EE-doh een-teh-ree-OHR
insulin	insulina	in-soo-LEE-nah
intestine	intestino	een-tehs-TEE-noh
iodine	yodo	YOH-doh
iris	iris	EE-rees
jaundice	ictericia	eek-teh-REE-see-ah
joint	coyunturas	ko-yoon-TOO-rahs
kidney	riñón	ree-NYOHN
knee	rodilla	roh-DEE-yah
kneecap	rótula	ROH-too-lah

English	Spanish	Spanish Pronunciation
laparoscopy	laparoscopía	lah-pah-rohs-KOH-pee-ah
larynx	laringe	lah-REEN-heh
leukorrhea	leucorrea	leh-oo-koh-RREH-ah
ligament	ligamento	lee-gah-MEHN-toh
light	luz	loos
liver	hígado	EE-gah-doh
lobe	lóbulo	LOH-boo-loh
lungs	pulmones	pool-MOH-nehs
lymph	linfa	LEEN-fah
lymph node	nódulo linfatico	NOH-doo-loh leen-FAH-tee-coh
lymphatic	linfático	leen-FAH-tee-coh
macular degeneration	degeneración macular	deh-heh-neh-rah-see-OHN mah-coo-LAHR
malignant	maligno	mah-LEEG-noh
mammogram	mamografía	mah-moh-grah-FEE-ah
masculine	masculino	mahs-koo-LEE-noh
menopause	menopausia	meh-noh-PAH-oo-see-ah
menstruation	menstruación	mehns-troo-ah-see-OHN
mouth	boca	BOH-kah
movement	movimiento	moh-bee-mee-EHN-toh
muscle	músculo	MOOS-koo-loh
myopia	miopía	mee-o-PEE-ah
nails	sarpullidos	sar-pooh-YEE-dohs
nerve	nervio	NER-bee-oh
newborn	recién nacida (feminine) recién nacido (masculine)	re-see-EHN nah-SEE-dah re-see-EHN nah-SEE-doh
nocturia	nocturia	nok-TOO-ree-ah
nose	nariz	nah-REES
nostril	orificio de la nariz	o-ree-FEE-see-oh deh lah nah-REES
obstruction	obstrucción	obs-trook-see-OHN
oliguria	oliguria	oh-lee-GOO-ree-ah
ophthalmoscopy	oftalmoscopía	ohf-tahl-mohs-coh-PEE-ah
otalgia	otalgía	oh-tahl-HEE-ah
otitis media	otitis media	oh-TEE-tees MEH-dee-ah
otoscope	otoscopio	oh-tohs-COH-pee-oh
otoscopy	otoscopía	oh-tohs-coh-PEE-ah
ovary	ovario	oh-BAH-ree-oh
pain	dolor	doh-LOHR

Continued

English	Spanish	Spanish Pronunciation
pancreas	páncreas	PAHN-kreh-ahs
paralysis	parálisis	pah-RAH-lee-sees
penis	pene	PEH-neh
perspiration	perspiración	pehr-spee-rah-see-OHN
pink	rosada (female)	roh-SAH-dah
	rosado (male)	roh-SAH-doh
pituitary	pituitaria	pee-too-ee-TAH-ree-ah
pneumonia	pulmonía	pool-moh-NEE-ah
pregnant	embarazada	ehm-bah-rah-SAH-dah
prostate	próstata	PROHS-tah-tah
protein	proteína	proh-teh-EE-nah
pulse	pulso	POOL-soh
rapid	rápida (feminine)	RAH-pee-dah
	rápido (masculine)	RAH-pee-doh
rectum	recto	REHK-toh
reduction	reducción	reh-dook-see-OHN
renal pelvis	pelvis renal	PEHL-bees reh-NAHL
retina	retina	reh-TEE-nah
retinitis	retinitis	reh-tee-NEE-tees
rhythm	ritmo	REET-moh
rib	costilla	coh-STEE-yah
sacrum	sacro	SAH-croh
sclera	esclera	es-KLEH-rah
seizure	convulsion	con-vuhl-see-OHN
	OR	
	ataque de apoplejía	ah-TAH-keh deh ah-pohp-leh-HEE-uh
sensation	sensación	sen-sah-see-OHN
sexual intercourse	coito	KOH-ee-toh
shoulder	hombro	OHM-broh
sigmoidoscopy	sigmoidoscopia	seeg-moh-ee-doh-SKOH-pee-ah
sinus	seno	SEH-noh
skin	piel	pee-EHL
slow	lenta (feminine)	LEHN-tah
	lento (masculine)	LEHN-toh
sore	llaga	YAH-gah
	OR	
	úlcera	OOL-seh-rah
spinal column	espina dorsal	ehs-PEE-nah dohr-SAHL

English	Spanish	Spanish Pronunciation
sprain	torcer	tohr-SEHR
sputum	esputo	ehs-POO-toh
sternum	esternón	ehs-tehr-NOHN
stiff	dura (feminine)	DOO-rah
	duro (masculine)	DOO-roh
stomach	estómago	es-TOH-mah-goh
stroke	ataque	ah-TAH-keh
stroke	ataque cerebral	ah-TAH-keh seh-reh-BRAHL
support	soporte	soh-POHR-teh
swallow	tragar	trah-GAHR
symptom	síntoma	SEEN-toh-mah
syncope	síncope	SEEN-coh-peh
teeth	diente	dee-EHN-teh
tendon	tendón	tehn-DOHN
testicle	testículo	tehs-TEE-koo-loh
thigh	muslo	MOOS-loh
thyroid	tiroides	tee-ROH-ee-dehs
tinnitus	tinitus	tee-NEE-toos
tissue	tejido	teh-HEE-doh
toe, finger	dedo	DEH-doh
tonsil	amígdala	ah-MEEG-dah-lah
trachea	tráquea	TRAH-keh-ah
ulcer	úlcera	OOL-seh-rah
ultrasonography	ultrasonografía	ool-trah-soh-noh-grah-FEE-ah
unconscious	inconsciente	een-kons-see-EHN-teh
ureter	uréter	oo-REH-tehr
urethra	uretra	oo-REH-trah
urinalysis	urinálisis	oo-ree-NAH-lee-sees
urinary	urinario	oo-ree-NAH-ree-oh
urinary tract infection	infección del tracto urinario	een-fek-see-OHN dehl TRAK-toh oo-ree-NAH-ree-oh
urinate	orinar	oh-ree-NAHR
urine	orina	oh-REE-nah
urology	urología	ooh-roh-loh-HEE-ah
uterus	útero	OO-teh-roh
vagina	vagina	bah-HEE-nah

Continued

English	Spanish	Spanish Pronunciation
valve	válvula	BAHL-boo-lah
varicose vein	vena varicosa	BEH-nah bah-ree-KOH-sah
vein	vena	BEH-nah
ventricle	ventrículo	behn-TREE-koo-loh
vertebrae	vértebra	BEHR-teh-brah
vision	visión	bee-see-OHN
voice	voz	bohs
vomit	vómito	BOH-mee-toh
wound	herida	eh-REE-dah
wrist	muñeca	moo-NYEH-kah
x-ray	rayos equis *OR* radiografía	RAH-yohs EH-kees rah-dee-oh-grah-FEE-yah
yellow	amarilla (feminine) amarillo (masculine)	ah-mah-REE-yah ah-mah-REE-yoh

INDEX

Note: An "f" following a page number indicates a figure; a "t" following a page number indicates a table.

A

Abbreviations, 613–621
  body structure, 50
  cardiovascular and lymphatic systems, 189
  digestive system, 255
  ear, 525
  endocrine system, 429
  eye, 525
  integumentary system, 84
  musculoskeletal system, 486
  nervous system, 429
  radiology, 50
  reproductive system, 366
  respiratory system, 132
  urinary system, 305
Abdomen, 402
  quadrants of, 45–46, 45f
Abdominal adhesions, 50f
Abdominal cavity, 45
Abdominopelvic cavity, 45
Abdominopelvic quadrants, 45–46, 45f
Abdominopelvic regions, 45f, 46–48
Abnormal condition, 224, 244, 253
Abrasion, 84
Abscess, 84
Accessory glands, 354
Accessory organs of digestion, 245–254
Achilles tendon, 459
Achromatopsia, 525
Acidosis, 133
Acne, 84, 85f
Acoustic, 518
Acoustic neuroma, 529
Acquired immunodeficiency syndrome
  (AIDS), 82, 84, 129, 193
Acromegaly, 404
Acute renal failure (ARF), 303
Acute respiratory distress syndrome, 133
Addison disease, 429
Adduction, 38
Adenocarcinoma, 295
Adenodynia, 295
Adenohypophysis, 402–403, 404
Adenoidectomy, 109
Adenoids, 109
Adenoma, 71, 295, 396
Adenopathy, 182
Adhesion, 50, 50f
Adipectomy, 71
Adipocele, 64, 76
Adipoid, 343
Adipoma, 71
Adipose tissue, 348
Adrenal cortex, 404, 411
Adrenalectomy, 396, 410
Adrenal glands, 287, 396, 410, 446
Adrenal hormones, 410, 411t
Adrenaline, 410
Adrenal medulla, 411
Adrenocorticotropic hormone (ACTH), 404,
  429
Adrenomegaly, 410

Adventitious breath sounds, 133
Aerohydrotherapy, 114
Aerophagia, 110, 112, 231
Aerophobia, 127
Aerotherapy, 114
Agglutination, 182
AIDS, 82, 84, 129, 193
Air pressure, 520
Albinism, 70, 78
Aldosteronism, 411
Alimentary canal, 217
Allograft, 91
Alopecia, 85
Alveolar, 109
Alveolus(i), 109, 121
Alzheimer disease, 431
Amblyopia, 509
Amniocentesis, 332, 372, 372f
Amnion, 332
Amniotic sac, 332
Amphiarthroses, 474
Amyotrophic lateral sclerosis (ALS), 431
Anacusis, 518, 529
Anal fistula, 257
Anaphylaxis, 182
Anastomosis, 54, 54f, 237
Anatomic position, 34
Androgen(s), 354
Androsterone, 354
Anesthesia, 363
Anesthetics, 438
Aneurysm, 157, 181, 181f
Aneurysmectomy, 426
Aneurysmorrhaphy, 157
Angina pectoris, 190
Angiocarditis, 184
Angiography, 157, 194
Angioma, 168
Angioplasty, 184, 198, 198f
Angiorrhaphy, 184
Angiorrhexis, 184
Anhidrosis, 74
Anisocoria, 508
Ankylosing spondylitis, 463, 490
Ankylosis, 464, 489
Anorchia, 369
Anorchism, 369
Anorexia, 220
Anosmia, 110
Anoxia, 134
Answer key, 558–603
Antacids, 263
Anterior, 34, 35, 36, 400, 401, 402, 458
Anterolateral, 36
Anteroposterior, 401–402
Antiarrhythmics, 202
Antibiotics, 92, 313
Anticoagulants, 180, 202
Anticonvulsants, 438
Antidiarrheals, 263
Antidiuretic hormone (ADH), 404
Antiemetics, 263
Antifungals, 92, 379

Antiglaucoma drugs, 535
Antihypertensives, 202
Antiparkinsonian agents, 438
Antipruritics, 92
Antipsychotics, 438
Antispasmodics, 313
Anuria, 300
Anus, 233, 239, 241
Aorta, 157, 162, 169, 181
Aortic aneurysm, 181
Aortic stenosis, 169
Aortic valve, 169, 171
Aortopathy, 169
Aortostenosis, 157
Aphasia, 419
Aplasia, 362
Apnea, 110, 124, 125
Appendectomy, 233, 255, 256f
Appendicitis, 233, 255
Appendix, 233, 255
Aqueous humor, 511
Arachnoid, 424
Arachnoid membrane, 422
Areola, 348
Arm bone, upper, 463
Arrhythmia, 164, 190
Arterial blood gas, 136
Arterial calculus, 167
Arterial hardening, 167
Arterial spasm, 167
Arteriole(s), 157, 169, 282
Arteriolith, 167
Arteriopathy, 168
Arteriorrhaphy, 168
Arteriosclerosis, 157, 158, 168, 169, 170, 178,
  179
Arteriospasm, 168, 170
Artery(ies), 157, 168, 169. *See also specific*
  arteries
  hardening of, 169, 170, 178, 179
Arthralgia, 475
Arthritis, 464, 474, 475–476
Arthrocentesis, 474, 475, 476, 492
Arthroclasia, 465
Arthrodesis, 465
Arthrodynia, 476
Arthropathy, 474
Arthroplasty, 475, 475f, 492
  total hip, 475, 475f
Arthroscope, 474
Arthroscopy, 474, 474f
Articulate, 474
Articulation, 483
Ascending colon, 238, 239
Ascites, 255, 256f
Aspermatism, 358
Aspermia, 355
Aspirate, 122
Asthma, 129, 130f
Astigmatism, 516f, 525
Atelectasis, 4, 110
Atheroma, 157
Atherosclerosis, 178, 179, 180, 191f

Athlete's foot, 224
Atrial, 162, 174
Atrial flutter, 164
Atrioventricular, 157, 174
Atrioventricular (AV) block, 191
Atrioventricular (AV) node, 174
Atrium, 157, 162, 163, 165, 174
Atrophy, 429
Audiogram, 532
Audiologist, 507, 522
Audiology, 522
Audiometer, 518, 532
Audiometry, 531
Auditory, 518
Auditory tube, 333, 518, 520
Auricle, 519
Autografts, 82, 91
Automatic external defibrillator, 199
Automatic implantable cardioverter-
    defibrillator, 199, 200f
Autorhythmicity, 457
Axillary dissection, 376
Axillary nodes, 181, 184
Axon terminal synapse, 418f
Azotemia, 281, 307
Azoturia, 305

B

Backbone, 463, 476, 482
Bacterium, 164, 165
Bacteriuria, 290
Balanitis, 355, 369
Baldness, 85
Balloon expander, 377
Bariatric surgery, 262, 262f
Barium enema, 260, 260f
Barium swallow, 260
Bartholin glands, 97, 345
Basal cell carcinoma, 80, 81f
Basal layer of skin, 64f, 68
Bedsore, 68
Bell palsy, 432
Belly side, 425
Benign prostatic hyperplasia (BPH), 359,
    360f, 377
Benign prostatic hypertrophy (BPH), 359,
    360f, 377
Benign, 295
Beta blockers, 202
Bilateral, 363
Bilateral vasectomy, evaluation, 384
    terminology, 383–384
Bile, 244, 247, 248
Bile duct, 244, 249, 252
Bile vessel, 244
Biliary colic, 251
Biopsy, 136, 350, 375
Blackhead, 73, 84
Black lung, 122
Bladder, 280, 289–295, 343
Bleeding, postmenopausal, 381–382
Blepharectomy, 514
Blepharoplasty, 514, 516
Blepharoplegia, 514
Blepharoptosis, 509, 516
Blepharospasm, 508, 514, 516
Blepharotomy, 514

Blood clot, 157, 180, 425, 426
Blood condition, 280
Blood flow, through heart, 166–171
Blood urea nitrogen (BUN), 307
Blood vessel(s), 156, 156f
    renal, 282
    widened, 157, 426
Body, cavities of, 42f, 44–45
    cellular level of, 27
    levels of structural organization in,
        28f
    movements of, 459, 460f
    organization of, 28f, 29–30
    planes of, 35f, 41–44
    regions of, 40
Body structure, 27–61
    word elements, 56–57
Bolus, 226
Bone cell, 465
Bone densitometry, 492
Bone density test, 492
Bone marrow, 419, 424, 425, 464, 471
Bone marrow aspiration biopsy, 197
Bone marrow transplant (BMT), 201
Bone reabsorption inhibitors, 493
Bone(s), 404, 409, 462, 465, 487–490.
    See also specific bones
    of lower extremities, 463–464
    of upper extremities, 463
    structure and function of, 455,
        466–472
    types of, 466–467
Bone scan, 492
Borborygmus, 255
Bowel movement, 225
Bowman capsule, 297
Bradycardia, 165, 177
Bradyphagia, 165
Bradypnea, 165
Brain, 420–422, 421f, 478
Brainstem, 421
Breast, 332, 347–349, 349f, 376–377,
    404
Breastbone, 463, 476
Breast cancer, 348, 350, 376
Breath sounds, 133
Bronchial, 128
Bronchial tree, 118
Bronchiectasis, 109
Bronchiole(s), 109, 118
Bronchiolitis, 109
Bronchitis, 120, 128, 129
Bronchodilators, 139, 140f
Bronchopneumonia, 128
Bronchoscope, 109
Bronchoscopy, 136, 137f, 144–146
Bronchospasm, 120
Bronchostenosis, 120
Bronchus(i), 109, 118, 119
Bruit, 190
Bulbourethral glands, 354, 358
Bulla, 88f
Bundle branches, 174
Bundle of His, 174
Bunion, 487, 487f
Bursae, 480
Butterfly rash, of systemic lupus
    erythematosus, 194f

C

C1-C5, 482
Calcaneodynia, 463
Calcaneum, 463, 476
Calcemia, 407, 409, 470
Calcitonin, 407
Calcium, 396, 407, 470
Calculus(i), 244, 248, 250, 281, 284, 358
Canal of Schlemm, 511, 526, 527f
Cancer (CA), 114, 230, 251
    of breast, 348, 350, 376
    of lung, 123, 135
    of pancreas, 251
    of prostate, 361–362, 377
    renal, 284
Candida albicans, 366
Candidiasis, 366
Capillaries, 169, 170
Carbon dioxide (CO2), 120, 121, 122
Carbuncle, 84, 85f
Carcinoma(s), 81, 230, 242
    papillary, 142, 143–144
Carcinophobia, 426
Carcinosarcoma of esophagus, evaluation,
    268
    terminology, 267
Cardiac, 34, 169, 179
Cardiac catheterization, 194, 195f, 206–207
    medical records, 206
Cardiac center, 422
Cardiac cycle, 176–181
Cardiac enzyme studies, 194
Cardiac muscle fibers, 457
Cardiac tamponade, 160
Cardiography, 195
Cardiologist, 155
    interventional, 155
    pediatric, 155
Cardiology, 155
Cardiomegaly, 157, 177
Cardiothoracic surgeon, 155
Cardiovascular system, 156f, 159–181
    abbreviations, 189
    diagnostic procedures, 194–197
    diseases and conditions, 190–193
    therapeutic procedures, 198–200
    word elements, 208–209
Cardioversion, 199
Cardium, 165
Carotid artery, 191f
    atherosclerosis of, 179f
    doppler ultrasonography of, 197f
Carotid endarterectomy, 200, 201f
Carpal tunnel syndrome, 487
Carpoptosis, 463
Carpus, 463, 476
Cartilage, 118, 456, 464, 469, 481
Cataract, 526
Cataract surgery, 533
Catheterization, 309, 310f
Caudal, 38
Cauterize, 54
Cecum, 239
Cell(s), 78–82, 411, 413, 425, 465
    body organization and, 31–32
Cellular necrosis, 82
Central nervous system (CNS), 417–418

Cephalad, 37
Cephalagia, 477
Cephalodynia, 477
Cephalometer, 478
Cerclage, 375
Cerebellum, 421, 421f
Cerebral, 421
Cerebral aneurysm, 181
Cerebral palsy, 432
Cerebrospinal, 419, 424
Cerebrospinal fluid (CSF), 422, 424, 429, 436, 436f
Cerebrotomy, 421
Cerebrovascular accident (CVA), 426
Cerebrum, 419, 426, 432
Cervical, 346, 463, 482
Cervical nerves, 422
Cervical nodes, 181, 184
Cervical vertebra(ae), 482
Cervicitis, 332, 345
Cervix, 345
Cervix uteri, 332, 345, 463
Cesarean section (CS, C-section), 352
Chemabrasion, 92
Chemical peel, 92
Chest plate, 480
Chest radiograph, 52f
Childbirth, 333
Chiropractic medicine, 454
Chiropractor, 454
Chlamydia, 351, 371
Cholangiography, 249
Cholangiole, 244
Cholecyst, 248, 250
Cholecystalgia, 251
Cholecystectomy, 244, 251
Cholecystitis, 248, 250, 251
Cholecystodynia, 251
Cholecystolith, 248
Cholecystolithiasis, 250, 251
Choledoch, 249
Choledochitis, 249
Choledocholith, 249
Choledocholithiasis, 249, 252f
Choledochoplasty, 249, 252
Choledochorrhaphy, 249
Choledochotomy, 244, 249
Cholelith, 244, 248, 250, 252f
Cholelithiasis, 244, 252f
Cholemesis, 247
Chondritis, 118, 469
Chondrocyte, 469
Chondrogenesis, 469
Chondroma, 118, 469
Chondropathy, 118
Chondroplasty, 118
Chondrotomy, 456
Chordae tendineae, 171
Choroid, 508, 512
Choroiditis, 512
Choroidopathy, 508, 512
Chromaffin cell tumor, 431
Chronic obstructive pulmonary disease (COPD), 129, 130f
Ciliary body, 512
Ciliated epithelium, 112
Circulation, 161
Circulatory system. See Cardiovascular system

Circumcision, 377
Circumscribed, 95
Cirrhosis, 256
Clitoris, 345
Close, 515
Closed angle glaucoma, 526
Closed fracture, 479
Clot(s), 425, 426
Clubfoot, 490, 490f
Clumping, 182
Coccygeal nerve, 422
Coccyx, 484
Cochlea, 520
Cochlear implant, 534
Colectomy, 233, 238
Colitis, 238, 258
Collecting tubule, 297
Colles fracture, 479
Colon, 233, 235f, 238, 242
Colonoscope, 242
Colonoscopy, 233, 241, 242, 242f, 261
Color blindness, 525
Colorrhaphy, 238
Colors, combining forms denoting, 78–85
Coloscopy, 241
Colostomy, 225, 238, 239f
Colotomy, 238
Colpalgia, 341
Colpitis, 340–341
Colpocele, 332
Colpocervical, 345
Colpocystocele, 343
Colpodynia, 341
Colpohysterectomy, 343
Colpopexy, 341
Colpoptosis, 341
Colporrhagia, 342
Colporrhaphy, 341
Colposcope, 332, 346, 372
Colposcopy, 262, 332, 346, 372, 373f
Colpospasm, 341
Combining form(s), body structure, 56
    cardiovascular system, 157–158, 173, 188
    creation of, 5–7
    denoting colors, 83
    digestive system, 222, 243, 244, 254
    ears, 518
    eyes, 508–509
    female reproductive system, 332–333
    integumentary system, 64–65
    lymphatic system, 182
    muscles, 455–457
    respiratory tract, 147
    skeletal, 463–465
    urinary system, 320
Combining vowel, 222
Comedo, 73, 84
Comminuted fracture, 479
Common bile duct, 244, 245, 247
Compact bone, 467
Complicated fracture, 479
Compound fracture, 479
Compound nevus, medical record, 95–96
Computed tomography (CT) scan, 52f, 53f, 136, 260, 308
Congestive heart failure (CHF), 192
Conjunctiva, 508, 514
Conjunctivitis, 508, 514

Connective tissue, 456
Continence, 303
Continuous positive airway pressure (CPAP), 124
Contraceptives, 379
Contraction, 177
Contracture, 487
Contusion, 86
Convergent strabismus, 528f, 529
Convulsion, 434
Copulatory organ, 354
Coreometer, 508
Cornea, 508, 511, 513
    hard, 73
Corneal transplant, 508, 533
Corneitis, 508
Coronal, 42, 43
Coronary, 157
Coronary artery bypass graft (CABG), 199, 199f
Coronary artery disease (CAD), 178, 178f
Corticosteroids, 92, 139
Cortisol, 429
Coryza, 134
Costalgia, 479
Costochondritis, 464
Cowper glands, 354, 358
Cranial cavity, 44, 45
Craniotomy, 438, 463
Cranium, 463, 476
Creatinine clearance, 307
Crepitation, 487
Crib death, 135
Crohn disease, 238, 258
Crooked, 464
Cross-eye, 528, 528f
Cross-sectional, 43
Croup, 133, 134
Crusting, 95
Cryosurgery, 91
Cryotherapy, 66
Cryptorchidism, 355, 369
C-section, 352
CT scan. see Computed tomography (CT) scan
Culture & sensitivity, 51
Curet, 340
Cushing syndrome, 411, 412f, 429
Cusp, 171
Cutaneous, 34, 64, 253
Cutaneous laser, 92
Cyanoderma, 78, 80
Cyanosis, 80, 110
Cyst, 85, 302, 488
Cystic, 247
Cystic duct, 246
Cystic fibrosis, 134
Cystitis, 290, 294
    evaluation, 316
    medical records, 315–316
    terminology, 315
Cystocele, 280, 291, 291f
Cystolith, 290
Cystolithiasis, 290
Cystolithotomy, 290
Cystorrhaphy, 290
Cystoscope, 292
Cystoscopy, 280, 292, 292f

Cystourethrography, 309
Cystourethroscope, 294
Cystourography, 309
Cytology, 78, 79
Cytotoxic T lymphocytes, 187

D

Dacryadenalgia, 517
Dacryadenitis, 518
Dacryorrhea, 509, 516
Deafness, 518, 522, 529
Debridement, 91
Decubitus ulcer, 89
Deep vein thrombosis, 190
Defibrillators, 199
Dementia, 431
Dentist, 219, 225
Dentistry, 225
Deoxygenated, 162
Dermabrasion, 92
Dermatitis, 68, 72
Dermatologist, 63, 68, 72
Dermatology, 63–67, 73
Dermatoma, 72
Dermatome, 82
Dermatomycosis, 65, 74
Dermatopathy, 68, 72
Dermatoplasty, 66, 72
Dermis, 64f, 67, 68
Dermoid, 66
Dermopathy, 75
Descending colon, 238
Diabetes mellitus, 97, 396, 397, 414, 430
    evaluation, 441–442
    terminology, 440–441
    type 1, 414, 430
    type 2, 414, 430
Diabetic retinopathy, 526
Diagnosis, 225
Diagnostic procedures, 604–605
Diagnostic suffixes, 18
Diagnostic terms, 51–54
Dialysis, 278, 281, 310
Diaphoresis, 66, 74, 97
Diaphragm, 42f, 44, 126, 127f, 457
Diaphysis, 465, 467
Diarrhea, 220, 240
Diarthroses, 474
Diastole, 176
Dictionary, 337
Digestion, 220, 231
Digestive system, 217–276, 218f
    abbreviations, 255
    accessory organs of, 245–254
    combining forms, 222, 243, 244, 254, 269
    diagnostic procedures, 260–261
    diseases and conditions, 255–260
    therapeutic terms, 262–263
    word elements, 269–270
Digital rectal examination (DRE), 374,
    375f
Dilation, 110
Dilation and curettage (D&C), 340, 340f,
    375
Diplopia, 509, 515, 529
Directional terms, 32–41
Diseases. *See specific disease*

Disk, ruptured, 484
Distal, 38, 301, 469
Distal epiphysis, 468, 470
Diuresis, 306
Diuretics, 202, 287, 313
Divergent strabismus, 528f, 529
Diverticula, 257
Diverticular disease, 257, 257f
Doppler ultrasonography, 197, 197f
Dorsal, 32, 33, 34
Dropped wrist, 463
Drug classifications, 607–612
Dual energy x-ray absorptiometry (DEXA),
    492
Duchenne dystrophy, 486
Duct, 158
Ductus deferens, 354, 358
Duodenectomy, 235, 237
Duodenorrhaphy, 237
Duodenoscopy, 228, 261
Duodenostomy, 233, 236
Duodenotomy, 236, 237
Duodenum, 228, 233, 234, 235, 236, 237,
    245, 247f
Dura matter, 422, 424
Dwarfisme, 398, 403
Dx, 97
Dysentery, 257
Dysmenorrhea, 346
Dyspepsia, 220, 231
Dysphagia, 220, 231
Dysplasia, 362
Dyspnea, 125
Dysrhythmia, 190
Dystocia, 333
Dysuria, 290, 294

E

Earache, 519
Ear canal, 519
Eardrum, 518, 519, 520
Ear irrigation, 534, 534f
Ear(s), 517–524
    abbreviations, 525
    diagnostic procedures, 532
    inner, 521f
    path of vibrations, 521f
    pathological terms, 529–530
    structures of, 520, 521f
    therapeutic procedures, 534–535
Ecchymosis, 86, 86f
ECG, 176
E chart, 531, 531f
Echo. *See* Ultrasonography (US)
Echocardiography, 195
Eclampsia, 368
Ectopic pregnancy, 366, 367f
Eczema, 85, 86f
Edema, 287, 298
Ejaculate, 355
Ejaculatory duct, 354
EKG, 176
Electrical, 174
Electricity, 174
Electrocardiogram, 158, 175f, 176, 177
Electrocardiograph, 158
Electrocardiography, 158, 176, 195

Electroencephalography (EEG), 436
Elements of medical words, 548–557
ELISA, 197
Embolus(i), 190, 425, 426
Emmetropia, 515, 516f
Emotional illness, 426–427
Emphysema, 129, 130f, 135
Empyema, 134
Encephalitis, 419, 420, 478
Encephalocele, 478
Encephaloma, 420, 478
Encephalomalacia, 478
Endarterectomy, 200
Endocardium, 158, 159, 160, 171
Endocrine glands, 394, 395f
Endocrine system, 393–417
    abbreviations, 429
    diagnostic procedures, 435
    diseases and conditions, 429–431
    medical and surgical procedures, 437
    word elements, 446–447
Endocrinologists, 393
Endocrinology, 393
Endometriosis, 366, 368f
Endometritis, 332
Endometrium, 332, 340
Endoscope, 228, 233, 261
Endoscopy, 51, 51f, 217, 228, 241, 261
Endotracheal intubation, 138, 139f
End-stage renal disease, 306
Enteral, 238
Enterectomy, 238
Enteritis, 97
Enterologist, 225
Enteropathy, 233
Enterorrhaphy, 238
ENT physician, 507–508
Enuresis, 306
Epidermis, 64f, 67, 68
Epididymides, 363
Epididymis, 354, 358
Epidural space, 424
Epigastric, 47, 230
Epiglottis, 134
Epiglottitis, 134
Epilepsy, 431, 434
Epinephrine, 410, 411
Episiotomy, 333
Epispadias, 370
Epistaxis, 134
Epithelium, ciliated, 112
Epstein-Barr virus, 193
Erectile agents, 379
Erectile dysfunction, 370
Erectile tissue, 354
Erythematous, 97
Erythrocyte(s), 79, 120
Erythrocytosis, 80
Erythroderma, 78
Erythropia, 515
Erythropoiesis, 468
Erythrosis, 80
Esophageal ulcers, 227
Esophagoplasty, 228, 252
Esophagoscope, 219
Esophagoscopy, 219
Esophagotome, 229
Esophagotomy, 229

Esophagus, 219, 224, 226, 228, 229, 252
   carcinoma of, 267, 268
Esotropia, 528f, 529
Estrogen hormone deficiency, 339
Estrogen(s), 338, 348, 379, 411
Eupnea, 125
Eustachian tube, 333, 336, 518, 520
Ewing sarcoma, 488
Excimer laser, 91
Excision, 123, 179, 244, 246, 251, 284, 333,
   347–348
Excoriations, 88f
Excretory urogram, 308
Exhalation, 127
Exhale, 121
Exophthalmic, 406
Exophthalmic goiter, 430
Exophthalmos, 404, 406, 406f
Exotropia, 528f, 529
Expansion, 110, 168
Expiration, 127
Extracapsular cataract extraction (ECCE),
   533
Extracorporeal shock-wave lithotripsy
   (ESWL), 255, 262, 285, 286f
Eyeball, 511, 511f
Eyelid(s), 508, 509, 514
Eye(s), 508–517
   abbreviations, 525
   bulging of, 404, 406, 406f, 407, 430
   diagnostic procedures, 530–531
   diseases and conditions, 525–528
   pathological terms, 525–528
   structures of, 511f, 513
   therapeutic procedures, 533

F

Fallopian tube(s), 333, 334, 336, 351–352,
   518, 520
Farsightedness, 515, 516f
Fascia, 455
Fascioplasty, 455
Fasting blood sugar (FBS), 225, 255, 435
Fat, 72
Fatty plaque, 157
Fatty tumor, 71
Fear, 427
Feces, 239, 255
Female, 332
Female reproductive system. *See* Reproductive
   system(s), female
Femoral, 463
Femur, 463, 467f, 476
Fiberoptic gastroscope, 219
Fibrillation, 164, 190
Fibroid of uterus, 367
Fibroma, 455
Fibrous tissue, 409
Fibrous tunic, 511
Fibula, 464, 476
Fibular, 464
Fingernail, structure of, 75, 75f
Fingers, bones of, 463
Fistula, 257, 341
Flat bones, 466–467
Floating kidney, 288
Flow, 219, 220, 222, 240

Fluoroscopy, 52
Flutter, 164
Follicle-stimulating hormone (FSH), 404
Foot, 465
Forced expiratory volume in one second
   (FEV1), 137
Forced vital capacity, 137
Foreskin, 361
Fovea, 512
Fracture(s), and repairs, 479, 481f
   types of, 479, 481f
Front, 35
Frontal, 35
Fulguration, 91
Fungus(i), 74, 128, 224
Furuncle, 84, 85f

G

Galactorrhea, 332
Gall, 244, 247, 248
Gallbladder, 244, 245, 247–251, 247f
Gallstone, 244, 248, 250
Gametes, 330
Ganglion cyst, 488
Gangrene, 82
Gastralgia, 220, 227
Gastrectomy, 229
Gastric ulcers, 227
Gastritis, 227, 230
Gastrocnemius muscle, 459
Gastroduodenostomy, 237
Gastrodynia, 220, 227
Gastroenteroanastomosis, 237
Gastroenterologist, 217, 225
Gastroenterology, 217–221
Gastroenterostomy, 237
Gastroesophageal reflux disease (GERD),
   257
Gastroileostomy, 237
Gastrointestinal, 225
Gastrointestinal system. *See* Digestive system
Gastrointestinal (GI) tract, 217, 218f
   lower, 234–245
   upper, 221–234, 223f
Gastrologist, 225, 253
Gastrology, 225
Gastromegaly, 220, 228, 253
Gastroplasty, 228, 262, 262f
Gastroscopy, 219, 228, 261
Gastrotome, 229
Gastrotomy, 229
Gigantism, 403
Gingivitis, 219, 226
Gland(s), 182
Glandular tissue, 348
Glans penis, 355, 361, 370
Glaucoma, 526, 527f, 531, 533
Glial cells, 418, 418f
Glioma(s), 418, 419
Glomerulonephritis, 286, 298
Glomerulopathy, 298
Glomerulosclerosis, 298
Glomerulus(i), 280, 297, 298
Glossary of medical word elements,
   548–557
Glucagon(s), 41, 411
Glucocorticoid hormone, 411

Glucocorticoids, 411, 429
Glucogenesis, 396, 413
Glucometer, 413
Glucose, 413
Glucose tolerance test (OGTT), 435
Glue, 419
Glycogen, 413
Glycogenesis, 413
Glycogenolysis, 413
Goiter, 406f, 430
Gold salts, 493
Gonadotropin(s), 355, 379
Gonads, 354, 355
Gonorrhea, 351, 371
Gout, 489
Graft, 82, 91
Grand mal seizures, 434
Graves disease, 404, 406, 406f, 407, 430
Gravida, 350–351
Greenstick fracture, 479
Growth, 362, 465
Growth hormone (GH), 398, 403, 404
Gums, 219, 225, 226
GYN, 346
Gynecologist, 332, 346
Gynecology (GYN), 329–330, 346
Gynecopathy, 346

H

Hair, 65, 75
Hair follicle, 64f
Hallux valgus, 487, 487f
Hand bones, 463, 476
Hard, 73
Hardening, 72, 298, 458
Hardening of arteries, 287
Head, 477–478
Hearing, 518, 522
Hearing loss, complete, 529
   conductive, 529
Heart, 157
   blood flow through, 166–171
   conduction pathway of, 174–176, 175f
   hormones and, 399
   internal structures of, 163f
   sounds of, 176–181
   structures of, 159, 161f, 172f
   valves and cusps of, 171, 172f
   walls, layers of, 159–160
Heart attack, 192, 205
Heart block, 191
Heart condition, 158
Heart failure (HF), 192
Heel bone, 464, 476
Hemangiectasis, 168
Hemangioma, 168
Hematemesis, 231, 339
Hematochezia, 258
Hematologist, 168, 339
Hematology, 168, 339
Hematoma, 86, 339
Hematopathy, 339
Hematosalpinx, 333
Hematuria, 302, 303
Hemiparesis, 419
Hemiplegia, 456, 459
Hemoccult test, 261

Hemodialysis, 310, 311f
Hemophobia, 128
Hemorrhage, 86, 181, 186, 339, 426
Hemorrhagic stroke, 426
Hemorrhoid, 258
Hemosalpinx, 333
Hemothorax, 135
Hepatectomy, 246
Hepatic duct, 246
Hepatitis B, 246
Hepatitis, 244, 246, 253
Hepatocyte, 246
Hepatodynia, 246
Hepatolith, 248
Hepatoma, 246
Hepatomegaly, 244, 246, 253
Hepatorrhaphy, 246
Hepatosis, 250
Hernia, 48, 76, 122, 233, 258, 258f, 280,
    281, 291
Herniated disk, 488, 488f
Herpes genitalis, 371
Herpes simplex virus type 2, 371
Heterograft, 91
Heteropsia, 509
Hidradenitis, 65, 74
Hidrosis, 74
High blood pressure. *See* Hypertension
Hirsutism, 87
Histiocytoma, 97
Histocompatibility testing, 198
HIV, 193. *See also* AIDS
Hives, 89
Hodgkin disease, 183, 193
Holter monitor, 195, 196f
Homeostasis, 63, 278, 394
Homograft, 91
Hordeolum, 526, 527f
Horizontal, 42, 43
Hormone replacement therapy (HRT), 339,
    438
Hormones, 338, 354, 394, 398–400, 399f
Horny tissue, 73, 509
Human immunodeficiency virus (HIV),
    193. *See also* AIDS
Human papillomavirus (HPV), 371
Humeral, 463
Humerus, 463, 476
Hunchback, 490, 491f
Huntington chorea, 431
Hydrocele, 361
Hydrocephalus, 419
Hydronephrosis, 301–302, 301f
Hydrotherapy, 114
Hydrothorax, 135
Hydroureter, 301
Hypercalcemia, 407, 409, 471
Hyperemesis, 220, 230
Hyperemia, 249
Hyperglycemia, 396, 414, 430
Hyperopia, 515, 516f
Hyperparathyroidism, 409
Hyperplasia, 362
Hypersalivation, 219, 223
Hypersecretion, 399, 400
Hypertension, 192, 286, 287, 298
    gestational, 368
Hyperthyroidism, 405, 430

Hypertrophy, 397
Hypertropia, 509
Hypocalcemia, 396, 407, 409, 470
Hypodermic, 65
Hypogastric region, 48
Hypogastric, 47
Hypoglossal, 219
Hypoglycemia, 414
Hypoglycemics, oral, 438
Hypophysis. *See* Pituitary gland
Hypopituitarism, 396
Hyposecretion, 399, 400
Hypospadias, 307
Hypothalamus, 402
Hypothyroidism, 430
Hypoxemia, 135
Hypoxia, 110, 135
Hysteralgia, 332
Hysterectomy, 332, 337, 337f, 368
Hysterocele, 338
Hysterodynia, 337
Hysteropathy, 337
Hysteropexy, 338
Hysteroplasty, 338
Hysteroptosis, 338
Hysterosalpingo-oophorectomy, 376
Hysteroscopy, 338
Hysterospasm, 337
Hysterotome, 352
Hysterotomy, 337, 352

I

Ichthyosis, 65
Ileectomy, 235
Ileitis, 238
Ileorrhaphy, 237
Ileostomy, 233, 236
Ileotomy, 236
Ileum, 233, 234, 235, 236, 237, 238
Immune, 182, 186
Immunity, 182, 186
Immunocompromised persons, 129
Immunogen, 182
Immunologist, 155
Immunology, 155
Impacted fracture, 479
Impetigo, 87
Impotence, 370
Incision and drainage (I&D), 91
Incomplete fracture, 479
Incontinence, 303
Increase, 80
Incus, 520
Indigestion, 220
Infarct, 180
Inferior, 36, 37, 38, 43, 45
Inferior vena cava (IVC), 166, 170
Inflammation, 51
Inflammatory bowel disease, 258
Influenza, 135
Inguinal, 47, 49
Inguinal hernia, 48
Inguinal nodes, 184
Inhalation, 127, 127f
Inhaler with spacer, 140f
Insulin, 411, 413, 414, 430
Insulin-dependent diabetes, 414, 430

Insulinoma, 430
Integumentary structures, 69f
Integumentary system, 63–105
    abbreviations, 84
    combining forms for, 100–104
    compound nevus, 95–96
    diagnostic procedures, 90
    diseases and conditions, 84–92
    prefixes for, 100–104
    psoriasis, 97–99
    suffixes for, 100–104
    therapeutic procedures, 91–92
    word elements, 100–104
Interatrial septum (IAS), 164
Intercostal muscles, 478
Interocular, 509
Interstitial nephritis, 307
Interstitial spaces, 181
Interventricular septum (IVS), 164
Intervertebral, 481–482
Intervertebral disk(s), 481–482
    degenerative disease of, evaluation, 497
    terminology, 495–496
Intestine, 290
Intravenous, 414
Intravenous fluorescein angiography
    (IVFA), 531
Intravenous pyelogram, 299
Intravenous pyelography (IVP), 298, 299,
    308
Intravenous urography, 308
Iridectomy, 533
Iridocele, 512
Iridoplegia, 509
Iris, 509, 512
Irregular bones, 466–467
Irritable bowel syndrome, 259
Ischemia, 192, 426
Islets of Langerhans, 411, 430

J

Jaundice, 249, 256
Jaw, 223
Jejunal feeding tube, 236
Jejunectomy, 235
Jejunorrhaphy, 233, 237
Jejunotomy, 236
Jejunum, 233, 234, 235, 236, 237
Joint(s), 464, 474–476, 487–489
Juvenile warts, 89

K

Kaposi sarcoma, 82, 193
Keratin, 68
Keratitis, 509, 513
Keratoma, 73
Keratoplasty, 509, 533
Keratorrhexis, 512
Keratosis, 65, 73
Ketosis, 430
Kidney dialysis, 278, 310
Kidney(s), 278, 279f, 280, 282–288, 283f,
    307–308, 404, 409, 414
Kidney stone(s), 284, 285f
Kidney transplantation, 306, 306f, 311
Killer cells, 187

Kneecap, 464, 476
KUB, 298
Kyphosis, 490, 491f

L

L1-L5, 484
Labia majora, 345
Labia minora, 345
Labor, 333
Labyrinth(s), 520, 521f
Lacrimal apparatus, 509
Lacrimation, 509
Lactation, 347, 348
Lactiferous duct, 348
Lactogen, 332
Lamina, 464
Laminectomy, 464
Laparoscope, 372, 373f
Laparoscopy, 244, 251, 372, 373f
Laparotomy, 262
Large intestine, 233, 234–240
Laryngectomy, 115
Laryngitis, 116
Laryngoscope, 109, 115, 116
Laryngoscopy, 116
Laryngostenosis, 115
Larynx, 109, 115, 119
Laser keratotomy, 513
Laser photocoagulation, 534
Laser, cutaneous, 92
Laser, excimer, 91
Laser-assisted in situ keratomileusis
    (LASIK), 534
Lateral, 32, 33, 36, 37
Laxatives, 263
Lazy-eye syndrome, 509
Leiomyoma, 368, 455
Lens of eye, 525
Leukemia, 79
Leukocyte(s), 79
Leukocytopenia, 79
Leukocytosis, 80
Leukoderma, 78, 89
Leukopoiesis, 468
Leukorrhea, 368
Lipectomy, 71
Lipid panel, 196
Lipocele, 76
Lipocyte(s), 64, 71
Lipoid, 343
Lipoma, 71
Liposuction, 71, 72
Lithectomy, 285
Lithiasis, 250, 281, 284
Lithotripsy, 262, 281, 285
Liver, 239, 244, 245, 246–247, 247f, 248,
    250, 413
LLQ, 46
Lobar, 123
Lobe(s), 123, 348, 400
Lobectomy, 123
Lobitis, 123
Lobotomy, 123
Loins, 48, 455
Long bone(s), 466–467, 467f
Loosening, 244
Lordosis, 491, 491f

Lou Gehrig disease, 431
Lower back, 48, 455
Lumbar nerves, 422
Lumbar puncture, 436, 436f
Lumbar vertebrae, 482
Lumbar, 47, 484
Lumboabdominal, 48
Lumbocostal, 455
Lumbodynia, 484
Lumpectomy, 350, 350f, 376
Lung cancer, 123, 135
Lung(s), 109, 112, 119, 122, 123, 136f, 162
Lunula, 75
LUQ, 46
Luteinizing hormone (LH), 404
Lymph, 182
Lymphadenitis, 182
Lymphangiectomy, 201
Lymphangiography, 197
Lymphangioma, 182
Lymphatic duct, 184
Lymphatic system, 156f, 182–189, 185f
    abbreviations, 189
    diagnostic procedures, 197–198
    diseases and conditions, 193–194
    structures of, 183–186
    therapeutic procedures, 201
    word elements, 182
Lymph capillaries, 181, 183
Lymph cells, 184
Lymph gland, 182
Lymph node(s), 181, 182, 184
Lymphocyte(s), 183, 184, 187
Lymphoid, 184
Lymphoid tissue, 182
Lymphoma, 183
Lymphopathy, 184
Lymphopoiesis, 182, 183
Lymphosarcoma, 193
Lymph vessel(s), 169, 182, 183, 184

M

Macrophage, 186
Macular degeneration, 526, 528f
Macule, 88f, 97
Magnetic resonance imaging (MRI), 52, 52f,
    137, 261, 437
Magnetoencephalography (MEG), 436
Malacia, 76, 118
Male reproductive system. See Reproductive
    system(s), male
Malignant, 230, 295
Malleus, 520
Mammary glands, 347–349, 349f
Mammogram, 332
Mammography, 348, 373
Mammoplasty, 348
Mania(a), 427
Masculinization, 354
Mastalgia, 348
Mastectomy, 348, 376, 377f
Mastodynia, 348
Mastopexy, 332, 348
Mastoplasty, 348
Matrix, 75
Meatorrhaphy, 294
Meatotomy, 294

Meatus, 280
Mediad, 37
Medial, 37
Median, 42, 43
Medical and surgical procedures, 605–606
Medical record(s)
    bilateral vasectomy, 383–384
    carcinosarcoma of esophagus, 267–268
    cardiac catheterization, 206
    cerebrovascular accident, 443–445
    compound nevus, 95–96
    cystitis, 315–316
    degenerative intervertebral disk disease,
        495–496
    diabetes mellitus, 440–442
    myocardial infarction, 204–206
    otitis media, 539–540
    papillary carcinoma, 143–144
    postmenopausal bleeding, 381–382
    psoriasis, 97–99
    rectal bleeding, 265–267
    retinal detachment, 537–539
    rotator cuff tear, 497–499
Medical specialties, 622–623
Medical word building, 1–25
Medical word elements, 548–557
Medical words, defining of, 14–15
Medulla, 422
Medullary cavity, 468
Megalocardia, 177, 228
Melanin, 70
Melanocyte(s), 70, 79, 80
Melanoderma, 78
Melanoma, 65, 70, 80, 95
Melanosis, 80
Menarche, 333
Ménière disease, 529
Meninges, 419, 424
Meningioma, 419, 424
Meningitis, 424
Meningocele, 419, 424, 434, 435f
Meningomyelocele, 434, 435f
Menorrhagia, 347
Menorrhea, 346, 347
Menses, 332, 333, 346, 369
Menstruation, 332, 333, 346–347, 369
Mental disorders, 426–427
Metacarpectomy, 463
Metacarpus, 463, 476
Metastasis, 130
Metastasize, 130
Metroplasty, 338
Microcardia, 177
Microscope, 120
Midsagittal, 42, 43
Mineralocorticoids, 411
Miotics, 535
Mitral valve, 167, 171
Mitral valve prolapse, 167, 192
Modified radical mastectomy, 376, 377f
Mohs surgery, 91
Mononucleosis, 193
Morbid obesity, 259
Motion sickness drugs, 535
Mouth, 219, 222, 224, 236, 238
MRI. See Magnetic resonance imaging
    (MRI)
Mucoid, 227, 343, 358

Mucous, 227, 343, 345, 359
Mucus, 343, 345, 359
Multigravida, 350
Multipara, 333
Multiple sclerosis, 432
Muscle fibers, 457–459
Muscle(s), 454, 457–461, 471
    body movements generated by, 454f, 460f
    disorders of, 486–487
    functions of, 454
Muscular, 455
Muscular dystrophy, 486
Musculoskeletal system, 453–506
    abbreviations, 486
    composition of, 454
    diagnostic procedures, 492
    therapeutic procedures, 492
    word elements, 500–501
Myalgia, 456, 458
Myasthenia, 456
Myasthenia gravis, 486
Mycosis, 74, 224
Mydriatics, 535
Myelalgia, 419
Myelin, 432
Myelitis, 424, 425
Myelocele, 434, 435f, 464
Myelogenesis, 471
Myelogram, 471, 472
Myeloma, 425
Myelomalacia, 425, 471
Myelopathy, 424
Myelotome, 424
Myocardial infarction (MI), 192, 205
    medical records, 204–206
Myocardium, 159, 160, 164
Myodynia, 458
Myogenesis, 458
Myopathy, 456, 458
Myopia, 515, 516f
Myoplasty, 458
Myorrhaphy, 456, 458
Myorrhexis, 455, 458
Myosarcoma, 456
Myosclerosis, 458
Myotomy, 458
Myringotomy, 518, 522, 529, 535
Myxedema, 430

N

Nail bed, 75
Nail body, 75
Nail root, 75
Nares, 111
Narrowing, 158, 241, 280, 286
Nasal, 109
Nasal cavity, 112
Nasogastric, 111
Nasogastric intubation, 263
Natal, 350
Navel, 47
Nearsightedness, 515, 516f
Nebulized mist treatment (NMT), 139, 140f
Neck of uterus, 332, 463
Necrectomy, 179
Necrophobia, 179, 427

Necrosis, 82, 179
Neonate, 350
Neonatologist, 329, 350
Neonatology, 329, 350
Neoplasms, 362
Nephralgia, 284
Nephrectomy, 284, 288
Nephritis, 284, 307
Nephrolithiasis, 284, 287
Nephrolithotomy, 286, 288
Nephrolith(s), 284, 287
Nephrologist, 277, 303
Nephrology, 277–278
Nephroma, 280
Nephromegaly, 284
Nephron(s), 282, 283f, 296–303, 297f
Nephropathy, 281
Nephropexy, 281, 288
Nephroptosis, 281, 288
Nephrorrhaphy, 288
Nephrosclerosis, 288
Nephroscope, 299
Nephroscopy, 299
Nephrosis, 288
Nephrotic syndrome, 286
Nephrotomy, 288
Nerve glue, 426
Nerve(s), 419, 422, 423f
Nervous system, 394, 417–438, 418f
    abbreviations, 429
    diseases and conditions, 432–435
    medical and surgical procedures, 438
    peripheral, 417–418
    sympathetic, 411
    word elements, 419, 446–447
Neuralgia, 425, 426
Neuritis, 425
Neuroblastoma, 432
Neurocyte, 426
Neuroglia, 418, 418f
Neuroglial tissue, 419
Neurohypophysis, 402–403
Neurologists, 393
Neurology, 393
Neurolysis, 419
Neuroma, 425
Neurons, 418, 418f, 425, 426, 458
Neuropathy, 425
Neuroses, 427
Neurosis, 427
Neurosurgeon, 394
Neurosurgery, 394
Nipple, 348
Nitrogenous compounds, 281
Nocturia, 302
Noncancerous, 295, 362
Non-Hodgkin lymphoma, 183, 193
Nonsteroidal antiinflammatory drugs (NSAIDs), 493
Norepinephrine, 411
Nose, 109, 111
Nosebleed, 134
Nourishment, 397
Nuclear, 34
Nuclear scan, 52f, 53
Nuclear stress test, 196
Nucleus, 31
Nucleus pulposus, 489

O

Obesity, 259
Obstetrician, 329
Obstetrics, 329–330, 346
Obstructive sleep apnea (OSA), 124, 125f
Odontalgia, 225
Offspring, 333
Oligomenorrhea, 369
Oligospermia, 358
Oliguria, 298, 302
Onychoma, 76
Onychomalacia, 65, 76
Onychomycosis, 76
Onychopathy, 76
Oophoritis, 352
Oophoroma, 333, 334, 352
Oophoropathy, 336, 416
Oophoropexy, 336
Oophoroplasty, 336
Oophorotomy, 416
Open angle glaucoma, 526
Open fracture, 479
Opening, 236, 238, 280
Ophthalmectomy, 514
Ophthalmodynia, 513
Ophthalmologist, 507, 513
Ophthalmology, 507
Ophthalmomalacia, 514
Ophthalmoplegia, 514
Ophthalmoscope, 509, 513
Ophthalmoscopy, 513
Optic, 509
Optician, 507
Optic nerve, 511
Optometrist, 507
Oral, 219, 221
Oral cavity, 221–226
Oral hypoglycemics, 438
Orbit, 511
Orchidectomy, 355
Orchiopexy, 355, 359, 369, 416
Orchioplasty, 359
Orchiorrhaphy, 359
Orthodontist, 219, 226
Orthopedics, 453, 465
Orthopedists, 453
Orthopnea, 125
Ostealgia, 469
Osteitis, 465, 469
Osteitis deformans, 489
Osteitis fibrosa cystica, 409
Osteoarthritis, 14, 476
Osteoarthropathy, 476
Osteoarthrosis, 476
Osteoblasts, 468
Osteoclast, 465
Osteocyte(s), 465, 468, 469
Osteodynia, 469
Osteogenesis, 468, 470
Osteomalacia, 465, 470
Osteomyelitis, 472, 472f
Osteopathic physician, 453
Osteopathy, 453, 469
Osteoporosis, 465, 470
Osteorrhaphy, 469
Osteosclerosis, 469
Osteotomy, 469
Otalgia, 519

Otitis externa, 529
Otitis media, 522, 525, 530
    evaluation, 540
    terminology, 539–540
Otodynia, 519
Otolaryngologists, 507
Otolaryngology, 507–508
Otoplasty, 523
Otorrhea, 518
Otosclerosis, 522
Otoscope, 522, 532
Otoscopy, 522, 532
Ovariorrhexis, 333, 347
Ovary(ies), 333, 334, 355, 376, 404, 415
Oviducts, 489
Ovulation, 334, 336
Ovum, 334, 336
Oxygen (O₂), 110, 120, 121, 122
Oxytocics, 379
Oxytocin, 404

P

Paget disease, 489
Palsy, 432
Pancreas, 244, 245, 246, 247f, 248, 251–
    253, 396, 411–415, 430
Pancreatectomy, 251
Pancreatic, 247
Pancreatic cancer, 251
Pancreatic duct, 247, 250
Pancreatic hormone(s), 413, 413t
Pancreatic tumor, 430
Pancreatitis, 396, 430
Pancreatolith, 248, 412
Pancreatolithiasis, 250, 412
Pancreatolysis, 244, 412
Pancreatoma, 412
Pancreatopathy, 412
Panhypopituitarism, 431
Papanicolaou (Pap) test, 372, 374
Papillary carcinoma, 143–144
    terminology, 143–144
Papule, 88f, 97
Para, 351, 409
Paralysis, 419, 432, 433f, 456, 459, 509
Paranasal, 112
Paraplegia, 432
Parathormone, 409, 409t
Parathyroidectomy, 396
Parathyroid glands, 396, 408–409
Parathyroid hormone (PTH), 409, 409t
Parkinson disease, 434
Parotid gland, 222
Partial paralysis, 419
Patella, 464, 476
Patellectomy, 464
Patency, 364
Patent ductus arteriosus, 192
Pathogens, 186, 351
Pathological, 241
Pathological suffixes, 19–21
PCP, 129
Pelvic cavity, 45
Pelvic girdle, 476
Pelvic inflammatory disease (PID), 351–352
Pelvimetry, 464
Pelvis, 464, 476

Penis, 354, 361
Peptic ulcer disease, 227
Percutaneous transluminal coronary angio-
    plasty (PTCA), 198, 198f
Pericardiectomy, 160
Pericardiocentesis, 160
Pericardiorrhaphy, 160
Pericarditis, 160
Pericardium, 159, 160
Perineorrhaphy, 333
Perineum, 333
Periodontist, 226
Periodontitis, 226
Periosteum, 467, 467f, 468
Peripheral nervous system (PNS), 417–418
Peristalsis, 227, 239
Peritoneal dialysis, 310, 311f
Peritonitis, 259
Peritonsillar, 109
Pertussis, 135
Petechia, 86
PET scan, 52f
Peyer patches, 181
Phacoemulsification, 533, 533f
Phagocyte, 182
Phalanges, 463, 476
Phalangitis, 463
Pharyngitis, 109, 115, 227
Pharyngocele, 115
Pharyngomycosis, 114
Pharyngoparalysis, 114
Pharyngoplasty, 115
Pharyngoplegia, 114
Pharyngospasm, 110, 115
Pharyngostenosis, 115
Pharyngotome, 115
Pharyngotomy, 115
Pharyngotonsillitis, 219
Pharynx, 109, 111, 114, 115, 219, 226, 518
Pheochromocytoma, 431
Phimosis, 370
Phlebitis, 157
Phleborrhaphy, 168
Phleborrhexis, 168
Phlebostenosis, 168
Phlebotomy, 168
Phobia(s), 426
Photophobia, 526
Phrenoptosis, 126
Phrenospasm, 126
Pia mater, 422, 424
PID, 351–352
Pilocystic, 75
Pilonidal, 65
Pineal gland, 415
Pinkeye, 508
Pituitary gland, 395f, 396, 399f, 400–404
Pituitary hormones, 404t
Plantar warts, 89
Platelet, 425
Pleura(ae), 109, 123, 480
Pleural effusion, 135
Pleuralgia, 109
Pleural rub, 133
Pleurisy, 109, 124
Pleuritic, 109
Pleuritis, 123
Pleurocele, 123

Pleurodynia, 124
Pleuropneumonia, 123
Plural suffixes, 21
Pneumatic otoscopy, 532
Pneumectomy, 109
Pneumocentesis, 122
Pneumoconiosis, 122
Pneumocystis i pneumonia, 129
Pneumomelanosis, 122
Pneumonectomy, 121, 122
Pneumonia, 109, 121, 128, 253
Pneumonitis, 121
Pneumonocele, 122
Pneumonomycosis, 128
Pneumonopathy, 122
Pneumonosis, 122
Pneumothorax, 135, 136f
Poliomyelitis, 434
Polycystic, 302
Polycystic kidney disease (PKD), 302
Polydipsia, 397, 415
Polyphagia, 415
Polyp(s), 259, 261
Polysomnography, 137, 138f
Polyuria, 281, 415
Pons, 421
Positron emission tomography (PET), 52f,
    437
Posterior, 34, 35, 36, 44, 253, 400, 401–402,
    458
Posteroanterior (PA), 402
Posteroinferior, 402
Posterolateral, 36, 402
Posterosuperior, 402
Postmenopausal, 347
Postmenopausal bleeding, evaluation, 382
    terminology, 381–382
Postmenopause, 339
Postnatal, 350
Postpartum, 329
Postprandial, 244
Postural drainage, 139
Potassium supplements, 313
Preeclampsia, 368
Prefixes, 23–25
Pregnancy, 333
Premenopausal, 347
Premenopause, 339
Prenatal, 333, 350
Presbycusis, 530
Pressure ulcer, 89, 89f
Pressure-equalizing (PE) tube, 522, 523f,
    529
Primigravida, 333, 350
Proctalgia, 240
Proctitis, 241
Proctocele, 233
Proctologist, 233
Proctoscopy, 241, 261
Proctospasm, 241
Progesterone, 338, 348
Programmed learning, 1–25
Prolactin, 404
Prolapsed disk, 488f, 489
Pronunciation, 9, 15
Prostate, 360f, 361
    biopsy of, 375
Prostate cancer, 361–362, 374

Prostatectomy, 361
Prostate gland, 354, 358, 359
Prostate-specific antigen (PSA) test, 361
Prostatic hyperplasia, 359, 360f, 377
Prostatitis, 361, 362, 363
Prostatocystitis, 361
Prostatocystotomy, 361
Prostatomegaly, 359
Protection, 182
Proteinuria, 286, 302
Proximal, 38, 470
Proximal epiphysis, 468, 470
Pruritis, 97
PSA test, 361
Pseudocyesis, 333
Psoriasis, 87, 87f
    medical record, 97–99
Psychiatric disorders, 426–427
Psychiatry, 427
Psychoses, 427
Psychotherapy, 427
Ptyalism, 219
Pulmonary, 34, 169
Pulmonary arteries, 162, 166
Pulmonary capillaries, 120
Pulmonary circulation, 166
Pulmonary function tests, 137
Pulmonary medicine, 107–111
Pulmonary trunk, 162
Pulmonary valve, 166, 171
Pulmonary veins, 162, 167
Pulmonologist, 107, 110
Pulmonology, 107–111
Pupil, 508, 513
Pupillary, 508
Purkinje fibers, 174
Purulent discharge, 518
Pustule, 73
P wave, 177
Pyelitis, 299
Pyelogram, 300, 308
Pyelography, 299, 308
Pyelonephritis, 299–300
Pyelopathy, 298
Pyeloplasty, 280, 300
Pylorotomy, 219
Pylorus, 219, 241
Pyoderma, 66
Pyonephrosis, 300
Pyorrhea, 300
Pyothorax, 110, 135
Pyuria, 290, 300, 302

Q
QRS wave, 177
Quadriplegia, 419, 432, 459

R
Radiation, 464
Radiation therapy, 471
Radiograph(s), 43, 52f, 54f, 401, 464
Radiography, 52f, 293, 373
Radiologist, 470, 471
Radiology, 44, 50, 401, 471
Radiotherapy, 471
Radius, 401, 464

Rales, 133
Raynaud phenomenon, 192
Reabsorption, 278
Reconstructive breast surgery, 377, 378f
Rectal bleeding, evaluation, 265–267
    terminology, 265–266
Rectalgia, 240
Rectitis, 240
Rectocele, 233, 291, 291f
Rectocolitis, 240
Rectoplasty, 240
Rectoscope, 360
Rectospasm, 241
Rectostenosis, 241
Rectovaginal, 240
Rectovaginal fistula, 342
Rectum, 233, 239, 241
Red blood cells (RBCs), 186
Reflux, 257
Refraction of eye, 516f
Renal, 280, 302, 308
Renal artery, 282
Renal artery stenosis, 286
Renal biopsy, 286
Renal calculi, 301
Renal cortex, 282, 297
Renal dialysis, 284
Renal failure, 303, 306
Renal hypertension, 286, 307
Renal medulla, 282, 297
Renal pelvis, 280, 300
Renal scan, nuclear, 308
Renal transplantation, 306, 306f, 311
Renal vein, 282
Reproductive system(s), 366
    diseases and conditions, 366–371
    female, 330–353, 331f, 335f
        diagnostic procedures, 372–374
        external structures, 345–347
        therapeutic procedures, 375–377, 378f
    male, 354–364, 354f
        diagnostic procedures, 359–360
        pathological terms, 366
        therapeutic procedures, 377
    word elements, 385–386
Respiration, 119, 121
Respiratory center, 422
Respiratory distress syndrome (ARDS),
    acute, 133
Respiratory system, 107–153
    combining forms of, 109–110
    diagnostic procedures, 136–137, 137f
    diseases and conditions, 133–136
    lower, 107, 108f, 109–110, 113f,
        118–130
    structures of, 107, 108f
    upper, 107, 108f, 109, 113f
    word elements, 147–148
Retina, 509, 512
Retinal detachment, 527
    evaluation, 538–539
    terminology, 537–538
Retinitis, 512
Retinopathy, 509, 512
Retrograde pyelography (RP), 299, 308
Retroversion, 333
Rheumatoid arthritis, 489, 489f
Rheumatoid factor, 492

Rheumatoid spondylitis, 489
Rheumatologist, 453
Rhinoplasty, 112
Rhinorrhagia, 112
Rhinorrhea, 112
Rhinotomy, 112
Rhonchi, 133
Ribs, 463, 476
Rickets, 470
Right atrium, 174
Ringworm, 89
Rinne test, 532, 532f
RLQ, 46
Roentgenology, 471
Rotator cuff, injuries to, 489
    tear of, evaluation, 497–499
    terminology, 497–498
Roux-en-Y gastric bypass (RGB), 262, 262f
Rupture, 333, 455, 458, 484

S
Sacral nerves, 422
Sacral vertebrae, 484
Sacrum, 484
Saliva, 219, 223
Salivary glands, 222
Salpingectomy, 333, 336, 352
Salpingitis, 520
Salpingocele, 336
Salpingopharyngeal, 518
Salpingoplasty, 336
Salpingoscope, 336, 520
Salpingoscopy, 336, 520
Salpingostenosis, 520
Scabies, 87
Scan, 52f
Schizophrenia, 427
Schwann cell, 418f
Sciatica, 434
Sclera, 287, 458, 509, 511
    of eye, 65
Scleritis, 509, 513
Scleroderma, 65, 72, 73
Scleromalacia, 513
Sclerosed, 98
Sclerosis, 73, 287, 458
Sclerotherapy, 200
Sclerotomy, 538
Scoliosis, 491, 491f
Scrotum, 355, 356
Sebaceous, 73, 85
Seborrhea, 65
Sebum, 65
Seizure, 434
Semen, 355, 357, 358
Semicircular canals, 520
Seminal fluid, 355, 358
Seminal vesicle(s), 354, 355, 358
Sensorineural hearing loss, 529
Sensory tunic, 511
Separation, 244
Septicemia, 51, 351
Septum(a), 164, 165
Sequestrectomy, 492
Sequestrum, 490
Serous otitis media, 530
Serum, 135

Sex hormones, 354, 411
Sexually transmitted diseases (STDs), 351, 371
Shin bone, 464
Shingles, 434
Short bones, 466–467
Sialitis, 222
Sialorrhea, 219, 222
Sigmoid, 233
Sigmoid colon, 233, 238, 239, 240, 241
Sigmoidectomy, 240, 242
Sigmoiditis, 240
Sigmoidoscope, 242
Sigmoidoscopy, 242, 242f, 261
Sigmoidotomy, 233
Simple mastectomy, 376
Sinoatrial node (SA), 174
Sinusitis, 98
Sinus rhythm, 177
Skeletal muscle fibers, 457
Skin, 63, 67–73, 78
    accessory organs of, 73–77
    disease of, 70
    inflammation of, 70
    structure of, 63, 64f
Skin graft, 91
Skin lesions, 87–89, 88f
Skin resurfacing, 92
Skin test, 90, 90f
Sleep apnea, 124, 125, 125f
Slit-lamp examination, 530
Small incision cataract surgery (SICS), 533, 533f
Small intestine, 233, 234–240, 235f, 238, 242
Smooth muscle fibers, 457
Snellen chart, 531, 531f
Spanish translations, 624–632
Spastic colon, 259
Specialists, 219
Spermatic cord, 355
Spermatocide, 355
Spermatocyte, 355, 358
Spermatogenesis, 357, 358
Spermatoid, 358
Spermatolith, 358
Spermatozoa, 355, 357, 358
Spermaturia, 358
Sperm cells, 355, 357, 358
Spermicide, 355, 379
Sperm transporting ducts, 354
Spina bifida, 434, 435f
Spina bifida cystica, 434
Spina bifida occulta, 434
Spinal cavity, 44, 45
Spinal cord, 422–426, 423f
Spinal cord compression, 491
Spinal nerves, 422, 423f
Spinal puncture, 436, 436f
Spinal tap, 436, 436f
Spirometry, 137, 138f
Spleen, 182, 186, 239
Splenomegaly, 182
Spondylolisthesis, 491
Squamous, 65
Stapedectomy, 522
Staphylococcus aureus, 369
Statins, 202
Steatitis, 64

Stenosis, 280
Sterility, 369
Sternocostal, 463
Sternum, 463, 476, 480
Stoma, 233, 236
Stomach, 111, 219, 226, 228, 229, 237, 242, 253
Stomatalgia, 222
Stomatitis, 221
Stomatodynia, 222
Stomatomycosis, 224
Stomatopathy, 219
Stomatoplasty, 219
Stone(s), 244, 248, 250, 281, 284, 358
Stool guaiac, 261
Strabismus, 528, 528f
Strain, 487
Stratum corneum, 64f, 68
Stress test, 196
Stricture, 115, 241
Stridor, 133
Stroke, 426
    evaluation, 444–445
    terminology, 443–444
Sty, 526, 528f
Subcostal, 463, 479
Subcutaneous, 71
Subcutaneous tissue(s), 69, 71
    structure of, 63, 64f
Subdural space, 424
Sublingual, 219, 224
Sublingual gland, 224
Subluxation, 489
Submandibular gland, 224
Submaxillary, 223
Sudden infant death syndrome, 136
Sudoresis, 65
Sudoriferous, 73, 74
Sudoriferous gland, 70
Suffixes, 16, 30, 56, 66, 147–148, 244, 320
    diagnostic, 18
    pathological, 19–21
    plural, 21
    surgical, 16–17
Superior vena cava (SVC), 166, 170
Suppurative otitis media, 530
Suprarenal glands, 287, 396, 410
Surgical suffixes, 16–17
Sweat gland, 74
Swimmer's ear, 519, 529
Symbols, 621
Sympathetic nervous system, 411
Synarthroses, 474
Syncope, 98
Synovial fluid, 475
Synthetic skin graft, 91
Syphilis, 371
Systemic circulation, 166
Systemic lupus erythematosus (SLE), 194, 194f
Systemic sclerosis, 73
Systole, 176

T
Tachycardia, 158, 165, 177
Tachyphagia, 165

Tachypnea, 165
Talipes, 490, 490f
Target organs, 394
Target tissues, 394
TB, 130, 135
T cells, 187
Tear gland, 517
Tendinitis, 455, 487
Tendon, 455, 459
Tendonitis, 455, 487
Tendoplasty, 455, 459
Tendotome, 459
Tendotomy, 459
Tenotomy, 455
Testalgia, 355
Testectomy, 357
Testicles, 355, 356, 357
Testis(es), 354, 355, 356, 361, 363–364, 369, 404, 414, 415–416
Testitis, 357
Testopathy, 356, 357
Testosterone, 355, 356
Thalamotomy, 438
Thermometer, 252
Thigh bone, 464, 476
Thoracentesis, 126, 126f, 135
Thoracic, 184, 483
Thoracic cavity, 45, 126
Thoracic duct, 184
Thoracic nerves, 422
Thoracic vertebrae, 482–483
Thoracocentesis, 126, 126f, 135
Thoracodynia, 110
Thoracopathy, 110
Thoracotomy, 126
Thrombectomy, 180
Thrombocyte, 425
Thrombogenesis, 180, 425
Thrombolysis, 180, 425
Thrombolytic therapy, 202
Thrombosis, 180
Thrombus(i), 157, 180, 425, 426
Thrush, 224
Thymectomy, 415
Thymoma, 182
Thymosin, 187
Thymus gland, 182, 186, 187
Thyroidectomy, 396, 409
Thyroid gland, 396, 404, 405
    in goiter, 406f
Thyroid hormones, 407t
Thyroidism, 253
Thyroidotome, 407
Thyroidotomy, 407
Thyroid-stimulating hormone (TSH), 404
Thyromegaly, 396, 405
Thyropathy, 405
Thyrotomy, 405
Thyrotoxicosis, 406, 406f, 430
Thyroxine (T4), 407, 430
Tibia, 464, 476
Tibial, 464
Tinea, 89
Tinnitus, 530
Tissue expander, 377, 378f
Tissue typing, 198
T lymphocytes, 187

Toes, bones of, 463
Tomography, 53
Tonic-clonic seizures, 434
Tonometry, 530f, 530
Tonsils, 109, 186
Tooth (Teeth), 219, 225
Toothache, 225
Torticollis, 487
Total hip arthroplasty, 475, 475f
Total mastectomy, 376
Toxic, 34, 252, 253, 396
Toxic goiter, 406, 406f, 430
Toxicologist, 396, 406
Toxicology, 252, 253, 406
Toxicopathy, 407
Toxicosis, 253
Toxic shock syndrome (TSS), 369
Toxin, 396
Trachea, 109, 118, 119
Tracheolaryngotomy, 119
Tracheomalacia, 118
Tracheopathy, 119
Tracheoplasty, 119
Tracheostenosis, 119
Tracheostomy, 109, 118, 119f
Tracheostomy tube, 119f
Tracheotomy, 119
Transdermal, 339
Transient ischemic attack, 435
Transmission, 65
Transrectal ultrasound (TRUS), 375
Transsphenoidal hypophysectomy, 437, 437f
Transurethral resection of prostate (TURP), 359–360, 360f, 377
Transverse colon, 238
Transverse rectus abdominis muscle (TRAM) flap, 377, 378f
Trichomoniasis, 371
Trichomycosis, 75
Trichopathy, 65, 75
Trichosis, 75
Tricuspid valve, 166, 171
Troponin I test, 196
Tubercles, 130
Tuberculosis (TB), 130, 135
Tumor(s), blood, 339
    fatty, 71
    ovarian, 334
    skin, 88f
Tuning fork test, 532
T wave, 177
Tympanic membrane, 519, 520
Tympanitis, 519
Tympanoplasty, 518, 535
Tympanostomy tubes, 535

U

Ulcer, 88f, 89, 227
Ulcerative colitis, 258
Ultrasonography (US), 52f, 53, 54f, 197, 253, 261, 309, 374, 375
Ultrasound. *See* Ultrasonography (US)
Umbilical, 34, 47, 48
Umbilical region, 48
Umbilicus, 47
Underproduction, 399

Upper GI series, 260
Upper respiratory infection (URI), 522
Uremia, 280, 307
Ureteral stent, 312, 312f
Ureterorrhaphy, 290
Ureterostenosis, 280
Ureterovaginal fistula, 341
Ureter(s), 279f, 280, 285f, 289–295
Urethra, 280, 289–295, 299, 354
Urethral, 294
Urethralgia, 293
Urethral stricture, 294
Urethrectomy, 293
Urethritis, 293, 371
Urethrocele, 280
Urethrocystitis, 293
Urethropexy, 293
Urethroplasty, 293
Urethrorectal, 294
Urethroscope, 294
Urethroscopy, 294
Urethrotomy, 312
Urinalysis, 309
Urinary, 280
Urinary incontinence, 303
Urinary system, 277–327, 279f, 283f
    abbreviations, 305
    diagnostic procedures, 307–309
    diseases and conditions, 305–307
    therapeutic terms, 309–311
    word elements, 320–321
Urinary tract, 280
Urinary tract infection (UTI), 293, 302
Urination, excessive, 302, 415
    scanty, 302
Urogram, 308
Urography, 308
Urologist, 277, 303, 330
Urology, 277, 330
Urticaria, 89, 90f
Uterine retroversion, 333
Uterine tubes, 351–352
Uteropexy, 338
Uteroplasty, 338
Uteroscopy, 338
Uterovaginal, 332
Uterus, 332, 333, 334, 337, 338, 352, 404
Uvea, 511

V

Vagina, 332, 334, 335f, 340–341, 341–343
Vaginal, 346
Vaginal fistula, 342
Vaginal hysterectomy, 343
Vaginitis, 341
Vaginocele, 332
Vaginoplasty, 341
Vaginoscope, 341
Vaginotomy, 341
Valve(s), 171–172, 171f, 172f
Valvuloplasty, 200
Varicocele, 355
Varicose veins, 158, 170
Varicosities, 170
Vascular, 158, 169

Vascular surgeon, 155
Vascular tunic, 512
Vas deferens, 158, 354, 355, 358
Vasectomy, 355, 363–364, 363f, 383–384
Vasectomy reversal, 364
Vasomotor center, 422
Vasospasm, 158
Vasovasostomy, 364
Vein(s), 157, 158, 167, 168, 171, 171f, 355
Vena cava(ae), 162
Venereal disease, 351, 371
Venosclerosis, 168
Venospasm, 168
Venotomy, 168
Venous, 157, 186
Ventral, 32, 33, 34
Ventricle(s), 158, 163
Ventricular, 158, 164
Ventriculotomy, 163
Venule, 169
Vermillion border, 95
Verruca, 89
Vertebra(ae), 463, 476, 480, 481, 482–484
Vertebral, 463
Vertebral arch, 464
Vertebral column, 463, 480, 482, 483f
Vertebrectomy, 480
Vertebrocostal, 480
Vertebrosternal, 480
Vertical banded gastroplasty, 262
Vertigo, 530
Vertigo drugs, 535
Vesicle, 88f
Vesicocele, 280
Vesicoenteric, 290
Vesicovaginal fistula, 341, 342f
Vesiculitis, 355
Vessel(s), 158, 184
    blood, 158
Vestibule, 520
Villi, 234
Visceral, 455
Vision, 509, 515
Visual acuity test, 531
Visual examination, 228, 233, 241
Vitamin D deficiency, 465, 470
Vitiligo, 89, 90f
Voice box, 109, 115
Voiding cystourography, 309
Volvulus, 260
Vomiting, 220, 247
Vulgaris, 98
Vulva, 330, 333, 345
Vulvitis, 345
Vulvopathy, 333, 345
Vulvouterine, 345

W

Wall-eye, 528f, 529
Wart, 89
Wax emulsifiers, 535
Weber test, 532
Western blot test, 197
Wheal, 88f, 89
Wheezes, 133

White blood cells, 79
Whooping cough, 135
Wilms tumor, 307
Windpipe, 109, 118
Woman, 332, 350
Womb. *See* Uterus
Word building, 1–25
    rules for, 10–13
Word roots, 4–5
Wrist bones, 463, 476

Writing, 253
Wryneck, 487

X

Xanthemia, 79
Xanthocyte, 79
Xanthoderma, 78
Xanthoma(s), 78, 79
Xanthopia, 515

Xanthosis, 80
Xenograft, 91
Xenophobia, 427
Xeroderma, 65, 76, 78
X-ray(s). *See* Radiograph(s)

Y

Yeasts, 74

RULES FOR SINGULAR AND PLURAL SUFFIXES

This table presents common singular suffixes, the rules for forming plurals, and examples of each.

Rule		Example	
Singular	Plural	Singular	Plural
-a	Retain a and add e.	pleura	pleurae
-ax	Drop x and add ces.	thorax	thoraces
-en	Drop en and add ina.	lumen	lumina
-is	Drop is and add es.	diagnosis	diagnoses
-ix	Drop ix and add ices.	appendix	appendices
-ex	Drop ex and add ices.	apex	apices
-ma	Retain ma and add ta.	carcinoma	carcinomata
-on	Drop on and add a.	ganglion	ganglia
-um	Drop um and add a.	bacterium	bacteria
-us	Drop us and add i.	bronchus	bronchi
-y	Drop y and add ies.	deformity	deformities